Neuroendocrinology: Recent Studies in Neuropeptide GPCRs

Neuroendocrinology: Recent Studies in Neuropeptide GPCRs

Edited by Dylan Edwards

STATES
ACADEMIC PRESS
www.statesacademicpress.com

States Academic Press,
109 South 5th Street,
Brooklyn, NY 11249, USA

Visit us on the World Wide Web at:
www.statesacademicpress.com

ISBN: 978-1-63989-371-3

Cataloging-in-Publication Data

Neuroendocrinology : recent studies in neuropeptide GPCRs / edited by Dylan Edwards.
p. cm.
Includes bibliographical references and index.
ISBN 978-1-63989-371-3
1. Neuroendocrinology. 2. Neuropeptides. 3. G proteins--Receptors. 4. Neurohormones. I. Edwards, Dylan.
QP356.4 .N48 2022
612.8--dc23

Table of Contents

Preface

Neuroendocrinology is the branch of physiology which deals with the study of interactions between the endocrine system and the nervous system. It encompasses the way brain regulates the hormonal activity in the body. To regulate the physiological processes of the human body, the endocrine and nervous systems often act together and the process is known as neuroendocrine integration. Neuroendocrine system is a system by which hypothalamus maintains homeostasis by regulating metabolism, energy utilization, eating and drinking behavior, reproduction, blood pressure and osmolarity. G protein-coupled receptors (GPCRs) are the neuropeptide targets via which the intracellular signaling transduction pathways are activated. This book is a valuable compilation of topics, ranging from the basic to the most complex advancements in the field of neuroendocrinology. It is an upcoming field of science that has undergone rapid development over the past few decades. This book is a resource guide for experts as well as students.

The researches compiled throughout the book are authentic and of high quality, combining several disciplines and from very diverse regions from around the world. Drawing on the contributions of many researchers from diverse countries, the book's objective is to provide the readers with the latest achievements in the area of research. This book will surely be a source of knowledge to all interested and researching the field.

In the end, I would like to express my deep sense of gratitude to all the authors for meeting the set deadlines in completing and submitting their research chapters. I would also like to thank the publisher for the support offered to us throughout the course of the book. Finally, I extend my sincere thanks to my family for being a constant source of inspiration and encouragement.

Editor

1

Development and aging of the kisspeptin–GPR54 system in the mammalian brain: what are the impacts on female reproductive function?

Isabelle Franceschini [1,2,3,4]* **and** ***Elodie Desroziers*** [1,2,3,4]†

[1] UMR85 Physiologie de la Reproduction et des Comportements, Institut National de Recherche Agronomique, Nouzilly, France
[2] UMR7247, Centre National de la Recherche Scientifique, Nouzilly, France
[3] Université François Rabelais de Tours, Tours, France
[4] Institut Français du Cheval et de l'Equitation, Nouzilly, France

Edited by:
Hubert Vaudry, University of Rouen, France

Reviewed by:
Manuel Tena-Sempere, University of Cordoba, Spain
Vance Trudeau, University of Ottawa, Canada

****Correspondence:***
Isabelle Franceschini, Centre INRA de Tours, Unité de Physiologie de la Reproduction et des Comportements, UMR 7247 INRA/CNRS/Univ. Tours/IFCE, 37380 Nouzilly, France.
e-mail: isabelle.franceschini@tours.inra.fr

The prominent role of the G protein coupled receptor GPR54 and its peptide ligand kisspeptin in the progression of puberty has been extensively documented in many mammalian species including humans. Kisspeptins are very potent gonadotropin-releasing hormone secretagogues produced by two main populations of neurons located in two ventral forebrain regions, the preoptic area and the arcuate nucleus. Within the last 2 years a substantial amount of data has accumulated concerning the development of these neuronal populations and their timely regulation by central and peripheral factors during fetal, neonatal, and peripubertal stages of development. This review focuses on the development of the kisspeptin–GPR54 system in the brain of female mice, rats, sheep, monkeys, and humans. We will also discuss the notion that this system represents a major target through which signals from the environment early in life can reprogram reproductive function.

Keywords: kisspeptin, GPR54, ontogenesis, neuron, differentiation, regulation, reproduction, environment

INTRODUCTION

The G protein coupled receptor GPR54 was initially cloned based on its high homology with the galanin receptor (Lee et al., 1999). Its peptide ligands were purified from human placenta (Ohtaki et al., 2001) and identified as the proteolysis products of a 145 amino acid protein encoded by the tumor suppressor gene *Kiss1* (Lee et al., 1996). These ligands have been termed kisspeptins and share a 10 amino acid long sequence at their amidated C terminal, a sequence that is sufficient to bind and activate GPR54 (Ohtaki et al., 2001). The importance of the kisspeptin–GPR54 system in reproductive function came to light in 2003 when it was discovered that some human families displaying hypogonadotropic hypogonadism and absence or delay in puberty bore mutations in the *GPR54* gene (de Roux et al., 2003; Seminara et al., 2003).

Kiss1 and *GPR54* have since been cloned from many mammalian species. Kisspeptin–GPR54 signaling predominantly acts at the level of the brain to control reproductive function (Oakley et al., 2009 for review). Kisspeptins are in fact the most potent gonadotropin-releasing hormone (GnRH) peptide secretagogue discovered to date (Messager et al., 2005). Kisspeptins are produced by two main populations of neurons, one within the preoptic area (POA) and one within the arcuate nucleus (ARC, or infundibulum in primates), that have been implicated in the regulations of the preovulatory GnRH surge and GnRH pulsatile release, respectively (**Figure 1**; Lehman et al., 2010 for review). Importantly, kisspeptin neurons express a large variety of hormonal receptors not expressed by GnRH neurons and may integrate and convey to GnRH neurons a large panel of information about the body, enabling adaptive outcomes on reproduction.

Within the last 2 years, a substantial amount of data has accumulated on the physiological regulation and function of the kisspeptin–GPR54 system in the developing brain and we consider it as timely and worthwhile to review this topic. In addition, we review recent evidence indicating that the kisspeptin–GPR54 system may represent a major target through which signals from the environment early in life can produce long-lasting defects on reproductive function. This review focuses on females and discusses data from mice, rats, sheep, monkeys, and humans in separate sections since marked differences exist between species and sexes relative to the developmental regulation of the kisspeptin–GPR54 system. For more detailed specific information on the neuroanatomy and regulation of the system in developing males or in adulthood, please refer to recent reviews on these subjects (Lehman et al., 2010; Clarke, 2011; Poling and Kauffman, 2013). Barely a decade has passed since the discovery of the importance of GPR54 in the development of reproductive function and, despite

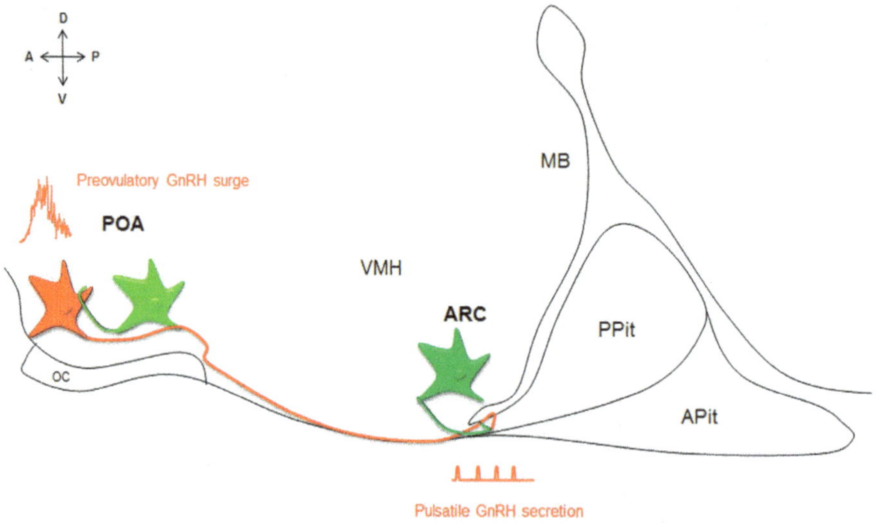

FIGURE 1 | Neuroanatomy of the kisspeptin–GPR54 system. Simplified scheme of a midsagittal section through the ventral forebrain, representing the neuroanatomy of the kisspeptin–GPR54 system. Two anatomically and phenotypically distinct populations of kisspeptin neurons (green) control GnRH (red) secretion: kisspeptin neurons in the POA drive GnRH surges and kisspeptin cells in the ARC modulate the tonic pulsatile release of GnRH. Both populations of kisspeptin neurons interact with GnRH neurons in part directly. A, anterior; P, posterior; D, dorsal; V, ventral; POA, preoptic area; ARC, arcuate nucleus; OC, optic chiasm, VMH, ventromedial hypothalamus; MB, mammillary bodies; APit, anterior pituitary; PPit, posterior pituitary.

the relative youth of the field, some consensus ideas and matters of controversies are starting to emerge with implications for important future directions.

A ROLE FOR THE KISSPEPTIN–GPR54 SYSTEM IN PUBERTY AND SEXUAL DIFFERENTIATION

The prominent involvement of central nervous system kisspeptin signaling in the maturation of reproductive function is strongly suggested from genetic association studies of developmental reproductive disorders in humans and from experimental data on a variety of animal models. These studies are detailed below for each species and summarized in **Table 1**.

MOUSE

In the mouse, targeted genetic disruption of *GPR54* (de Roux et al., 2003; Funes et al., 2003; Seminara et al., 2003) or of *Kiss1* (d'Anglemont de Tassigny et al., 2007; Lapatto et al., 2007) produce a similar hypogonadotropic hypogonadism phenotype, suggesting that kisspeptins represent the main ligands for this receptor. This major effect on the development of reproductive function does not appear to involve a reduction of GnRH peptide levels in the brain nor a reduction in GnRH neuronal numbers (Seminara et al., 2003; d'Anglemont de Tassigny et al., 2007; Lapatto et al., 2007) but involves an impairment in tonic GnRH release (Dungan et al., 2007). *In vitro* studies further suggest that central kisspeptins can already signal developing GnRH neurons well before birth. Nasal placodes from embryonic day (E) 11.5 mouse embryos can be explanted *in vitro* to produce a GnRH neuronal network that releases GnRH in a pulsatile manner (Constantin et al., 2009a). If kisspeptins are applied to these cultures, it increases both GnRH pulse frequency and pulse amplitude (Constantin et al., 2009a). Kisspeptins have also been shown to promote neurite outgrowth of GnRH neurons from embryonic POA explants, suggesting their participation in morphogenetic events (Fiorini and Jasoni, 2010). Notably, developmental strategies leading to the maturation of the GnRH system through puberty appear remarkably plastic at early stages of mouse development. For instance, if kisspeptin neurons are conditionally ablated with a toxin during the juvenile stage, mice display hypogonadism, persistent diestrus, and infertility but this is not the case if these cells are congenitally ablated indicating that strong compensatory mechanisms can occur earlier in development (Mayer and Boehm, 2011). *GPR54* deletion has also been found to inhibit defeminization/masculinization of brain circuits and behavior in males (Kauffman et al., 2007a) without interfering with the perinatal testosterone surge (Poling and Kauffman, 2012). In particular, *GPR54* knock-out males display a pattern of kisspeptin expression in the POA and an olfactory-mediated partner preference behavior characteristic of females (Kauffman et al., 2007a). By contrast, no behavioral deficits have yet been reported in female *GPR54* knock-out mice (Kauffman et al., 2007a). Nevertheless, a major neuroendocrine effect has been found since these females become unable to perform a surge of luteinizing hormone (LH) under estrogen positive feedback conditions in adulthood (Clarkson et al., 2008), raising the possibility that the development of female-specific brain circuits may be impacted by this genetic deletion. Further investigations on the impact of the kisspeptin–GPR54 system on the sexual differentiation of the brain and behaviors in females remain an important future direction.

RAT

The involvement of the kisspeptin–GPR54 system in the central maturation of rat reproductive function has been explored with great precision by the group of Tena-Sempere since 2004 (Navarro et al., 2004a,b; Castellano et al., 2005, 2006). These studies used various modes of administration of synthetic forms of kisspeptins at different stages of development, followed by the

Table 1 | Summary of studies showing a role of kisspeptin–GPR54 system in the development of female reproductive function.

Approaches	Species	Reference	Manipulation	Period of manipulation	Time of analysis	Physiological impact	Hypothalamic analysis
Genetic	Human	Seminara et al. (2003), de Roux et al. (2003), Nimri et al. (2011)	GPR54 mutations (loss of function)	Congenital	Adult	IHH	
		Teles et al. (2008)	GPR54 mutations (gain of function)		Child	ICPP	
		Silveira et al. (2010)	Kiss1 mutations	Congenital	Child	IHH and ICPP	
		Topaloglu et al. (2012)			Child and Adult	IHH	
	Mouse	Seminara et al. (2003)	GPR54-KO	Congenital	Peripubertal to adult	HH, puberty delayed, no estrus cycle	No change in GnRH content (RIA)
		Funes et al. (2003)			Peripubertal to adult	HH, infertility	
		Lapatto et al. (2007)			Peripubertal to adult	HH, puberty delayed, no estrus cycle	
		Dungan et al. (2007)			Peripubertal to adult	HH, low circulating LH even after ovariectomy	No change in GnRH cell numbers
		Clarkson et al. (2008)			Peripubertal to adult	Compromised ability to mount LH surges	
		Lapatto et al. (2007)	Kiss1-KO	Congenital	Peripubertal to adult	HH, puberty delayed, no estrus cycle	
		d'Anglemont de Tassigny et al. (2007)			Peripubertal to adult	HH, puberty delayed, low circulating LH levels	No change in GnRH content (RIA), GnRH cell numbers and median eminence fiber density
		Mayer and Boehm (2011)	Kiss1 cell ablation Kiss1-DTA	Congenital	Prepubertal (P20) and adult	HH, estrus cycle present but less regular than control	Decrease in Kiss1 mRNA in ARC and kisspeptin-immunoreactive cell numbers in POA
			Kiss1 conditional cell ablation	Prepubertal (P20)	Pubertal (P40) and adult	No estrus cycle: persistent diestrous, infertility	

(Continued)

Table 1 | Continued

Approaches	Species	Reference	Manipulation	Period of manipulation	Time of analysis	Physiological impact	Hypothalamic analysis
Pharmacological	Rat	Matsui et al. (2004)	Kp s.c. injection (acute)	Prepubertal (P25)	Prepubertal (P25)	Increase in circulating LH	Effect abolished by GnRH receptor antagonist
		Navarro et al. (2004b)	Kp i.c.v. injection (acute)	Prepubertal (P25)	Prepubertal (P25)	Increase in circulating LH, decrease in circulating prolactin	
		Navarro et al. (2004a)	Kp i.c.v. injections (chronic)	Prepubertal (P26–P31)	Prepubertal (P26–P31)	Puberty advanced, increase of uterus weight, increase in circulating LH and E2	LH-releasing effect abolished by GnRH receptor antagonist
		Castellano et al. (2006)	Kp i.p. injection (acute)	Neonatal (P5), Prepubertal (P15 and P25)	Neonatal (P5), Prepubertal (P15 and P25)	Increase in circulating LH but significant only at P15	
		Pineda et al. (2010)	GPR54-antagonist i.c.v. infusion	Prepubertal (from P30 to P36)	Prepubertal (P36)	Puberty delayed	
	Sheep	Redmond et al. (2011a)	Kp i.v. injection	Prepubertal (28W)	Prepubertal (28W)	Increase in LH pulsatility (frequency and amplitude) and circulating E2	
	Monkey	Guerriero et al. (2012a)	Kp i.c.v. injection	Prepubertal (52–81W) and pubertal (112–175W)	Prepubertal (52–81W) and pubertal (112–175W)		Increase in GnRH pulsatile release GNRH-response to kp increases at puberty
			GPR54-antagonist i.c.v. injection	Prepubertal (52–81W) and pubertal (112–175W)	Prepubertal (52–81W) and pubertal (112–175W)		Decrease in GnRH pulsatile release only at prepubertal stage
		Roseweir et al. (2009)	GPR54-antagonist i.c.v. injection	Pubertal (132W)	Pubertal (132W)		Decrease in GnRH pulsatile release and basal GnRH (microdialysis)

IHH, idiopathic hypogonadotropic hypogonadism; ICPP, idiopathic central precocious puberty; HH, hypogonadotropic hypogonadism; s.c., sub cutaneous; i.v., intravenous; i.p., intraperitoneal; i.c.v., intracerebroventricular; RIA, radioimmunoassay; POA, preoptic area; ARC, arcuate nucleus; ME, median eminence; GnRH, gonadotropin-releasing hormone; LH, luteinizing hormone; E2, estradiol; P, postnatal day; W, weeks.

monitoring of endocrine and physiological changes. In prepubertal female rats, kisspeptins, whether administered centrally or peripherally, induce an immediate elevation of circulating LH levels and this effect can be abolished by central administration of a GnRH receptor antagonist (Matsui et al., 2004; Navarro et al., 2004a). The GnRH-releasing activity of kisspeptins was directly tested on hypothalamic explants derived from female rats of various postnatal stages and found similar between the neonatal, infantile, and juvenile stages (Castellano et al., 2006). Repeated intracerebroventricular injections during the late juvenile period are able to increase uterus weight, circulating levels of LH and estradiol, and to advance the age of vaginal opening, a peripheral landmark of puberty onset in rodents (Navarro et al., 2004a). Conversely, central infusion of a GPR54 antagonist to peripubertal female rats decreases uterus and ovary weights without affecting total body weights and delays puberty onset (Pineda et al., 2010). Taken together, these observations provide convincing evidence that prepubertal kisspeptins are both necessary and sufficient for triggering various indices of female puberty in this species.

SHEEP

The functional relevance of the kisspeptin–GPR54 system in the maturation of female reproductive function has been well characterized during the last decade in mice and rats, as detailed in the preceding sections; however it was not until 2011 that this aspect has been explored in species other than rodents such as sheep and monkeys. In ewes, chronic hourly intravenous injections of kisspeptins during the prepubertal period stimulated a pulsatile release of LH within 15 min following injections, increasing both pulse frequencies and amplitudes (Redmond et al., 2011a). Mean circulating levels of LH and estradiol were increased and a surge like release of LH developed in some lambs 17 h post treatment. These animals were however unable to develop a long-lasting luteal phase as attested by circulating progesterone levels and did not achieve regular estrus cyclicity, suggesting that the reproductive neuroendocrine axis was not yet fully mature (Redmond et al., 2011a).

MONKEY

In female monkeys, it has recently become possible to directly monitor the GnRH-releasing activity of kisspeptins *in vivo* (Guerriero et al., 2012a). The GnRH-releasing response to kisspeptin infusion directly within the medial basal hypothalamus and stalk median eminence is dose dependent and greater in pubertal than prepubertal females (Guerriero et al., 2012a). Conversely, mean GnRH levels are diminished following central infusion with a GPR54 antagonist at both developmental stages (Roseweir et al., 2009; Guerriero et al., 2012a). This provides convincing evidence that a GPR54-mediated mechanism is required for the reactivation of GnRH release at puberty in the female monkey.

HUMAN

The fundamental role of the kisspeptin–GPR54 system in Pubertal development was initially discovered by two independent groups that identified loss of function mutations in the *GPR54* gene within human families with idiopathic hypogonadotropic hypogonadism (IHH) (de Roux et al., 2003; Seminara et al., 2003). Mutations of the *GPR54* gene have since been found in other families with IHH associated with various levels of GnRH deficiency (Nimri et al., 2011; Wahab et al., 2011). A very recent report also discovered an inactivating mutation of the *Kiss1* gene associated with IHH (Topaloglu et al., 2012). Idiopathic central precocious puberty (ICPP) is another developmental reproductive disorder that has been associated with either *GPR54* mutations (Teles et al., 2008), *Kiss1* mutations (Silveira et al., 2010), or polymorphisms (Luan et al., 2007a,b). Taken together, these pathologies attest for the critical role played by kisspeptin signaling in the development of the human hypothalamic–pituitary–gonadal axis.

DEVELOPMENTAL CHANGES OF KISSPEPTIN–GPR54 COINCIDE WITH CHANGES IN LH SECRETION THROUGHOUT LIFE

MOUSE

Recent evidence points to an early onset of *Kiss1* and *GPR54* expression in the mouse nervous system. For instance, *Kiss1* mRNA has been detected in the mediobasal hypothalamus of the mouse as early as embryonic day (E) 13, by reverse transcription polymerase chain reaction (Fiorini and Jasoni, 2010). At this early developmental stage, *in situ* hybridization further identified *GPR54* mRNA in some GnRH neurons along the nasal portion of their migratory route (Constantin et al., 2009b). Furthermore, *in vitro* studies suggest that GnRH neurons are already able to respond to kisspeptins by enhanced secretion during prenatal life (Constantin et al., 2009a,b). However, the presence of the kisspeptin protein remains to be shown in mouse embryos.

Postnatally, *Kiss1*-expressing cells can already be detected in the ARC a few hours only after birth, using *in situ* hybridization (Poling and Kauffman, 2012). *Kiss1* mRNA levels increase in this region at the time of puberty but only in hypogonadal hpg mice, which are deficient in GnRH receptor signaling and hence display very low levels of sex steroids (Gill et al., 2010, 2012). In wild type mice, it appears that *Kiss1* expression in the ARC is strongly repressed postnatally by circulating estradiol and no developmental changes have yet been detected in this region at the *Kiss1* transcript or kisspeptin protein level (Clarkson and Herbison, 2006; Gill et al., 2010, 2012). Of interest, however, is the significant increase in neurokinin B (NKB; another GnRH secretagogue expressed by kisspeptin neurons) transcript levels that has been observed in this nucleus prior to puberty onset (Gill et al., 2012). In the POA, expression of *Kiss1* appears to develop later than in the ARC, between postnatal day 8 and 10 (Semaan et al., 2010) and increases thereafter until puberty is reached (Gill et al., 2010). Similarly, a peripubertal increase in the number of POA kisspeptin-immunoreactive neurons has been shown (Clarkson and Herbison, 2006; Clarkson et al., 2009; Gill et al., 2010; Mayer et al., 2010). This increase has been correlated with the development of the capacity for GnRH/LH surges (Clarkson et al., 2009). Another interesting feature observed in the development of this system is a peripubertal increase in the proportion of GnRH neurons closely apposed to kisspeptin-immunoreactive fibers, suggesting a postnatal morphological maturation of kisspeptin circuitry associated with puberty (Clarkson and Herbison, 2006). Furthermore, a longitudinal analysis of transgenic mice in which

LacZ has been introduced in the *GPR54* locus identified a prepubertal rise in the percentage of GnRH neurons expressing *GPR54* (Herbison et al., 2010). These different changes observed in the female POA at the time of puberty may be related to the increase in circulating LH levels that precedes puberty onset in the mouse (Michael et al., 1980; Gill et al., 2012). In any case, debate still persists about the relative importance of ARC versus POA kisspeptin neurons in triggering the onset of puberty in the female mouse.

RAT

A recent study in the rat has provided strong foundation for our understanding of the embryonic stages of kisspeptin neuron development. Using a BrdU pulse chasing approach, we have established that the neurogenesis period of ARC kisspeptin cells in the female rat hypothalamus begins at about E12.5, peaks around E15.5, and is not yet over at E17.5 (Desroziers et al., 2012a). Using immunohistochemistry, we further show that some cells in the developing ARC already synthesize kisspeptins from about E14.5 (Desroziers et al., 2012a; **Figure 2**). The number of kisspeptin-immunoreactive cells in the fetal ARC increases between E14.5 and E18.5 which coincides with the time when GnRH fibers reach the portal vessels of the median eminence and circulating LH levels reach their maximum in the rat fetus (Ugrumov et al., 1985; Huhtaniemi, 1995). At E18.5, close appositions between kisspeptin- and GnRH-immunoreactive fibers can be detected in the median eminence (**Figure 2D**), consistent with the hypothesis that kisspeptins already control GnRH release prenatally. The number of kisspeptin-immunoreactive cells, as well as hypothalamic *Kiss1* mRNA levels, decrease at the end of gestation (Desroziers et al., 2012a). The mechanism of action and physiological relevance of this decrease have yet to be fully elucidated.

During postnatal development, *Kiss1* expression continues to be tightly regulated as shown in the pioneering study by Navarro et al. (2004b). In particular, real-time quantitative RT-PCR of *Kiss1* and *GPR54* content in the hypothalamus revealed a transient decline in the expression levels of both genes during the infantile period, followed by an increase around the time of puberty (Navarro et al., 2004b). These changes have since been spatially refined by studying the respective expression of these genes either by RT-PCR on tissue punches (Knox et al., 2009; Takase et al., 2009; Lederman et al., 2010; Li et al., 2012) or by *in situ* hybridization (Cao and Patisaul, 2011; Takumi et al., 2011; Patisaul et al., 2012). In the ARC, *Kiss1* expression is relatively high during the neonatal and early infantile period but decreases during the third postnatal week (Cao and Patisaul, 2011; Takumi et al., 2011). A decline in the density of kisspeptin-immunoreactive fibers has also been measured during that period of time (Desroziers et al., 2012b). These observations may be correlated to the reported transient activation of LH secretion during early postnatal life (Döhler and Wuttke, 1975). *Kiss1* expression in the ARC increases again at puberty (Knox et al., 2009; Takase et al., 2009; Takumi et al., 2011). This increase has been associated with an increase in basal

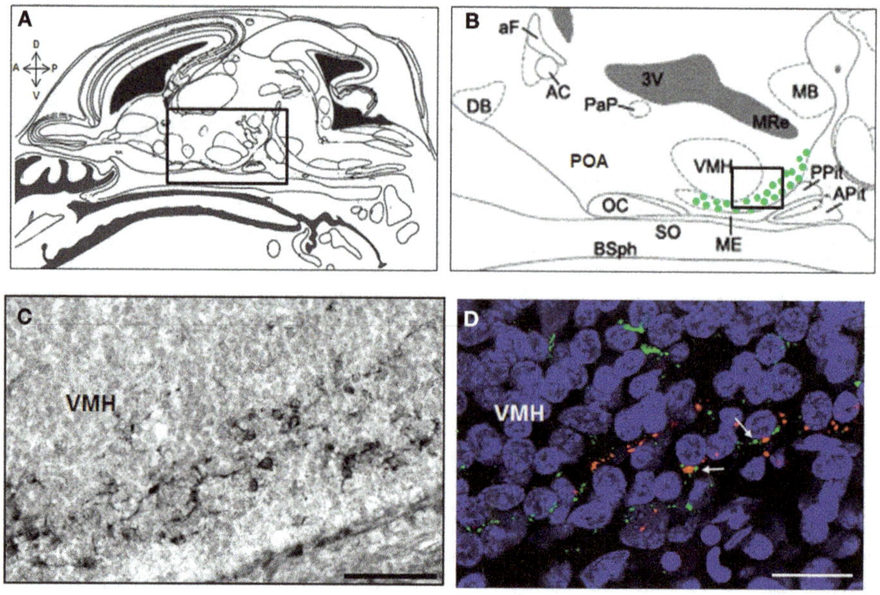

FIGURE 2 | Kisspeptin-immunoreactive cells and fibers in the ARC and median eminence at embryonic day E18.5 in rats. Schematic mid sagittal view of embryonic head at E18.5 **(A)** (adapted from Paxinos and Ashwell, 2008) with a higher resolution of the embryonic hypothalamus **(B)** [corresponding to the box in **(A)**] depicting the area were kisspeptin-immunoreactive cells were detected (green dots). Numerous kisspeptin-immunoreactive cells were detected in the ARC at embryonic day (E) 18.5 as shown on this immunoperoxidase-labeled brain section with anti-kisspeptin AC067 **(C)** [corresponding to the box in **(B)**]. In the median eminence, close appositions (white arrows) between kisspeptin fibers (green) and GnRH fibers (red) were detected as shown in this confocal optical section of a slice double immunofluorescence-labeled for kisspeptin (sheep anti-5-18 kisspeptin 52 # AC067, Desroziers et al., 2012a) and GnRH (rabbit anti-2-10 GnRH # 19900, Caldani et al., 1988) and counterstained with Hoechst nuclear marker **(D)**. A, anterior; P, posterior; D, dorsal; V, ventral; DB, diagonal band of Broca; aF, anterior fornix; AC, anterior commissure; PaP, paraventricular nucleus; 3V, third ventricle; OC, optic chiasma; POA, preoptic area; SO, supraoptic nucleus; ME, median eminence; VMH, ventro-medial hypothalamus; MB, mammillary bodies; Pit, pituitary; Apit, anterior pituitary; Ppit, posterior pituitary; BSph, sphenoid bones; MRe, mammillary recess. Scale bars: 100 μm **(C)** and 20 μm **(D)**.

circulating LH levels (Takase et al., 2009). Similarly, kisspeptin-immunoreactive cell numbers and fiber densities increase in the ARC during the peripubertal period (Desroziers et al., 2012b). As in mice, *Kiss 1* expression in the POA of rats is detected later than in the ARC, starting during the second postnatal week (Cao and Patisaul, 2011), and continues to increase until the fifth postnatal week (Desroziers et al., 2010; Takumi et al., 2011). By contrast to mice, however, no kisspeptin-immunoreactive cells has been detected so far in the POA throughout rat postnatal life, unless colchicine was administered (Takase et al., 2009; Desroziers et al., 2010, 2012b; Lederman et al., 2010). A very recent study on Sprague Dawley rats has enabled the peripubertal changes in *Kiss1* and *GPR54* expression in the ARC and POA to be assessed with greater time resolution and in relation to changes in the frequency of LH pulses (Li et al., 2012). No changes in *GPR54* expression are observed during this developmental time window but *Kiss1* mRNA levels significantly increase prior to puberty onset, first in the ARC and later in the POA. Notably, these changes are accompanied by an increase in LH pulse frequencies (Li et al., 2012). Our recent analysis of kisspeptin-immunoreactive fiber density across each of these two regions similarly suggest a sequential activation of kisspeptin-immunoreactivity at the time of puberty, first in the ARC, and second in the POA (Desroziers et al., 2012b). Collectively, these findings provide strong support for an important role of kisspeptins produced by ARC neurons in triggering puberty in female rats. During pubertal progression, this would be followed by an estrogen-dependent amplification system of GnRH release mediated by kisspeptins neurons of the POA.

In adult cycling females, the number of *Kiss1*-expressing cells varies across the estrous cycle, in opposite phases between the ARC and the POA (Smith et al., 2006a). Changes in *Kiss1* expression have also been evaluated across aging. In the rat, unlike in humans, reproductive senescence is associated with a decrease in the frequency and amplitude of GnRH/LH pulses and a progressive disappearance of GnRH/LH surges (Scarbrough and Wise, 1990). Consistently, a significantly lower number of kisspeptin-immunoreactive cells are detected in the POA of middle-aged rats compared to young rats, under estradiol positive feedback conditions (Lederman et al., 2010).

Thus, in the rat, *Kiss1* expression appears tightly regulated throughout the reproductive life cycle, not only in the POA, but also in the ARC where it is already detected prenatally. The developmental profile of *Kiss1* expression in the ARC and POA differ significantly. This may be related to different roles played by the two kisspeptin cell populations in the control of GnRH pulse amplitude and frequency.

SHEEP

Studies of the kisspeptin–GPR54 system in sheep have focused on two critical periods of development, the prenatal period and the peripubertal period. *Kiss1* expression has been detected by RT-PCR in the hypothalamus of 110 day old sheep fetuses (birth occurring around gestational day 145 in this species) both in rostral and caudal hypothalamic slices including the POA and ARC, respectively (Bellingham et al., 2009). This is a time when LH is already secreted in a GnRH-dependent, pulsatile manner (Matwijiw and Faiman, 1987). Thus, it is tempting to speculate that kisspeptins already provide tonic drive to GnRH neuronal activity *in utero*. *Kiss1* expression has further been studied by *in situ* hybridization in an estradiol-supplemented ovariectomized model of puberty (Redmond et al., 2011b). In this study, puberty was preceded by an elevation in the number of *Kiss1*-expressing neurons both in the POA and ARC. However, it is the increase in *Kiss1* expression levels in the ARC more specifically that could be correlated with an increase in LH pulse frequency (Redmond et al., 2011b). In intact ewes, the number of kisspeptin-immunoreactive cells in the ARC was shown to increase at puberty, concomitantly to an increase in LH pulse frequency but not pulse amplitude (Nestor et al., 2012). Over that same period of time, the proportion of GnRH neurons with close appositions of kisspeptin-immunoreactive fibers increase (Nestor et al., 2012), as previously reported in mice (Clarkson and Herbison, 2006). Whether this reflects a postnatal morphological plasticity of the system, or is related to enhanced *Kiss1* expression remains to be investigated. Taken together, these findings point to a potential relationship between postnatal changes in the kisspeptin–GPR54 system and the increase of LH secretion accompanying ovine puberty.

MONKEY

In the female monkey, hypothalamic *Kiss1* and *GPR54* expression levels have been monitored across puberty and aging. Real-time quantitative RT-PCR of *Kiss1* and *GPR54* mRNA levels in the mediobasal hypothalamus revealed that both of these transcripts significantly increase at puberty (Shahab et al., 2005). More recently, using an *in vivo* microdialysis method, the team of Ei Terasawa was able to show an increase in kisspeptin pulsatile release within the stalk median eminence during puberty (Guerriero et al., 2012b). During late puberty, *in vivo* secretion of kisspeptin is pulsatile and in almost perfect synchrony with GnRH pulses, a finding consistent with a possible role of kisspeptins in the tuning of GnRH pulsatility at puberty (Keen et al., 2008). Notably, no changes in the POA have yet been reported across monkey physiology. With aging, *Kiss1* and *GPR54* mRNA levels increase in the mediobasal hypothalamus but remain unchanged in the POA (Kim et al., 2009; Eghlidi et al., 2010). By analogy, LH pulsatile secretion increases in aging monkeys but these are still able to generate GnRH/LH surges (Gore et al., 2004). Collectively, these observations suggest that GnRH release in the monkey continues to be under the tight regulatory control of ARC and POA kisspeptins late in postnatal life.

HUMAN

A very recent study detected kisspeptin and GPR54 immunoreactivities in the hypothalamus of second trimester human fetuses (Guimiot et al., 2012). Kisspeptin-immunoreactivity declined at the end of gestation, as previously observed in rats (Desroziers et al., 2012a). A causal link between this decline and the decline in circulating levels of gonadotropins that was monitored in cord blood between the 30th week of prenatal life and birth was suggested (Guimiot et al., 2012). Postnatal analysis of *Kiss1* expression or kisspeptin-immunoreactivity in human brains has only been reported in post-pubertal subjects (Rometo et al., 2007; Hrabovszky et al., 2010, 2011). *Kiss1* expression in the infundibular nucleus has been shown to increase after menopause in women (Rometo et al., 2007). This increase may be related to the increase in GnRH/LH secretion characterizing human reproductive senescence (Kermath and Gore, 2012 for review). Again, these findings are consistent with the hypothesis that GnRH secretion in women continues to be regulated by kisspeptins late in life.

In conclusion, analogies can be found in each species between fluctuations in GnRH/LH levels and fluctuations in some aspects of the kisspeptin–GPR54 system, supporting the view that kisspeptin signaling in the brain controls GnRH secretion throughout life, including prenatally (**Figure 3**). The regulatory mechanism by which these changes in the kisspeptin–GPR54 system operate will be the focus of the following section.

ENDOGENOUS REGULATORS OF KISSPEPTIN–GPR54 DURING DEVELOPMENT

DEVELOPMENTAL REGULATION OF THE KISSPEPTIN–GPR54 SYSTEM BY GONADAL STEROIDS

Ever since the discovery that *Kiss1* expression is under tight regulation of estrogen receptor signaling (Smith et al., 2005) and that kisspeptin neurons express numerous sex steroid receptors in adult mice, rats, and sheep (Smith et al., 2005, 2006a, 2007; Franceschini et al., 2006; Adachi et al., 2007; Clarkson et al., 2008; Cheng et al., 2010), numerous studies have investigated the regulation of the kisspeptin–GPR54 system by gonadal steroids across development (**Table 2**).

Mouse

Female mice display a much greater number of kisspeptin-immunoreactive cells in the POA than male mice (Clarkson and Herbison, 2006) even after gonadectomy (González-Martínez et al., 2008), suggestive of organizational effects of sex steroids on this cell population during development. This sexual dimorphism appears to develop between postnatal days 10 and 12, that is shortly after the first *Kiss1*-expressing cells can be detected in this region (Semaan et al., 2010). It does not appear to involve bax-mediated apoptosis (Semaan et al., 2010) but differential transcription patterns of the *Kiss1* gene governed by sex-specific epigenetic mechanisms during development (Semaan et al., 2012). For instance, the methylation pattern of the *Kiss1* gene in the POA (but not the ARC) significantly differs at several CpG sites between males and females (Semaan et al., 2012). The contribution of estrogen signaling to the sexual differentiation of the kisspeptin cell population of the POA has mostly been explored by the means of genetic manipulations. Mice genetically deficient in alpha-fetoprotein (AFP-knock-out) have excess estradiol signaling in the brain during the perinatal period. Female AFP-knock-out mice develop as few kisspeptin cells in the POA as males and their circulating LH levels are not increased by estradiol and progesterone-induced positive feedback conditions (González-Martínez et al., 2008). Thus, it may be that estradiol signaling in the brain at the time of the perinatal testosterone surge may be in part responsible for the defeminization/masculinization of the POA kisspeptin cell population in males. Interestingly, transgenic reduction of developmental sex steroid hormone signaling in a variety of mouse models also results in a marked decrease in the adult number of kisspeptin-immunoreactive neurons in the POA (Clarkson et al., 2009; Bakker et al., 2010; Gill et al., 2010; Mayer et al., 2010). For example, in the adult hypogonadal hpg mice, the number of kisspeptin-immunoreactive cells in the POA is reduced by half and it is not possible to increase this number by estradiol administration as it is for wild type mice (Gill et al., 2010). In aromatase knock-out (ArKO) mice which completely lack the capacity to synthesize estrogens, the number of kisspeptin-immunoreactive cells in the POA is also significantly reduced compared to wild type mice (Clarkson et al., 2009), even under identical positive feedback conditions (Bakker et al., 2010). In the same vein, ArKO mice, whether ovariectomized or treated with estradiol and/or progesterone to mimic positive feedback conditions, display fewer *Kiss1*-expressing cells in the POA compared to wild type mice (Szymanski and Bakker, 2012), consistent with the hypothesis that postnatal estrogens may reprogram *Kiss1*

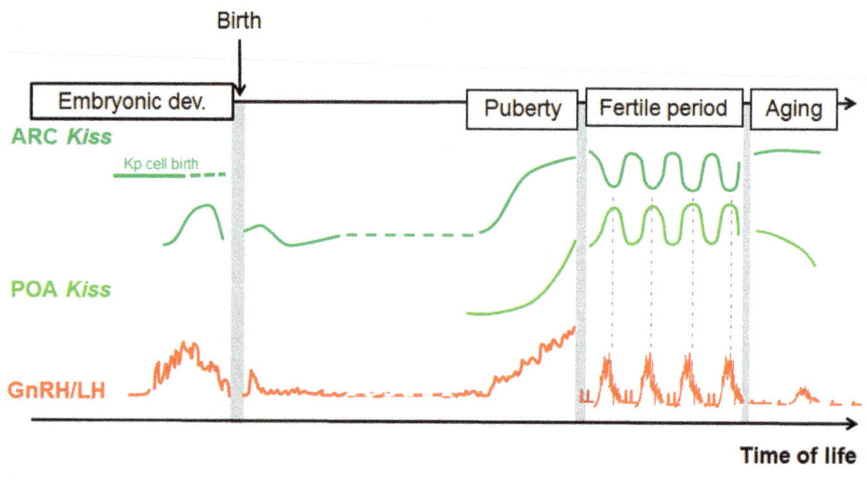

FIGURE 3 | Parallel developmental changes in *Kiss1* mRNA and circulating LH levels in rats. Hypothetical scheme highlighting the parallel that can be made between Kiss1 expression in the POA and ARC and the profile of GnRH/LH release across different time windows of rat development (separated from each other by grey bars on the scheme because analyzed in separate studies). POA, preoptic area; ARC, arcuate nucleus; Kp, kisspeptin; LH, luteinizing hormone.

Table 2 | Summary of studies showing an effect of sex steroids on the kisspeptin–GPR54 system throughout female development.

Approaches	Species	Reference	Treatment	Period of treatment	Time of analysis	Hypothalamic impact	Physiological impact
Transgenetical reduction in sex steroid signalization	Mouse	González-Martínez et al. (2008)	Genetic deletion of alpha-fetoprotein (AFP-KO mice)	Late embryonic and neonatal period	Adult	Decrease in kp-ir cell numbers in the POA	Infertility
		Gill et al. (2010)	Mutation of GnRH receptor, resulting in reduced sex steroid signaling (Hpg mice)	Congenital	Peripubertal (P10, P30, P45) and adult	Decrease in Kiss1 mRNA and kp-ir cell numbers in the POA, increase of Kiss1 mRNA in the ARC	Absence of vaginal opening, infertility
		Mayer et al. (2010)	Targeted genetic deletion of estrogen receptor alpha in kisspeptin cells	Congenital	Peripubertal (P15, P25, P35) and adult	Decrease in kp-ir cell numbers in the POA, increase in Kiss1 mRNA in the ARC	Advanced vaginal opening
		Clarkson et al. (2009), Bakker et al. (2010)	Genetic deletion of aromatase (ARKO: mice)	Congenital	Adult	Ovariectomy decreases Kiss1 mRNA and kp-ir cell numbers in the POA	Infertility
Gonadectomy ± sex steroid replacement	Mouse	Kauffman et al. (2009)	Ovariectomy	Prepubertal (PI4 and PI8) and adult	Prepubertal (P18) and adult	Decrease in Kiss1 cell numbers in the POA, increase in Kiss1 cell numbers in the ARC	Increase in circulating LH
		Clarkson et al. (2009)	Ovariectomy ± E2	Prepubertal (P15–P30 or P22–P30)	Prepubertal (P30)	Ovariectomy decreases kp-ir cell numbers in the POA. Effect reversed by E2 treatment	Increase in circulating LH. Circulating LH restored by E2
	Rat	Takase et al. (2009)	Ovariectomy ± E2	Prepubertal (P15–P21, P20–P26)	Peripubertal (P21, P26, P31, P36–41)	Ovariectomy suppresses the peripubertal increase in Kiss1 mRNA in the POA and ARC. Effect reversed by E2 treatment	Ovariectomy suppresses the peripubertal increase in circulating LH. Effect reversed by E2 treatment
		Takumi et al. (2012a)	Ovariectomy	Prepubertal (P14–P18)	Prepubertal (P18)	Decrease in Kiss1 cell numbers in the POA and ARC	
	Sheep	Nestor et al. (2012)	Ovariectomy	Pre- (20–24W) and post-pubertal (>36W)	Pre- (20–24W) and post-pubertal (>36W)	Increase in kp-ir cell numbers in the ARC, specifically at prepubertal stage	Increase in LH pulse frequency in prepubertal stage

(Continued)

Table 2 | Continued

Approaches	Species	Reference	Treatment	Period of treatment	Time of analysis	Hypothalamic impact	Physiological impact
	Monkey	Guerriero et al. (2012b)	Ovariectomy ± E2	Prepubertal (52–81 W) and pubertal (112–175 W)	Prepubertal (52–81 W) and pubertal (112–175 W)		Ovariectomy increases kp release specifically at pubertal stage. Effect reversed by E2 treatment
Pharmacological	Rat	Dickerson et al. (2011b)	EB injection	Embryonic (E16–E18)	Neonatal (P1) and adult	Decrease in kp-ir fiber density in the POA (adult)	Advanced vaginal opening, decrease in circulating LH
		Gore et al. (2011)	EB injection	Embryonic and neonatal (E19–P7)	Adult	Decrease in Kiss1 mRNA in the POA	Decrease in circulating E2, irregular estrus cycle
		Cao et al. (2012)	EB injection	Neonatal (P0–P2)	Neonatal (P4) and infantile (P10)	Decrease in Kiss1 mRNA from P4 in the ARC and from P10 in the POA	
		Navarro et al. (2004b), Navarro et al. (2009)	EB injection	Neonatal (P1)	Peripubertal (P30) and adult	Decrease in hypothalamic Kiss1 mRNA	Decrease in circulating LH
		Losa et al. (2011), Losa-Ward et al. (2012), Patisaul et al. (2012)	EB or E2 injection	Neonatal (P0–P3)	Peripubertal (from P17 to P33)	Decrease in Kiss1 mRNA and kp-ir in the POA and ARC	Advanced vaginal opening
		Kauffman et al. (2007b)	TP injection	Neonatal (P1)	Adult	Decrease in Kiss1 cell numbers in the POA but not in the ARC	Decrease in circulating LH
		Bateman and Patisaul (2008), Patisaul et al. (2009), Patisaul et al. (2012)	EB injection	Neonatal (P0–P3)	Adult	Decrease in kp-ir in the POA and ARC	Irregular estrus cycles, decrease in circulating LH
	Sheep	Cheng et al. (2010)	TP injection	End of gestation	Adult	No change in kp-ir cell numbers in the POA and ARC	Increase in circulating LH and LH pulse frequency

POA, preoptic area; ARC, arcuate nucleus; GnRH, gonadotropin-releasing hormone; LH, luteinizing hormone; kp-ir, kisspeptin-immunoreactive; EB, estradiol benzoate; TP, testosterone propionate; E2, estradiol; E, embryonic day; P, postnatal day; W, weeks.

transcription in the POA. Furthermore, while odors from male urine are able to induce c-fos expression in a good proportion of POA kisspeptin cells in wild type female mice, this proportion is markedly reduced in the ArKO mice (Bakker et al., 2010). Data from experimental gonadectomy and estradiol replacement during development suggest that estrogens stimulate kisspeptin expression in the POA before puberty (Clarkson et al., 2009). These authors proposed that this estrogen-dependent increase of kisspeptin expression in the POA may facilitate the emergence of pulsatile gonadotropin secretion necessary for puberty onset, as well as the preovulatory estrogen-dependent surge (Clarkson et al., 2009). However, it was recently shown that ArKO mice maintain the ability to mount an LH surge when treated with hormones mimicking positive feedback conditions in adulthood, questioning the absolute requirement of the full female-typical (estrogen induced) complement of POA kisspeptin neurons in generating GnRH/LH surge (Szymanski and Bakker, 2012).

In the mouse ARC, the sexual dimorphism of the kisspeptin cell population is not as obvious as in the POA. In this nucleus, female mice display a greater number of *Kiss1*-expressing cells than males on the day of birth but this difference is no longer visible during infancy or in adulthood (Kauffman et al., 2009; Poling and Kauffman, 2012). By gonadectomizing the mice at different stages of development, Kauffman et al. (2009) revealed an important gonadal hormone-independent sex difference in the number of ARC *Kiss1* cells during the infantile period. Prepubertal gonadal hormones appear to exert a greater repressive action on ARC *Kiss1* expression in females than in males (Kauffman et al., 2009). Of interest, this strong downregulation of *Kiss1* expression in the prepubertal female ARC most likely occurs through Erα signaling within kisspeptin cells themselves and may be of physiological relevance in the timing of puberty (Mayer et al., 2010). Indeed, female mice with a targeted deletion of *Esr1* within kisspeptin cells not only display enhanced *Kiss1* expression in the ARC at the juvenile stage but also a dramatic advance in the timing of vaginal opening. Moreover, circulating LH levels in these genetically modified mice are higher than in control mice (Mayer et al., 2010). These authors proposed that the prepubertal repressive action of estrogen signaling on *Kiss1* expression in the ARC represents an essential break to the central activation of the gonadotropic axis, preventing premature puberty onset (Mayer et al., 2010).

Collectively, these findings suggest that in the mouse, estrogen signaling may exert organizational effects on the kisspeptin cell population of the POA during the perinatal period in males and during the prepubertal period in females. Further studies are needed to elucidate the developmental origin of the sexual dimorphism observed at the level of ARC kisspeptin cell population. In particular, it is still unclear whether the sex-specific pattern of *Kiss1* expression detected in the absence of gonadal hormones during infancy in this nucleus is conditioned by a sex-specific and gonad-independent developmental program or by an organizational effect of the perinatal testosterone surge.

Rat

The number of POA *Kiss1*-expressing cells is greater in female rats than in male rats under identical estrogen positive feedback conditions, suggesting that, like in mice, developmental sex steroids may have important organizational effects on this cell population (Kauffman et al., 2007b; Homma et al., 2009). The importance of the perinatal period in this process is suggested from several studies using gain or loss of function approaches. Male pups neonatally orchidectomized develop a female-specific pattern of *Kiss1* expression in the POA (Homma et al., 2009; Takumi et al., 2012a). Conversely, female pups exposed to synthetic estrogens or aromatizable androgens such as estradiol benzoate or testosterone propionate during the perinatal period display a male-specific pattern of *Kiss1* expression or kisspeptin-immunoreactivity in adulthood (Navarro et al., 2004b; Kauffman et al., 2007b; Homma et al., 2009; Dickerson et al., 2011a).

By contrast to the POA, similar numbers of *Kiss1*-expressing cells and similar levels of *Kiss1* transcripts have been detected in the ARC of gonadectomized male and female rats (Adachi et al., 2007; Kauffman et al., 2007b; Homma et al., 2009). Furthermore, the downregulating effect of estradiol on *Kiss1* transcription in this nucleus appears similar in both sexes (Adachi et al., 2007; Kauffman et al., 2007b; Homma et al., 2009). In the ARC of intact adult rats, however, several studies have shown that females display more *Kiss1*-expressing cells or kisspeptin-immunoreactivity than males (Iijima et al., 2011; Takumi et al., 2011; Desroziers et al., 2012b). A real-time quantitative RT-PCR analysis of *Kiss1* transcript content in the ARC also points to the fact that the sex difference in *Kiss1* transcript levels is more or less visible, depending on the stage of the estrus cycle (Adachi et al., 2007). This sex difference develops during the neonatal period (Cao and Patisaul, 2011; Desroziers et al., 2012b) and its amplitude appears to fluctuate across postnatal development (Cao and Patisaul, 2011; Takumi et al., 2011; Desroziers et al., 2012b), presumably reflecting different developmental fluctuations in circulating gonadal hormones between males and females, as well as sex-specific developmental changes in the sensitivity of ARC kisspeptin cells to these hormones. For instance, data from experimental ovariectomy and estradiol replacement across different developmental time windows suggest that the regulatory action of estrogen signaling on *Kiss1* expression may change at the time of female puberty, leading to a developmental increase of *Kiss1* mRNA levels in both regions, and to an increase in circulating LH levels (Takase et al., 2009). Accordingly, we recently measured a peripubertal increase in kisspeptin-immunoreactivity within both regions at a time when peripheral estradiol levels were relatively constant (Desroziers et al., 2012b).

Another period of life when the sensitivity of kisspeptin cells to the feedback action of ovarian hormones appears to change is during aging. Middle-aged female rats that are gonadectomized and supplemented with estradiol benzoate and progesterone to mimic positive feedback conditions display an attenuated rise in the number of kisspeptin-immunoreactive cells in the POA as compared to young females under the same conditions (Lederman et al., 2010). By contrast, the repressive action of these gonadal hormones on ARC *Kiss1* mRNA and kisspeptin levels appears unaffected by aging (Lederman et al., 2010).

Collectively, these results suggest that estrogen signaling during the neonatal period organizes sex differences in *Kiss1* expression in the POA and that the sensitivity of both kisspeptin cell populations to estrogen signaling is dynamic across the lifespan of female rats.

Sheep

Female sheep display a greater number of kisspeptin-immunoreactive cells than male sheep not only in the POA but also in the ARC (Cheng et al., 2010). This sex difference in the ARC is also observed in pubertal sheep after gonadectomy, suggesting that it may result from organizational effects of gonadal steroids (Nestor et al., 2012). In this precocious species, sexual differentiation of the neuroendocrine circuits controlling reproductive function is mainly under the organizational influence of prenatal androgens during fetal life. Accordingly, female sheep treated prenatally with androgens display a lower responsiveness of the GnRH system to the negative feedback influence of progesterone. This translates into increased LH pulse frequencies and mean concentrations in peripheral blood (Cheng et al., 2010). However, this prenatal androgenization does not alter the number of kisspeptin-immunoreactive cells in the ARC nor in the POA. Rather, it is the number of cells immunoreactive for dynorphin or NKB, two other neuropeptides co-expressed with kisspeptins in the ARC, that is reduced compared to control females (Cheng et al., 2010). It may be that a greater exposure to androgens is required (dose and length) or that the influence of sex-specific genetic factors prevail in the sexual differentiation of the ovine kisspeptin system. Around the time of puberty, the negative feedback action of gonadal hormones on ARC kisspeptin-immunoreactivity diminishes parallel to an increase in LH pulse frequencies, suggesting, as in the rat, that a change in the sensitivity of ARC kisspeptin cells to the negative feedback action of estradiol signaling may initiate puberty onset (Nestor et al., 2012).

Monkey

There is to our knowledge no published information of a clear sexual dimorphism of the kisspeptin system in the monkey. In the female monkey, the positive and negative feedback action of estradiol on the kisspeptin–GPR54 system have been studied at the time of puberty (Guerriero et al., 2012b) and during aging (Eghlidi et al., 2010). Prepubertal ovariectomy does not prevent the peripubertal rise in kisspeptin pulsatile release within the median eminence. In fact, the repressive action of estradiol on this release appears to develop later, once puberty has already started (Guerriero et al., 2012b). Ovariectomy and short-term estradiol replacement appears to have little effect on ARC *Kiss1* expression levels in young monkeys (Eghlidi et al., 2010). By contrast, long-term ovariectomy (mimicking the loss of ovarian steroid negative feedback that occurs during perimenopause) significantly increases ARC *Kiss1* expression levels. *Kiss1* expression levels can be restored to normality by short-term estradiol supplementation (Eghlidi et al., 2010). Collectively, these results minimize the role played by estradiol signaling in the upregulation of kisspeptin release at puberty in the female monkey but suggest a role of this signaling in the upregulation of *Kiss1* expression in the ARC with aging.

Human

Little is known in humans about the impact of sex steroids on the developing kisspeptin–GPR54 system. In adult women, the number of kisspeptin-immunoreactive neurons is greater than in men both in the infundibular nucleus and in the POA (Hrabovszky et al., 2010). However, the involvement of developmental sex steroids in this dimorphism is yet to be defined.

DEVELOPMENTAL REGULATION OF KISSPEPTIN NEURONS BY OTHER FACTORS

In the adult, there exists neuroanatomical, electrophysiological, and/or pharmacological evidence that the kisspeptin–GPR54 system may be the target of a variety of other hormones, neurotransmitters, and neuropeptides (**Figure 4**, squared by dotted lines). These include leptin (Smith et al., 2006b; Backholer et al., 2010), corticosterone (Kinsey-Jones et al., 2009), prolactin (Li et al., 2011), melanocortin hormone (Cravo et al., 2011), pheromones (Bakker et al., 2010), melatonin (Revel et al., 2006), ghrelin (Forbes et al., 2009), melanin-concentrating hormone (Wu et al., 2009; Cravo et al., 2011), corticotropin-releasing hormone (Takumi et al., 2012b), vasopressin (Vida et al., 2010), glutamate (Ducret et al., 2010), GABA (García-Galiano et al., 2012a), dopamine (Goodman et al., 2012), NKB (Navarro et al., 2011), and RFRP3 (Rizwan et al., 2012). However, only a few of these molecular factors have yet been identified as potential actors in the developmental regulation of the kisspeptin–GPR54 system (**Figure 4**, squared by full lines).

Leptin

Among hormonal factors, leptin, a well known permissive factor for pubertal maturation, is a potential upstream regulator of the kisspeptin–GPR54 system. Leptin deficient ob/ob mice display a marked reduction of *Kiss1* expression in the ARC and in the number of kisspeptin-immunoreactive cells in the POA but it is not yet known when exactly during development this effect starts (Quennell et al., 2011). The gonadotropin response of prepubertal rats to acute central administration of kisspeptin is preserved in different models of leptin deficiencies such as after central immunoneutralization of leptin or food restriction and in leptin resistant Zucker rats, indicating that leptin must act upstream of kisspeptin signaling (Navarro et al., 2004a; Castellano et al., 2011). In prepubertal rats under different food regimens, a positive correlation has been found between circulating leptin levels and hypothalamic *Kiss1* and *GPR54* mRNA levels (Iwasa et al., 2010a; Castellano et al., 2011). Pharmacological manipulations of mTOR, a transducer of leptin's effect on energy homeostasis, suggested that this signaling pathway is essential for activating *Kiss1* transcription in the ARC at puberty onset (Roa et al., 2009). However, administration of leptin was able to restore hypothalamic levels of *GPR54* but not *Kiss1* mRNA in prepubertal rats displaying reduced levels of both *GPR54* and *Kiss1* mRNA after 24 h food deprivation (Iwasa et al., 2010a). The precise site of leptin's action in the brain during the pubertal transition period may vary between species and remains a matter of debate (Elias and Purohit, 2013).

Neuropeptides

Among neuropeptides potentially regulating the kisspeptin–GPR54 system during development, a particular attention has been paid to NKB. Indeed, human genetic studies have associated loss of function mutations on either TAC3 or TACR3 genes (encoding NKB and its receptor NK3R respectively) with hypogonadism and infertility, similar to the phenotypes of *Kiss1* or *GPR54* mutants

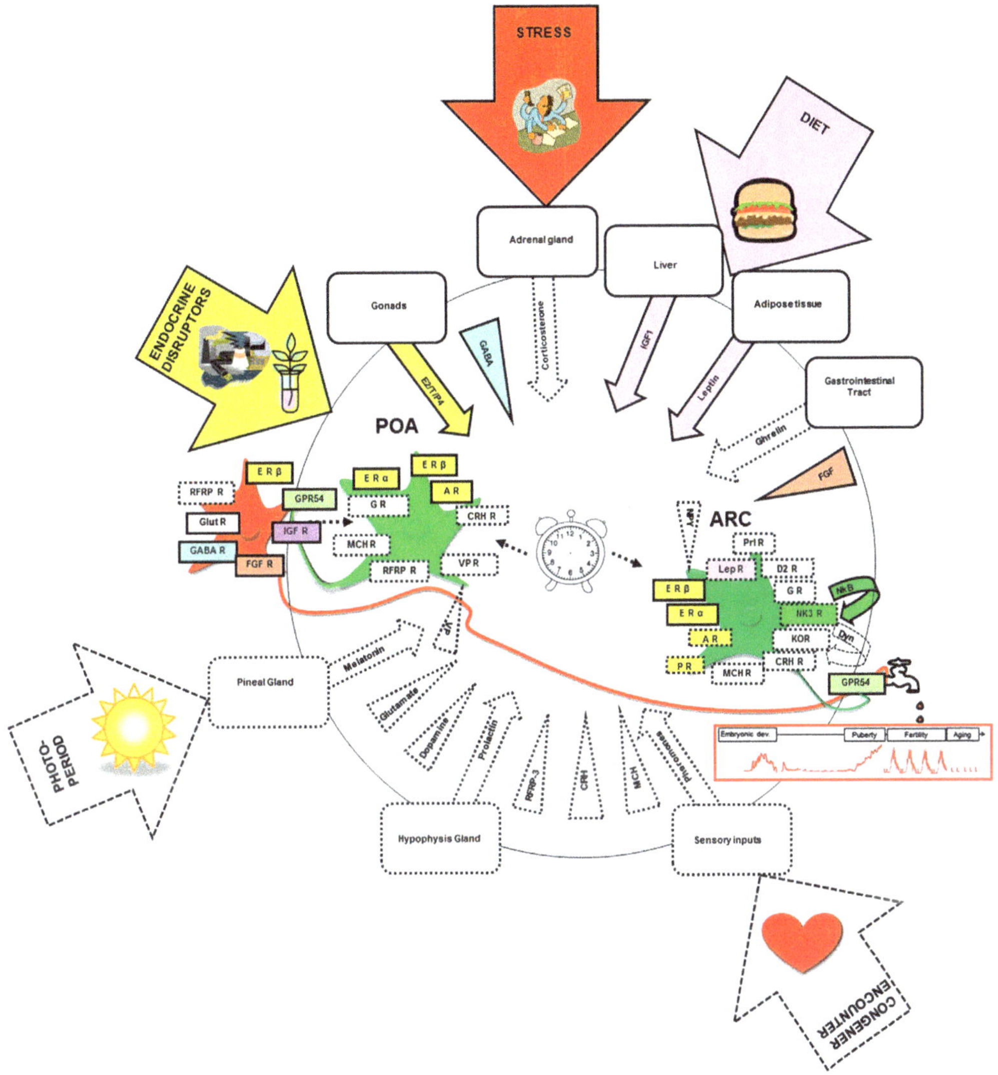

FIGURE 4 | Neural, hormonal, and environmental factors regulating the kisspeptin–GPR54 system. Scheme summarizing the different factors that have been shown to regulate the kisspeptin–GPR54 system only during adulthood (squared by dashed lines) or also during development (squared by full lines and colored). Hormonal factors are codified by an arrow and central factors by a triangle. Molecular factors have been included whose receptors have been found on some kisspeptin neurons, factors found within fibers in close apposition to kisspeptin neurons, factors eliciting c-fos expression, or an electrophysiological response within kisspeptin neurons or changing *Kiss1* or *GPR54* mRNA levels, kisspeptin or GPR54 immunoreactivities, or the number of Kiss1/kisspeptin expressing cells when exogenously administered. Of note this synthetic scheme combines data from mice, rats, sheep, and monkeys and therefore occults potential species differences that may exist in these regulations. It is hypothesized that the developmental pattern of GnRH release (red graph below the tap) is shaped by interactions of these different neural and hormonal factors with an intrinsic differentiation program of the system (central clock). The developing kisspeptin–GPR54 system is particularly vulnerable to some environmental factors like endocrine disruptors, diet, and stress which can alter GnRH secretion and reproductive function on the long-term. POA, preoptic area; ARC, arcuate nucleus; E2, estradiol; T, testosterone; P4, progesterone; ER, estrogen receptor; AR, androgen receptor; PR, progestin receptor; IGF, insulin-like growth factor; IGF-R, insulin-like growth factor receptor; FGF, fibroblast growth factor; FGF-R, fibroblast growth factor receptor; GABA-R, GABA receptor; RFRP3, RF-amides related peptide-3; RFRP3-R, RFRP3 receptor; LepR, leptin receptor; Prl-R, Prolactin receptor; NKB, neurokinin B; NK3R, NKB receptor; Glut-R, glutamate receptor; VP, vasopressin; VP-R, vasopressin receptor; MCH, melanocortin; MCH-R, MCH receptor; Dyn, dynorphin; KOR, kappa-opioid receptor (Dyn-receptor); GR, Glucocorticoid receptor; CRH, corticotrophin-releasing hormone; CRH R, corticotrophin-releasing hormone receptor; D2-R, dopamine-receptor. The illustrations in the arrows were obtained from Clipart Microsoft Word®.

(Topaloglu et al., 2009). Interestingly, NKB receptors have been found on kisspeptin neurons of the ARC, which also co-express NKB, but not on GnRH neurons (Navarro et al., 2012). In prepubertal hpg mice, administration of a specific NK3R antagonist showed that NKB does not control *Kiss1* expression (Gill et al., 2012). Instead, there is increasing evidence that this neuropeptide stimulates kisspeptin release. For instance, the LH releasing activity of the NKB agonist senktide is abolished in *GPR54* knock-out mice (García-Galiano et al., 2012b), in the presence of a GPR54 antagonist in prepubertal rats (Grachev et al., 2012) or after

GPR54 desensitizing in agonadal juvenile monkeys (Ramaswamy et al., 2011). A model has recently been proposed where NKB would participate in the initiation of pulses of kisspeptin release by synchronizing ARC kisspeptin neuronal activity through an autofeedback loop (Navarro, 2012).

Another neuropeptide that may cross-talk with the kisspeptin–GPR54 system during development is RFRP3. This mammalian ortholog of GnIH is already found closely apposed to a large proportion of GnRH neurons in prepubertal rats (Losa-Ward et al., 2012) where it may act by decreasing the GnRH neuronal response to kisspeptins as previously shown by electrophysiological recordings on brain slices from adult mice (Wu et al., 2009). In addition, RFRP3 may act upstream of kisspeptin neurons in light of a recent study in hamster where this peptide has been proposed to convey a melatoninergic signal to GnRH neurons through regulation of *Kiss1* transcription (Ancel et al., 2012).

Growth factors

The developing kisspeptin–GPR54 system may also be the target of growth factors: mice harboring deficiencies in FGF8 and/or FGFR-1 display a greater number of kisspeptin-immunoreactive cells in the POA at some stages of peripubertal development specifically, suggesting that FGF signaling pathways may control kisspeptin cell numbers or act on the *Kiss1* gene at transcriptional or post-transcriptional levels (Tata et al., 2012). Another growth factor that may be implicated during development of kisspeptin neurons is IGF1. Female rats that receive an intracerebroventricular administration of IGF1 during the prepubertal period display increased *Kiss1* mRNA levels in the POA specifically. This effect can be abolished by the administration of an IGF1 receptor antagonist and appears dependent on the presence of gonadal estrogens (Hiney et al., 2009). This contrasts with results obtained in adulthood where the same antagonist produces no effect on *Kiss1* expression, suggesting that the IGF1 receptor response of kisspeptin neurons may change as development proceeds (Todd et al., 2007).

GABA

In the female rhesus monkey, a very recent study demonstrated the fundamental role of GABA signaling in restraining kisspeptin release prior to puberty. $GABA_A$ receptor antagonist administration during the prepubertal period but not during the pubertal period stimulates kisspeptin release in the medial basal hypothalamus (Kurian et al., 2012). In the same study, the use of a GPR54 antagonist suggested that kisspeptin neurons may relay inhibitory GABA signals to GnRH neurons prior to puberty. In addition, the response of GnRH neurons to kisspeptins can be modulated by GABA signaling in adult mice and rats and it will be interesting to further explore when during development this cross-talk is established (Pielecka-Fortuna and Moenter, 2010; García-Galiano et al., 2012a).

Transcription factors

The concept has recently been put forward that puberty is controlled by regulatory gene networks composed of multiple functional modules operating with overlaps of partially redundant pathways (Ojeda et al., 2010). In this context, there has been a great interest in positioning the *Kiss1* gene within a framework of puberty-associated identified transcription factors. *In vitro* promoter assays in human cell lines suggest that the *Kiss1* gene is regulated by a set trans-activators and repressors involved in the system-wide control of mammalian puberty, among which TTF1, CUX1-p200, EAP1, YY1, and CUX1-p110 (Mueller et al., 2011). It will be of great interest to confirm the relevance of these findings *in vivo*.

THE DEVELOPING KISSPEPTIN–GPR54 SYSTEM AS TARGET OF ENVIRONMENTAL DISRUPTORS OF REPRODUCTION

ENDOCRINE DISRUPTORS

A variety of endocrine disrupting chemicals (EDCs) have recently been shown to disrupt the orderly progression of the female reproductive life cycle in association with changes in the development of the kisspeptin–GPR54 system. Most studies reporting alterations of the kisspeptin–GPR54 system by EDCs have been performed in rats. For example, estradiol benzoate, genistein, and polychlorinated bisphenyls (PCBs), if administered during rat perinatal development, have each been shown to advance vaginal openings and accelerate reproductive senescence, associated with a reduction in hypothalamic kisspeptin-immunoreactivity in adulthood (both at the level of the POA and ARC). This reduction in kisspeptin-immunoreactivity is observed after normalization of sex steroid circulating levels and is associated with a decline in the proportion of GnRH neurons being activatable by hormonal stimuli mimicking estradiol positive feedback conditions (Bateman and Patisaul, 2008; Dickerson et al., 2011a; Patisaul et al., 2012). Long Evans rats administered with estradiol benzoate or genistein during the first 4 days of life have further been analyzed for kisspeptin-immunoreactivity around puberty (Losa et al., 2011). A significant reduction in kisspeptin-immunoreactivity (both at the level of the POA and ARC) was detected in these EDC-treated animals compared to control rats. A recent *in situ* hybridization analysis shows that female Long Evans rats neonatally administered with estradiol benzoate display lower *Kiss1* hybridization signals than controls in both brain regions during the pubertal transition period (Patisaul et al., 2012). This reduction has been evidenced as early as postnatal day 4 in the ARC and postnatal day 10 in the POA (Cao et al., 2012), suggesting that the *Kiss1* gene may represent an early target of this endocrine disruptor in the hypothalamus. By postnatal day 10, sex differences in *Kiss1* mRNA signal in the ARC are no longer observed following neonatal administration of estradiol benzoate (Cao et al., 2012). Interestingly, this study also suggests that a neonatal exposure to estradiol benzoate can induce a rapid downregulation of *Esr1* and *Esr2* transcript levels in various hypothalamic nuclei, including the POA and ARC (Cao et al., 2012). Of note, other hypothalamic targets of estradiol benzoate have recently been evidenced in the POA of newborn Sprague Dawley rats that had been exposed *in utero* to this endocrine disruptor, using a 48 gene TaqMan PCR-based array (Dickerson et al., 2011b). For instance, on the first day of postnatal life, the gene encoding prodynorphin was shown to be upregulated and genes encoding subtypes of NMDA and GABA receptors downregulated in the POA (Dickerson et al., 2011b). A similar result was obtained following prenatal PCB exposure (Dickerson et al., 2011b). At the age of 2 months, 4 POA genes out of 48 appear significantly reduced to male levels in the EDC-exposed females, including the androgen receptor, NMDA receptor 2b, IGF1, and TGFβ1. It is noteworthy that all four of these genes play roles in hypothalamic development, including in the regulation of GnRH and kisspeptin neurons (Hiney et al., 2009; Oakley et al., 2009; Kurian et al., 2012). However, no changes in *Kiss1* expression levels could be detected in this study, despite the reduction in kisspeptin-immunoreactivity observed (Dickerson et al., 2011a). This may be due to a methodological limitation or to a different regulation between the mRNA and the protein. The same approach has been used to examine the molecular consequences in the POA of the aged female progeny, of a perinatal exposure to estradiol benzoate, a treatment that results in an acceleration of reproductive aging in Fisher rats (Gore et al., 2011). A complex regulatory neural/glial network of 17 genes controlling reproductive function appears upregulated in the POA by this perinatal estradiol benzoate treatment, including sex steroid hormone receptors, GABA and glutamate receptor subunits, growth factors, neuropeptide receptors, and a transcription factor. The *Kiss1* gene appears significantly downregulated and *Esr1* upregulated, relative to controls. Interestingly, an increase in methylation at some CpG sites in the *Esr1*gene is observed, suggesting that early exposure to this endocrine disruptor can induce lifelong epigenetic changes in this gene (Gore et al., 2011). It will be of great interest to further assess whether endocrine disruptors can also interfere with epigenetic marks on the *Kiss1* gene (Semaan et al., 2012) and to position *Kiss1* within this identified network of EDC-sensitive hypothalamic genes.

Bisphenol A (BPA), another endocrine disruptor with both estrogenic and anti-androgenic activities, may also target the kisspeptin–GPR54 system during development. However, studies are sparser and often incomplete, making it difficult to draw a clear picture of its mechanism of action. Administration of high (but not low) doses of BPA to neonatal female Long Evans rat results in adulthood in decreased kisspeptin-immunoreactivity in the ARC, independently of the steroidogenic milieu (Patisaul et al., 2009). If administered at high doses to neonatal Wistar rats, BPA induces a decrease in *Kiss1* hypothalamic expression levels, as well as a decrease in kisspeptin-immunoreactivity in the ARC at puberty (Navarro et al., 2009; Losa-Ward et al., 2012). If administered at low doses to neonatal Wistar rats, it advances the time of vaginal opening without any changes in kisspeptin-immunoreactivity being detectable in the ARC or POA at puberty. Finally, a low dose neonatal administration to Long Evans rats has recently been shown to decrease *Kiss1* hybridization signals in the POA as early as P10 (Cao et al., 2012). In CD1 mice, a lifelong-exposure to high doses of BPA results in an increase rather than a decrease in hypothalamic *Kiss1* mRNA levels (Xi et al., 2011). Furthermore, BPA-exposed mice display higher levels of circulating estradiol than control mice (Xi et al., 2011). Similarly, a perinatal exposure of female CD1 mice to extremely low levels of BPA results in an increase in the number of kisspeptin-immunoreactive cells in the POA (Panzica et al., 2011). These opposite effects of BPA between mice and rats illustrate the species-specificity of the effect of endocrine disruptors in general.

The consequences of real life exposure to EDCs was furthermore assessed in a farm animal species, the sheep. The fetuses (110 day old) of pregnant ewes exposed from the first day of conception to sewage sludge containing common endocrine disruptors display lower *Kiss1* mRNA levels in the ARC and in the POA relative to control animals maintained on pasture treated with conventional inorganic fertilizers (Bellingham et al., 2009). The physiological and behavioral outcomes of this exposure remains to be assessed.

Whether there is a causal link between disruption of the kisspeptin–GPR54 system and the different reproductive defects engendered by these EDCs remains to be fully investigated. Many recent studies on neuroendocrine disruption of reproductive function have focused on analysis of the kisspeptin–GPR54 system as potential target but it is clear that developmental exposure to some endocrine disruptors can advance the time of vaginal opening independently of kisspeptin signaling (Witham et al., 2012). This may in some cases derive from direct peripheral effects of the EDC or through interferences with other steroid-sensitive neural circuits regulating GnRH secretion. For example, neonatal exposure of female rats to low levels of BPA was recently found to advance the time of vaginal opening and has been associated to a decrease in the number of RFRP3-immunoreactive neurons and in the proportion of GnRH neurons displaying RFRP3-immunoreactive fiber appositions (Losa-Ward et al., 2012). On the other hand, no changes in kisspeptin-immunoreactivity could be detected (Losa-Ward et al., 2012).

DIET

It has been known for a long time that diet can have a strong impact on reproductive function, including on the timing of puberty onset. This observation has led several laboratories to investigate a potential regulatory role of diet on the development of the kisspeptin–GPR54 system. In mice, a high fat diet given from the time of weaning can induce infertility in the DJA strain but not in the C57/Bl6 strain. Accordingly, this food regimen results in adulthood in a decrease of ARC and POA *Kiss1* expression specifically in the DJA strain (Quennell et al., 2011). Mouse nutrition has also been manipulated during early postnatal development by varying litter sizes during lactation from postnatal day 4 until weaning and this was shown to produce long-lasting changes in kisspeptin-immunoreactivity and in physiological parameters (Caron et al., 2012). Under-nourished pups raised in large litters during lactation display delayed puberty onset and reduced fertility index and this has been associated with a decrease in the density of fibers double labeled for kisspeptin and NKB in medial preoptic nuclei (Caron et al., 2012). DiI anterograde tracing studies suggest that this results from a neonatal impairment of kisspeptin neural projections from the ARC toward the medial preoptic nucleus (Caron et al., 2012).

In rats, chronic undernutrition from the time of weaning onward (Castellano et al., 2005; Navarro et al., 2012) diminishes hypothalamic *Kiss1* mRNA levels around puberty. This is associated with delayed onset of vaginal opening, and decreased circulating levels of LH, effects that can be rescued by prepubertal chronic daily central administration of either kisspeptin (Castellano et al., 2005) or senktide, a NKB agonist (Navarro et al., 2012). Chronic undernutrition exclusively during the fetal period (Iwasa et al., 2010b) or during lactation (Castellano et al., 2011) is sufficient to induce long-term changes, at least until the pubertal period: puberty onset is again delayed and hypothalamic *Kiss1* mRNA levels are decreased. Neuroanatomical analysis further showed a decrease in the number of kisspeptin immunoreactive cells in the ARC following undernutrition during lactation (Castellano et al., 2011). Conversely, overnutrition by litter size manipulation during lactation increases hypothalamic *Kiss1* mRNA levels at the pubertal transition period, advances puberty onset, and increases kisspeptin-immunoreactive fiber density in the POA (Castellano et al., 2011). High fat diet from the time of weaning can also advance puberty onset and results in an increase in *Kiss1* mRNA levels in the ARC prior to vaginal opening, followed by a decrease in the POA (Li et al., 2012).

STRESS

The functioning of the hypothalamic–pituitary–gonadal axis can also be altered by stressful experiences early in life. Female rats that are exposed to an immunological stress before 7 days of postnatal life exhibit a significant delay in puberty-associated with decreased *Kiss1* but not *GPR54* expression in the POA (Knox et al., 2009). Thus, kisspeptin neurons may represent important cellular relays through which stress-related factors impact the reactivation of GnRH pulsatile release at puberty. Notably, corticotropin-releasing factor receptors and glucocorticoid receptors have recently been detected by immunohistochemistry in kisspeptin neurons of the ARC in adulthood (Takumi et al., 2012b), implying a possible direct effect of stress-related factors on kisspeptin neurons. It will be interesting to determine when during development expression of these receptors start.

CONCLUSION

Loss and gain of function studies during development have now provided compelling evidence that kisspeptin signaling in the brain is essential for the maturation of reproductive function through puberty in several mammalian species including humans. Upregulation of *Kiss1* transcription both in the ARC and POA appears to play a major role in the onset and progression through puberty in several mammalian species. Numerous potential regulators of *Kiss1* transcription during development have been identified and light has also recently been shed on developmental regulators of kisspeptin release, including NKB and GABA. Nevertheless, a lively debate still persists on the respective roles played by the ARC and POA populations of kisspeptin neurons in puberty onset, progression, and completion. For example, *Kiss1* expression or kisspeptin-immunoreactivity does not appear to increase in the ARC at the time of puberty in mice, as opposed to rats, sheep, and monkeys for which positive correlations have been found between *Kiss1* mRNA levels in the ARC and LH pulse frequencies. On the other hand, the mouse is the only species for which an upregulation of *GPR54* expression has been described in GnRH neurons during female postnatal development. Since studies using different species often rely on different approaches with different sensitivities, it may be hazardous at this stage to put these different observations at the account of true species differences. Clearly, further investigations using a variety of complementary approaches on each animal model are needed in order to identify and ascertain species-specific processes in the developmental regulation and function of the kisspeptin–GPR54 system.

Numerous studies have shown that the kisspeptin–GPR54 system is particularly sensitive to gonadal steroids. In fact, all species studied develop a clear sexual dimorphism in the pattern of *Kiss1* expression in the POA (with greater expression in females) but the precise roles of developmental sex steroids in this process have so far only been studied in mice and rats using different yet complementary approaches. Estrogen receptor signaling appears to exert important organizational effects during the perinatal and peripubertal periods that may involve epigenetic regulations of the *Kiss1* and/or *Esr1* genes. In mice, rats, sheep, and humans, sex differences in the amounts of *Kiss1* expression and/or kisspeptin-immunoreactivity have also been detected in the ARC at some points of development (different depending on species) but the respective roles played by organizational and activational effects of sex steroids in these sex differences remain to be fully analyzed and documented. In mice, rats, and sheep, different yet dynamic sensitivities of male and female ARC kisspeptin cells to circulating sex steroids have been highlighted at the time of puberty. It seems clear that estrogen signaling can exert both organizational and activational effects on the kisspeptin–GPR54 system albeit at times of development and at cellular levels that can greatly vary between species and strains. More detailed studies on the mechanism of action of sex steroids on the development of the kisspeptin–GPR54 system with its neuroendocrine and behavioral consequences should be conducted in the future.

Moreover, studies in rodents suggest that kisspeptin cells may be reprogrammed during development by environmental threats including endocrine disruptors, diet, and stress, with long-term often deleterious effects on reproductive function. Therefore, it remains important to decipher for each species the critical periods of plasticity of the kisspeptin–GPR54 system and to better understand the molecular and cellular mechanisms involved in its developmental programing. Most recently, it has been shown in rats and humans that kisspeptins are already synthesized in some ARC cells well before birth. The physiological significance of these observations have yet to be revealed but one likely hypothesis is that kisspeptins already regulate tonic GnRH release prenatally, hence contributing to early maturation processes of the gonads and possibly to sexual differentiation of some brain circuits. The embryonic period of progenitor cell proliferation and neurogenesis has recently been identified for the ARC kisspeptin neurons of rat. This represents an important first step in the exploration of the morphogenetic processes shaping this neuronal system during early development. In a translational perspective, these studies should help the development of predictive cellular models for assessing the danger of environmental chemicals on reproductive function.

ACKNOWLEDGMENTS

Authors are very grateful to Drs. Alain Caraty, Yves Tillet, and Anne Duittoz for valuable discussions and assistance in performing the research presented in this review, to the anonymous referees that have stimulated improvements of this review article and to Laura Szymanski for carefully checking the English of this manuscript. The work presented herein was supported by the Institut National de Recherche Agronomique (INRA), Centre National de la Recherche Scientifique (CNRS), Université of Tours, and by grants from the French National Research Agency (ANR) and Région Centre. Elodie Desroziers was recipient of a Ph.D. fellowship from the INRA and Région Centre.

REFERENCES

Adachi, S., Yamada, S., Takatsu, Y., Matsui, H., Kinoshita, M., Takase, K., et al. (2007). Involvement of anteroventricular periventricular metastin/kisspeptin neurons in estrogen positive feedback action on luteinizing hormone release in female rats. *J. Reprod. Dev.* 53, 367–378.

Ancel, C., Bentsen, A. H., Sébert, M. E., Tena-Sempere, M., Mikkelsen, J. D., and Simonneaux, V. (2012). Stimulatory effect of RFRP-3 on the gonadotrophic axis in the male Syrian hamster: the exception proves the rule. *Endocrinology* 153, 1352–1363.

Backholer, K., Smith, J. T., Rao, A., Pereira, A., Iqbal, J., Ogawa, S., et al. (2010). Kisspeptin cells in the ewe brain respond to leptin and communicate with neuropeptide Y and proopiomelanocortin cells. *Endocrinology* 151, 2233–2243.

Bakker, J., Pierman, S., and González-Martínez, D. (2010). Effects of aromatase mutation (ArKO) on the sexual differentiation of kisspeptin neuronal numbers and their activation by same versus opposite sex urinary pheromones. *Horm. Behav.* 57, 390–395.

Bateman, H. L., and Patisaul, H. B. (2008). Disrupted female reproductive physiology following neonatal exposure to phytoestrogens or estrogen specific ligands is associated with decreased GnRH activation and kisspeptin fiber density in the hypothalamus. *Neurotoxicology* 29, 988–997.

Bellingham, M., Fowler, P. A., Amezaga, M. R., Rhind, S. M., Cotinot, C., Mandon-Pepin, B., et al. (2009). Exposure to a complex cocktail of environmental endocrine-disrupting compounds disturbs the kisspeptin/GPR54 system in ovine hypothalamus and pituitary gland. *Environ. Health Perspect.* 117, 1556–1562.

Caldani, M., Batailler, M., Thiéry, J. C., and Dubois, M. P. (1988). LHRH-immunoreactive structures in the sheep brain. *Histochemistry* 89, 129–139.

Cao, J., Mickens, J. A., McCaffrey, K. A., Leyrer, S. M., and Patisaul, H. B. (2012). Neonatal bisphenol A exposure alters sexually dimorphic gene expression in the postnatal rat hypothalamus. *Neurotoxicology* 33, 23–36.

Cao, J., and Patisaul, H. B. (2011). Sexually dimorphic expression of hypothalamic estrogen receptors α and β and Kiss1 in neonatal male and female rats. *J. Comp. Neurol.* 519, 2954–2977.

Caron, E., Ciofi, P., Prevot, V., and Bouret, S. G. (2012). Alteration in neonatal nutrition causes perturbations in hypothalamic neural circuits controlling reproductive function. *J. Neurosci.* 32, 11486–11494.

Castellano, J. M., Bentsen, A. H., Sánchez-Garrido, M. A., Ruiz-Pino, F., Romero, M., Garcia-Galiano, D., et al. (2011). Early metabolic programming of puberty onset: impact of changes in postnatal feeding and rearing conditions on the timing of puberty and development of the hypothalamic kisspeptin system. *Endocrinology* 152, 3396–3408.

Castellano, J. M., Navarro, V. M., Fernández-Fernández, R., Castaño, J. P., Malagón, M. M., Aguilar, E., et al. (2006). Ontogeny and mechanisms of action for the stimulatory effect of kisspeptin on gonadotropin-releasing hormone system of the rat. *Mol. Cell. Endocrinol.* 257–258, 75–83.

Castellano, J. M., Navarro, V. M., Fernández-Fernández, R., Nogueiras, R., Tovar, S., Roa, J., et al. (2005). Changes in hypothalamic KiSS-1 system and restoration of pubertal activation of the reproductive axis by kisspeptin in undernutrition. *Endocrinology* 146, 3917–3925.

Cheng, G., Coolen, L. M., Padmanabhan, V., Goodman, R. L., and Lehman, M. N. (2010). The kisspeptin/neurokinin B/dynorphin (KNDy) cell population of the arcuate nucleus: sex differences and effects of prenatal testosterone in sheep. *Endocrinology* 151, 301–311.

Clarke, I. J. (2011). Control of GnRH secretion: one step back. *Front. Neuroendocrinol.* 32, 367–375.

Clarkson, J., Boon, W. C., Simpson, E. R., and Herbison, A. E. (2009). Postnatal development of an oestradiol-kisspeptin positive feedback mechanism implicated in puberty onset. *Endocrinology* 150, 3214–3220.

Clarkson, J., d'Anglemont de Tassigny, X., Moreno, A. S., Colledge, W. H., and Herbison, A. E. (2008). Kisspeptin-GPR54 signaling is essential for preovulatory gonadotropin-releasing hormone neuron activation and the luteinizing hormone surge. *J. Neurosci.* 28, 8691–8867.

Clarkson, J., and Herbison, A. E. (2006). Postnatal development of kisspeptin neurons in mouse hypothalamus; sexual dimorphism and projections to gonadotropin-releasing hormone neurons. *Endocrinology* 147, 5817–5825.

Constantin, S., Caraty, A., Wray, S., and Duittoz, A. H. (2009a). Development of gonadotropin-releasing hormone-1 secretion in mouse nasal explants. *Endocrinology* 150, 3221–3227.

Constantin, S., Caligioni, C. S., Stojilkovic, S., and Wray, S. (2009b). Kisspeptin-10 facilitates a plasma membrane-driven calcium oscillator in gonadotropin-releasing hormone-1 neurons. *Endocrinology* 150, 1400–1412.

Cravo, R. M., Margatho, L. O., Osborne-Lawrence, S., Donato, J. Jr., Atkin, S., Bookout, A. L., et al. (2011). Characterization of Kiss1 neurons using transgenic mouse models. *Neuroscience* 173, 37–56.

d'Anglemont de Tassigny, X., Fagg, L. A., Dixon, J. P., Day, K., Leitch, H. G., Hendrick, A. G., et al. (2007). Hypogonadotropic hypogonadism in mice lacking a functional Kiss1 gene. *Proc. Natl. Acad. Sci. U.S.A.* 104, 10714–10719.

de Roux, N., Genin, E., Carel, J. C., Matsuda, F., Chaussain, J. L., and Milgrom, E. (2003). Hypogonadotropic hypogonadism due to loss of function of the KiSS1-derived peptide receptor GPR54. *Proc. Natl. Acad. Sci. U.S.A.* 100, 10972–10976.

Desroziers, E., Droguerre, M., Bentsen, A. H., Robert, V., Mikkelsen, J. D., Caraty, A., et al. (2012a). Embryonic development of kisspeptin neurones in rat. *J. Neuroendocrinol.* 24, 1284–1295.

Desroziers, E., Mikkelsen, J. D., Duittoz, A., and Franceschini, I. (2012b). Kisspeptin-immunoreactive changes in a sex- and hypothalamic-region-specific manner across rat postnatal development. *J. Neuroendocrinol.* 24, 1154–1165.

Desroziers, E., Mikkelsen, J., Simonneaux, V., Keller, M., Tillet, Y., Caraty, A., et al. (2010). Mapping of kisspeptin fibres in the brain of the pro-oestrous rat. *J. Neuroendocrinol.* 22, 1101–1112.

Dickerson, S. M., Cunningham, S. L., Patisaul, H. B., Woller, M. J., and Gore, A. C. (2011a). Endocrine disruption of brain sexual differentiation by developmental PCB exposure. *Endocrinology* 152, 581–594.

Dickerson, S. M., Cunningham, S. L., and Gore, A. C. (2011b). Prenatal PCBs disrupt early neuroendocrine development of the rat hypothalamus. *Toxicol. Appl. Pharmacol.* 252, 36–46.

Döhler, K. D., and Wuttke, W. (1975). Changes with age in levels of serum gonadotropins, prolactin and gonadal steroids in prepubertal male and female rats. *Endocrinology* 97, 898–907.

Ducret, E., Gaidamaka, G., and Herbison, A. E. (2010). Electrical and morphological characteristics of anteroventral periventricular nucleus kisspeptin and other neurons in the female mouse. *Endocrinology* 151, 2223–2232.

Dungan, H. M., Gottsch, M. L., Zeng, H., Gragerov, A., Bergmann, J. E., Vassilatis, D. K., et al. (2007). The role of kisspeptin-GPR54 signaling in the tonic regulation and surge release of gonadotropin-releasing hormone/luteinizing hormone. *J. Neurosci.* 27, 12088–12095.

Eghlidi, D. H., Haley, G. E., Noriega, N. C., Kohama, S. G., and Urbanski, H. F. (2010). Influence of age and 17beta-oestradiol on kisspeptin, neurokinin B, and prodynorphin gene expression in the arcuate-median eminence of female rhesus macaques. *Endocrinology* 151, 3783–3794.

Elias, C. F., and Purohit, D. (2013). Leptin signaling and circuits in puberty and fertility. *Cell Mol. Life Sci.* 70, 841–862.

Fiorini, Z., and Jasoni, C. L. (2010). A novel developmental role for kisspeptin in the growth of gonadotrophin-releasing hormone neurites to the median eminence in the mouse. *J. Neuroendocrinol.* 22, 1113–1125.

Forbes, S., Li, X. F., Kinsey-Jones, J., and O'Byrne, K. (2009). Effects of ghrelin on kisspeptin mRNA expression in the hypothalamic medial preoptic area and pulsatile luteinising hormone secretion in the female rat. *Neurosci. Lett.* 460, 143–147.

Franceschini, I., Lomet, D., Cateau, M., Delsol, G., Tillet, Y., and Caraty, A. (2006). Kisspeptin immunoreactive cells of the ovine preoptic area and arcuate nucleus co-express estrogen receptor alpha. *Neurosci. Lett.* 401, 225–230.

Funes, S., Hedrick, J. A., Vassileva, G., Markowitz, L., Abbondanzo, S., Golovko, A., et al. (2003). The KiSS-1 receptor GPR54 is essential for the development of the murine reproductive system. *Biochem. Biophys. Res. Commun.* 312, 1357–1363.

García-Galiano, D., Pineda, R., Roa, J., Ruiz-Pino, F., Sánchez-Garrido, M. A., Castellano, J. M., et al. (2012a). Differential modulation of gonadotropin responses to kisspeptin by aminoacidergic, peptidergic, and nitric oxide neurotransmission. *Am.

J. Physiol. Endocrinol. Metab. 303, E1252–E1263.

García-Galiano, D., van Ingen Schenau, D., Leon, S., Krajnc-Franken, M. A., Manfredi-Lozano, M., Romero-Ruiz, A., et al. (2012b). Kisspeptin signaling is indispensable for neurokinin B, but not glutamate, stimulation of gonadotropin secretion in mice. *Endocrinology* 153, 316–328.

Gill, J. C., Navarro, V. M., Kwong, C., Noel, S. D., Martin, C., Xu, S., et al. (2012). Increased neurokinin B (tac2) expression in the mouse arcuate nucleus is an early marker of pubertal onset with differential sensitivity to sex steroid-negative feedback than kiss1. *Endocrinology* 153, 4883–4893.

Gill, J. C., Wang, O., Kakar, S., Martinelli, E., Carroll, R. S., and Kaiser, U. B. (2010). Reproductive hormone-dependent and -independent contributions to developmental changes in kisspeptin in GnRH-deficient hypogonadal mice. *PLoS ONE* 5:e11911. doi:10.1371/journal.pone.0011911

González-Martínez, D., De Mees, C., Douhard, Q., Szpirer, C., and Bakker, J. (2008). Absence of gonadotropin-releasing hormone 1 and Kiss1 activation in alpha-fetoprotein knockout mice: prenatal estrogens defeminize the potential to show preovulatory luteinizing hormone surges. *Endocrinology* 149, 2333–2340.

Goodman, R. L., Maltby, M. J., Millar, R. P., Hileman, S. M., Nestor, C. C., Whited, B., et al. (2012). Evidence that dopamine acts via kisspeptin to hold GnRH pulse frequency in check in anestrous ewes. *Endocrinology* 153, 5918–5927.

Gore, A. C., Walker, D. M., Zama, A. M., Armenti, A. E., and Uzumcu, M. (2011). Early life exposure to endocrine-disrupting chemicals causes lifelong molecular reprogramming of the hypothalamus and premature reproductive aging. *Mol. Endocrinol.* 25, 2157–2168.

Gore, A. C., Windsor-Engnell, B. M., and Terasawa, E. (2004). Menopausal increases in pulsatile gonadotropin-releasing hormone release in a nonhuman primate (*Macaca mulatta*). *Endocrinology* 145, 4653–4659.

Grachev, P., Li, X. F., Lin, Y. S., Hu, M. H., Elsamani, L., Paterson, S. J., et al. (2012). GPR54-dependent stimulation of luteinizing hormone secretion by neurokinin B in prepubertal rats. *PLoS ONE* 7:e44344. doi:10.1371/journal.pone.0044344

Guerriero, K. A., Keen, K. L., Millar, R. P., and Terasawa, E. (2012a). Developmental changes in GnRH release in response to kisspeptin agonist and antagonist in female rhesus monkeys (*Macaca mulatta*): implication for the mechanism of puberty. *Endocrinology* 153, 825–836.

Guerriero, K. A., Keen, K. L., and Terasawa, E. (2012b). Developmental increase in kisspeptin-54 release in vivo is independent of the pubertal increase in oestradiol in female rhesus monkeys (*Macaca mulatta*). *Endocrinology* 153, 1887–1897.

Guimiot, F., Chevrier, L., Dreux, S., Chevenne, D., Caraty, A., Delezoide, A. L., et al. (2012). Negative fetal FSH/LH regulation in late pregnancy is associated with declined kisspeptin/KISS1R expression in the tuberal hypothalamus. *J. Clin. Endocrinol. Metab.* 97, E2221–E2229.

Herbison, A. E., de Tassigny, X., Doran, J., and Colledge, W. H. (2010). Distribution and postnatal development of Gpr54 gene expression in mouse brain and gonadotropin-releasing hormone neurons. *Endocrinology* 151, 312–321.

Hiney, J. K., Srivastava, V. K., Pine, M. D., and Les Dees, W. (2009). Insulin-like growth factor-I activates KiSS-1 gene expression in the brain of the prepubertal female rat. *Endocrinology* 150, 376–384.

Homma, T., Sakakibara, M., Yamada, S., Kinoshita, M., Iwata, K., Tomikawa, J., et al. (2009). Significance of neonatal testicular sex steroids to defeminize anteroventral periventricular kisspeptin neurons and the GnRH/LH surge system in male rats. *Biol. Reprod.* 81, 1216–1225.

Hrabovszky, E., Ciofi, P., Vida, B., Horvath, M. C., Keller, E., Caraty, A., et al. (2010). The kisspeptin system of the human hypothalamus: sexual dimorphism and relationship with gonadotropin-releasing hormone and neurokinin B neurons. *Eur. J. Neurosci.* 31, 1984–1998.

Hrabovszky, E., Molnár, C. S., Sipos, M. T., Vida, B., Ciofi, P., Borsay, B. A., et al. (2011). Sexual dimorphism of kisspeptin and neurokinin B immunoreactive neurons in the infundibular nucleus of aged men and women. *Front. Endocrinol. (Lausanne)* 2:80. doi:10.3389/fendo.2011.00080

Huhtaniemi, I. (1995). Molecular aspects of the ontogeny of the pituitary-gonadal axis. *Reprod. Fertil. Dev.* 7, 1025–1035.

Iijima, N., Takumi, K., Sawai, N., and Ozawa, H. (2011). An immunohistochemical study on the expressional dynamics of kisspeptin neurons relevant to GnRH neurons using a newly developed anti-kisspeptin antibody. *J. Mol. Neurosci.* 43, 146–154.

Iwasa, T., Matsuzaki, T., Murakami, M., Kinouchi, R., Gereltsetseg, G., Fujisawa, S., et al. (2010a). Sensitivities of mRNA expression levels of Kiss1 and its receptor, Kiss1r, to nutritional status are changed during the developmental period in female rats. *J. Endocrinol.* 207, 195–202.

Iwasa, T., Matsuzaki, T., Murakami, M., Fujisawa, S., Kinouchi, R., Gereltsetseg, G., et al. (2010b). Effects of intrauterine undernutrition on hypothalamic Kiss1 expression and the timing of puberty in female rats. *J. Physiol. (Lond.)* 588, 821–829.

Kauffman, A. S., Navarro, V. M., Kim, J., Clifton, D. K., and Steiner, R. A. (2009). Sex differences in the regulation of Kiss1/NKB neurons in juvenile mice: implications for the timing of puberty. *Am. J. Physiol. Endocrinol. Metab.* 297, E1212–E1221.

Kauffman, A. S., Park, J. H., McPhie-Lalmansingh, A. A., Gottsch, M. L., Bodo, C., Hohmann, J. G., et al. (2007a). The kisspeptin receptor GPR54 is required for sexual differentiation of the brain and behavior. *J. Neurosci.* 127, 8826–8835.

Kauffman, A. S., Gottsch, M. L., Roa, J., Byquist, A. C., Crown, A., Clifton, D. K., et al. (2007b). Sexual differentiation of Kiss1 gene expression in the brain of the rat. *Endocrinology* 148, 1774–1783.

Keen, K. L., Wegner, F. H., Bloom, S. R., Ghatei, M. A., and Terasawa, E. (2008). An increase in kisspeptin-54 release occurs with the pubertal increase in luteinizing hormone-releasing hormone-1 release in the stalk-median eminence of female rhesus monkeys in vivo. *Endocrinology* 149, 4151–4157.

Kermath, B. A., and Gore, A. C. (2012). Neuroendocrine control of the transition to reproductive senescence: lessons learned from the female rodent model. *Neuroendocrinology* 96, 1–12.

Kim, W., Jessen, H. M., Auger, A. P., and Terasawa, E. (2009). Postmenopausal increase in KiSS-1, GPR54, and luteinizing hormone releasing hormone (LHRH-1) mRNA in the basal hypothalamus of female rhesus monkeys. *Peptides* 30, 103–110.

Kinsey-Jones, J. S., Li, X. F., Knox, A. M., Wilkinson, E. S., Zhu, X. L., Chaudhary, A. A., et al. (2009). Down-regulation of hypothalamic kisspeptin and its receptor, Kiss1r, mRNA expression is associated with stress-induced suppression of luteinising hormone secretion in the female rat. *J. Neuroendocrinol.* 21, 20–29.

Knox, A. M., Li, X. F., Kinsey-Jones, J. S., Wilkinson, E. S., Wu, X. Q., Cheng, Y. S., et al. (2009). Neonatal lipopolysaccharide exposure delays puberty and alters hypothalamic Kiss1 and Kiss1r mRNA expression in the female rat. *J. Neuroendocrinol.* 21, 683–689.

Kurian, J. R., Keen, K. L., Guerriero, K. A., and Terasawa, E. (2012). Tonic control of kisspeptin release in prepubertal monkeys: implications to the mechanism of puberty onset. *Endocrinology* 153, 3331–3336.

Lapatto, R., Pallais, J. C., Zhang, D., Chan, Y. M., Mahan, A., Cerrato, F., et al. (2007). Kiss1-/- mice exhibit more variable hypogonadism than Gpr54-/- mice. *Endocrinology* 148, 4927–4936.

Lederman, M. A., Lebesgue, D., Gonzalez, V. V., Shu, J., Merhi, Z. O., Etgen, A. M., et al. (2010). Age-related LH surge dysfunction correlates with reduced responsiveness of hypothalamic anteroventral periventricular nucleus kisspeptin neurons to oestradiol positive feedback in middle-aged rats. *Neuropharmacology* 58, 314–320.

Lee, D. K., Nguyen, T., O'Neill, G. P., Cheng, R., Liu, Y., Howard, A. D., et al. (1999). Discovery of a receptor related to the galanin receptors. *FEBS Lett.* 446, 103–107.

Lee, J. H., Miele, M. E., Hicks, D. J., Phillips, K. K., Trent, J. M., Weissman, B. E., et al. (1996). KiSS-1, a novel human malignant melanoma metastasis-suppressor gene. *J. Natl. Cancer Inst.* 88, 1731–1737.

Lehman, M. N., Merkley, C. M., Coolen, L. M., and Goodman, R. L. (2010). Anatomy of the kisspeptin neural network in mammals. *Brain Res.* 1364, 90–102.

Li, F. X., Lin, Y. S., Kinsey-Jones, J. S., and O'Byrne, K. T. (2012). High-fat diet increases LH pulse frequency and kisspeptin-neurokinin B expression in puberty-advanced female rats. *Endocrinology* 153, 4422–4431.

Li, Q., Rao, A., Pereira, A., Clarke, I. J., and Smith, J. T. (2011). Kisspeptin cells in the ovine arcuate nucleus express prolactin receptor but not melatonin receptor. *J. Neuroendocrinol.* 23, 871–882.

Losa, S. M., Todd, K. L., Sullivan, A. W., Cao, J., Mickens, J. A., and

Patisaul, H. B. (2011). Neonatal exposure to genistein adversely impacts the ontogeny of hypothalamic kisspeptin signaling pathways and ovarian development in the peripubertal female rat. *Reprod. Toxicol.* 31, 280–289.

Losa-Ward, S. M., Todd, K. L., McCaffrey, K. A., Tsutsui, K., and Patisaul, H. B. (2012). Disrupted organization of RFamide pathways in the hypothalamus is associated with advanced puberty in female rats neonatally exposed to bisphenol A. *Biol. Reprod.* 87, 28.

Luan, X., Yu, H., Wei, X., Zhou, Y., Wang, W., Li, P., et al. (2007a). GPR54 polymorphisms in Chinese girls with central precocious puberty. *Neuroendocrinology* 86, 77–83.

Luan, X., Zhou, Y., Wang, W., Yu, H., Li, P., Gan, X., et al. (2007b). Association study of the polymorphisms in the KISS1 gene with central precocious puberty in Chinese girls. *Eur. J. Endocrinol.* 157, 113–118.

Matsui, H., Takatsu, Y., Kumano, S., Matsumoto, H., and Ohtaki, T. (2004). Peripheral administration of metastin induces marked gonadotropin release and ovulation in the rat. *Biochem. Biophys. Res. Commun.* 320, 383–388.

Matwijiw, I., and Faiman, C. (1987). Control of gonadotropin secretion in the ovine fetus: the effects of a specific gonadotropin-releasing hormone antagonist on pulsatile luteinizing hormone secretion. *Endocrinology* 121, 347–351.

Mayer, C., Acosta-Martinez, M., Dubois, S. L., Wolfe, A., Radovick, S., Boehm, U., et al. (2010). Timing and completion of puberty in female mice depend on estrogen receptor alpha-signaling in kisspeptin neurons. *Proc. Natl. Acad. Sci. U.S.A.* 107, 22693–22698.

Mayer, C., and Boehm, U. (2011). Female reproductive maturation in the absence of kisspeptin/GPR54 signaling. *Nat. Neurosci.* 14, 704–710.

Messager, S., Chatzidaki, E. E., Ma, D., Hendrick, A. G., Zahn, D., Dixon, J., et al. (2005). Kisspeptin directly stimulates gonadotropin-releasing hormone release via G protein-coupled receptor 54. *Proc. Natl. Acad. Sci. U.S.A.* 102, 1761–1766.

Michael, S. D., Kaplan, S. B., and MacMillan, B. T. (1980) Peripheral plasma concentrations of LH, FSH, prolactin and GH from birth to puberty in male and female mice. *J. Reprod. Fertil.* 59, 217–222.

Mueller, J. K., Dietzel, A., Lomniczi, A., Loche, A., Tefs, K., Kiess, W., et al. (2011). Transcriptional regulation of the human KiSS1 gene. *Mol. Cell. Endocrinol.* 342, 8–19.

Navarro, V. M. (2012). New insights into the control of pulsatile GnRH release: the role of Kiss1/neurokinin B neurons. *Front. Endocrinol. (Lausanne)* 3:48. doi:10.3389/fendo.2012.00048

Navarro, V. M., Castellano, J. M., McConkey, S. M., Pineda, R., Ruiz-Pino, F., Pinilla, L., et al. (2011). Interactions between kisspeptin and neurokinin B in the control of GnRH secretion in the female rat. *Am. J. Physiol. Endocrinol. Metab.* 300, E202–E210.

Navarro, V. M., Fernández-Fernández, R., Castellano, J. M., Roa, J., Mayen, A., Barreiro, M. L., et al. (2004a). Advanced vaginal opening and precocious activation of the reproductive axis by KiSS-1 peptide, the endogenous ligand of GPR54. *J. Physiol. (Lond.)* 561, 379–386.

Navarro, V. M., Castellano, J. M., Fernández-Fernández, R., Barreiro, M. L., Roa, J., Sanchez-Criado, J. E., et al. (2004b). Developmental and hormonally regulated messenger ribonucleic acid expression of KiSS-1 and its putative receptor, GPR54, in rat hypothalamus and potent luteinizing hormone-releasing activity of KiSS-1 peptide. *Endocrinology* 145, 4565–4574.

Navarro, V. M., Ruiz-Pino, F., Sánchez-Garrido, M. A., García-Galiano, D., Hobbs, S. J., Manfredi-Lozano, M., et al. (2012). Role of neurokinin B in the control of female puberty and its modulation by metabolic status. *J. Neurosci.* 15, 2388–2397.

Navarro, V. M., Sánchez-Garrido, M. A., Castellano, J. M., Roa, J., García-Galiano, D., Pineda, R., et al. (2009). Persistent impairment of hypothalamic KiSS-1 system after exposures to estrogenic compounds at critical periods of brain sex differentiation. *Endocrinology* 150, 2359–2367.

Nestor, C. C., Briscoe, A. M., Davis, S. M., Valent, M., Goodman, R. L., and Hileman, S. M. (2012). Evidence of a role for kisspeptin and neurokinin B in puberty of female sheep. *Endocrinology* 153, 2756–2765.

Nimri, R., Lebenthal, Y., Lazar, L., Chevrier, L., Phillip, M., Bar, M., et al. (2011). A novel loss-of-function mutation in GPR54/KISS1R leads to hypogonadotropic hypogonadism in a highly consanguineous family. *J. Clin. Endocrinol. Metab.* 96, E536–E545.

Oakley, A. E., Clifton, D. K., and Steiner, R. A. (2009). Kisspeptin signaling in the brain. *Endocr. Rev.* 30, 713–743.

Ohtaki, T., Shintani, Y., Honda, S., Matsumoto, H., Hori, A., Kanehashi, K., et al. (2001). Metastasis suppressor gene KiSS-1 encodes peptide ligand of a G-protein-coupled receptor. *Nature* 411, 613–617.

Ojeda, S. R., Dubay, C., Lomniczi, A., Kaidar, G., Matagne, V., Sandau, U. S., et al. (2010). Gene networks and the neuroendocrine regulation of puberty. *Mol. Cell. Endocrinol.* 324, 3–11.

Panzica, G. C., Bo, E., Martini, M. A., Miceli, D., Mura, E., Viglietti-Panzica, C., et al. (2011). Neuropeptides and enzymes are targets for the action of endocrine disrupting chemicals in the vertebrate brain. *J. Toxicol. Environ. Health B Crit. Rev.* 14, 449–472.

Patisaul, H. B., Losa-Ward, S. M., Todd, K. L., McCaffrey, K. A., and Mickens, J. A. (2012). Influence of ERβ selective agonism during the neonatal period on the sexual differentiation of the rat hypothalamic-pituitary-gonadal (HPG) axis. *Biol. Sex Differ.* 3, 2.

Patisaul, H. B., Todd, K. L., Mickens, J. A., and Adewale, H. B. (2009). Impact of neonatal exposure to the ERalpha agonist PPT, bisphenol-A or phytoestrogens on hypothalamic kisspeptin fiber density in male and female rats. *Neurotoxicology* 30, 350–357.

Paxinos, G., and Ashwell, K. W. S. (eds). (2008). *Atlas of the Developing Rat Nervous System*, 3rd Edn. San Diego, CA: Academic Press.

Pielecka-Fortuna, J., and Moenter, S. M. (2010). Kisspeptin increases gamma-aminobutyric acidergic and glutamatergic transmission directly to gonadotropin-releasing hormone neurons in an estradiol-dependent manner. *Endocrinology* 151, 291–300.

Pineda, R., Garcia-Galiano, D., Roseweir, A., Romero, M., Sanchez-Garrido, M. A., Ruiz-Pino, F., et al. (2010). Critical roles of kisspeptins in female puberty and preovulatory gonadotropin surges as revealed by a novel antagonist. *Endocrinology* 151, 722–730.

Poling, M. C., and Kauffman, A. S. (2012). Sexually dimorphic testosterone secretion in prenatal and neonatal mice is independent of kisspeptin-Kiss1r and GnRH signaling. *Endocrinology* 149, 4151–4157.

Poling, M. C., and Kauffman, A. S. (2013). Organizational and activational effects of sex steroids on kisspeptin neuron development. *Front. Neuroendocrinol.* 34, 3–17.

Quennell, J. H., Howell, C. S., Roa, J., Augustine, R. A., Grattan, D. R., and Anderson, G. M. (2011). Leptin deficiency and diet-induced obesity reduce hypothalamic kisspeptin expression in mice. *Endocrinology* 152, 1541–1550.

Ramaswamy, S., Seminara, S. B., and Plant, T. M. (2011). Evidence from the agonadal juvenile male rhesus monkey (*Macaca mulatta*) for the view that the action of neurokinin B to trigger gonadotropin-releasing hormone release is upstream from the kisspeptin receptor. *Neuroendocrinology* 94, 237–245.

Redmond, J. S., Macedo, G. G., Velez, I. C., Caraty, A., Williams, G. L., and Amstalden, M. (2011a). Kisspeptin activates the hypothalamic-adenohypophyseal-gonadal axis in prepubertal ewe lambs. *Reproduction* 141, 541–548.

Redmond, J. S., Baez-Sandoval, G. M., Spell, K. M., Spencer, T. E., Lents, C. A., Williams, G. L., et al. (2011b). Developmental changes in hypothalamic Kiss1 expression during activation of the pulsatile release of luteinising hormone in maturing ewe lambs. *J. Neuroendocrinol.* 23, 815–822.

Revel, F. G., Saboureau, M., Masson-Pévet, M., Pévet, P., Mikkelsen, J. D., and Simonneaux, V. (2006). Kisspeptin mediates the photoperiodic control of reproduction in hamsters. *Curr. Biol.* 16, 1730–1735.

Rizwan, M. Z., Poling, M. C., Corr, M., Cornes, P. A., Augustine, R. A., Quennell, J. H., et al. (2012). RFamide-related peptide-3 receptor gene expression in GnRH and kisspeptin neurons and GnRH-dependent mechanism of action. *Endocrinology* 153, 3770–3779.

Roa, J., Garcia-Galiano, D., Varela, L., Sánchez-Garrido, M. A., Pineda, R., Castellano, J. M., et al. (2009). The mammalian target of rapamycin as novel central regulator of puberty onset via modulation of hypothalamic Kiss1 system. *Endocrinology* 150, 5016–5026.

Rometo, A. M., Krajewski, S. J., Voytko, M. L., and Rance, N. E. (2007). Hypertrophy and increased kisspeptin gene expression in the hypothalamic infundibular nucleus of postmenopausal women and ovariectomized monkeys. *J. Clin. Endocrinol. Metab.* 92, 2744–2750.

Roseweir, A. K., Kauffman, A. S., Smith, J. T., Guerriero, K. A., Morgan, K., Pielecka-Fortuna, J., et al. (2009). Discovery of potent kisspeptin antagonists delineate physiological mechanisms of gonadotropin regulation. *J. Neurosci.* 29, 3920–3929.

Scarbrough, K., and Wise, P. M. (1990). Age-related changes in pulsatile luteinizing hormone release precede the transition to estrous acyclicity and depend upon estrous cycle history. *Endocrinology* 126, 884–890.

Semaan, S. J., Dhamija, S., Kim, J., Ku, E. C., and Kauffman, A. S. (2012). Assessment of epigenetic contributions to sexually-dimorphic kiss1 expression in the anteroventral periventricular nucleus of mice. *Endocrinology* 153, 1875–1886.

Semaan, S. J., Murray, E. K., Poling, M. C., Dhamija, S., Forger, N. G., and Kauffman, A. S. (2010). BAX-dependent and BAX-independent regulation of Kiss1 neuron development in mice. *Endocrinology* 151, 5807–5817.

Seminara, S. B., Messager, S., Chatzidaki, E. E., Thresher, R. R., Acierno, J. S. Jr., Shagoury, J. K., et al. (2003). The GPR54 gene as a regulator of puberty. *N. Engl. J. Med.* 349, 1614–1627.

Shahab, M., Mastronardi, C., Seminara, S. B., Crowley, W. F., Ojeda, S. R., and Plant, T. M. (2005). Increased hypothalamic GPR54 signaling: a potential mechanism for initiation of puberty in primates. *Proc. Natl. Acad. Sci. U.S.A.* 102, 2129–2134.

Silveira, L. G., Noel, S. D., Silveira-Neto, A. P., Abreu, A. P., Brito, V. N., Santos, M. G., et al. (2010). Mutations of the KISS1 gene in disorders of puberty. *Clin. Endocrinol. Metab.* 95, 2276–2280.

Smith, J. T., Clay, C. M., Caraty, A., and Clarke, I. J. (2007). KiSS-1 messenger ribonucleic acid expression in the hypothalamus of the ewe is regulated by sex steroids and season. *Endocrinology* 148, 1150–1157.

Smith, J. T., Cunningham, M. J., Rissman, E. F., Clifton, D. K., and Steiner, R. A. (2005). Regulation of Kiss1 gene expression in the brain of the female mouse. *Endocrinology* 146, 3686–3692.

Smith, J. T., Popa, S. M., Clifton, D. K., Hoffman, G. E., and Steiner, R. A. (2006a). Kiss1 neurons in the forebrain as central processors for generating the preovulatory luteinizing hormone surge. *J. Neurosci.* 26, 6687–6694.

Smith, J. T., Acohido, B. V., Clifton, D. K., and Steiner, R. A. (2006b). KiSS-1 neurones are direct targets for leptin in the ob/ob mouse. *J. Neuroendocrinol.* 18, 298–303.

Szymanski, L., and Bakker, J. (2012). Aromatase knockout mice show normal steroid-induced activation of gonadotrophin-releasing hormone neurones and luteinising hormone surges with a reduced population of kisspeptin neurones in the rostral hypothalamus. *J. Neuroendocrinol.* 24, 1222–1233.

Takase, K., Uenoyama, Y., Inoue, N., Matsui, H., Yamada, S., Shimizu, M., et al. (2009). Possible role of oestrogen in pubertal increase of Kiss1/kisspeptin expression in discrete hypothalamic areas of female rats. *J. Neuroendocrinol.* 21, 527–537.

Takumi, K., Iijima, N., Iwata, K., Higo, S., and Ozawa, H. (2012a). The effects of gonadal steroid manipulation on the expression of Kiss1 mRNA in rat arcuate nucleus during postnatal development. *J Physiol Sci* 62, 453–460.

Takumi, K., Iijima, N., Higo, S., and Ozawa, H. (2012b). Immunohistochemical analysis of the colocalization of corticotropin-releasing hormone receptor and glucocorticoid receptor in kisspeptin neurons in the hypothalamus of female rats. *Neurosci. Lett.* 2012 531, 40–45.

Takumi, K., Iijima, N., and Ozawa, H. (2011). Developmental changes in the expression of kisspeptin mRNA in rat hypothalamus. *J. Mol. Neurosci.* 43, 138–145.

Tata, B. K., Chung, W. C., Brooks, L. R., Kavanaugh, S. I., and Tsai, P. S. (2012). Fibroblast growth factor signaling deficiencies impact female reproduction and kisspeptin neurons in mice. *Biol. Reprod.* 86, 119.

Teles, M. G., Bianco, S. D., Brito, V. N., Trarbach, E. B., Kuohung, W., Xu, S., et al. (2008). A GPR54-activating mutation in a patient with central precocious puberty. *N. Engl. J. Med.* 358, 709–715.

Todd, B. J., Fraley, G. S., Peck, A. C., Schwartz, G. J., and Etgen, A. M. (2007). Central insulin-like growth factor 1 receptors play distinct roles in the control of reproduction, food intake, and body weight in female rats. *Biol. Reprod.* 77, 492–503.

Topaloglu, A. K., Reimann, F., Guclu, M., Yalin, A. S., Kotan, L. D., Porter, K. M., et al. (2009). TAC3 and TACR3 mutations in familial hypogonadotropic hypogonadism reveal a key role for Neurokinin B in the central control of reproduction. *Nat. Genet.* 41, 354–358.

Topaloglu, A. K., Tello, J. A., Kotan, L. D., Ozbek, M. N., Yilmaz, M. B., Erdogan, S., et al. (2012). Inactivating KISS1 mutation and hypogonadotropic hypogonadism. *N. Engl. J. Med.* 366, 629–635.

Ugrumov, M. V., Ivanova, I. P., Mitskevich, M. S., Liposits, Z., Sétáló, G., and Flerkó, B. (1985). Axovascular relationships in developing median eminence of perinatal rats with special reference to luteinizing hormone-releasing hormone projections. *Neuroscience* 16, 897–906.

Vida, B., Deli, L., Hrabovszky, E., Kalamatianos, T., Caraty, A., Coen, C. W., et al. (2010). Evidence for suprachiasmatic vasopressin neurones innervating kisspeptin neurones in the rostral periventricular area of the mouse brain: regulation by oestrogen. *J. Neuroendocrinol.* 22, 1032–1039.

Wahab, F., Quinton, R., and Seminara, S. B. (2011). The kisspeptin signaling pathway and its role in human isolated GnRH deficiency. *Mol. Cell. Endocrinol.* 346, 29–36.

Witham, E. A., Meadows, J. D., Shojaei, S., Kauffman, A. S., and Mellon, P. L. (2012). Prenatal exposure to low levels of androgen accelerates female puberty onset and reproductive senescence in mice. *Endocrinology* 153, 4522–4532.

Wu, M., Dumalska, I., Morozova, E., van den Pol, A., and Alreja, M. (2009). Melanin-concentrating hormone directly inhibits GnRH neurons and blocks kisspeptin activation, linking energy balance to reproduction. *Proc. Natl. Acad. Sci. U.S.A.* 106, 17217–17222.

Xi, W., Lee, C. K., Yeung, W. S., Giesy, J. P., Wong, M. H., Zhang, X., et al. (2011). Effect of perinatal and postnatal bisphenol A exposure to the regulatory circuits at the hypothalamus-pituitary-gonadal axis of CD-1 mice. *Reprod. Toxicol.* 31, 409–417.

2

A closer look at the role of urotensin II in the metabolic syndrome

Pierre-Olivier Barrette and Adel Giaid Schwertani*

Division of Cardiology, Department of Medicine, McGill University Health Center, Montreal, QC, Canada

Edited by:
Hubert Vaudry, University of Rouen, France

Reviewed by:
Lan Ma, Fudan University, China
Leo T. Lee, The University of Hong Kong, Hong Kong

*Correspondence:
Adel Giaid Schwertani, Division of Cardiology, Department of Medicine, McGill University Health Center, 1650 Cedar Avenue, Room C9-166, Montreal, QC, Canada H3G 1A4.
e-mail: adel.giaid@mcgill.ca

Urotensin II (UII) is a vasoactive peptide that was first discovered in the teleost fish, and later in mammals and humans. UII binds to the G protein coupled receptor GPR14 (now known as UT). UII mediates important physiological and pathological actions by interacting with its receptor. The metabolic syndrome (MetS) is described as cluster of factors such as obesity, dyslipidemia, hypertension, and insulin resistance (IR), further leading to development of type 2 diabetes mellitus and cardiovascular diseases. UII levels are upregulated in patients with the MetS. Evidence directly implicating UII in every risk factor of the MetS has been accumulated. The mechanism that links the different aspects of the MetS relies primarily on IR and inflammation. By directly modulating both of these factors, UII is thought to play a central role in the pathogenesis of the MetS. Moreover, UII also plays an important role in hypertension and hyperlipidemia thereby contributing to cardiovascular complications associated with the MetS.

Keywords: metabolic syndrome, insulin resistance, inflammation, obesity, dyslipidemia, hypertension, diabetes

UROTENSIN II

The peptide Urotensin II (UII) was first identified in the teleost fish *Gillichthys mirabilis* (Pearson et al., 1980). Homologs of this peptide were subsequently found in mammals and humans (Pearson et al., 1980; Conlon et al., 1996; Ames et al., 1999; Coulouarn et al., 1999). Although the amino acid sequence of these homologs changes depending on the species, a cyclic sequence of six amino acids is conserved (Cys-Phe-Trp-Lys-Tyr-Cys). It is believed that this sequence is responsible for the biological activity of the peptide (Conlon et al., 1990). UII acts as a vasoactive peptide by binding to the G protein coupled receptor GPR14, better known as UT (Ames et al., 1999; Liu et al., 1999). A recent study has shown that UII vasoconstrictive effects are mediated by calcium influx via STIM1 and Orai-1 (Domínguez-Rodríguez et al., 2012). Human UII (hUII) and its receptor have been found in cardiac and vascular tissues, spinal cord, central nervous system, kidney, liver, and pancreas (Maguire et al., 2000; Matsushita et al., 2001). UII is also present in the blood plasma in picomolar concentrations (Matsushita et al., 2001). However, it tends to act mainly in an autocrine and paracrine fashion rather than as a hormone (Yoshimoto et al., 2004). Even though the relation between UII and its receptor was made in 1999, the physiological and pathological roles of UII are only beginning to be unraveled. In a healthy state, the binding of UII with UT is known to play an important role in the control of vascular tone, blood pressure, and insulin release (Douglas and Ohlstein, 2000; Douglas et al., 2000; Loirand et al., 2008). UII has been identified as the most potent vasoactive peptide known to date, being more potent vasoconstrictor than endothelin-1 and angiotensin-II (Ames et al., 1999; Douglas and Ohlstein, 2000; Maguire et al., 2000). UII also controls the function of vascular smooth-muscle cells (VSMCs) through the release of endothelial-cell-derived vasodilators such as nitric oxide (Gibson, 1987; Gardiner et al., 2001; Stirrat et al., 2001). The role of UII in pathological states is still debated. Many studies have shown increased levels of UII and its receptor in diverse cardiovascular and metabolic diseases such as type 2 diabetes mellitus, renal dysfunction, atherosclerosis, systematic and essential hypertension, obesity, congestive heart failure, myocardial infarction, cardiac fibrosis, hypertrophy, and remodeling (Reviewed in Hassan et al., 2003; Ross et al., 2010; Gruson et al., 2012). The elevated levels of UII in disease states suggest that UII is expressed either as a protective response to pathologies or as a pathological agent. Some studies claim that temporary elevation of UII levels may lower cardiovascular disease risk factors in end-stage renal disease (Mallamaci et al., 2005; Zoccali et al., 2006), myocardial infarction (Babińska et al., 2012) and restore endothelial function (Zoccali and Mallamaci, 2008). On the other hand, other studies have demonstrated that UII acts as a pathological agent inducing cardiac hypertrophy in synergy with angiotensin II by phosphorylation of the Akt kinase (Chanalaris et al., 2005; Gruson et al., 2010b, 2012).

METABOLIC SYNDROME

As mentioned above, the metabolic syndrome (MetS) consists of a set of risk factors, such as obesity, hyperlipidemia, hypertension, hyperglycemia, and insulin resistance (IR), leading to the development of type 2 diabetes, cardiovascular diseases, non-alcoholic fatty liver disease, and renal impairment (Grundy, 1999; Cho, 2011). The relation between these risk factors and complications seems to be mostly attributed to IR (Eckel et al., 2010), which is why the syndrome was first defined as an IR syndrome (Reaven, 1988). Since then, the National Cholesterol Education Program (NCEP)-Adult Treatment Panel III, the World Health Organization (WHO) and the International Diabetes Federation (IDF) set up some criteria for the clinical definition of MetS.

A recent study using data from the 2003–2006 National Health and Nutrition Examination Survey and the NCEP/IDF MetS criteria, revealed that the prevalence of MetS was 34.3% among all adults in the US (Ford et al., 2010). However, high prevalence of MetS is not only restricted to the Western world. MetS seems to be highly prevalent in sub-Saharan Africa, Middle-East, South America, and South Asian Countries (Misra and Khurana, 2008). Central obesity is considered the main precursor to MetS (Cameron et al., 2008). According to the WHO, the global obese population increased from 200 million in 1995 to 300 million in 2000. The WHO has also determined that the obesity epidemic is also spreading in developing countries with over 115 million people suffering from obesity-related illnesses (Misra and Khurana, 2008; WHO, 2008). Popkin and Doak (1998) have also reported increasing obesity prevalence in the United States, Latin America, Europe, and Asia, which confirms the worldwide epidemic proportions of obesity and overweight. In addition, the Aerobic Center Longitudinal Study, which included 33,230 cancer-free men followed for 14 years, showed 56% enhanced risk of cancer mortality for men affected by MetS (Jaggers et al., 2009). The direct implication of the syndrome in CVD, type 2 diabetes, non-alcoholic fatty liver, and cancer, as well as an increasing prevalence of obesity and decreased physical inactivity in Western societies makes the MetS a major health preoccupation (NCEP, 2002)

Recent researches have shown that UII has an impact on the risk factors as well as the overall pathogenesis of the MetS (Ong et al., 2008). A study using the American Heart Association/National Heart, Lung, and Blood Institute criteria for MetS revealed that MetS patients show higher plasma levels of UII (Gruson et al., 2010a). Our group also demonstrated an increase in UII plasma levels in mice when all risk factors of MetS are present (You et al., 2012). Moreover, we recently found that UII gene deletion in mice (UIIKO) significantly decreased body mass, visceral fat, blood pressure, and increased insulin and glucose tolerance when compared to wild-type mice (You et al., 2012). Even though there is a clear association between MetS and UII, it is still unclear whether the peptide plays a role in the initiation of the disease, or if the elevated plasma levels of UII are a result of the syndrome. This review aims to give a closer look at the implication of UII in the risk factors and pathways involved in the development of the MetS.

INSULIN RESISTANCE (IR)

Insulin plays a major role in glucose and lipid metabolism such as adipose tissue triglyceride lipolysis, lipoprotein lipase activity, muscle and adipose tissue glucose absorption, muscle and liver glycogen synthesis, and endogenous glucose production (Cornier et al., 2008). When cells react poorly to an insulin stimulus, they are defined as IR. The latter is known to be the link between the individual components of MetS (Eckel et al., 2010). For instance, it seems that IR correlates positively with atherosclerosis (Fernández-Real and Ricart, 2003) and coronary artery disease (CAD; Juhan-Vague et al., 1991), and also an indirect cause of hyperinsulinemia (Reaven, 2003), dyslipidemia, hyperglycemia, and hypertension (Sowers, 2004) through an increase in free fatty acid (FFA) synthesis in adipose tissue (Boden and Shulman, 2002) and a chronic inflammatory response (Fernández-Real and Ricart, 2003).

The IR Atherosclerosis Study (IRAS) and the Atherosclerosis Risk in Communities Study showed that insulin sensitivity (measured with an intravenous glucose tolerance test) correlates negatively with intimal-medial thickness of the carotid artery (Howard et al., 1996). Subsequent studies also found a significant correlation between carotid intimal-media thickening and IR and hyperinsulinemia (Golden et al., 2002; Zavaroni et al., 2006). Intimal-media thickness has been shown to be a significant predictor of myocardial infarction and coronary death (Hodis et al., 1998). As a result, IR is a major risk factor in developing cardiovascular complications. Indeed, IR has been associated with increased plasma levels of plasminogen activator inhibitor 1 (PAI-1; Juhan-Vague et al., 1991). Increased levels of PAI-1 are known to impair fibrinolysis, which leads to progression of coronary atherosclerosis in glucose intolerant patients (Bavenholm et al., 1998) and increased risk of myocardial reinfarction within 3 years in less than 45-year-old men (Hamsten et al., 1985, 1987; Gram et al., 1987; Juhan-Vague et al., 1991) as well as increased risk of CAD (Juhan-Vague et al., 1991). UII is known to increase expression of PAI-1 in vascular SMC (Djordjevic et al., 2005), hence UII may contribute to atherosclerosis through PAI-1 inhibition of fibrinolysis.

Free fatty acids play an important role in MetS by having direct effects on dyslipidemia, hypertension (Fagot-Campagna et al., 1998), IR (Boden, 1997), and pancreatic β-cell dysfunction (Sako and Grill, 1990; Unger, 1995; McGarry and Dobbins, 1999; Boden and Shulman, 2002). Impaired insulin action in adipose tissue tends to increase FFAs concentrations in the plasma by reducing the insulin inhibition of adipose tissue triglyceride lipolysis (Randle et al., 1963; Randle, 1998; Kahn and Flier, 2000; Cornier et al., 2008). On the other hand, FFAs induce IR in skeletal muscles (DeFronzo et al., 1985) and liver by inhibiting insulin suppression of glycogenolysis (Boden et al., 2002), which results in a vicious cycle increasing IR, FFA levels, and promotion of hyperglycemia. Furthermore, higher plasma glucose and FFA levels tend to increase insulin secretion in the pancreas (Boden and Shulman, 2002), thus leading to hyperinsulinemia. Such high plasma insulin levels promote hypertension (Welborn et al., 1966; Reaven, 2003), which is another risk factor of MetS. An increase in FFA levels also predicts development of type 2 diabetes (Paolisso et al., 1995; Charles et al., 1997). In the liver, higher FFA levels increase low density lipoprotein (LDL) and triglyceride production, while lowering high density lipoprotein (HDL) production (Brinton et al., 1991; Muramaki et al., 1995).

The direct effects of UII on lipid mobilization and FFA release are somewhat contradictory. In the coho salmon, administration of UII stimulated the activity of triacylglycerol lipase and the release of FFAs in the liver (Sheridan and Bern, 1986; Sheridan et al., 1987). On the contrary, UII injection in dogfish showed no significant increase in FFA release or plasma triglyceride concentrations (Conlon et al., 1994). We recently found that UII gene deletion in mice fed high fat diet significantly reduced serum levels of FFAs in comparison with wild-type (You et al., 2012). In light of our own findings and those of others linking UII to IR and glucose metabolism (Silvestre et al., 2001, 2004; Ong et al., 2006; You et al., 2012), we suggest that UII may mediate lipid mobilization and FFA indirectly through IR. However, the direct influence of UII in lipid metabolism still requires further research.

The role of UII in the MetS seems to be closely related to insulin activity and the overall glucose metabolism in the pancreas (**Figure 1**). In fact, UII and UT are both expressed in rat pancreatic islets, where their interaction seems to inhibit glucose-mediated insulin release (Silvestre et al., 2001, 2004). Also, when high concentrations of UII are administrated to the rat pancreas, glucose and arginine induced insulin response are blocked (Silvestre et al., 2001, 2004). Some UII and UT gene haplotypes are known to be associated with IR (Ong et al., 2006), impaired glucose tolerance (Ong et al., 2006), β-cell pancreatic function, and type 2 diabetes (Sun et al., 2002; Zhu et al., 2002; Wenyi et al., 2003; Suzuki et al., 2004; Tan et al., 2006; Sáez et al., 2011). UII upregulation in plasma and skeletal muscle in type 2 diabetes mellitus is coherent with this association (Totsune et al., 2003; Wang et al., 2009). In addition, UII increases glucose-6-phosphatase activity in salmon liver, which tends to reduce glycogen content and increase glucose levels, leading to hyperglycemia. Our recent study has demonstrated that UII gene knockout in mice reduced serum glucose and insulin, and increased glucose and insulin tolerance in comparison with wild-type mice (You et al., 2012).

INFLAMMATORY RESPONSE IN THE MetS

It is well known that IR and MetS are both associated with an inflammatory response (Sutherland et al., 2004). The relationship between IR and inflammation seems to be bidirectional; IR promotes an inflammatory response and vice versa (Fernández-Real and Ricart, 2003), resulting in a vicious circle increasing risk of MetS incidence. An acute-phase inflammatory response is not only linked with IR (Fernández-Real et al., 2001; Festa et al., 2002; Grimble, 2002; Leinonen et al., 2003), but also with type 2 diabetes (McMillan, 1989; Arnalich et al., 2000; Festa et al., 2002; Leinonen et al., 2003), obesity (Laimer et al., 2002; Leinonen et al., 2003), and the overall MetS (Chan et al., 2002; Das, 2002). The activity of inflammatory markers such as C-reactive protein, tumor necrosis factor-alpha (TNF-α), Interleukin-18 (IL-18) and PAI-1 increases as the presence of MetS risk factors increase (Cornier et al., 2008).

Tumor necrosis factor-alpha prevents the action of insulin in cultured cells and in animal models (Hotamisligil et al., 1993, 1994, 1996) by inducing serine phosphorylation of the insulin receptor substrate-1, which reduces the tyrosine kinase activity

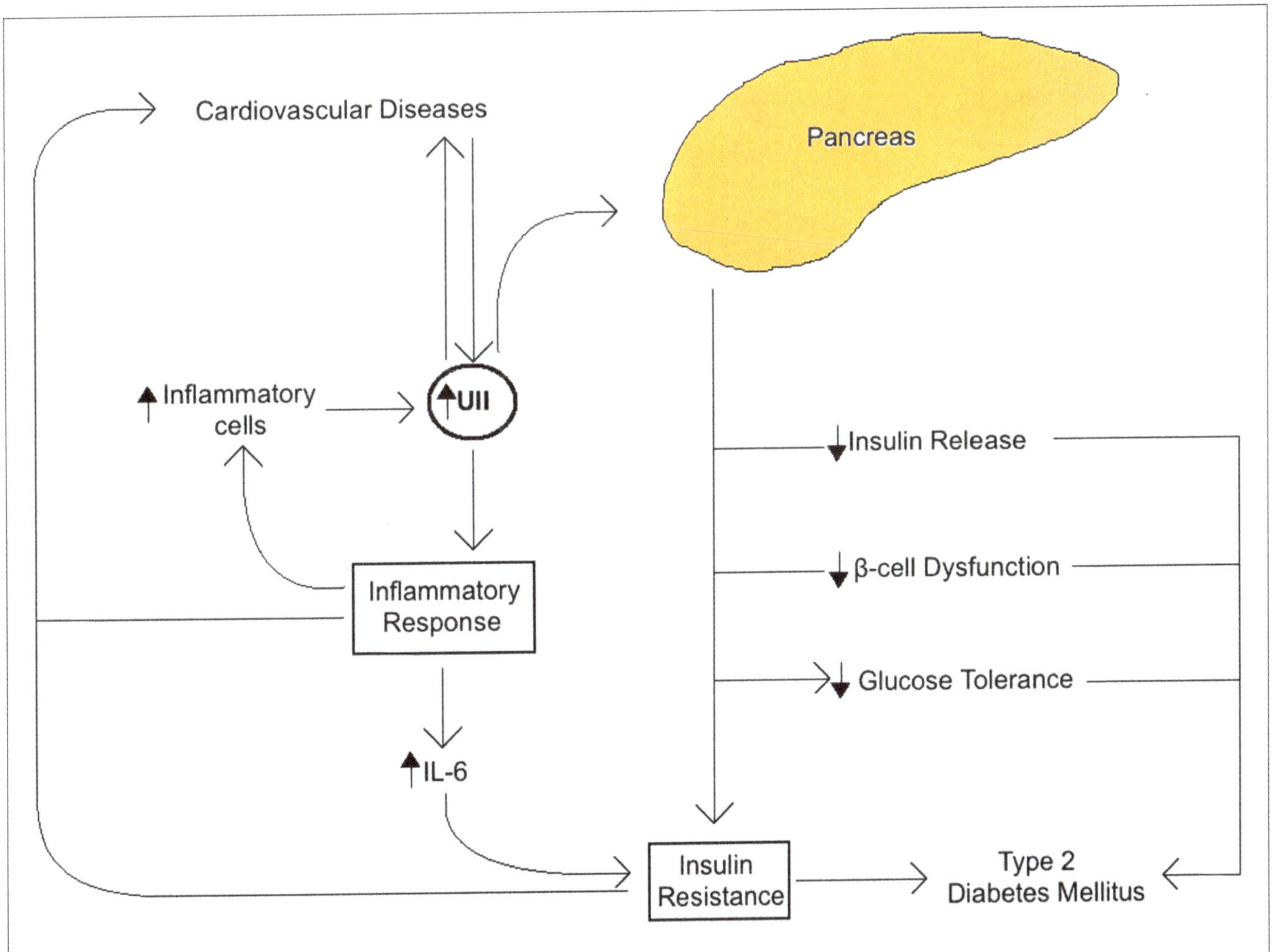

FIGURE 1 | Summary of the role of Urotensin II (UII) on insulin activity and glucose metabolism associated with the metabolic syndrome. UII expressed in the pancreas acts directly to impair glucose tolerance, reduce glucose-mediated insulin release, impair pancreatic β-cell function, and block insulin response resulting in IR and increased risk of type 2 diabetes and cardiovascular diseases.

of the insulin receptor (Hotamisligil et al., 1996), resulting in IR. Furthermore, TNF-α stimulates the production of endothelin-1 (Kahaleh and Fan, 1997) and angiotensin (Brasier et al., 1996) *in vitro*, which are directly involved in vasoconstriction and thus may lead to increased hypertension. Indeed, there is a positive correlation between TNF-α, systolic blood pressure, and IR (Dörffel et al., 1999). TNF-α also stimulates VLDL production (Grunfeld and Feingold, 1992) and decreases HDL cholesterol (Jovinge et al., 1998). Dyslipidemia in mice is significantly related to increased TNF-α levels (Fleet et al., 1992).

Elevated levels of the inflammatory cytokine IL-6 are associated with obesity, IR (Fried et al., 1998; Bastard et al., 2000; Fernández-Real et al., 2001; Kern et al., 2001; Bastard et al., 2002), and type 2 diabetes (Pradhan et al., 2001; Vozarova et al., 2003). IL-6 also plays a role in the pathology of dyslipidemia by decreasing LPL activity in adipocytes (Greenberg et al., 1992) which increases hepatic triglyceride levels (Nonogaki et al., 1995). In man, IL-6 correlates with increased FFA (Stouthard et al., 1995), fasting triglycerides, and VLDL (Fernández-Real et al., 2000), and decreased HDL cholesterol (Zuliani et al., 2007). This cytokine may also have an impact on hypertension by stimulating the sympathetic and central nervous system (Besedovsky and Del Rey, 1996; Papanicolaou et al., 1996), and angiotensin expression (Takano et al., 2000).

The central role of the inflammatory response in MetS is also related to UII and UT expression (**Figure 2**). Inflammatory cells including lymphocytes, macrophages, monocytes, and foam cells express UII and UT mRNA (Bousette et al., 2004). Lymphocytes are by far the largest producers of UII, whereas monocytes and macrophages produce the highest levels of UT. Moreover, inflammatory markers such as TNF-α, lipopolysaccharide, and interferon-γ are all known to induce UT expression *in vitro* (Segain et al., 2007). These findings suggest that an inflammatory response to MetS and its components may increase UII levels by increasing inflammatory cells production of the peptide. On the other hand, UII is known to contribute to the inflammatory response by inducing the release of inflammatory cytokines like IL-6 in cardiomyocytes (Sano et al., 2000; Tzanidis et al., 2003; Johns et al., 2004; Russell and Molenaar, 2004). UII mediates aortic inflammation by stimulating the release of leukotriene C (LTC_4), a lipid inflammatory mediator, from aortic adventitial fibroblasts through 5-lipoxygenase pathway (Dong

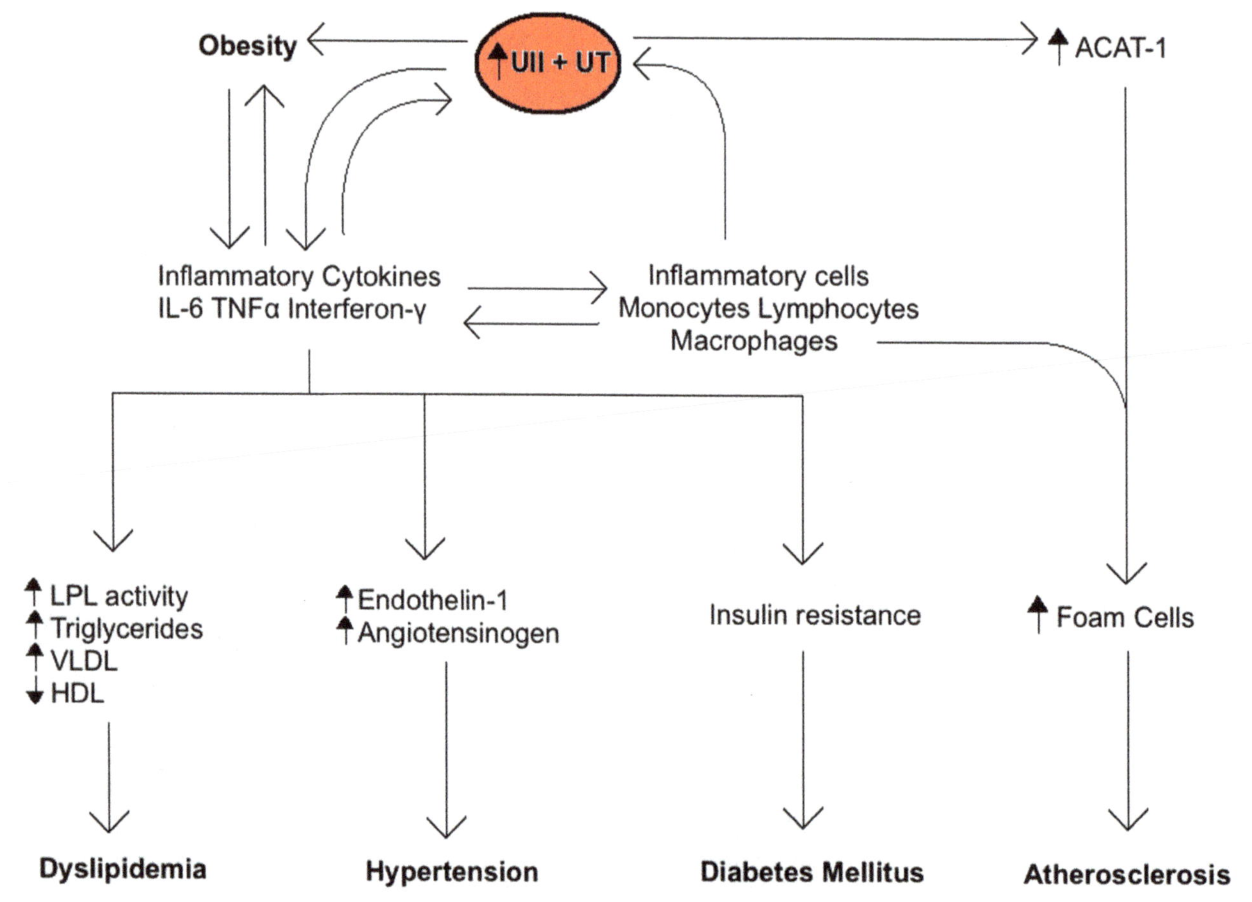

FIGURE 2 | Summary of the role of Urotensin II (UII) on the inflammatory response associated with the metabolic syndrome. Inflammatory cytokines increase UII and UT expression and vice-versa, resulting in a positive feedback. The ensuing chronic inflammation is directly involved in the development of obesity, insulin resistance, dyslipidemia, hypertension, and atherosclerosis.

et al., 2012). LTC_4 plays a key role in the pathogenesis of atherosclerosis as a chemoattractant and activator for monocytes in the vascular endothelium. It is also known to initiate contraction of smooth muscle cells in the adjacent medial tissues of the vasculature (Dong et al., 2012). In addition, we have recently shown that UII gene deletion in mice fed a high fat diet reduces the serum levels of inflammatory cytokines including monocyte chemoattractant protein-1, monokine induced by γ-interferon, and keratinocyte chemoattractant when compared to wild-type mice (You et al., 2012).

UII, HYPERTENSION, AND CARDIOVASCULAR DISEASES

The MetS is identified as a clustering of risk factors that perpetuate cardiovascular diseases. Since UII has been shown to play a role in the pathogenesis of atherosclerosis (Maguire et al., 2004; Hassan et al., 2005; Papadopoulos et al., 2009), congestive heart failure (Hassan et al., 2003), myocardial ischemia (Zhang et al., 2002; Zhou et al., 2003), ventricular hypertrophy, and fibrosis (Sano et al., 2000; Tzanidis et al., 2003; Johns et al., 2004; Russell and Molenaar, 2004), it is therefore reasonable to suggest that induction of UII in the MetS may contribute to the cardiovascular abnormalities associated with this syndrome.

Atherosclerosis is the main cause of morbidity and mortality in cardiovascular diseases and cause of death in the Western world (Libby et al., 2009). Atherosclerosis is known to induce UT and UII overexpression in mice aortic tissues (Douglas et al., 2002; Bousette et al., 2004; Wang et al., 2006; Libby et al., 2009). In mice overexpressing UT receptor (UT^+), aortic atherosclerosis lesion formation is significantly increased (Papadopoulos et al., 2009), whereas lesion formation is decreased in UIIKO mice with an atherosclerotic background (APOE; You et al., 2012). UII is known to promote vascular remodeling by mediating VSMC proliferation and migration inside the intima, a process directly involved in atherogenesis (Sauzeau et al., 2001; Watanabe et al., 2001a,b; Tamura et al., 2003; Albertin et al., 2009; Iglewski and Grant, 2010). It has been suggested that vascular endothelial growth factor (VEGF), a major angiogenic protein, could be responsible for UII-mediated vascular remodeling. Even though UII does not affect VEGF expression in human endothelium (Albertin et al., 2009), recent evidence has shown that UII induces secretion of VEGF in the adventitia in synergy with angiotensin II (Song et al., 2012). VEGF stimulates proliferation of endothelial and smooth muscles cells while also stimulating proliferation and migration of adventitial fibroblasts in the intima (Sartore et al., 2001; Stenmark et al., 2006; Zhang et al., 2008). In addition, UII contributes to the inflammatory response in atherosclerosis by acting as a chemoattractant for monocytes (Segain et al., 2007) and increasing IL-6 expression in cardiomyocytes (Sano et al., 2000; Tzanidis et al., 2003; Johns et al., 2004; Russell and Molenaar, 2004). UII interacts with UT receptors on the surface of macrophages to promote expression of ACAT-1 (Watanabe et al., 2005). ACAT-1 is known to accelerate foam cells formation, which has a major impact on atherosclerotic lesion development (Watanabe et al., 2005). Another main effect of UII on atherosclerosis is the increased expression of NADPH oxidase, which is a main source of reactive oxygen species (ROS; Djordjevic et al., 2005; Tsoukas et al., 2011). ROS are central in the early initiation of atherosclerosis by converting LDL into oxidized-LDL (Djordjevic et al., 2005). NADPH oxidase-derived superoxide inactivates nitric oxide, resulting in impaired endothelial dependant vasodilatation (Zou et al., 2004) and hypertension (Lassègue and Clempus, 2003).

Urotensin II also contributes to essential (Matsushita et al., 2001) and secondary (Heller et al., 2002) hypertension by inducing vascular remodeling. Increased blood pressure in cats (Behm et al., 2004), rats (Lin et al., 2003), and sheep (Watson et al., 2003) with UII administration is coherent with these findings. In humans, plasma UII correlates positively with systolic blood pressure, independently of an atherosclerotic background (Cheung et al., 2004). Indeed, the UII gene (UTS2) is associated with essential hypertension (Yi et al., 2006) and myocardial infarction (Nishihama et al., 2007; Oguri et al., 2009). In a chronic heart failure or essential hypertension state, UII loses its dilatory function (Lim et al., 2004; Sondermeijer et al., 2005).

UII, OBESITY, AND HYPERLIPIDEMIA

Obesity seems to be a main cause of IR in both men and women (Carey et al., 1996; Cornier et al., 2008; Stefan et al., 2008). Moreover, it seems that physical activity and a diet rich in monounsaturated or hydrogenated fat leads to an impairment of insulin sensitivity (Mayer-Davis et al., 1998; Vessby et al., 2001; Han et al., 2002). Obesity is also known as a chronic inflammatory state; it induces release of proinflammatory cytokines and adipokines (Yudkin et al., 1999; Festa et al., 2001; Engström et al., 2003; Trayhurn and Wood, 2004). As a result, the pathologic role of inflammation in IR and MetS may be enhanced by obesity. However, some suggest that obesity may be, on the opposite, an outcome of inflammation (Das, 2001). Obesity may contribute to increase local IR in the adipocytes as well as in other tissue such as the liver and skeletal muscles (Cornier et al., 2008; Gregor and Hotamisligil, 2011).

Plasma UII correlates positively with body weight in humans independently of atherosclerotic background (Cheung et al., 2004). Adipokines (dipeptidyl peptidase-4, endocan, insulin-like growth factor-binding proteins), known to play a role in diabetes mellitus and obesity (Janke et al., 2006; Neumiller et al., 2010; Ruan and Lai, 2010) were reduced in UII/ApoE double knockout mice in comparison with ApoEKO (You et al., 2012). Reduction of body mass, visceral fat, visceral adipocytes diameter, serum LDL, triglycerides, as well as increase in HDL is also observed with UII gene deletion in mice (You et al., 2012; **Figure 3**). A reduction in hepatic cholesterol esterification is also observed in UIIKO mice (Kiss et al., 2011). These results are attributed to a reduction in cholesterol and apolipoprotein B production by hepatocytes (Kiss et al., 2011). Furthermore, Jiang et al. (2008) found that the UII gene (UTS2) regulates fat accumulation in humans.

CONCLUSION

The mechanism that links the various components of MetS relies primarily on IR and inflammation (Sutherland et al., 2004; Eckel et al., 2010). The ability of UII to modulate both of these factors suggests an important role for the peptide in the pathogenesis of the MetS. Other risk factors mediated by UII, such as obesity, may tend to initiate the positive feedback cycle, which contributes to

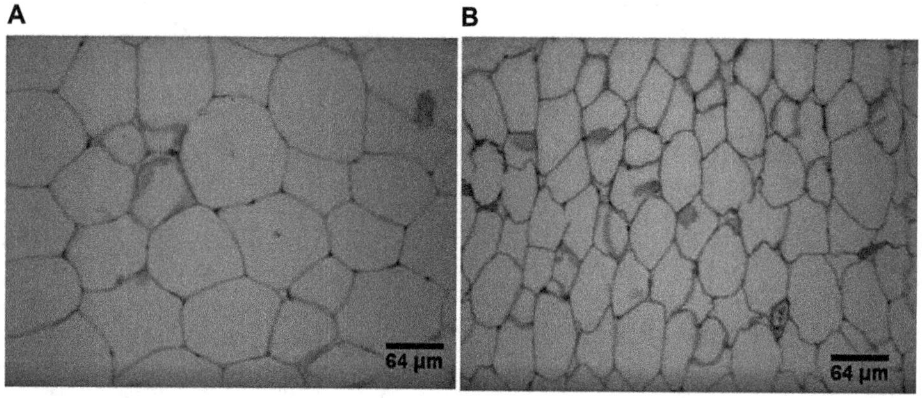

FIGURE 3 | Hematoxylin and eosin staining of visceral adipose tissue sections in wild-type mice (A) and UIIKO mice (B). Adipocytes of UIIKO mice appear smaller than wild-type mice.

the development of MetS. In fact, genetic manipulation or the use of UT receptor antagonists seems to have a positive effect on every risk factor of the MetS (You et al., 2012). However, it is still unclear whether UII is important in the initiation or only in the progression and further complications of the disease. The biological activities of UII, and the recent reports of increased serum levels of UII in patients with the MetS suggest that pharmacological manipulation of the UII pathway as a possible future treatment of the syndrome.

ACKNOWLEDGMENTS

We acknowledge the support of the Canadian Institute of Health Research and the Heart and Stroke Foundation of Quebec. We also thank Zhipeng You for his technical help.

REFERENCES

Albertin, G., Guidolin, D., Sorato, E., Spinazzi, R., Mascarin, A., Oselladore, B., et al. (2009). Pro-angiogenic activity of Urotensin-II on different human vascular endothelial cell populations. *Regul. Pept.* 157, 64–71.

Ames, R. S., Sarau, H. M., Chambers, J. K., Willette, R. N., Aiyar, N. V., Romanic, A. M., et al. (1999). Human urotensin-II is a potent vasoconstrictor and agonist for the orphan receptor GPR14. *Nature* 401, 282–286.

Arnalich, F., Hernanz, A., Lopez-Maderuelo, D., Peña, J. M., Camacho, J., Madero, R., et al. (2000). Enhanced acute-phase response and oxidative stress in older adults with type II diabetes. *Horm. Metab. Res.* 32, 407–412.

Babińska, M., Holecki, M., Prochaczak, F., Owczarek, A., Kokocińska, D., Chudek., J., et al. (2012). Is plasma urotensin II concentration an indicator of myocardial damage in patients with acute coronary syndrome? *Arch. Med. Sci.* 8, 449–454.

Bastard, J. P., Jardel, C., Bruckert, E., Blondy, P., Capeau, J., Laville, M., et al. (2000). Elevated levels of interleukin 6 are reduced in serum and subcutaneous adipose tissue of obese women after weight loss. *J. Clin. Endocrinol. Metab.* 85, 3338–3342.

Bastard, J. P., Maachi, M., Van Nhieu, J. T., Jardel, C., Bruckert, E., Grimaldi, A., et al. (2002). Adipose tissue IL-6 content correlates with resistance to insulin activation of glucose uptake both in vivo and in vitro. *J. Clin. Endocrinol. Metab.* 87, 2084–2089.

Bavenholm, P., de Faire, U., Landou, C., Efendic, S., Nilsson, J., Wilman, B., et al. (1998). Progression of coronary artery disease in young male post-infarction patients is linked to disturbances of carbohydrate and lipoprotein metabolism and to impaired fibrinolytic function. *Eur. Heart J.* 19, 402–410.

Behm, D. J., Doe, C. P., Johns, D. G., Maniscalco, K., Stankus, G. P., Wibberley, A., et al. (2004). Urotensin-II: a novel systemic hypertensive factor in the cat. *Naunyn Schmiedebergs Arch. Pharmacol.* 369, 274–280.

Besedovsky, H. O., and Del Rey, A. (1996). Immune-neuro-endocrine interactions. *Endocr. Rev.* 17, 64–102.

Boden, G. (1997). Role of fatty acids in the pathogenesis of insulin resistance and NIDDM. *Diabetes* 46, 3–10.

Boden, G., and Shulman, G. I. (2002). Free fatty acids in obesity and type 2 diabetes: defining their role in the development of insulin resistance and β-cell dysfunction. *Eur. J. Clin. Invest.* 32(Suppl. 3), 14–23.

Boden, G., Cheung, P., Stein, T. P., Kresge, K., and Mozzoli, M. (2002). FFA cause hepatic insulin resistance by inhibiting insulin suppression of glycogenolysis. *Am. J. Physiol. Endocrinol. Metab.* 283, E12–E19.

Bousette, N., Patel, L., Douglas, S. A., Ohlstein, E. H., and Giaid, A. (2004). Increased expression of urotensin II and its cognate receptor GPR14 in atherosclerotic lesions of the human aorta. *Atherosclerosis* 176, 117–123.

Brasier, A. R., Li, J., and Wimbish, K. A. (1996). Tumor necrosis factor activates angiotensinogen gene expression by the Rel A transactivator. *Hypertension* 27, 1009–1017.

Brinton, E. A., Eisenberg, S., and Breslow, J. L. (1991). Increased apo A-I and apo A-II fractional catabolic rate in patients with low high density lipoprotein-cholesterol levels with or without hypertriglyceridemia. *J. Clin. Invest.* 87, 536–544.

Cameron, A. J., Boyko, E. J., Sicree, R. A., Zimmet, P. Z., Söderberg, S., Alberti, K. G., et al. (2008). Central obesity as a precursor to the metabolic syndrome in the AusDiab study and Mauritius. *Obesity (Silver Spring)* 16, 2707–2716.

Carey, D. G., Jenkins, A. B., Campbell, L. V., Freund, J., and Chisholm, D. J. (1996). Abdominal fat and insulin resistance in normal and overweight women: direct measurements reveal a strong relationship in subjects at both low and high risk of NIDDM. *Diabetes* 45, 633–638.

Chan, J. C., Cheung, J. C., Stehouwer, C. D., Emeis, J. J., Tong, P. C., Ko, G. T., et al. (2002). The central roles of obesity-associated dyslipidaemia, endothelial activation and cytokines in the metabolic syndrome—an analysis by structural equation modelling. *Int. J. Obes. Relat. Metab. Disord.* 26, 994–1008.

Chanalaris, A., Lawrence, K. M., Townsend, P. A., Davidson, S., Jamshidi, Y., Stephanou, A., et al. (2005). Hypertrophic effects of urocortin homologous peptides are mediated via activation of the Akt pathway. *Biochem. Biophys. Res. Commun.* 328, 442–448.

Charles, M. A., Eschwege, E., Thicult, N., Claude, J. R., Warnet, J. M., Rosselin, G. E., et al. (1997). The role of non-esterified fatty acids in the deterioration of glucose tolerance in Caucasian subjects: results of the Paris Prospective Study. *Diabetologia* 40, 1101–1106.

Cheung, B. M., Leung, R., Man, Y. B., and Wong, L. Y. (2004). Plasma concentration of urotensin II is raised in hypertension. *J. Hypertens.* 22, 1341–1344.

Cho, L. W. (2011). Metabolic syndrome. *Singapore Med. J.* 52, 779–785.

Conlon, J. M., Agius, L., George, K., Alberti, M. M., and Hazon, N. (1994).

Effects of dogfish urotensin II on lipid mobilization in the fasted dogfish, *Scyliorhinus canicula*. *Gen. Comp. Endocrinol.* 93, 177–180.

Conlon, J. M., Arnold-Reed, D., and Balment, R. J. (1990). Post-translational processing of prepro-urotensin II. *FEBS Lett.* 266, 37–40.

Conlon, J. M., Yano, K., Waugh, D., and Hazon, N. (1996). Distribution and molecular forms of urotensin II and its role in cardiovascular regulation in vertebrates. *J. Exp. Zool.* 275, 226–238.

Cornier, M. A., Dabelea, D., Hernandez, T. L., Lindstrom, R. C., Steig, A. J., Stob, N. R., et al. (2008). The metabolic syndrome. *Endocr. Rev.* 29, 777–822.

Coulouarn, Y., Jégou, S., Tostivint, H., Vaudry, H., and Lihrmann, I. (1999). Cloning, sequence analysis and tissue distribution of the mouse and rat urotensin II precursors. *FEBS Lett.* 457, 28–32.

Das, U. N. (2001). Is obesity an inflammatory condition? *Nutrition* 17, 953–966.

Das, U. N. (2002). Is metabolic syndrome X an inflammatory condition? *Exp. Biol. Med.* 227, 989–997.

DeFronzo, R. A., Gunnarsson, R., Björkman, O., Olsson, M., and Wahren, J. (1985). Effects of insulin on peripheral and splanchnic glucose metabolism in noninsulin-dependent (type II) diabetes mellitus. *J. Clin. Invest.* 76, 149–155.

Djordjevic, T., BelAiba, R. S., Bonello, S., Pfeilschifter, J., Hess, J., and Görlach, A. (2005). Human urotensin II is a novel activator of NADPH oxidase in human pulmonary artery smooth muscle cells. *Arterioscler. Thromb. Vasc. Biol.* 25, 519–525.

Domínguez-Rodríguez, A., Díaz, I., Rodríguez-Moyano, M., Caderón-Sánchez, E., Antonio, R. J., Ordóñez, A., et al. (2012). Urotensin-II signalling mechanism in rat coronary artery: role of STIM1 and Orai1-dependant store operated calcium influx in vasoconstriction. *Arterioscler. Thromb. Vasc. Biol.* 35, 1325–1332.

Dong, X., Ye, X., Song, N., Zhao, J., Di, B., Peng, F., et al. (2012). Urotensin II promotes the production of LTC(4) in rat aortic adventitial fibroblasts through NF-κB-5-LO pathway by p38 MAPK and ERK activations. *Heart Vessels* doi: 10.1007/s00380-012-0291-0 [Epub ahead of print].

Dörffel, Y., Lätsch, C., Stuhlmüller, B., Schreiber, S., Scholze, S., Burmester, G. R., et al. (1999). Preactivated peripheral blood monocytes in patients with essential hypertension. *Hypertension* 34, 113–117.

Douglas, S. A., and Ohlstein, E. H. (2000). Human urotensin-II, the most potent mammalian vasoconstrictor identified to date, as a therapeutic target for the management of cardiovascular disease. *Trends Cardiovasc. Med.* 131, 1262–1274.

Douglas, S. A., Sulpizio, A. C., Piercy, V., Sarau, H. M., Ames, R. S., Aiyar, N. V., et al. (2000). Differential vasoconstrictor activity of human urotensin-II in vascular tissue isolated from the rat, mouse, dog, pig, marmoset and cynomolgus monkey. *Br. J. Pharmacol.* 131, 1262–1274.

Douglas, S. A., Tayara, L., Ohlstein, E. H., Halawa, N., and Giaid, A. (2002). Congestive heart failure and expression of myocardial urotensin II. *Lancet* 359, 1990–1997.

Eckel, R. H., Alberti, K. G., Grundy, S. M., and Zimmet, P. Z. (2010). The metabolic syndrome. *Lancet* 375, 181–183.

Engström, G., Hedblad, B., Stavenow, L., Lind, P., Janzon, L., and Lindgärde, F. (2003). Inflammation-sensitive plasma proteins are associated with future weight gain. *Diabetes* 52, 2097–2101.

Fagot-Campagna, A., Balkau, B., Simon, D., Warnet, J. M., Claude, J. R., Ducimetiere, P., et al. (1998). High free fatty acid concentration: an independent risk factor for hypertension in the Paris Prospective Study. *Int. J. Epidemiol.* 27, 808–813.

Fernández-Real, J. M., Broch, M., Vendrell, J., Richart, C., and Ricart, W. (2000). Interleukin 6 gene polymorphism and lipid abnormalities in healthy subjects. *J. Clin. Endocrinol. Metab.* 85, 1334–1339.

Fernández-Real, J. M., Vayreda, M., Richart, C., Gutiérrez, C., Broch, M., Vendrell, J., et al. (2001). Circulating interleukin 6 levels, blood pressure and insulin sensitivity in apparently healthy men and women. *J. Clin. Endocrinol. Metab.* 86, 1154–1159.

Fernández-Real, J. M., and Ricart, W. (2003). Insulin resistance and chronic cardiovascular inflammatory syndrome. *Endocr. Rev.* 24, 278–301.

Festa, A., D'Agostino, R. Jr., Williams, K., Karter, A. J., Mayer-Davis, E. J., Tracy, R. P., et al. (2001). The relation of body fat mass and distribution to markers of chronic inflammation. *Int. J. Obesity* 25, 1407–1415.

Festa, A., D'Agostino, R., Tracy, R. P., and Haffner, S. M. (2002). Elevated levels of acute-phase proteins and plasminogen activator inhibitor-1 predict the development of type 2 diabetes. The insulin resistance atherosclerosis study. *Diabetes* 51, 1131–1137.

Fleet, J. C., Clinton, S. K., Salomon, R. N., Loppnow, H., and Libby, P. (1992). Atherogenic diets enhance endotoxin-stimulated interleukin-1 and tumor necrosis factor gene expression in rabbit aortae. *J. Nutr.* 122, 294–305.

Ford, E. S., Li, C., and Zhao, G. (2010). Prevalence and correlates of metabolic syndrome based on a harmonious definition among adults in the US. *J. Diabetes* 2, 180–193.

Fried, S. K., Bunkin, D. A., and Greenberg, A. S. (1998). Omental and subcutaneous adipose tissues of obese subjects release interleukin-6: depot difference and regulation by glucocorticoid. *J. Clin. Endocrinol. Metab.* 83, 847–850.

Gardiner, S. M., March, J. E., Kemp, P. A., Davenport, A. P., and Bennett, T. (2001). Depressor and regionally selective vasodilator effects of human urotensin II in conscious rats. *Br. J. Pharmacol.* 132, 1625–1629.

Gibson, A. (1987). Complex effects of *Gillichthys* urotensin II on rat aortic strips. *Br. J. Pharmacol.* 91, 205–212.

Golden, S. H., Folsom, A. R., Coresh, J., Sharrett, A. R., Szklo, M., and Brancati, F. (2002). Risk factor groupings related to insulin resistance and their synergistic effects on subclinical atherosclerosis: the atherosclerosis risk in communities study. *Diabetes* 51, 3069–3076.

Gram, J., Jespersen, J., Kluft, C., and Rijken, D. C. (1987). On the usefulness of fibrinolysis variables in the characterization of a risk group for myocardial reinfarction. *Acta. Med. Scand.* 221, 149–153.

Greenberg, A. S., Nordan, R. P., McIntosh, J., Calvo, J. C., Scow, R. O., and Jablons, D. (1992). Interleukin-6 reduces lipoprotein lipase activity in adipose tissue of mice in vivo and in 3T3-L1 adipocytes: a possible role for interleukin-6 in cancer cachexia. *Cancer. Res.* 52, 4113–4116.

Gregor, M. F., and Hotamisligil, G. S. (2011). Inflammatory mechanisms in obesity. *Annu. Rev. Immunol.* 23, 415–445.

Grimble, R. F. (2002). Inflammatory status and insulin resistance. *Curr. Opin. Clin. Nutr. Metab. Care* 5, 551–559.

Grundy, S. M. (1999). Hypertriglyceridemia, insulin resistance, and the metabolic syndrome. *Am. J. Cardiol.* 83, 25–29.

Grunfeld, C., and Feingold, K. R. (1992). Role of cytokines in inducing hyperlipidemia. *Diabetes* 41(Suppl. 2), 97–101.

Gruson, D., Rousseau, M. F., Ketelslegers, J. M., and Hermans, M. P. (2010a). Raised plasma urotensin II in type 2 diabetes patients is associated with the metabolic syndrome phenotype. *J. Clin. Hypertens. (Greenwich)* 12, 653–660.

Gruson, D., Ginion, A., Decroly, N., Lause, P., Vanoverschelde, J. L., Ketelslegers, J. M., et al. (2010b). Urotensin II induction of adult cardiomyocytes hypertrophy involves the Akt/GSK-3beta signaling pathway. *Peptides* 31, 1326–1333.

Gruson, D., Ginion, A., Lause, P., Ketelslegers, J. M., Thissien, J. P., and Bertrand, L. (2012). Urotensin II and urocortin trigger the expression of myostatin, a negative regulator of cardiac growth, in cardiomyocytes. *Peptides* 33, 351–353.

Hamsten, A., Wiman, B., Defaire, U., and Blomback, M. (1985). Increased plasma level of a rapid inhibitor of tissue plasminogen activator in young survivors of myocardial infarction. *N. Engl. J. Med.* 313, 1557–1563.

Hamsten, A., Defaire, U., Walldius, G., Dahlen, G., Szamosi, A., Landov, C., et al. (1987). Plasminogen activator inhibitor in plasma: risk factor for recurrent myocardial infarction. *Lancet* 2, 3–9.

Han, S. N., Leka, L. S., Lichtenstein, A. H., Ausman, L. M., Schaefer, E. J., and Meydani, S. N. (2002). Effect of hydrogenated and saturated, relative to polyunsaturated, fat on immune and inflammatory responses of adults with moderate hypercholesterolemia. *J. Lipid. Res.* 43, 445–452.

Hassan, G. S., Chouiali, F., Saito, T., Hu, F., Douglas, S. A., Ao, Z., et al. (2003). Effect of human urotensin-II infusion on hemodynamics and cardiac function. *Can. J. Physiol. Pharmacol.* 81, 125–128.

Hassan, G. S., Douglas, S. A., Ohlstein, E. H., and Giaid, A. (2005). Expression of urotensin-II in human coronary atherosclerosis. *Peptides* 26, 2462–2472.

Heller, J., Schepke, M., Neef, M., Woitas, R., Rabe, C., and Sauerbruch, T. (2002). Increased urotensin II plasma levels in patients with cirrhosis and portal hypertension. *J. Hepatol.* 37, 767–772.

Hodis, H. N., Mack, W. J., LaBree, L., Selzer, R. H., Liu, C. R., Liu, C. H., et al. (1998). The role of carotid arterial intima-media thickness in predicting clinical coronary events. *Ann. Intern. Med.* 128, 262–269.

Hotamisligil, G. S., Budavari, A., Murray, D., and Spiegelman, B. M. (1994). Reduced tyrosine kinase activity of the insulin receptor in obesity-diabetes. *J. Clin. Invest.* 94, 1543–1549.

Hotamisligil, G. S., Peraldi, P., Budavari, A., Ellis, R., White, M. F., and Spiegelman, B. M. (1996). IRS-1-mediated inhibition of insulin receptor tyrosine kinase activity in TNF-α and obesity-induced insulin resistance. *Science* 271, 665–668.

Hotamisligil, G. S., Shargill, N. S., and Spiegelman, B. M. (1993). Adipose expression of tumor necrosis factor-α: direct role in obesity-linked insulin resistance. *Science* 259, 87–91.

Howard, G., O'Leary, D. H., Zaccaro, D., Haffner, S., Rewers, M., Hamman, R., et al. (1996). Insulin sensitivity and atherosclerosis. *Circulation* 93, 1809–1817.

Iglewski, M., and Grant, S. R. (2010). Urotensin II-induced signaling involved in proliferation vascular smooth muscle cells. *Vasc. Health Risk. Manag.* 6, 723–734.

Jaggers, J. R., Sui, X., Hooker, S. P., LaMonte, M. J., Matthews, C. E., Hand, G. A., et al. (2009). Metabolic syndrome and risk of cancer mortality in men. *Eur. J. Cancer* 45, 1831–1838.

Janke, J., Engeli, S., Gorzelniak, K., Feldpausch, M., Heintze, U., Böhnke, J., et al. (2006). Adipose tissue and circulating endothelial cell specific molecule-1 in human obesity. *Horm. Metab. Res.* 38, 28–33.

Jiang, Z., Michal, J. J., Tobey, D. J., Wang, Z., Macneil, M. D., and Magnuson, N. S. (2008). Comparative understanding of UTS2 and UTS2R genes for their involvement in type 2 diabetes mellitus. *Int. J. Biol. Sci.* 4, 96–102.

Johns, D. G., Ao, Z., Naselsky, D., Herold, C. L., Maniscalco, K., Sarov-Blat, L., et al. (2004). Urotensin- II-mediated cardiomyocyte hyper- trophy: effect of receptor antagonism and role of inflammatory mediators. *Arch. Pharmacol.* 370, 238–250.

Jovinge, S., Hamsten, A., Tornvall, P., Proudler, A., Bavenholm, P., Ericsson, C. G., et al. (1998). Evidence for a role of tumor necrosis factor in disturbances of triglyceride and glucose metabolism predisposing to coronary heart disease. *Metabolism* 47, 113–118.

Juhan-Vague, I., Alessi, M. C., and Vague, P. (1991). Increased plasma plasminogen activator inhibitor 1 levels. A possible link between insulin resistance and atherothrombosis. *Diabetologia* 34, 457–462.

Kahaleh, M. B., and Fan, P. S. (1997). Effect of cytokines on the production of endothelin by endothelial cells. *Clin. Exp. Rheumatol.* 15, 163–167.

Kahn, B. B., and Flier, J. S. (2000). Obesity and insulin resistance. *J. Clin. Invest.* 106, 473–481.

Kern, P. A., Ranganathan, S., Li, C., Wood, L., and Ranganathan, G. (2001). Adipose tissue tumor necrosis factor and interleukin-6 expression in human obesity and insulin resistance. *Am. J. Physiol. Endocrinol. Metab.* 280, E745–E751.

Kiss, R. S., You, Z., Genest, J. Jr., Behm, D. J., and Giaid, A. (2011). Urotensin II differentially regulates macrophage and hepatic cholesterol homeostasis. *Peptides* 32, 956–963.

Laimer, M., Ebenbichler, C. F., Kaser, S., Sandhofer, A., Weiss, H., Nehoda, H., et al. (2002). Markers of chronic inflammation and obesity: a prospective study on the reversibility of this association in middle-aged women undergoing weight loss by surgical intervention. *Int. J. Obes. Relat. Metab. Disord.* 26, 659–662.

Lassègue, B., and Clempus, R. E. (2003). Vascular NAD(P)H oxidases: specific features, expression, and regulation. *Am. J. Physiol. Regul. Integr. Comp. Physiol.* 285, 277–297.

Leinonen, E., Hurt-Camejo, E., Wiklund, O., Hulten, L. M., Hiukka, A., and Taskinen, M. R. (2003). Insulin resistance and adiposity correlate with acute-phase reaction and soluble cell adhesion molecules in type 2 diabetes. *Atherosclerosis* 166, 387–394.

Libby, P., Ridket, P. M., Hansson, G. K., and Leducq Transatlantic Network on Atherothrombosis. (2009). Inflammation in atherosclerosis: from pathophysiology to practice. *J. Am. Coll. Cardiol.* 54, 2129–2138.

Lim, M., Honisett, S., Sparkes, C. D., Komesaroff, P., Kompa, A., and Krum, H. (2004). Differential effect of urotensin II on vascular tone in normal subjects and patients with chronic heart failure. *Circulation* 109, 1212–1214.

Lin, Y., Tsuchihashi, T., Matsumura, K., Fukuhara, M., Ohya, Y., Fujii, K., et al. (2003). Central cardiovascular action of urotensin II in spontaneously hypertensive rats. *Hypertens. Res.* 26, 839–845.

Liu, Q., Pong, S. S., Zeng, Z., Zhang, Q., Howard, A. D., Williams, D. L., et al. (1999). Identification of urotensin II as the endogenous ligand for the orphan G-protein-coupled receptor GPR14. *Biochem. Biophys. Res. Commun.* 266, 174–178.

Loirand, G., Rolli-Derkinderen, M., and Pacaud, P. (2008). Urotensin II and atherosclerosis. *Peptides* 29, 778–782.

Maguire, J. J., Kuc, R. E., and Davenport, A. P. (2000). Orphan-receptor ligand human urotensin II: receptor localization in human tissues and comparison of vasoconstrictor responses with endothelin-1. *Br. J. Pharmacol.* 131, 441–446.

Maguire, J. J., Kuc, R. E., Wiley, K. E., Kleinz, M. J., and Davenport, A. P. (2004). Cellular distribution of immunoreactive urotensin-II in human tissues with evidence of increased expression in atherosclerosis and a greater constrictor response of small compared to large coronary arteries. *Peptides* 25, 1767–1774.

Mallamaci, F., Pizzini, P., Tripepi, G., and Zoccali, C. (2005). Urotensin II in end-stage renal disease: an inverse correlate of sympathetic function and cardiac natriuretic peptides. *J. Nephrol.* 18, 727–732.

Matsushita, M., Shichiri, M., Imai, T., Iwashina, M., Tanaka, H., Takasu, N., et al. (2001). Co-expression of urotensin II and its receptor (GPR14) in human cardiovascular and renal tissues. *J. Hypertens.* 19, 2185–2190.

Mayer-Davis, E. J., D'Agostino, R. Jr., Karter, A. J., Haffner, S. M., Rewers, M. J., Saad, M., et al. (1998). Intensity and amount of physical activity in relation to insulin sensitivity: the Insulin Resistance Atherosclerosis Study. *JAMA* 279, 669–674.

McGarry, J. D., and Dobbins, R. L. (1999). Fatty acids, lipotoxicity and insulin secretion. *Diabetologia* 42, 128–138.

McMillan, D. E. (1989). Increased levels of acute-phase serum proteins in diabetes. *Metabolism* 38, 1042–1046.

Misra, A., and Khurana, L. (2008). Obesity and the metabolic syndrome in developing countries. *J. Clin. Endocrinol. Metab.* 93(Suppl. 1), S9–S30.

Muramaki, T., Michelagnoli, S., Longhi, R., Gianfranceschi, G., Pazzucconi, F., Calabresi, L., et al. (1995). Triglycerides are major determinants of cholesterol esterification/transfer and HDL remodelling in human plasma. *Atherioscler. Throm. Vasc. Biol.* 15, 1819–1828.

National Cholesterol Education Program (NCEP) Expert Panel on Detection, Evaluation, and Treatment of High Blood Cholesterol in Adults (Adult Treatment Panel III). (2002). Third Report of the National Cholesterol Education Program (NCEP) Expert Panel on Detection, Evaluation, and Treatment of High Blood Cholesterol in Adults (Adult Treatment Panel III) final report. *Circulation* 106, 3143–3421.

Neumiller, J. J., Wood, L., and Campbell, R. K. (2010). Dipeptidyl peptidase-4 inhibitors for the treatment of type 2 diabetes mellitus. *Pharmacotherapy* 30, 463–484.

Nishihama, K., Yamada, Y., Matsuo, H., Segawa, T., Watanabe, S., Kato, K., et al. (2007). Association of gene polymorphisms with myocardial infarction in individuals with or without conventional coronary risk factors. *Int. J. Mol. Med.* 19, 129–141.

Nonogaki, K., Fuller, G. M., Fuentes, N. L., Moser, A. H., Staprans, I., and Grunfeld, C. (1995). Interleukin-6 stimulates hepatic triglyceride secretion in rats. *Endocrinology* 136, 2143–2149.

Oguri, M., Kato, K., Yokoi, K., Itoh, T., Yoshida, T., Watanabe, S., et al. (2009). Association of genetic variants with myocardial infarction in Japanese individuals with metabolic syndrome. *Atherosclerosis* 206, 486–493.

Ong, K. L., Wong, L. Y., and Cheug, B. M. (2008). The role of urotensin II in the metabolic syndrome. *Peptides* 29, 859–867.

Ong, K. L., Wong, L. Y., Man, Y. B., Leung, R. Y., Song, Y. Q., Lam, K. S., et al. (2006). Haplotypes in the urotensin II gene and urotensin II receptor gene are associated with insulin resistance and impaired glucose tolerance. *Peptides* 27, 1659–1667.

Paolisso, G., Tataranni, P. A., Foley, J. E., Bogardus, C., Howard, B. V., and Ravussin, E. (1995). A high concentration of fasting plasma non-esterified fatty acids is a risk factor for the development of NIDDM. *Diabetologia* 38, 1213–1217.

Papadopoulos, P., Bousette, N., Al-Ramli, W., You, Z., Behm, D. J., Ohlstein, E. H., et al. (2009). Targeted overexpression of the human urotensin receptor transgene in smooth muscle cells: effect of UT antagonism in ApoE knockout mice fed with Western Diet. *Atherosclerosis* 204, 395–404.

Papanicolaou, D. A., Petrides, J. S., Tsigos, C., Bina, S., Kalogeras, K. T., Wilder, R., et al. (1996). Exercise stimulates interleukin-6 secretion: inhibition by glucocorticoids and correlation with catecholamines. *Am. J. Physiol.* 271, E601–E605.

Pearson, D., Shively, J. E., Clark, B. R., Geschwind, I. I., Barkley, M., Nishioka, R. S., et al. (1980). Urotensin II antagonist peptide in the caudal neurosecretory system of fishes. *Proc. Natl. Acad. Sci. U.S.A.* 77, 5021–5024.

Popkin, B. M., and Doak, C. M. (1998). The obesity epidemic is a worldwide phenomenon. *Nutr. Rev.* 56, 106–114.

Pradhan, A. D., Manson, J. E., Rifai, N., Buring, J. E., and Ridker, P. M. (2001). C-reactive protein, interleukin 6, and risk of developing type 2 diabetes mellitus. *JAMA* 286, 327–334.

Randle, P. J. (1998). Regulatory interactions between lipids and carbohydrates: the glucose fatty acid cycle after 35 years. *Diabetes Metab. Rev.* 14, 263–283.

Randle, P. J., Garland, P. B., Hales, C. N., and Newsholme, E. A. (1963). The glucose fatty-acid cycle. Its role in insulin sensitivity and the metabolic disturbances of diabetes mellitus. *Lancet* 1, 785–789.

Reaven, G. M. (1988). Banting lecture 1988. Role of insulin resistance in human disease. *Diabetes* 37, 1595–1607.

Reaven, G. M. (2003). Insulin resistance/compensatory hyperinsulinemia, essential hypertension, and cardiovascular disease. *J. Clin. Endocrinol. Metab.* 88, 2399–2403.

Ross, B., McKendy, K., and Giaid, A. (2010). Role of urotensin II in health and disease. *Am. J. Physiol. Regul. Integr. Comp. Physiol.* 298, R1156–R1172.

Ruan, W., and Lai, M. (2010). Insulin-like growth factor binding protein: a possible marker for the metabolic syndrome? *Acta. Diabetol.* 47, 5–14.

Russell, F. D., and Molenaar, P. (2004). Investigation of signalling pathways that mediate the inotropic effect of urotensin-II in human heart. *Cardiovasc. Res.* 63, 673–681.

Sáez, M. E., Smani, T., Ramírez-Lorca, R., Díaz, I., Serrano-Ríos, M., Ruiz, A., et al. (2011). Association analysis of urotensin II gene (UTS2) and flanking regions with biochemical parameters related to insulin resistance. *PLoS ONE* 6:e19327. doi: 10.1371/journal.pone.0019327

Sako, Y., and Grill, V. E. (1990). A 48-hour lipid infusion in the rat time-dependently inhibits glucose-induced insulin secretion and B cell oxidation through a process likely coupled to fatty acid oxidation. *Endocrinology* 127, 1580–1589.

Sano, M., Fukuda, K., Kodama, H., Pan, J., Saito, M., Matsuzaki, J., et al. (2000). Interleukin-6 family of cytokines mediate angiotensin II-induced cardiac hypertrophy in rodent cardiomyocytes. *J. Biol. Chem.* 275, 29717–22923.

Sartore, S., Chiavegato, A., Faggin, E., Franch, R., Puato, M., Ausoni, S., et al. (2001). Contribution of adventitial fibroblasts to neointima formation and vascular remodeling: from innocent bystander to active participant. *Circ. Res.* 89, 1111–1121.

Sauzeau, V., Le Mellionnec, E., Bertoglio, J., Scalbert, E., Pacaud, P., and Loirand, G. (2001). Human urotensin II-induced contraction and arterial smooth muscle cell proliferation are mediated by RhoA and Rho-kinase. *Circ. Res.* 88, 1102–1104.

Segain, J. P., Rolli-Derkinderen, M., Gervois, N., Raingeard de la Blétière, D., Loirand, G., and Pacaud, P. (2007). Urotensin II is a new chemotactic factor for UT-expressing monocytes. *J. Immunol.* 179, 901–909.

Sheridan, M. A., and Bern, H. A. (1986). Both somatostatin and the caudal neuropeptide, urotensin II, stimulate lipid mobilization from coho salmon liver incubated in vitro. *Regul. Pept.* 14, 333–344.

Sheridan, M. A., Plisetskaya, E. M., Bern, H. A., and Gorbman, A. (1987). Effects of somatostatin-25 and urotensin II on lipid and carbohydrate metabolism of coho salmon, *Oncorhynchus kisutch*. *Gen. Comp. Endocrinol.* 66, 405–414.

Silvestre, R. A., Egido, E. M., Hernández, R., Leprince, J., Chatenet, D., Tollemer, H., et al. (2004). Urotensin-II is present in pancreatic extracts and inhibits insulin release in the perfused rat pancreas. *Eur. J. Endocrinol.* 151, 803–809.

Silvestre, R. A., Rodríguez-Gallardo, J., Egido, E. M., and Marco, J. (2001). Inhibition of insulin release by urotensin II – a study on the perfused rat pancreas. *Horm. Metab. Res.* 33, 379–381.

Sondermeijer, B., Komp, A., Komesaroff, P., and Krum, H. (2005). Effects of exogenous urotensin-II on vascular tone in skin microcirculation of patients with essential hypertension. *Am. J. Hypertens.* 22, 1341–1344.

Song, N., Ding, W., Chu, S., Zhao, J., Dong, X., Di, B., et al. (2012). Urotensin II stimulates vascular endothelial growth factor secretion from advential fibroblasts in synergy with angiotensin II. *Circ. J.* 76, 1267–1273.

Sowers, J. R. (2004). Insulin resistance and hypertension. *Am. J. Physiol. Heart Circ. Physiol.* 286, H1597–H1602.

Stefan, N., Kantartzis, K., Machann, J., Schick, F., Thamer, C., Rittig, K., et al. (2008). Identification and characterization of metabolically benign obesity in humans. *Arch. Intern. Med.* 168, 1609–1616.

Stenmark, K. R., Davie, N., Frid, M., Gerasimovskaya, E., and Das, M. (2006). Role of the adventitia in pulmonary vascular remodelling. *Physiology (Bethesda)* 21, 134–145.

Stirrat, A., Gallagher, M., Douglas, S. A., Ohlstein, E. H., Berry, C., Kirk, A., et al. (2001). Potent vasodilator responses to human urotensin-II in human pulmonary and abdominal resistance arteries. *Am. J. Physiol. Heart Circ. Physiol.* 280, H925–H928.

Stouthard, J. M., Romijn, J. A., Van der Poll, T., Endert, E., Klein, S., Bakker, P. J., et al. (1995). Endocrinologic and metabolic effects of interleukin-6 in humans. *Am. J. Physiol.* 268, E813–E819.

Sun, H. X., Du, W. N., Zuo, J., Wu, G. D., Shi, G. B., Shen, Y., et al. (2002). The association of two single nucleotide polymorphisms in PRKCZ and UTS2 respectively with type 2 diabetes in Han people of northern China. *Zhongguo Yi Xue Ke Xue Yuan Xue Bao* 24, 223–227.

Sutherland, J. P., McKinley, B., and Eckel, R. H. (2004). The metabolic syndrome and inflammation. *Metab. Synd. Relat. Disord.* 2, 82–104.

Suzuki, S., Wenyi, Z., Hirai, M., Hinokio, Y., Suzuki, C., Yamada, T., et al. (2004). Genetic variations at urotensin II and urotensin II receptor genes and risk of type 2 diabetes mellitus in Japanese. *Peptides* 25, 1803–1808.

Takano, M., Itoh, N., Yayama, K., Yamano, M., Ohtani, R., and Okamoto, H. (2000). Interleukin 6 as a mediator responsible for inflammation-induced increase in plasma angiotensinogen. *Biochem. Pharmacol.* 45, 201–206.

Tamura, K., Okazaki, M., Tamura, M., Isozumi, K., Tasaki, H., and Nakashima, Y. (2003). Urotensin II-induced activation of extracellular signal-regulated kinase in cultured vascular smooth muscle cells: involvement of cell adhesion-mediated integrin signalling. *Life Sci.* 72, 1049–1060.

Tan, Y. J., Fan, Z. T., and Yang, H. X. (2006). Role of urotensin II gene in the genetic susceptibility to gestational diabetes mellitus in northern Chinese women. *Zhonghua Fu Chan Ke Za Zhi* 41, 732–735.

Totsune, K., Takahashi, K., Arihara, Z., Sone, M., Ito, S., and Murakami, O. (2003). Increased plasma urotensin II levels in patients with diabetes mellitus. *Clin. Sci.* 104, 1–5.

Trayhurn, P., and Wood, I. S. (2004). Adipokines: inflammation and the pleiotropic role of white adipose tissue. *Br. J. Nutr.* 92, 347–355.

Tsoukas, P., Kane, E., and Giaid, A. (2011). Potential clinical implications of the urotensin II receptor antagonists. *Front. Pharmacol.* 2:38. doi: 10.3389/fphar.2011.00038

Tzanidis, A., Hannan, R. D., and Thomas, W. G. (2003). Direct actions of urotensin II on the heart implications for cardiac fibrosis and hypertrophy. *Circ. Res.* 93, 246–253.

Unger, R. H. (1995). Lipotoxicity in the pathogenesis of obesity-dependant NIDDM. Genetic and clinical implications. *Diabetes* 44, 863–870.

Vessby, B., Unsitupa, M., Hermansen, K., Riccardi, G., Rivellese, A. A., Tapsell, L. C., et al. (2001). Substituting dietary saturated for monounsaturated fat impairs insulin sensitivity in healthy men and women: the KANWU Study. *Diabetologia* 44, 312–319.

Vozarova, B., Fernandez-Real, J. M., Knowler, W. C., Gallart, L., Hanson, R. L., Gruber, J. D., et al. (2003). The interleukin-6 (174) G/C promoter polymorphism is associated with type-2 diabetes mellitus in Native Americans and Caucasians. *Hum. Genet.* 112, 409–413.

Wang, H. X., Zeng, X. J., Liu, Y., Wang, J., Lu, L. Q., Hao, G., et al. (2009). Elevated expression of urotensin II and its receptor in skeletal muscle of diabetic mouse. *Regul. Pept.* 154, 85–90.

Wang, Z. J., Shi, L. B., Xiong, Z. W., Zhang, L. F., Meng, L., Bu, D. F., et al. (2006). Alteration of vascular urotensin II receptor in mice with apolipoprotein E gene knockout. *Peptides* 27, 858–863.

Watanabe, T., Pakala, R., and Katagiri, T. (2001a). Synergistic effect of urotensin II with mildly oxidized LDL on DNA synthesis in vascular smooth muscle cells. *Circulation* 104, 16–18.

Watanabe, T., Pakala, R., and Katagiri, T. (2001b). Synergistic effect of urotensin II with serotonin on vascular smooth muscle cell proliferation. *J. Hypertens.* 19, 2191–2196.

Watanabe, T., Suguro, T., Kanome, T., Sakamoto, Y., Kodate, S., Hagiwara, T., et al. (2005). Human urotensin II accelerates foam cell formation in human monocyte-derived macrophage. *Hypertension* 46, 738–744.

Watson, A. M., Lambert, G. W., Smith, K. J., and May, C. N. (2003). Urotensin II acts centrally to increase epinephrine and ACTH release and cause potent inotropic and chronotropic actions. *Hypertension* 42, 373–379.

Welborn, T. A., Breckenridge, A., Rubinstein, A. H., Dollery, C. T., and Fraser,

T. R. (1966). Serum-insulin in essential hypertension and in peripheral vascular disease. *Lancet* 1, 1336–1337.

Wenyi, Z., Suzuki, S., Hirai, M., Hinokio, Y., Tanizawa, Y., Matsutani, A., et al. (2003). Role of urotensin II gene in genetic susceptibility to Type 2 diabetes mellitus in Japanese subjects. *Diabetologia* 46, 972–976.

World Health Organization. (2008). *Controlling the Global Obesity Epidemic.* Available at: http://www.who.int/nutrition/topics/obesity/en/index.html [accessed August 2012].

Yi, L., Gu, Y. H., Wang, X. L., An, L. Z., Xie, X. D., Shao, W., et al. (2006). Association of ACE, ACE2 and UTS2 polymorphisms with essential hypertension in Han and Dongxiang populations from north-western China. *J. Int. Med. Res.* 34, 272–283.

Yoshimoto, T., Matsushita, M., and Hirata, Y. (2004). Role of urotensin II in peripheral tissue as an autocrine/paracrine growth factor. *Peptides* 25, 1775–1781.

You, Z., Genest, J. Jr., Barrette, P. O., Hafiane, A., Behm, D. J., D'Orleans-Juste, P., et al. (2012). *Arterioscler. Thromb. Vasc. Biol.* 32, 1809–1816.

Yudkin, J. S., Stehouwer, C. D., Emeis, J. J., and Coppack, S. W. (1999). C-reactive protein in healthy subjects: associations with obesity, insulin resistance, and endothelial dysfunction: a potential role for cytokines originating from adipose tissue? *Artherioscler. Thromb. Vasc. Biol.* 19, 972–978.

Zavaroni, I., Ardigò, D., Zuccarelli, A., Pacetti, E., Piatti, P. M., Monti, L., et al. (2006). Insulin resistance/compensatory hyperinsulinemia predict carotid intimal media thickness in patients with essential hypertension. *Nutr. Metab. Cardiovasc. Dis.* 16, 22–27.

Zhang, Y., Li, J., Cao, J., Chen, J., Yan, J., Zhang, Z., et al. (2002). Effect of chronic hypoxia on contents of urotensin II and its functional receptors in rat myocardium. *Heart Vessels* 16, 64–68.

Zhang, Y. G., Li, J., Li, Y. G., and Wei, R. H. (2008). Urotensin II induces phenotypic differentiation, migration and collagen synthesis of adventitial fibroblasts from rat aorta. *J. Hypertens.* 26, 1119–1126.

Zhou, P., Wu, S. Y., Yu, C. F., Wang, H., Tang, C. S., Lin, L., et al. (2003). Effects of urotensin II on isolated rat hearts under normal perfusion and ischemia reperfusion. *Sheng Li Xue Bao* 55, 442–448.

Zoccali, C., Mallamaci, F., Tripepi, G., Cutrupi, S., Pizzini, P., and Malatino, L. (2006). Urotensin II is an inverse predictor of incident cardiovascular events in end-stage renal disease. *Kidney Int.* 69, 1253–1258.

Zoccali, C., and Mallamaci, F. (2008). Urotensin II: a cardiovascular and renal update. *Curr. Opin. Nephrol. Hypertens.* 17, 199–204.

Zhu, F., Ji, L., and Luo, B. (2002). The role of urotensin II gene in the genetic susceptibility to type 2 diabetes in Chinese population. *Zhonghua Yi Xue Za Zhi* 82, 1473–1475.

Zhu, Y., Zhu, Y., and Moore, P. (2006). The role of urotensin II in cardiovascular and renal physiology and diseases. *Br. J. Pharmacol.* 148, 884–901.

Zou, M. H., Cohen, R. A., and Ullrich, V. (2004). Peroxynitrite and vascular endothelial dysfunction in diabetes mellitus. *Endothelium* 11, 89–97.

Zuliani, G., Volpato, S., Ble, A., Bandinelli, S., Corsi, A. M., Lauretani, F., et al. (2007). High interleukin-6 plasma levels are associated with low HDL-C levels in community-dwelling older adults: the In Chianti study. *Atherosclerosis* 192, 384–390.

3

Neuropeptide W

Fumiko Takenoya[1,2], Haruaki Kageyama[1,3], Satoshi Hirako[1], Eiji Ota[1], Nobuhiro Wada[1], Tomoo Ryushi[1,4] and Seiji Shioda[1]*

[1] Department of Anatomy, Showa University School of Medicine, Tokyo, Japan
[2] Department of Exercise and Sports Physiology, Hoshi University School of Pharmacy and Pharmaceutical Science, Tokyo, Japan
[3] Faculty of Health Care, Kiryu University, Gunma, Japan
[4] Department of Sports and Health Science, Daito Bunka University, Saitama, Japan

Edited by:
Jae Y. Seong, Korea University, South Korea

Reviewed by:
Willis Samson, Saint Louis University, USA
Herbert Herzog, Garvan Institute, Australia

***Correspondence:**
Seiji Shioda, Department of Anatomy, Showa University School of Medicine, 1-5-8 Hatanodai, Shinagawa-ku, Tokyo 142-8555, Japan.
e-mail: shioda@med.showa-u.ac.jp

Neuropeptide W (NPW), which was first isolated from the porcine hypothalamus, exists in two forms, consisting of 23 (NPW23) or 30 (NPW30) amino acids. These neuropeptides bind to one of two NPW receptors, either NPBWR1 (otherwise known as GPR7) or NPBWR2 (GPR8), which belong to the G protein-coupled receptor family. GPR7 is expressed in the brain and peripheral organs of both humans and rodents, whereas GPR8 is not found in rodents. GPR7 mRNA in rodents is widely expressed in several hypothalamic regions, including the paraventricular, supraoptic, ventromedial, dorsomedial, suprachiasmatic, and arcuate nuclei. These observations suggest that GPR7 plays a crucial role in the modulation of neuroendocrine function. The intracerebroventricular infusion of NPW has been shown to suppress food intake and body weight and to increase both heat production and body temperature, suggesting that NPW functions as an endogenous catabolic signaling molecule. Here we summarize our current understanding of the distribution and function of NPW in the brain.

Keywords: food intake, hypothalamus, brain mapping, peptides, CPCRs

INTRODUCTION

In 1995, O'Dowd et al. (1995) used oligonucleotides based on the opioid receptor as well as the structurally related somatostatin receptor to identify two genes, GPR7 (NPBWR1) and GPR8 (NPBWR2), which were predicted to encode two G protein-coupled receptors (GPCRs) in the human brain. NPBWR1 mRNA expression is demonstrated in the human and rodent brain, whereas the NPBWR2 gene is detected in the human and rabbit, but not the rodent, brain (Lee et al., 1999). In 2002, Shimomura et al. (2002) identified the endogenous ligand for NPBWR1-2 by exposing Chinese Hamster Ovary (CHO) cells to porcine hypothalamic extracts with monitoring changes in the level of cAMP. Moreover, when cell lines that expressed either NPBWR1 or NPBWR2 were incubated with the hypothalamic extracts, forskolin-induced cAMP production was inhibited. These receptors were coupled to the heterotrimeric Gi protein-mediated receptors (Shimomura et al., 2002). Further structural analysis of the ligands responsible for the inhibition of cAMP production led to the identification of a novel peptide, neuropeptide W (NPW). Shimomura et al. identified mature peptide sequences of both 23 and 30 residues from porcine, rat, and human prepro NPW (**Figure 1**). NPW is named after the tryptophan residues appearing at both its N- and C-terminals in its two mature forms: NPW30 (the 30 amino acid form) and NPW23 (consisting of 23 amino acids, which are identical to the N-terminal 23 residues of NPW30) (**Figure 1**). At the same time, the human gene for NPW was identified by Tanaka et al. (2003), who also cloned the mouse gene and reported restricted expression in specific neurons in the mid-brain and brainstem. Similarly, Brezillon et al. (2003) identified the shorter 23 amino acid form of the peptide, which they termed L8 that was derived by proteolytic processing from the longer peptide. The prepropeptide was designated prepro-G protein-coupled receptor 8 ligand.

DISTRIBUTION OF NPW

Based on RT-PCR analysis, Brezillon et al. (2003) have reported that NPW mRNA is highly expressed in the substantia nigra and spinal cord, and moderately expressed in the hippocampus, amygdala, hypothalamus corpus callosum, cerebellum, and dorsal root ganglia in the human central nervous system. In rodents, *in situ* hybridization histochemistry has revealed that NPW mRNA is expressed in a few restricted brain regions, including the rat periaqueductal gray (PAG), Edinger-Westphal nucleus (EW), and dorsal raphe nucleus (Baker et al., 2003; Tanaka et al., 2003; Kitamura et al., 2006), while Kitamura et al. (2006) have reported that it is confined to specific nuclei in the rat midbrain and brainstem. However, based on RT-PCR analysis, we have reported that NPW mRNA is expressed in the rat hypothalamic paraventricular nucleus (PVN), ventromedial nucleus (VMH), arcuate nucleus (ARC), and lateral hypothalamus (LH) (Takenoya et al., 2010), with another study also reporting the expression of NPW in various areas of the rat brain (Dun et al., 2003). Immunohistochemical studies have shown that NPW-like immunoreactive (NPW-LI) neuronal cell bodies mainly observed in the hypothalamic areas, ARC and posterior pituitary gland, with a lower level in the PVN. Interestingly, NPW-LI cells appear to be more numerous in the male than the female hypothalamus (Dun et al., 2003). In another study, Kitamura et al. (2006) reported a heavy localization of NPW-LI cell bodies in the midbrain, including the PAG and EW. Furthermore, we first

	1	2	3	4	5	6	7	8	9	10	11	12	13	14	15	16	17	18	19	20	21	22	23	24	25	26	27	28	29	30
	▼																						NPW23 ▼							NPW23 ▼
Human	W	Y	K	H	V	A	S	P	R	Y	H	T	V	G	R	A	A	G	L	L	M	G	L	R	R	S	P	Y	L	W
Porcine	W	Y	K	H	T	A	S	P	R	Y	H	T	V	G	R	A	A	G	L	L	M	G	L	R	R	S	P	Y	M	W
Rat	W	Y	K	H	V	A	S	P	R	Y	H	T	V	G	R	A	S	G	L	L	M	G	L	R	R	S	P	Y	L	W
Mouse	W	Y	K	H	V	A	S	P	R	Y	H	T	V	G	R	A	S	G	L	L	M	G	L	R	R	S	P	Y	Q	W

FIGURE 1 | Sequence comparison of NPW-23 and NPW-30. Human, porcine rat and mouse NPW-23 and NPW-30 sequences are aligned. A gray area indicates a common amino acid sequence of both NPW-23 and NPW-30.

identified the presence of NPW-LI cell bodies and their processes in the PVN, VMH, and amygdala at the electron microscopic level (Takenoya et al., 2009). Moreover, NPW-LI nerve fibers were abundantly distributed in the midbrain and limbic system, including the CeA and BST, suggests that NPW may play a role in the regulation of fear and anxiety as well as in feeding behavior (Dun et al., 2003; Hondo et al., 2008; Takenoya et al., 2009, 2010).

In the peripheral tissues, NPW is expressed in the trachea, as well as in lymphoblastic leukemia in the fetal kidney and colorectal adenocarcinoma (Brezillon et al., 2003). Rat adrenocortical cells are also shown to produce NPW (Hondo et al., 2008), as have noradrenalin-containing cells in the rat adrenal medulla (Seki et al., 2008) and gastric antral G cells in rats and mice (Mondal et al., 2006), with expression of NPW in the rat stomach mucosa being regulated by nutritional status, glucocorticoids, and thyroid hormones (Caminos et al., 2008). Hochol et al. (2006) have reported expression of NPW in the thyroid and parathyroid glands, pancreatic islets, adrenal glands, ovary, and testis of the rat, while Rucinski et al. (2007) have demonstrated NPW immunoreactivity in all of the cells of the pancreatic islets, including the A, B, and D cells, and PP cells. In contrast, Dezaki et al. (2008) found NPW immunoreactivity in the B cells, but not in the A or D cells. In addition, NPW mRNA is expressed in the urogenital system, including the kidney, testis, uterus, ovary, and placenta (Fujii et al., 2002). Based on RT-PCR analysis, we have confirmed the presence of NPW mRNA in the pituitary gland, adrenal gland, and stomach (Seki et al., 2008). These observations suggest that NPW may play an important role in the regulation of the endocrine system in response to stress, as well as in the activation of the hypothalamus-pituitary-adrenal (HPA) axis (Niimi and Murao, 2005; Seki et al., 2008).

DISTRIBUTION OF NPBWR1-2

In humans, RT-PCR analysis has demonstrated that NPBWR1 mRNA is highly expressed in the amygdala, hippocampus, neocortex, and hypothalamus (Lee et al., 1999). *In situ* hybridization histochemical studies have demonstrated that NPBWR1 mRNA is present in the rat hypothalamus, including the ARC, VMH, PVN, and DMH, with Ishii et al. (2003) reported that NPBW1 knockout mice exhibit hyperphagia and develop adult-onset obesity. Singh et al. (2004) used [125I]-NPW receptor autoradiography and demonstrated a significant expression of NPBW1 in the rat amygdala and hypothalamus, as well as in the BST, medial preoptic area (MPA), PAG, superficial gray layer of the superior colliculus, and subfornical organ. In general, NPBWR1 is most commonly expressed at high levels in the amygdala (Singh et al., 2004; Kitamura et al., 2006; Skrzypski et al., 2012). Although the BST shows the highest level of NPBWR1 expression in small mammals, this phenomenon has not been demonstrated in humans. Kitamura et al. (2006) have reported that NPBWR1 is most abundantly expressed in the rat CeA and BST, which may indicate that NPBWR1 is involved in the regulation of stress, emotion, fear, and anxiety. On the other hand, NPBWR1-2 mRNAs are also localized in the pituitary and adrenal glands (in both the adrenal cortex and adrenal medulla) (Mazzocchi et al., 2005). These observations suggest that NPBWR1-2 may be involved in responding to stress via the HPA axis (Mazzocchi et al., 2005; Niimi and Murao, 2005). Ziolkowska et al. (2009) recently examined the expression and function of the NPW, NPB, and NPBWR1 system in cultured rat calvaria osteoblast-like cells, with their results suggesting a direct effect on this cell proliferation. NPB has been identified in larger mammals, as well as in rabbits, but has not been described in either rats or mice. RT-PCR analysis has shown that NPBWR2 mRNA is highly expressed in the human amygdala, hippocampus, pituitary gland, adrenal gland, and testis, as well as in the cortical cells in the adrenal gland (Mazzocchi et al., 2005).

REGULATION OF FEEDING AND ENERGY METABOLISM BY NPW

NPBWR1 knockout mice are hyperphagic and show decreased energy expenditure, suggesting that NPW may act as a modulator of feeding. icv infusion of NPW in male rats has been shown to increase food intake during the first 2 h in the light phase (Shimomura et al., 2002). Similarly, Levine et al. (2005) have reported that injection of NPW into the PVN increases food intake. These results suggest that NPW acts as an acute orexigenic peptide. However, Mondal et al. (2003) have reported that both forms of NPW suppress dark-phase and fasting-induced food intake, indicating that the effect of NPW on feeding differs depending on whether animals are maintained in a light or dark phase.

We have carried out a series of neuroanatomical studies to examine the neural relationship between NPW and other neuropeptides involved in the regulation of feeding. Very close neuronal interactions were observed between NPW-containing nerve fibers and orexin- or melanin-concentrating hormone-containing neuronal cell bodies and nerve fibers in the rat brain (Takenoya et al., 2005), while Levine et al. (2005) demonstrated that c-Fos expression was induced in orexin-containing neurons in the perifornical region of the LH after intracerebroventricular (icv) infusion of NPW. Interestingly, we also identified NPW-LI cell bodies in the VMH, which is known as a center for satiety (Takenoya et al., 2010). Leptin acts on neurons in the VMH, thereby reducing food intake, and Date et al. (2010) have recently reported that NPW-LI neurons and leptin receptors are colocalized in this region of the brain. NPW expression is also significantly up-regulated in *ob/ob* and *db/db* mice. Therefore, NPW may play important roles in feeding and energy metabolism, functioning as a substitute for leptin (Date et al., 2010) (**Figure 2**). Furthermore, NPW reduces food intake via the melanocortin-4-receptor signaling pathway, suggesting that it may activate POMC-containing neurons and inhibit NPY-containing neurons to control feeding regulation in the ARC (Date et al., 2010) (**Figure 2**).

Very recently, Skrzypski et al. (2012) have demonstrated that NPB and NPW regulate the expression and secretion of leptin and resistin, and increase lipolysis in isolated rat adipocytes. When NPW was administered to rats, the authors could not detect enhanced locomotor activity, but did observe increased O_2 consumption and increased CO_2 production, as well as an increase in body temperature (Mondal et al., 2003). Interestingly, Mondal et al. (2006) have reported that the levels of NPW isolated from rat stomach antral cells are lower in fasted animals, increasing once the animals have been re-fed. In contrast, female NPBWR1 −/− mice do not display hyperphagic activity compared with wild-type mice (Ishii et al., 2003). In addition, Dun et al. (2003) reported the existence of differences between male and female rats with respect to the distribution of NPW.

NEUROENDOCRINE FUNCTION OF NPW

Immunohistochemical studies have reported that NPBWR1 is expressed in the PVN, pituitary gland, and adrenal medulla in the human, mouse and rat (O'Dowd et al., 1995; Lee et al., 1999; Brezillon et al., 2003; Tanaka et al., 2003), particularly in the parvocellular subdivisions of the PVN and the posterior pituitary. However, NPW has not been reported to influence the release of other anterior pituitary hormones. These neuroendocrine effects of NPW are not directly mediated through NPWBR1 on the pituitary gland cells, but may occur indirectly through controlling the release of the hypothalamic hormone,

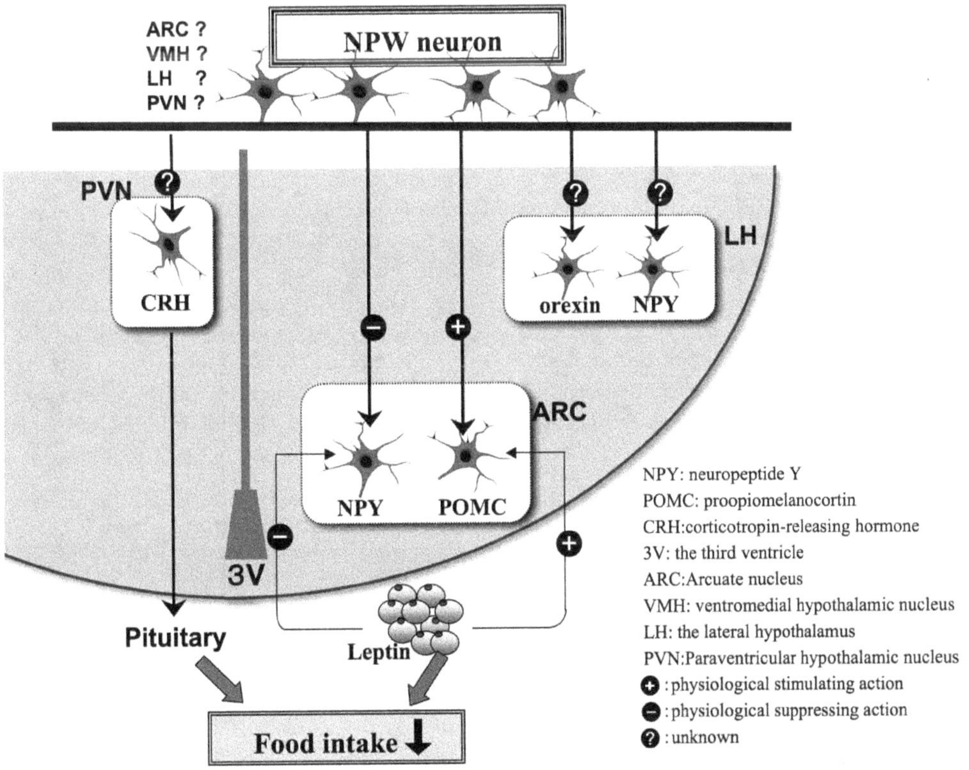

FIGURE 2 | Schematic illustration based on the findings of morphological and physiological studies of appetite regulation in the hypothalamus by NPW neurons and feeding-related peptides in hypothalamus. The plus or minus indicates stimulatory (+) or inhibitory (−) effects, respectively.

Table 1 | Physiological effect of NPW in Rat.

Effect		References
Food intake	↑	Shimomura et al. (2002), Levine et al. (2005)
	↓	Mondal et al. (2003)
Body weight	↑	Tanaka et al. (2003)
Heart rate	↑	Yu et al. (2007a)
Arterial blood pressure (ABP)	↑	Yu et al. (2007b)
ACTH	↑	Hochol et al. (2007), Yogo et al. (2012)
Prolactin	↑	Baker et al. (2003), Samson et al. (2004)
Growth hormone	↓	Baker et al. (2003), Samson et al. (2004)
Parathyroid hormone	↑	Hochol et al. (2006)
Corticosterome	↑	Baker et al. (2003), Taylor et al. (2005)
Testosterone	↑	Hochol et al. (2006)
Estradiol	↑	Hochol et al. (2006)

The plus or minus indicates stimulatory (↑) or inhibitory (↓) effects, respectively.

corticotrophin-releasing factor (CRF) (Brezillon et al., 2003; Samson et al., 2004). Colocalization of NPW with urocortin, a stress-related neuropeptide of the CRF family, has also been demonstrated in the EW.

On the other hand, icv infusion of NPW23 stimulates prolactin release in the rat (Shimomura et al., 2002), and an *in vitro* study has reported that log molar NPW23 concentrations, significantly alter prolactin, growth hormone and ACTH release from dispersed rat anterior pituitary cells (Baker et al., 2003). In addition, *in vivo* studies have revealed that icv infusion of NPW23 stimulates an increase in plasma prolactin levels (Baker et al., 2003). icv infusion of NPW23 also results in a significant, elevation in plasma corticosterone levels, suggesting that NPW plays a role in the hypothalamic response to stress. However, growth hormone levels in plasma are inhibited by icv infusion of this peptide. These findings suggest that NPW is the endogenous ligand for GPR7 and/or GPR8 and acts as a mediator of neuroendocrine function (Shimomura et al., 2002; Baker et al., 2003). Moreover, Taylor et al. (2005) have reported that the infusion of NPW activates the HPA axis, as demonstrated by changes in plasma corticosterone levels in conscious rats; NPW increases plasma corticosterone levels but does not stimulate the release of oxytocin or vasopressin in the peripheral circulation, or alter blood pressure or heart rate. Furthermore, icv infusion of a CRF antagonist does not significantly reduce corticosterone levels, although CRF antagonist pretreatment significantly reduces the capacity of centrally administered NPW to increase corticosterone levels (Taylor et al., 2005). Using electrophysiological studies with whole-cell patch recording of hypothalamic slice preparations, Taylor et al. (2005) have also shown that NPW depolarizes and increases the spike frequency of the majority of putative neuroendocrine PVN neurons. Furthermore, the response of these cells in the presence of tetrodotoxin confirmed that NPW was acting post-synaptically (Taylor et al., 2005).

Niimi and Murao (2005) have reported that double immunostaining for both NPW and c-Fos is significantly increased in response to stress. Immobilization stress increases parasympathetic outflow, whereas cold stress is primarily considered to increase sympathetic outflow, suggesting that NPW may participate in the regulation of both the sympathetic and parasympathetic branches of the autonomic nervous system. In the PVN, vasopressin- expressing neurons are known to be involved in the production of hormonal outputs in response to endocrine and autonomic stress (Ulrich-Lai and Herman, 2009). Kawasaki et al. (2006) have reported that centrally administered NPW activates magnocellular neurosecretory neurons in the SO and PVN, and significantly increases plasma arginine-vasopressin and plasma oxytocin levels. Price et al. (2008) have reported that the inhibition of growth hormone release due to the central effects of NPW results from activation of arcuate somatostatin neurons, which could produce inhibition of neurons expressing growth hormone releasing hormone. These findings suggest that endogenous NPW may play a physiologically relevant role in the neuroendocrine response to stress in the brain (**Table 1**).

ACKNOWLEDGMENTS

This study was supported in part by the Ministry of Education, Culture, Sports, Science and Technology of Japan via a Grant-in-Aid for Scientific Research (C) to Fumiko Takenoya (23500863) and to Haruaki Kageyama (21590222). Support was also received from the Ministry of Education, Culture, Sports, Science and Technology of Japan via a Grant-in-Aid for Exploratory Research to Seiji Shioda (21659059) and by a High-Technology Research Center project grant from the Ministry of Education, Culture, Sports, Science and Technology of Japan (to Seiji Shioda).

REFERENCES

Baker, J. R., Cardinal, K., Bober, C., Taylor, M. M., and Samson, W. K. (2003). Neuropeptide W acts in brain to control prolactin, corticosterone, and growth hormone release. *Endocrinology* 144, 2816–2821.

Brezillon, S., Lannoy, V., Franssen, J. D., Le Poul, E., Dupriez, V., Lucchetti, J., et al. (2003). Identification of natural ligands for the orphan G protein-coupled receptors GPR7 and GPR8. *J. Biol. Chem.* 278, 776–783.

Caminos, J. E., Bravo, S. B., Garcia-Rendueles, M. E., Ruth Gonzalez, C., Garces, M. F., Cepeda, L. A., et al. (2008). Expression of neuropeptide W in rat stomach mucosa: regulation by nutritional status, glucocorticoids and thyroid hormones. *Regul. Pept.* 146, 106–111.

Date, Y., Mondal, M. S., Kageyama, H., Ghamari-Langroudi, M., Takenoya, F., Yamaguchi, H., et al. (2010). Neuropeptide W: an anorectic peptide regulated by leptin and metabolic state. *Endocrinology* 151, 2200–2210.

Dezaki, K., Kageyama, H., Seki, M., Shioda, S., and Yada, T. (2008). Neuropeptide W in the rat pancreas: potentiation of glucose-induced insulin release and Ca2+ influx through L-type Ca2+ channels in beta-cells and localization in islets. *Regul. Pept.* 145, 153–158.

Dun, S. L., Brailoiu, G. C., Yang, J., Chang, J. K., and Dun, N. J. (2003). Neuropeptide W-immunoreactivity in the hypothalamus and pituitary of the rat. *Neurosci. Lett.* 349, 71–74.

Fujii, R., Yoshida, H., Fukusumi, S., Habata, Y., Hosoya, M., Kawamata, Y., et al. (2002). Identification of a neuropeptide modified with bromine as an endogenous ligand for GPR7. *J. Biol. Chem.* 277, 34010–34016.

Hochol, A., Belloni, A. S., Rucinski, M., Ziolkowska, A., Di Liddo, R., Nussdorfer, G. G., et al. (2006). Expression of neuropeptides B and W and their receptors in endocrine glands of the rat. *Int. J. Mol. Med.* 18, 1101–1106.

Hochol, A., Tortorella, C., Ricinski, M., Ziolkowska, A., Nussdorfer, G. G., and Malendowicz, L. K. (2007).

Effects of neuropeptides B and W on the rat pituitary-adrenocortical axis: *in vivo* and *in vitro* studies. *Int. J. Mol. Med.* 19, 207–211.

Hondo, M., Ishii, M., and Sakurai, T. (2008). The NPB/NPW neuropeptide system and its role in regulating energy homeostasis, pain, and emotion. *Results Probl. Cell Differ.* 46, 239–256.

Ishii, M., Fei, H., and Friedman, J. M. (2003). Targeted disruption of GPR7, the endogenous receptor for neuropeptides B and W, leads to metabolic defects and adult-onset obesity. *Proc. Natl. Acad. Sci. U.S.A.* 100, 10540–10545.

Kawasaki, M., Onaka, T., Nakazato, M., Saito, J., Mera, T., Hashimoto, H., et al. (2006). Centrally administered neuropeptide W-30 activates magnocellular neurosecretory cells in the supraoptic and paraventricular nuclei with neurosecretion in rats. *J. Endocrinol.* 190, 213–223.

Kitamura, Y., Tanaka, H., Motoike, T., Ishii, M., Williams, S. C., Yanagisawa, M., et al. (2006). Distribution of neuropeptide W immunoreactivity and mRNA in adult rat brain. *Brain Res.* 1093, 123–134.

Lee, D. K., Nguyen, T., Porter, C. A., Cheng, R., George, S. R., and O'Dowd, B. F. (1999). Two related G protein-coupled receptors: the distribution of GPR7 in rat brain and the absence of GPR8 in rodents. *Brain Res. Mol. Brain Res.* 71, 96–103.

Levine, A. S., Winsky-Sommerer, R., Huitron-Resendiz, S., Grace, M. K., and de Lecea, L. (2005). Injection of neuropeptide W into paraventricular nucleus of hypothalamus increases food intake. *Am. J. Physiol. Regul. Integr. Comp. Physiol.* 288, R1727–R1732.

Mazzocchi, G., Rebuffat, P., Ziolkowska, A., Rossi, G. P., Malendowicz, L. K., and Nussdorfer, G. G. (2005). G protein receptors 7 and 8 are expressed in human adrenocortical cells, and their endogenous ligands neuropeptides B and w enhance cortisol secretion by activating adenylate cyclase- and phospholipase C-dependent signaling cascades. *J. Clin. Endocrinol. Metab.* 90, 3466–3471.

Mondal, M. S., Yamaguchi, H., Date, Y., Shimbara, T., Toshinai, K., Shimomura, Y., et al. (2003). A role for neuropeptide W in the regulation of feeding behavior. *Endocrinology* 144, 4729–4733.

Mondal, M. S., Yamaguchi, H., Date, Y., Toshinai, K., Kawagoe, T., Tsuruta, T., et al. (2006). Neuropeptide W is present in antral G cells of rat, mouse, and human stomach. *J. Endocrinol.* 188, 49–57.

Niimi, M., and Murao, K. (2005). Neuropeptide W as a stress mediator in the hypothalamus. *Endocrine* 27, 51–54.

O'Dowd, B. F., Scheideler, M. A., Nguyen, T., Cheng, R., Rasmussen, J. S., Marchese, A., et al. (1995). The cloning and chromosomal mapping of two novel human opioid-somatostatin-like receptor genes, GPR7 and GPR8, expressed in discrete areas of the brain. *Genomics* 28, 84–91.

Price, C. J., Samson, W. K., and Ferguson, A. V. (2008). Neuropeptide W influences the excitability of neurons in the rat hypothalamic arcuate nucleus. *Neuroendocrinology* 88, 88–94.

Rucinski, M., Nowak, K. W., Chmielewska, J., Ziolkowska, A., and Malendowicz, L. K. (2007). Neuropeptide W exerts a potent suppressive effect on blood leptin and insulin concentrations in the rat. *Int. J. Mol. Med.* 19, 401–405.

Samson, W. K., Baker, J. R., Samson, C. K., Samson, H. W., and Taylor, M. M. (2004). Central neuropeptide B administration activates stress hormone secretion and stimulates feeding in male rats. *J. Neuroendocrinol.* 16, 842–849.

Seki, M., Kageyama, H., Takenoya, F., Hirayama, M., Kintaka, Y., Inoue, S., et al. (2008). Neuropeptide W is expressed in the noradrenalin-containing cells in the rat adrenal medulla. *Regul. Pept.* 145, 147–152.

Shimomura, Y., Harada, M., Goto, M., Sugo, T., Matsumoto, Y., Abe, M., et al. (2002). Identification of neuropeptide W as the endogenous ligand for orphan G-protein-coupled receptors GPR7 and GPR8. *J. Biol. Chem.* 277, 35826–35832.

Singh, G., Maguire, J. J., Kuc, R. E., Fidock, M., and Davenport, A. P. (2004). Identification and cellular localisation of NPW1 (GPR7) receptors for the novel neuropeptide W-23 by [1251]-NPW radioligand binding and immunocytochemistry. *Brain Res.* 1017, 222–226.

Skrzypski, M., Pruszynska-Oszmalek, E., Rucinski, M., Szczepankiewicz, D., Sassek, M., Wojciechowicz, T., et al. (2012). Neuropeptide B and W regulate leptin and resistin secretion, and stimulate lipolysis in isolated rat adipocytes. *Regul. Pept.* 176, 51–56.

Takenoya, F., Hirayama, M., Kageyama, H., Funahashi, H., Kita, T., Matsumoto, H., et al. (2005). Neuronal interactions between galanin-like-peptide- and orexin- or melanin-concentrating hormone-containing neurons. *Regul. Pept.* 126, 79–83.

Takenoya, F., Kageyama, H., Shiba, K., Date, Y., Nakazato, M., and Shioda, S. (2010). Neuropeptide W: a key player in the homeostatic regulation of feeding and energy metabolism? *Ann. N.Y. Acad. Sci.* 1200, 162–169.

Takenoya, F., Kageyama, H., Shiba, K., Endo, K., Nonaka, N., Date, Y., et al. (2009). Distribution of neuropeptide W in the rat brain. *Neuropeptides* 44, 99–106.

Tanaka, H., Yoshida, T., Miyamoto, N., Motoike, T., Kurosu, H., Shibata, K., et al. (2003). Characterization of a family of endogenous neuropeptide ligands for the G protein-coupled receptors GPR7 and GPR8. *Proc. Natl. Acad. Sci. U.S.A.* 100, 6251–6256.

Taylor, M. M., Yuill, E. A., Baker, J. R., Ferri, C. C., Ferguson, A. V., and Samson, W. K. (2005). Actions of neuropeptide W in paraventricular hypothalamus: implications for the control of stress hormone secretion. *Am. J. Physiol. Regul. Integr. Comp. Physiol.* 288, R270–R275.

Ulrich-Lai, Y. M., and Herman, J. P. (2009). Neural regulation of endocrine and autonomic stress responses. *Nat. Rev. Neurosci.* 10, 397–409.

Yogo, K., Oki, Y., Iino, K., Yamashita, M., Shibata, S., Hayashi, C., et al. (2012). Neuropeptide W stimulates adrenocorticotrophic hormone release via corticotrophin-releasing factor but not via arginine vasopressin. *Endocr. J.* 59, 547–554.

Yu, N., Chu, C., Kunitake, T., Kato, K., Nakazato, M., and Kannan, H. (2007a). Cardiovascular actions of central neuropeptide W in conscious rats. *Regul. Pept.* 138, 82–86.

Yu, N. S., Kunitake, T., Kato, K., Nakazato, M., and Kannan, H. (2007b). Effects of intracerebroventricular administration of neuropeptide W30 on neurons in the hypothalamic paraventricular nucleus in the conscious rat. *Neurosci. Lett.* 26, 140–145.

Ziolkowska, A., Rucinski, M., Tyczewska, M., and Malendowicz, L. K. (2009). Neuropeptide, B (NPB) and neuropeptide W (NPW) system in cultured rat calvarial osteoblast-like (ROB) cells: NPW and NPB inhibit proliferative activity of ROB cells. *Int. J. Mol. Med.* 24, 781–787.

4

Gonadotropin-inhibitory hormone action in the brain and pituitary

Takayoshi Ubuka, You Lee Son, Yasuko Tobari and Kazuyoshi Tsutsui*

Laboratory of Integrative Brain Sciences, Department of Biology, Center for Medical Life Science, Waseda University, Tokyo, Japan

Edited by:
Hubert Vaudry, University of Rouen, France

Reviewed by:
Lance Kriegsfeld, University of California, USA
José A. Muñoz-Cueto, University of Cadiz, Spain

***Correspondence:**
Kazuyoshi Tsutsui, Laboratory of Integrative Brain Sciences, Department of Biology, Center for Medical Life Science, Waseda University, 2-2 Wakamatsu-cho, Shinjuku-ku, Tokyo 162-8480, Japan.
e-mail: k-tsutsui@waseda.jp

Gonadotropin-inhibitory hormone (GnIH) was first identified in the Japanese quail as a hypothalamic neuropeptide inhibitor of gonadotropin secretion. Subsequent studies have shown that GnIH is present in the brains of birds including songbirds, and mammals including humans. The identified avian and mammalian GnIH peptides universally possess an LPXRFamide (X = L or Q) motif at their C-termini. Mammalian GnIH peptides are also designated as RFamide-related peptides from their structures. The receptor for GnIH is the G protein-coupled receptor 147 (GPR147), which is thought to be coupled to $G_{\alpha i}$ protein. Cell bodies of GnIH neurons are located in the paraventricular nucleus (PVN) in birds and the dorsomedial hypothalamic area (DMH) in mammals. GnIH neurons in the PVN or DMH project to the median eminence to control anterior pituitary function. GPR147 is expressed in the gonadotropes and GnIH suppresses synthesis and release of gonadotropins. It was further shown in immortalized mouse gonadotrope cell line (LβT2 cells) that GnIH inhibits gonadotropin-releasing hormone (GnRH) induced gonadotropin subunit gene transcriptions by inhibiting adenylate cyclase/cAMP/PKA-dependent ERK pathway. GnIH neurons also project to GnRH neurons in the preoptic area, and GnRH neurons express GPR147 in birds and mammals. Accordingly, GnIH may inhibit gonadotropin synthesis and release by decreasing the activity of GnRH neurons as well as directly acting on the gonadotropes. GnIH also inhibits reproductive behavior possibly by acting within the brain. GnIH expression is regulated by a nocturnal hormone melatonin and stress in birds and mammals. Accordingly, GnIH may play a role in translating environmental information to inhibit reproductive physiology and behavior of birds and mammals. Finally, GnIH has therapeutic potential in the treatment of reproductive cycle and hormone-dependent diseases, such as precocious puberty, endometriosis, uterine fibroids, and prostatic and breast cancers.

Keywords: gonadotropin-inhibitory hormone, gonadotropin-releasing hormone, gonadotropins, reproductive behavior, melatonin, stress, GPR147, RFamide-related peptide

INTRODUCTION

The decapeptide gonadotropin-releasing hormone (GnRH) is the primary factor responsible for the hypothalamic control of gonadotropin secretion. GnRH was first isolated from mammals (Matsuo et al., 1971; Burgus et al., 1972) and subsequently from birds (King and Millar, 1982; Miyamoto et al., 1982, 1984) and other vertebrates (for reviews, see Millar, 2003, 2005). Gonadal sex steroids and inhibin can modulate gonadotropin secretion. However, no hypothalamic neuropeptide inhibitor of gonadotropin secretion was known in vertebrates, although dopamine has been reported as an inhibitor of gonadotropin secretion in several fish groups. In 2000, a previously unidentified hypothalamic neuropeptide was shown to inhibit gonadotropin release from the cultured quail anterior pituitary gland and it was named gonadotropin-inhibitory hormone (GnIH; Tsutsui et al., 2000). Although it is now known that GnIH and its receptor are also expressed in the gonads of birds (Bentley et al., 2008; Maddineni et al., 2008; McGuire and Bentley, 2010; McGuire et al., 2011) and mammals (Zhao et al., 2010; Singh et al., 2011a,b; Li et al., 2012) including humans (Oishi et al., 2012), this review highlights the discovery of GnIH in the quail brain and the progress of GnIH research investigating its function in the brain and pituitary of birds and mammals. We also briefly review recent progresses in the study of GnIH peptides in fish and humans.

DISCOVERY OF GnIH IN BIRDS

Gonadotropin-inhibitory hormone was first discovered in the brain of Japanese quail, *Coturnix japonica*, while searching a novel RFamide peptide in birds. RFamide peptides, which have an Arg-Phe-NH_2 motif at its C-terminus, were first isolated in invertebrate species in the late 1970s. The first RFamide peptide, Phe-Met-Arg-Phe-NH_2 (FMRFamide), was a cardioexcitatory molecule isolated from the ganglia of the venus clam *Macrocallista nimbosa* (Price and Greenberg, 1977). After the discovery of FMRFamide peptide, numerous RFamide peptides that act as neurotransmitters, neuromodulators, and peripheral hormones have been identified in various invertebrates, including cnidarians, nematodes, annelids, molluscs, and arthropods. Subsequent immunohistochemical studies in vertebrates suggested the presence of RFamide peptides in the central nervous system. It was revealed that some of the FMRFamide-immunoreactive (-ir) neurons projected close to the pituitary gland, suggesting a role in the regulation of pituitary function in vertebrates.

Tsutsui et al. (2000) have isolated a novel RFamide peptide from 500 brains of the Japanese quail by high-performance liquid chromatography (HPLC) and a competitive enzyme-linked immunosorbent assay using an antibody raised against the dipeptide Arg-Phe-NH_2. The isolated peptide had a novel dodecapeptide structure, SIKPSAYLPLRFamide. Its C-terminus was identical to chicken LPLRFamide that was reported to be the first RFamide peptide isolated in vertebrates (Dockray et al., 1983), which is likely to be a degraded fragment of the dodecapeptide. The isolated peptide was localized in the hypothalamo-hypophyseal system, and shown to decrease gonadotropin release from cultured quail anterior pituitary glands (Tsutsui et al., 2000). This RFamide peptide was therefore named GnIH (Tsutsui et al., 2000).

Following the isolation of GnIH in the quail brain, the precursor polypeptide for GnIH was determined (Satake et al., 2001). A cDNA that encoded GnIH precursor polypeptide was identified by a combination of 3′ and 5′ rapid amplification of cDNA ends (3′/5′ RACE; Satake et al., 2001). The GnIH precursor consisted of 173 amino acid residues that encoded one GnIH and two GnIH-related peptides (GnIH-RP-1 and GnIH-RP-2) possessing an LPXRFamide (X = L or Q) sequence at their C-termini (**Figure 1**). These peptide sequences were flanked by a glycine C-terminal amidation signal and a single basic amino acid on each end as an endoproteolytic site (**Figure 1**). GnIH-RP-2 was also identified as a mature peptide by mass spectrometry in quail (**Figure 1**; Satake et al., 2001). GnIH was further isolated as mature peptides in European starlings (Ubuka et al., 2008a) and zebra finch (Tobari et al., 2010) within the class of birds (**Figure 1**; for reviews, see Tsutsui and Ukena, 2006; Tsutsui et al., 2007, 2010a,b, 2012; Tsutsui, 2009; Tsutsui and Ubuka, 2012).

IDENTIFICATION OF GnIH IN MAMMALS

In mammals, cDNAs that encode GnIH orthologs, LPXRFamide peptides, have been investigated by a gene database search (Hinuma et al., 2000; for a review, see Tsutsui and Ubuka, 2012). Mammalian LPXRFamide peptides are also designated as RFamide-related peptides (RFRP) from its structure. Although human, macaque, and bovine LPXRFamide precursor cDNAs encoded three RFRPs (RFRP-1, -2, and -3), only RFRP-1 and RFRP-3 possessed a C-terminal LPXRFamide (X = L or Q) motif, and RFRP-2 had C-terminal RSamide or RLamide sequences (**Figure 1**). On the other hand, rodents do not have RFRP-2 sequence in their precursors (see the precursor sequences of rat and hamster in **Figure 1**). Although the positions that encode GnIH-RP-1/RFRP-1 or GnIH/RFRP-2 in the precursor polypeptides were conserved between birds and mammals (only RFRP-1 in rodents), the positions of GnIH-RP-2 and RFRP-3 in their precursor polypeptides were different between birds and mammals (**Figure 1**).

The LPXRFamide motif at the C-terminus is followed by glycine as an amidation signal and arginine or lysine as endoproteolytic basic amino acids in mammals as well as birds (**Figure 1**). Endogenous LPXRFamide peptides can also be cleaved at basic amino acids at their N-termini. However, there were some exceptions in the cleavage site at the N-terminal, such as that of Siberian hamster RFRP-1 (**Figure 1**). Up until now, bovine RFRP-1 (Fukusumi et al., 2001) and -3 (Yoshida et al., 2003), rat RFRP-3 (Ukena et al., 2002), Siberian hamster RFRP-1 and -3 (Ubuka et al., 2012a), macaque RFRP-3 (Ubuka et al., 2009b), and human RFRP-1 and -3 (Ubuka et al., 2009c) are identified as mature peptides in mammals (**Figure 1**; for reviews, see Tsutsui and Ukena, 2006; Tsutsui et al., 2007, 2010a,b, 2012; Tsutsui, 2009; Tsutsui and Ubuka, 2012).

GnIH RECEPTOR

Bonini et al. (2000) have identified two G protein-coupled receptor (GPCR) for neuropeptide FF (NPFF), and designated them as NPFF1 (identical to GPR147) and NPFF2 (identical to GPR74). Hinuma et al. (2000) have also reported a specific receptor for RFRP and named it OT7T022, which was identical to GPR147. The binding affinities for GPR147 and GPR74 and the efficacies on signal transduction pathway were examined, using various analogs of RFRPs and NPFF. RFRPs showed a higher affinity for GPR147, whereas NPFF had potent agonistic activity for GPR74 (Bonini et al., 2000; Liu et al., 2001). Taken together, GPR147 (NPFF1, OT7T022) was suggested to be the receptor for RFRP (mammalian GnIH). **Figure 2** shows the predicted two-dimensional structure of human GPR147 from its nucleotide sequence (AB040104; Ubuka et al., 2008b, 2009c). It was shown that RFRPs suppress the production of cAMP in ovarian cells of Chinese hamster transfected with GPR147 cDNA, suggesting that GPR147 couples to $G_{\alpha i}$ protein (Hinuma et al., 2000).

To elucidate the mode of action of GnIH in birds, Yin et al. (2005) have identified GnIH receptor (GnIH-R) in the quail diencephalon and characterized its expression and binding activity. First, a cDNA encoding a putative GnIH-R was cloned by a combination of 3′/5′ RACE using PCR primers designed from the sequence of the receptor for RFRPs (GPR147). The crude membrane fraction of COS-7 cells transfected with the putative GnIH-R cDNA specifically bound GnIH and GnIH-RPs in a concentration-dependent manner, indicating that GPR147 is GnIH-R (Yin et al., 2005). GnIH-R also bound with high affinities to GnIH, GnIH-RPs and RFRPs, which have LPXRFamide (X = L or Q) motif at their C-termini. In contrast, C-terminal non-amidated GnIH failed to bind the receptor. Accordingly, the C-terminal LPXRFamide (X = L or Q) motif seems to be critical for its binding to GnIH-R (Yin et al., 2005; for reviews, see Tsutsui and Ukena, 2006; Tsutsui et al., 2007, 2010a,b, 2012; Tsutsui, 2009; Tsutsui and Ubuka, 2012). It was suggested that there is no functional difference among GnIH and GnIH-RPs because GnIH-R bound GnIH and GnIH-RPs with similar affinities (Yin et al., 2005). However, further studies are required to investigate if GnIH and GnIH-RPs work additively or synergistically to achieve their effects on the cells that express GnIH-R.

DISTRIBUTION OF GnIH CELLS AND FIBERS IN THE BRAIN

LOCATION OF GnIH NEUNONS IN THE BRAIN

The location of GnIH precursor mRNA was first investigated by Southern blot analysis of the RT-PCR products of GnIH precursor cDNA. Within the samples from telencephalon, diencephalon, mesencephalon, and cerebellum, GnIH precursor mRNA was only expressed in the quail diencephalon (Satake et al., 2001). *In situ*

```
Human        MEIISSKLFILLTLATSSLLTSNIFCADELVMSNLHSKE-NYDKYSEPRGYP--KGERSL  57
Macaque      MEIISSKLFILLTLATSSLLTSNISCADELMMSSLHNKE-NYDKYSEPRGYP--KRERSL  57
Bovine       MEIISLKRFILLMLATSSLLTSNIFCTDESRMPNLYSKK-NYDKYSEPRGDLGWEKERSL  59
Rat          MEIISSKRFILLTLATSSFLTSNTLCSDELMMPHFHSKE-GYGKYYQLRGIPKGVKERSV  59
Hamster      MEIISSKRFILLTLATSSLLTSNIFCTEELMMPHFHSKE-KEDKYSQPTGISKGEKERSV  59

Sparrow      MKVISTKKFILFALATVVFLTSNSMCLNEAMKSRLQSREDNDDKDYEIKDNILEEKQRSL  60
Zebra finch  MKVISNKKLILFALATVVFLTSNSMCLNEPMKSRLQSREDNDDKYYEIKDNILEEKQRSL  60
Starling     MKVILTQKFILFALAAVVLLTSNSMCLNEPMKPRLQSREDNDDKYYEIKDNILEEKQRSL  60
Quail        MEIISTQKFILLTLATVAFLTPHGACLDELMKSSLESREDDDDKYYETKDSILEEKQRSL  60

                                                RFRP-1           RFRP-2
Human        NFEELKDWGPKNVIKMSTPAVNKMPHSFANLPLRFGRNVQEERSAGATANLPLRSGRNME 117
Macaque      NFEELKDWGPKNVIKMSTPAVNKMPHSVTNLPLRFGRTTEEERSTGAIANLPLRSGRNME 117
Bovine       TFEEVKDWAPK--IKMNKPVVNKMPPSAANLPLRFGRNMEEERSTRAMAHLPLRLGKNRE 117
Rat          TFQELKDWGAKKDIKMSPAPANKVPHSAANLPLRFGRNIEDRRSP--------RARANME 111
Hamster      SFQEVKDWGAKNVIKMSPAPANKVPHSAANLPLRFGRTLEEDRST--------RARTNME 111

Sparrow      NFEEMEDWGSKDIIKMNPFTASKMPNSVANLPLRFGRNYPEERSIKPFSNLPLRFGRAFG 120
Zebra finch  NFEEMEDWRSKDIIKMNPFAASKMPNSVANLPLRFGRNYPEERSIKPFSNLPLRFGRAFG 120
Starling     NFDEMEDWGSKDIIKMNPFTVSKMPNSVANLPLRFGRNYPEERSIKPFANLPLRFGRAFG 120
Quail        NFEEMKDWGSKNFMKVNTPTVNKVPNSVANLPLRFGRSNPEERSIKPSAYLPLRFGRAFG 120
                                            GnIH-RP-1            GnIH

                   RFRP-3
Human        VSLVRRVPNLPQRFGRTTTAKSVCRMLSDLCQGSMHSPCANDLFYSMTCQHQEIQNPDQK 177
Macaque      VSLVRQVLNLPQRFGRTTTAKSVCRTLSDLCQGSLHSPCANDLFYSMTCQHQEIQNPDQK 177
Bovine       DSLSRWVPNLPQRFGRTTTAKSITKTLSNLLQQSMHSPSTNGLLYSMACQPQEIQNPGQK 177
Rat          AGTMSHFPSLPQRFGR-TTARRITKTLAGLPQKSLHSLASSELLYAMTRQHQEIQSPGQE 170
Hamster      ARTLSRVPSLPQRFGR-TTARSIPKTLSHLLQRFLHSMATSEVLNAMTCQHGEIQSPGGK 170

Sparrow      ENTPNHSPRVSHRLERSPLVKGSSQSLLNLPQRFGKSLAVNLPRDIQEFEPGI------- 173
Zebra finch  ENIRNHAPKVSHRLERSPLVKGSSQSLLNLPQRFGKSLPVNLPRDVEEFEPGI------- 173
Starling     ENIPNHAPKVLHRLGRSPLLKGSSQSLLNLPQRFGKSLVFNLPQDIQESEPGI------- 173
Quail        ESLSRRAPNLSNRSGRSPLARSSIQSLLNLPQRFGKSVPISLSQGVQESEPGM------- 173
                                          GnIH-RP-2

Human        QSRRLLFKKIDDAELKQEK--------------                            196
Macaque      RSRRLVFQKMDDAELKQEK--------------                            196
Bovine       NLRRRGFQKIDDAELKQEK--------------                            196
Rat          QPRKRVFTETDDAERKQEKIGNLQPVLQGAMKL                            203
Hamster      QPRRQAFMETDDEEGKHEK--------------                            189
```

FIGURE 1 | The alignment of GnIH (RFRP) precursor polypeptides of birds and mammals. The amino acid sequence of GnIH, GnIH-RP-1, GnIH-RP-2, RFRP-1, RFRP-3 with Gly (G) as an amidation signal and Arg (R) or Lys (K) as an endoproteolytic basic amino acid at the C-termini are shown in bold. Identified mature peptides are underlined. Endoproteolytic basic amino acid (R or K) at the N-termini are also shown in bold. A broken line indicates the putative human RFRP-2 sequence. Accession numbers are human (NM_022150), macaque (NM_001130827), bovine (NM_174168), rat (NM_023952), Siberian hamster (JF727837), white-crowned sparrow (AB128164), zebra finch (AB522971), European starling (EF486798) and Japanese quail (AB039815).

hybridization for GnIH precursor mRNA further showed that cells expressing GnIH mRNA were clustered in the paraventricular nucleus (PVN) in the hypothalamus (Ukena et al., 2003). Immunohistochemistry using GnIH antibody has revealed that clusters of GnIH-ir neurons were expressed in the PVN in quail (Tsutsui et al., 2000; Ubuka et al., 2003). GnIH expressing cell bodies were also clustered in the PVN in other birds (Bentley et al., 2003; Osugi et al., 2004; Ubuka et al., 2008a).

In mammals, expression of precursor mRNA of RFRP (mammalian GnIH) was only detected in the dorsomedial hypothalamic

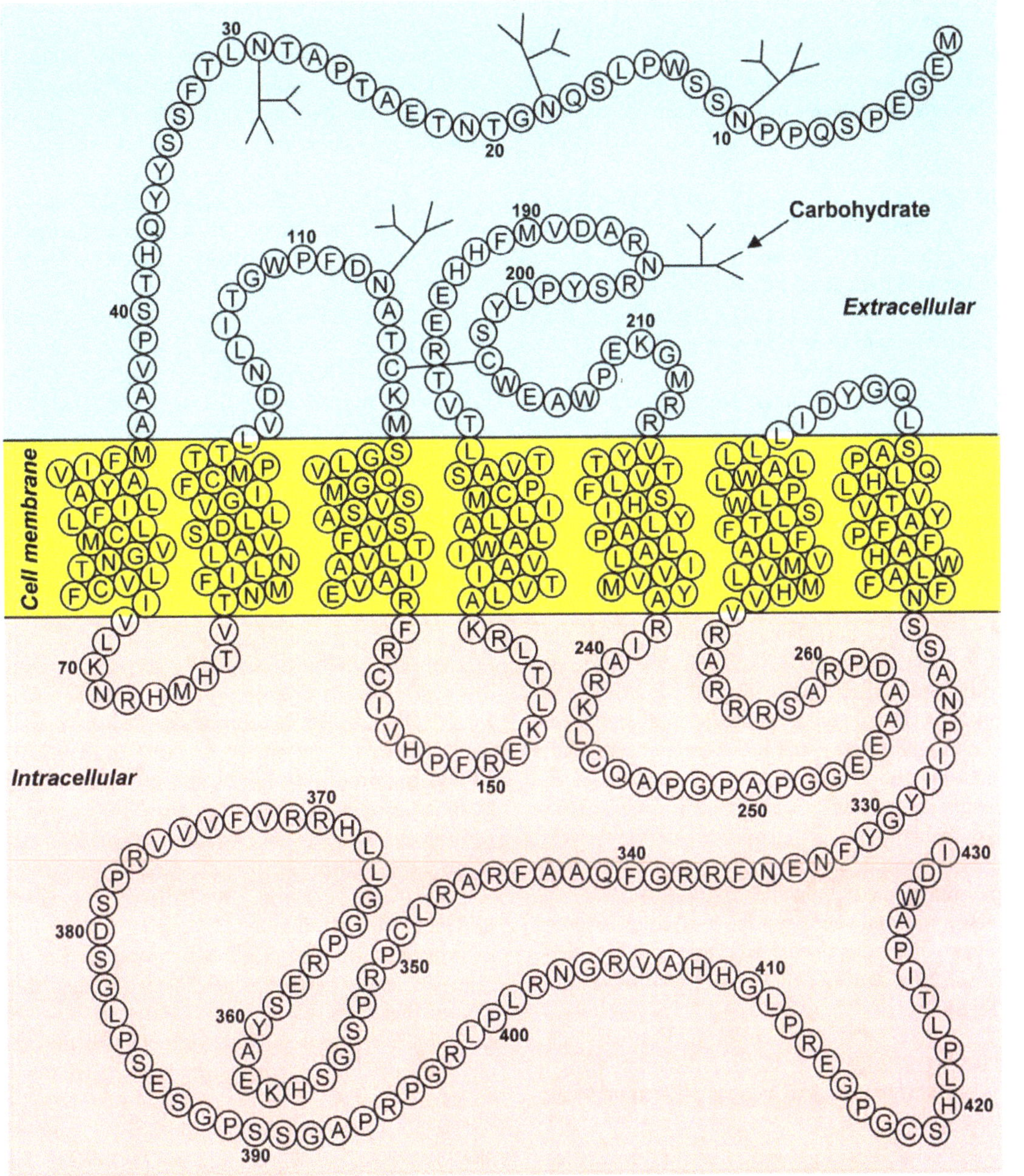

FIGURE 2 | Two-dimensional representation of the receptor (GPR147) for human GnIH (RFRP). The transmembrane region was predicted using SOSUI (Hirokawa et al., 1998). Glycosylation and disulfide bridge sites were predicted by GPCRDB (Horn et al., 1998). The accession number is AB040104. Adapted from Ubuka et al. (2008b).

area (DMH) in the mouse and hamster brains by *in situ* hybridization (Kriegsfeld et al., 2006; Ubuka et al., 2012a). In the rat brain, RFRP precursor mRNA was expressed in the periventricular nucleus (PerVN), and the portion between the dorsomedial nucleus (DMN) and the ventromedial nucleus (VMN) of the hypothalamus (Hinuma et al., 2000; Legagneux et al., 2009). The majority of RFRP mRNA expressing neuronal cell bodies were localized in the intermediate periventricular nucleus (IPe) of the hypothalamus in the macaque (Ubuka et al., 2009b), and in the DMN and PVN in the sheep (Clarke et al., 2008).

GnIH INNERVATION IN THE BRAIN

Although a dense population of GnIH neuronal cell bodies was only found in the PVN in quail, GnIH-ir neuronal fibers were widely distributed in the diencephalic and mesencephalic regions (Ukena et al., 2003). Dense networks of GnIH-ir fibers were found in the ventral paleostriatum, septal area, preoptic area (POA), median eminence, optic tectum, and the dorsal motor nucleus of the vagus. GnIH-ir neuronal fibers were also widely distributed in the diencephalic and mesencephalic regions in European starlings (Ubuka et al., 2008a) and white-crowned sparrows (Ubuka et al.,

2012b). Thus, it was hypothesized that GnIH may participate not only in the regulation of pituitary function, but also in behavioral and autonomic mechanisms in birds.

GnIH-ir neuronal fibers were also widely distributed in the diencephalic and mesencephalic regions in rodents. Dense GnIH-ir fibers were observed in the lateral septal nucleus, medial POA, amygdala, arcuate nucleus (ARC); moderate GnIH-ir fibers were observed in the paraventricular thalamic nucleus, the paraventricular hypothalamic nucleus, and the central gray in Siberian hamsters (Ubuka et al., 2012a). Dense GnIH-ir fibers were also observed in limbic and hypothalamic structures in rats (Johnson et al., 2007). Accordingly, it was hypothesized that GnIH may also participate in behavioral and autonomic mechanisms in mammals.

Innervation of GnIH neuronal fibers was intensively investigated in the rhesus macaque brain (Ubuka et al., 2009b). Abundant GnIH-ir fibers were observed in the nucleus of the stria terminalis in the telencephalon; habenular nucleus, PVN of the thalamus, POA, PVN of the hypothalamus, IPe, ARC of hypothalamus, median eminence and dorsal hypothalamic area in the diencephalon; medial region of the superior colliculus, central gray substance of the midbrain and dorsal raphe nucleus in the midbrain; and parabrachial nucleus in the pons. GnIH-ir fibers were observed in close proximity to GnRH-I, dopamine, pro-opiomelanocortin, and GnRH-II neurons in the POA, IPe, ARC of hypothalamus, and central gray substance of midbrain, respectively. Qi et al. (2009) have shown that RFRP (mammalian GnIH) cells project to neuropeptide Y and pro-opiomelanocortin neurons in the ARC, orexin and melanin-concentrating hormone neurons in the lateral hypothalamic area, as well as orexin cells in the DMN and corticotrophin-releasing hormone and oxytocin cells in the PVN, GnRH neurons in the POA in sheep. GnIH neurons might thus regulate these important neural systems in addition to directly regulating pituitary gonadotropin release (Ubuka et al., 2009b; for reviews, see Tsutsui, 2009; Tsutsui et al., 2010a,b, 2012; Tsutsui and Ubuka, 2012; **Figure 3**).

GnIH ACTION IN THE BRAIN

MODULATION OF THE ACTIVITY OF GnRH AND KISSPEPTIN NEURONS BY GnIH

Immunohistochemical studies using light and confocal microscopy indicated that GnIH (RFRP)-ir axon terminals are in probable contact with GnRH neurons in birds (Bentley et al., 2003), rodents (Kriegsfeld et al., 2006; Ubuka et al., 2012a), monkeys (Ubuka et al., 2009b), and humans (Ubuka et al., 2009c). Thus, there is potential for the direct regulation of the activity of GnRH neurons by GnIH (RFRP) neurons (**Figure 3**).

Ubuka et al. (2008a) investigated the interaction of GnIH neuronal fibers and GnRH neurons in the European starling brain. It is generally accepted that birds possess at least two forms of GnRH in their brains. One form is GnRH-I which is thought to be released at the median eminence to stimulate the secretion of gonadotropins from the anterior pituitary (King and Millar, 1982; Miyamoto et al., 1982; Sharp et al., 1990; Ubuka and Bentley, 2009, 2011; Ubuka et al., 2009a). The second form of GnRH is GnRH-II (Miyamoto et al., 1984; Millar, 2003), which is thought to influence reproductive behaviors in birds (Maney et al., 1997) and mammals (Temple et al., 2003; Barnett et al., 2006). Double-label immunocytochemistry showed GnIH axon terminals on GnRH-I and GnRH-II neurons in the songbird brain (Bentley et al., 2003; Ubuka et al., 2008a). *In situ* hybridization of starling GnIH-R mRNA combined with GnRH immunocytochemistry further showed the expression of GnIH-R mRNA in GnRH-I and GnRH-II neurons (Ubuka et al., 2008a; **Figure 3**).

Double-label immunocytochemistry also showed GnIH axon terminals on GnRH neurons in the Siberian hamster brain (Ubuka et al., 2012a) and GPR147 was expressed in GnRH neurons (Ubuka et al., 2012a). Central administration of GnIH inhibits the release of gonadotropin in white-crowned sparrows (Bentley et al., 2006), Syrian hamsters (Kriegsfeld et al., 2006), rats (Johnson et al., 2007), and Siberian hamsters (Ubuka et al., 2012a) in a manner similar to peripheral administration of GnIH (Osugi et al., 2004; Kriegsfeld et al., 2006; Ubuka et al., 2006). Accordingly, GnIH may inhibit the secretion of gonadotropins by decreasing the activity of GnRH neurons in addition to directly regulating pituitary gonadotropin secretion (**Figure 3**).

Direct application of RFRP-3 to GnRH cells in cultured mouse brain slices decreased firing rate in a subpopulation of cells, further indicating a direct action of RFRP-3 on GnRH neurons (Ducret et al., 2009). In addition, RFRP-3 inhibited firing of kisspeptin-activated vGluT2 (vesicular glutamate transporter 2)-GnRH neurons as well as of kisspeptin-insensitive GnRH neurons (Wu et al., 2009). More recent data have confirmed a role for RFRP-3 using an antagonist, RF9, against GnIH-R. Central administration of RF9 to rats and mice led to marked increases in gonadotropin concentrations, providing a pronounced role of RFRP-3 as a key regulator of the reproductive axis in mammals (Pineda et al., 2010).

Recently, Rizwan et al. (2012) have investigated (1) whether RFRP-3 can directly inhibit LH secretion without inhibiting GnRH neurons; (2) whether RFRP-3 neurons project to GnRH neurons and rostral periventricular kisspeptin neurons in mice, and (3) whether GPR147 and GPR74 are expressed by these neurons. Intravenous treatment with the GPR147 antagonist RF9 increased plasma LH concentrations in castrated male rats but was unable to do so in the presence of the GnRH antagonist cetrorelix. Approximately 26% of GnRH neurons of male and diestrous female mice were apposed by RFRP-3 fibers, and 19% of kisspeptin neurons of proestrous female mice were apposed by RFRP-3 fibers. They further showed that 33% of GnRH neurons and 9–16% of rostral periventricular kisspeptin neurons expressed GPR147, whereas GPR74 was not expressed in either population. These data show that RFRP-3 can act on GnRH neurons as well as kisspeptin neurons to modulate reproduction in rodents (**Figure 3**).

EFFECT OF CENTRAL ADMINISTRATION OF GnIH ON BEHAVIORS OF BIRDS AND MAMMALS

Central administration of GnIH or RFRP-3 to the third ventricle of the brain inhibited reproductive behavior of females in white-crowned sparrows (Bentley et al., 2006) or of males in rats (Johnson et al., 2007). It was known that GnRH-II enhances copulation solicitation in estrogen-primed female white-crowned sparrows exposed to the song of males (Maney et al., 1997).

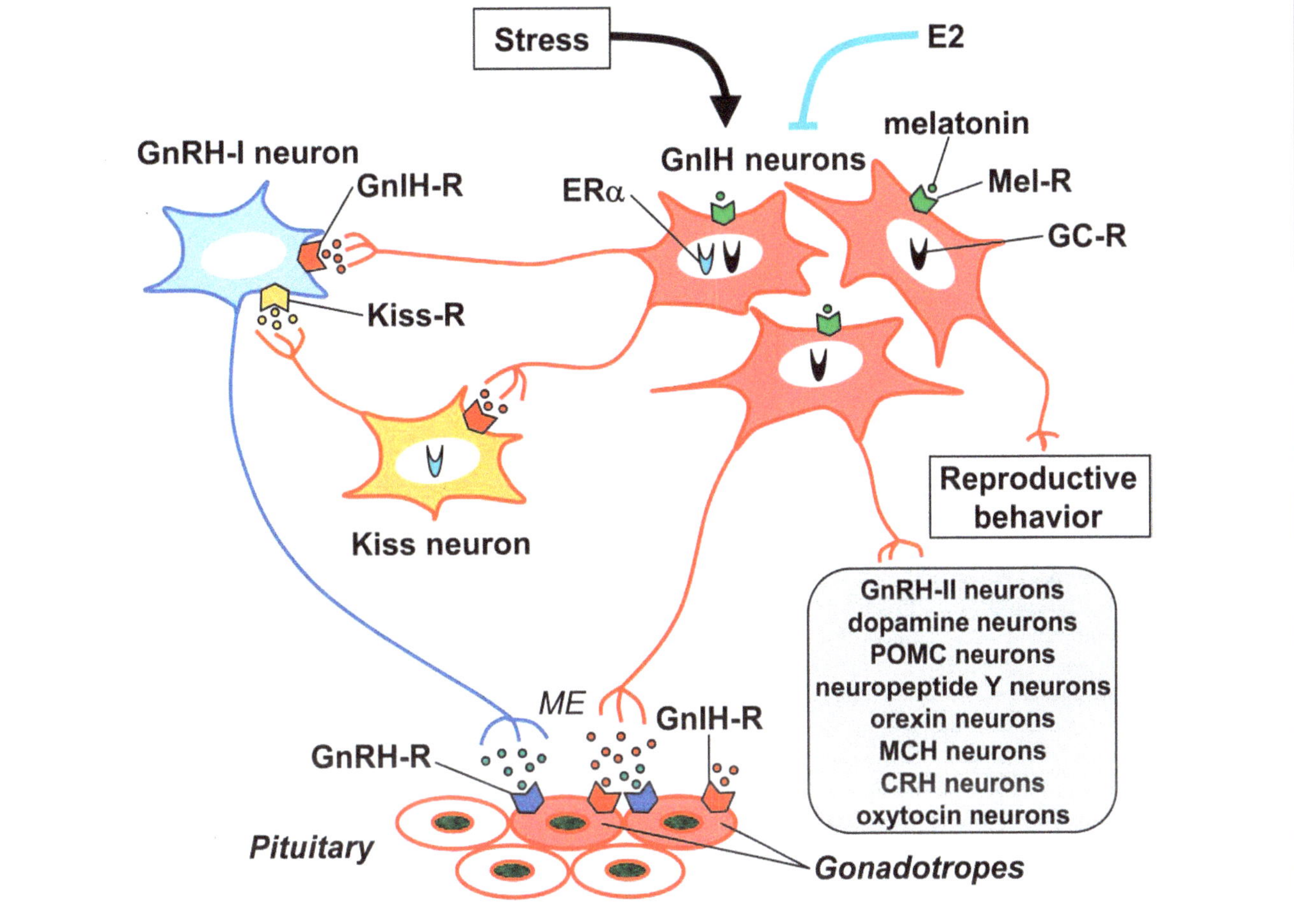

FIGURE 3 | Schematic model of GnIH (RFRP) action in the brain and pituitary. GnIH (RFRP) neurons in the brain project their axons to GnRH-I neurons as well as to the median eminence (ME). GnIH receptor (GnIH-R; GPR147) is expressed on GnRH-I neurons as well as gonadotropes. GnIH may thus inhibit gonadotropin synthesis and release by inhibiting the activity of GnRH-I neurons as well as directly inhibiting the pituitary gonadotrope. GnIH (RFRP) neurons may also regulate GnRH-I neurons by regulating the activity of kisspeptin (Kiss) neurons that project to GnRH-I neurons. There are also reports showing that GnIH (RFRP) neurons project their axons to GnRH-II, dopamine, pro-opiomelanocortin (POMC), neuropeptide Y, orexin, melanin-concentrating hormone (MCH), corticotrophin-releasing hormone (CRH) and oxytocin neurons in the brain. GnIH (RFRP) inhibits reproductive behaviors of birds and mammals by possibly acting within the brain. The expression of GnIH (RFRP) is regulated by melatonin, stress, and estradiol-17β (E2). Expressions of melatonin receptor (Mel-R), glucocorticoid receptor (GC-R), or estrogen receptor α (ERα) in GnIH (RFRP) neurons were shown in several species. These mechanisms of action of GnIH (RFRP) on gonadotropin secretion or regulatory mechanism of GnIH (RFRP) expression may vary between species, sexes, and developmental stages.

Because of the putative contact of GnIH neurons with GnRH-II neurons in white-crowned sparrows (Bentley et al., 2003), Bentley et al. (2006) investigated the effect of GnIH administration on copulation solicitation in females of this species. A centrally-administered physiological dose of GnIH inhibited copulation solicitation in estrogen-primed female white-crowned sparrows exposed to the song of males. Johnson et al. (2007) investigated the effect of central administration of RFRP-3 on reproductive behaviors of male rats. Behavioral tests indicated that RFRP-3 dose-dependently suppressed all facets of male sexual behavior. In contrast, immunoneutralization of RFRP in the rat brain increased male sexual behaviors. These results suggest that GnIH and RFRP inhibit reproductive behavior by inhibiting GnRH neuronal activities or by acting directly within the brain (**Figure 3**).

To identify the mechanism of GnIH neurons in the regulation of behavior, Ubuka et al. (2012b) investigated the effect of RNA interference (RNAi) of the GnIH gene on the behavior of white-crowned sparrows, a highly social songbird species. Administration of small interfering RNA against GnIH precursor mRNA into the third ventricle of male and female birds reduced resting time, spontaneous production of complex vocalizations, and stimulated brief agonistic vocalizations. GnIH RNAi further enhanced song production of short duration in male birds when they were challenged by playbacks of novel male songs. These behaviors resembled those of breeding birds during territorial defense. The overall results suggest that GnIH gene silencing induces arousal. In addition, the activities of male and female birds were negatively correlated with GnIH mRNA expression in the PVN. Density of GnIH neuronal fibers in the ventral tegmental area was decreased by GnIH RNAi treatment in female birds, and the number of GnRH neurons that received close appositions of GnIH neuronal fiber terminals was negatively correlated with the activity of male birds. In summary, GnIH may decrease arousal level resulting in the inhibition of specific motivated behavior, such as in reproductive contexts (Ubuka et al., 2012b).

Central administrations of GnIH or RFRP-3 can also stimulate feeding behavior in chicken or rats (Tachibana et al., 2005; Johnson et al., 2007; Murakami et al., 2008). There is a recent report showing that central administration of RFRP-3 can stimulate adrenocorticotropic hormone and oxytocin release, and induce anxiety behavior in rats (Kaewwongse et al., 2011). The fact that RFRP-ir fibers project to various neurons in the brain, such as dopamine and/or pro-opiomelanocortin neurons in the rat, sheep, and macaque (Qi et al., 2009; Ubuka et al., 2009b; **Figure 3**) suggests multiple functions of GnIH or RFRP in the brain.

GnIH ACTION IN THE PITUITARY

Dense population of GnIH-ir fibers at the median eminence (ME) in quail (Tsutsui et al., 2000; Ukena et al., 2003) as well as in other birds (Bentley et al., 2003; Osugi et al., 2004; Ubuka et al., 2008a), suggested a direct action of GnIH in the regulation of pituitary function in birds (**Figure 3**). The fact that GnIH inhibits synthesis and/or release of gonadotropins from cultured quail and chicken anterior pituitary gland provides strong support for this function (Tsutsui et al., 2000; Ciccone et al., 2004). Peripheral administration of GnIH also inhibits gonadotropin synthesis and/or release in birds (Osugi et al., 2004; Ubuka et al., 2006). In mammals, abundant RFRP-ir fibers were observed in the ME of sheep (Clarke et al., 2008), macaque (Ubuka et al., 2009b), and humans (Ubuka et al., 2009c). As GnIH in birds, RFRP-3 inhibits gonadotropin synthesis and/or release from cultured pituitaries in sheep (Sari et al., 2009) and cattle (Kadokawa et al., 2009). Peripheral administration of RFRP-3 also inhibits gonadotropin release in sheep (Clarke et al., 2008), rats (Murakami et al., 2008), and cattle (Kadokawa et al., 2009). It was further shown that GnIH-R (GPR147) mRNA is expressed in gonadotropes in the human pituitary (Ubuka et al., 2009c). Taken together, it is likely that GnIH and RFRP-3 directly act on the pituitary to inhibit gonadotropin secretion from the pituitary at least in these avian and mammalian species (**Figure 3**).

Recently, Smith et al. (2012) measured the concentration of RFRP-3 in hypophyseal portal blood in ewes during the non-breeding (anestrous) season and during the luteal and follicular phases of the estrous cycle in the breeding season. Pulsatile RFRP-3 secretion was observed in the portal blood of all animals. Mean RFRP-3 pulse amplitude and pulse frequency were higher during the non-breeding season. RFRP-3 was virtually undetectable in peripheral blood plasma. To determine the role of secreted RFRP-3, Smith et al. (2012) further examined its effects on GnRH-stimulated LH secretion in hypothalamo–pituitary-disconnected ewes, and a significant reduction in the LH response to GnRH was observed by RFRP-3 administration. These data show that RFRP-3 is secreted into portal blood to act on pituitary gonadotropes, reducing the action of GnRH in sheep (Smith et al., 2012).

On the contrary it was suggested that GnIH or RFRP-3 may not act directly on the pituitary in some birds and rodents, because there are relatively few or no GnIH (RFRP)-ir fibers in the ME of Rufous-winged sparrows (Small et al., 2007), hamsters (Kriegsfeld et al., 2006; Ubuka et al., 2012a), and rats (Rizwan et al., 2009). Rizwan et al. (2009) have injected a retrograde tracer Fluoro-Gold intraperitoneally in rats. The majority of GnRH neurons were labeled but essentially no RFRP neurons were labeled. In contrast, intracerebral injections of Fluoro-Gold into the rostral POA resulted in the labeling of 75 ± 5% of RFRP cell bodies. These observations suggested that RFRP-3 is not a hypophysiotropic neuroendocrine hormone in rats (Rizwan et al., 2009). However, there are also studies indicating that RFRP-3 can act directly to inhibit gonadotropin release from the pituitary of rats (Murakami et al., 2008). More extensive studies, analyzing peptide release into the hypophyseal portal blood, fiber projections by retrograde labeling, etc., are needed to elucidate the hypophysiotropic action of GnIH in various animals (for reviews, see Tsutsui et al., 2007, 2010a,b, 2012; Tsutsui, 2009; Tsutsui and Ubuka, 2012).

Since GPR147 couples to $G_{\alpha i}$ to inhibit adenylyl cyclase (AC; Hinuma et al., 2000), GPR147 (GnIH-R) activation may reduce intracellular cAMP levels, and reduce the activities of cAMP-dependent protein kinase (PKA) and mitogen-activated protein kinase (MAPK) signaling cascade. On the other hand, GnRH receptor (GnRH-R) couples with $G_{\alpha q/11}$ to activate phospholipase C (PLC), which results in the production of inositol tri-phosphate (IP3) and diacylglycerol (DAG). In turn, IP3 and DAG increase intracellular Ca^{2+} and activate the protein kinase C (PKC) pathway and MAPK signaling. GnRH-R was also reported to be coupled to $G_{\alpha s}$ to stimulate AC/cAMP/PKA pathway. A recent study using immortalized mouse gonadotrope cell line (LβT2 cells) has demonstrated that the inhibitory action of mouse RFRPs on gonadotropin gene expression is mediated by an inhibition of AC/cAMP/PKA-dependent extracellular signal-regulated kinase (ERK) pathway (Son et al., 2012). In the sheep, RFRP-3 can inhibit both GnRH-induced intracellular Ca^{2+} increase and ERK phosphorylation, impacting GnRH-induced gonadotropin release and synthesis (Sari et al., 2009). In the chicken, activation of GnRH-R can activate AC and stimulate cAMP responsive element (CRE) binding protein. GnIH may partly inhibit this GnRH-induced CRE activation, thus impacting gene transcription (Shimizu and Bédécarrats, 2010).

REGULATION OF GnIH EXPRESSION

EFFECT OF MELATONIN

Identification of the regulatory mechanisms governing GnIH expression is important in understanding the physiological role of the GnIH system. Photoperiodic mammals rely on the annual cycle of changes in nocturnal secretion of melatonin to drive their reproductive responses (Bronson, 1990). In contrast, a dogma has existed that birds do not use seasonal changes in melatonin secretion to time their reproductive effort, and a role for melatonin in birds has remained enigmatic (Wilson, 1991; Juss et al., 1993). Despite the accepted dogma, there is strong evidence that melatonin is involved in the regulation of several seasonal processes, including gonadal activity and gonadotropin secretion (Ohta et al., 1989; Guyomarc'h et al., 2001; Rozenboim et al., 2002). Ubuka et al. (2005) hypothesized that melatonin may be involved in the induction of GnIH expression, thus influencing gonadal activity. The action of melatonin on the expression of GnIH was studied in quail, a highly photoperiodic bird species. Because the pineal gland and eyes are the major sources of melatonin in the quail (Underwood et al., 1984), Ubuka et al. (2005) analyzed the effects of pinealectomy (Px) combined with orbital enucleation (Ex; Px plus Ex) on the expression of GnIH precursor mRNA and GnIH peptide. Subsequently, melatonin was administered to Px plus Ex birds. Px plus Ex decreased the expression of GnIH precursor mRNA and the content of mature GnIH peptide in the hypothalamus. Melatonin administration to Px plus Ex birds caused a dose-dependent increase in the expression of GnIH precursor mRNA and the production of mature peptide. They also investigated the expression of melatonin receptor in GnIH neurons. *In situ* hybridization combined with immunocytochemistry for GnIH revealed that the mRNA of Mel1c, a melatonin receptor subtype, was expressed in GnIH-ir neurons in the PVN. Autoradiography of melatonin receptors further revealed specific binding of melatonin in the PVN. Accordingly, melatonin appears to act directly on GnIH neurons through its receptor to induce expression of GnIH (Ubuka et al., 2005; **Figure 3**).

Chowdhury et al. (2010) further investigated the role of melatonin in the regulation of GnIH release and the negative correlation of GnIH release with LH release in quail. Melatonin administration dose-dependently increased GnIH release from hypothalamic explants *in vitro*. A clear diurnal change in GnIH release was observed in quail, and this change was negatively correlated with changes in plasma LH concentrations. GnIH release during the dark period was greater than that during the light period in explants from quail exposed to long-day (LD) photoperiods. Conversely, plasma LH concentrations decreased during the dark period. In contrast to LD, GnIH release increased under short-day (SD) photoperiods, when the duration of nocturnal secretion of melatonin increases. These results indicate that melatonin may play a role in stimulating not only GnIH expression but also GnIH release, thus inhibiting plasma LH concentrations in quail (**Figure 3**).

A similar, but opposite, action of melatonin on the inhibition of the expression of RFRP was shown in Syrian and Siberian hamsters, both photoperiodic mammals (Revel et al., 2008; Mason et al., 2010; Ubuka et al., 2012a). The level of RFRP mRNA and the number of RFRP-ir cell bodies were reduced in sexually quiescent Syrian and Siberian hamsters acclimated to SD photoperiod, compared to sexually active animals maintained under LD photoperiod. The photoperiodic variation of RFRP expression was abolished in Px hamsters and injections of LD hamsters with melatonin reduced the expression of RFRP down to SD levels, indicating a dependence upon melatonin (Revel et al., 2008; Ubuka et al., 2012a). There are also reports showing that the expression of RFRP precursor mRNA is regulated by melatonin in sheep (Dardente et al., 2008) and rats (Gingerich et al., 2009). These results demonstrate that the expression of GnIH and RFRP is photoperiodically modulated via a melatonin-dependent process (**Figure 3**).

Quail is a LD breeder, which activates its reproductive activity in LD and suppresses its reproductive activity in SD. It is understandable that the expression of GnIH is stimulated by a nocturnal hormone melatonin and SD when the duration of melatonin secretion is long. Accordingly, it was hypothesized that the increase of GnIH expression may inhibit reproductive activity in SD in quail (Ubuka et al., 2005). The opposite but similar thoughts can be applied to sheep. Sheep is a SD breeder that activates its reproductive activity in SD and suppresses its reproductive activity in LD. It is also understandable that the expression of RFRP is inhibited by a nocturnal hormone melatonin and SD when the duration of melatonin secretion is long. Accordingly, it was hypothesized that the increase of RFRP expression may inhibit reproductive activity in LD in sheep (Dardente et al., 2008). On the other hand, it was difficult to understand the inhibitory effect of melatonin or SD on RFRP expression in hamsters, because hamsters are LD breeders (Revel et al., 2008; Mason et al., 2010). However, recent report has shown that RFRP may have a stimulatory effect on gonadotropin secretion in SD in Siberian hamsters (Ubuka et al., 2012a). Long duration of melatonin secretion in SD may need to decrease RFRP expression to inhibit reproductive activities of Siberian hamsters in SD. Another recent work in male Syrian hamsters suggested that GnIH might be excitatory in LD as well (Ancel et al., 2012). Long duration of melatonin secretion in SD may decrease RFRP expression to inhibit reproductive activities and short duration of melatonin secretion in LD may increase RFRP expression to stimulate reproductive activities of Syrian hamsters in LD (Ancel et al., 2012). Further studies are required to understand the role of melatonin controlling GnIH and RFRP expression in seasonal breeders.

EFFECT OF STRESS

Stress leads to reproductive dysfunction in many species, including rodents and humans. Calisi et al. (2008) hypothesized that stress effects upon reproduction are mediated via the hypothalamic GnIH system in birds. They examined the effects of capture-handling stress in the hypothalamus of male and female adult house sparrows. There were more GnIH-positive neurons in fall birds versus those sampled in spring, and a significant increase in GnIH-positive neurons was seen in stressed birds in spring. These data imply an influence of stress upon the GnIH system that changes over the annual cycle of reproduction (**Figure 3**).

Kirby et al. (2009) showed that both acute and chronic immobilization stress lead to an up-regulation of the expression of RFRP in the DMH of adult male rats and that this increase in RFRP is associated with inhibition of downstream HPG activity. They also showed that adrenalectomy blocks the stress-induced increase in RFRP expression. Immunohistochemistry revealed that 53% of RFRP cells express receptors for glucocorticoids (GCs), suggesting that adrenal GCs can mediate the stress effect through direct action on RFRP cells. These data show that stress-induced increases in adrenal GCs cause an increase in RFRP that contributes to hypothalamic suppression of reproductive function (**Figure 3**).

Papargiris et al. (2011) tested if GnIH (RFRP) mediates the inhibitory effect of stress on LH secretion in ovariectomized ewes using a psychosocial stressor, isolation/restraint. Isolation/restraint stress increased plasma cortisol concentrations and decreased plasma LH concentrations. However, there was no significant effect of stress on RFRP peptide or mRNA levels, with no difference between control or stressed ewes. Furthermore, there was no difference in the number of RFRP-ir cells double-labeled for Fos between control and stressed ewes and there was no difference in the cellular expression of RFRP mRNA between groups. Accordingly, GnIH (RFRP) may not mediate the effects of stress on LH secretion in ewes or the effect of stress may depend on the presence of gonadal sex steroids.

EFFECT OF SEX STEROIDS

Estrogen secreted by the ovary feedbacks to the brain and pituitary to regulate gonadotropin secretion (Herbison, 1998; Petersen et al., 2003). Wintermantel et al. (2006) found that estrogen positive feedback to generate the preovulatory gonadotropin surge was normal in estrogen receptor (ER) β knockout mice, but absent in ERα mutant mice. Because GnRH neurons do not express ERα, estrogen positive feedback upon GnRH neurons must be indirect. RFRP (mammalian GnIH) neuronal system may be involved in estrogen feedback signaling to GnRH neurons because RFRP neurons in rodents express ERα and respond with c-Fos expression to an acute administration of estradiol-17β (E2; Kriegsfeld et al., 2006; **Figure 3**).

The role of RFRP-3 in regulating ovulatory function was investigated in female hamsters (Gibson et al., 2008). The cellular activity of RFRP neurons was suppressed at the time of the LH surge, suggesting removal of negative feedback by RFRP-3 at this time. The SCN, the master circadian clock triggering ovulation in rodents, projects to a large proportion of RFRP neurons, providing a mechanism for timing removal of negative drive on the GnRH system. Activities of the SCN, GnRH, and RFRP neurons were coordinated with ovulation (Gibson et al., 2008). Li et al. (2012) investigated the expression patterns in the reproductive axis of the female pig across the estrous cycle. The hypothalamic levels of both RFRP and its receptor mRNA were lowest in estrus and peaked in the proestrus and diestrus phases. Smith et al. (2010) examined Kiss1 and RFRP mRNA throughout the menstrual cycle of a female primate, rhesus macaque. Kiss1-expressing cells were found in the POA and ARC, and RFRP-expressing cells were located in the PVN/DMN. Kiss1 expression in the caudal ARC and POA was higher in the late follicular phase of the cycle (just before the GnRH/LH surge) than in the luteal phase. RFRP expression was also higher in the late follicular phase suggesting that RFRP fine tunes GnRH/LH surge in primates. There are also reports showing the correlation of RFRP expression and testicular activities of male mice (Sethi et al., 2010a,b).

Molnár et al. (2011) investigated the possibility that RFRP neurons are involved in estrogen feedback signaling to the reproductive axis in mice. They compared the expression of RFRP mRNA of ovariectomized mice, with and without E2 replacement. Subcutaneous administration of E2 via silastic capsules for 4 days significantly down-regulated RFRP mRNA expression. In ovariectomized mice, low levels of ERα immunoreactivity were detectable in 18.7 ± 3.8% of RFRP neurons, whereas RFRP neurons did not exhibit ERβ immunoreactivity. The estrogenic down-regulation of RFRP expression may contribute to estrogen positive feedback to the reproductive axis. However, whether E2 regulates RFRP neurons directly or indirectly remains an open question because ERα immunoreactivity is present only in a subset of RFRP cells (**Figure 3**).

Poling et al. (2012) examined changes in RFRP neurons in mice of both sexes during development and under different adulthood hormonal milieus. They identified two interspersed subpopulations of RFRP cells (high RFRP-expressing, HE; low RFRP-expressing, LE), which have unique developmental and steroidal regulation characteristics. The number of LE cells robustly decreased during postnatal development, whereas HE cell number increased significantly before puberty. In adults, they found that E2 and testosterone moderately repress RFRP expression in both HE and LE cells, whereas the non-aromatizable androgen dihydrotestosterone has no effect. They determined that approximately 25% of RFRP neurons coexpress ERα in each sex, whereas RFRP cells do not express androgen receptor in either sex, regardless of hormonal milieu. They detected coexpression of GPR147 but no coexpression of GPR74 in GnRH neurons of both intact and gonadectomized males and females. RFRP-3 may thus exert its effects on reproduction either directly, via GPR147 in a subset of GnRH neurons, and/or indirectly, via upstream regulators of GnRH (**Figure 3**).

RECENT PROGRESS IN GnIH STUDIES ON FISH AND HUMANS

We have described the progress of GnIH research investigating its function in the brain and pituitary of birds and mammals. Recently, there were important progresses in the study of GnIH peptides in fish and humans as we briefly summarize them below.

A cDNA encoding three GnIH orthologs, LPXRFamide peptides, was cloned from the goldfish brain by a combination of 3′/5′ RACE (Sawada et al., 2002). Mass spectrometric analyses revealed that a tridecapeptide (SGTGLSATLPQRFamide) is expressed in the brain as an endogenous ligand. Immunoreactive cell bodies were restricted to the nucleus posterioris periventricularis and the nervus terminalis and immunoreactive fibers were distributed in several brain regions including the nucleus lateralis tuberis pars posterioris and pituitary (Sawada et al., 2002). Amano et al. (2006) analyzed the hypophysiotropic activity of the three goldfish LPXRFamide peptides (gfLPXRFa-1, -2, and -3) in sockeye salmon. gfLPXRFa-ir cell bodies were detected in the nucleus posterioris periventricularis of the hypothalamus and immunoreactive fibers were distributed in various brain regions and the pituitary in sockeye salmon. gfLPXRFamide peptides stimulated the release of FSH, LH, and GH from cultured pituitary cells (Amano et al., 2006). In contrast, Zhang et al. (2010) have identified the orthologous GnIH genes in zebrafish, stickleback, medaka, and Takifugu. The zebrafish GnIH precursor contained three putative LPXRFamide peptides. Intraperitoneal administration of the mature zebrafish LPXRFa-3 (zfLPXRFa-3) significantly reduced the basal serum LH level in goldfish (Zhang et al., 2010).

Moussavi et al. (2012) examined the effects of synthetic gfLPXRFamide peptides on pituitary LHβ and FSHβ subunit, and gfLPXRFamide peptide receptor (gfLPXRFa-R) mRNA levels and LH secretion in goldfish. Intraperitoneal injections of gfLPXRFa-3 increased pituitary LHβ and FSHβ mRNA levels at early to late gonadal recrudescence, but reduced serum LH and pituitary gfLPXRFa-R mRNA levels, respectively, at early to mid-recrudescence and later stages of recrudescence. Static incubation with gfLPXRFa-3 elevated LH secretion from dispersed pituitary cell cultures from prespawning fish, but not at other recrudescent stages. gfLPXRFa-3 suppressed LHβ mRNA levels at early recrudescence and prespawning but elevated LHβ at mid-recrudescence, and consistently attenuated FSHβ mRNA in a dose-specific manner *in vitro*. These results indicate that the effect of gfLPXRFa-3 depends on maturational status and administration route in goldfish (Moussavi et al., 2012).

Recently, the mature peptide structures of human GnIH peptides (human RFRP-1 and RFRP-3) were identified by mass spectrometry (Ubuka et al., 2009c). Because the structure of human RFRP-3 was identical to the structure of sheep RFRP-3, physiological functions of human RFRP-3 were studied in the sheep. It was shown that sheep/human RFRP-3 inhibits gonadotropin synthesis and release *in vitro* (Sari et al., 2009) and gonadotropin release *in vivo* (Clarke et al., 2008; Smith et al., 2012). In view of its potent inhibition of gonadotropin secretion, human RFRP-3 (human GnIH) has the potential of an alternative or adjunct therapeutic agent to inhibit endogenous levels of gonadotropins and steroid hormones in humans. Thus, RFRP has therapeutic potential in the treatment of hormone-dependent diseases, such as precocious puberty, endometriosis, uterine fibroids, benign prostatic hyperplasia, and prostatic and breast cancers.

ACKOWLEDGMENTS

This work was supported by Grants-in-Aid for Scientific Research from the Ministry of Education, Science and Culture, Japan (22132004 and 22227002 to Kazuyoshi Tsutsui).

REFERENCES

Amano, M., Moriyama, S., Iigo, M., Kitamura, S., Amiya, N., Yamamori, K., et al. (2006). Novel fish hypothalamic neuropeptides stimulate the release of gonadotrophins and growth hormone from the pituitary of sockeye salmon. *J. Endocrinol.* 188, 417–423.

Ancel, C., Bentsen, A. H., Sébert, M. E., Tena-Sempere, M., Mikkelsen, J. D., and Simonneaux, V. (2012). Stimulatory effect of RFRP-3 on the gonadotrophic axis in the male Syrian hamster: the exception proves the rule. *Endocrinology* 153, 1352–1363.

Barnett, D. K., Bunnell, T. M., Millar, R. P., and Abbott, D. H. (2006). Gonadotropin-releasing hormone II stimulates female sexual behavior in marmoset monkeys. *Endocrinology* 147, 615–623.

Bentley, G. E., Jensen, J. P., Kaur, G. J., Wacker, D. W., Tsutsui, K., and Wingfield, J. C. (2006). Rapid inhibition of female sexual behavior by gonadotropin-inhibitory hormone (GnIH). *Horm. Behav.* 49, 550–555.

Bentley, G. E., Perfito, N., Ukena, K., Tsutsui, K., and Wingfield, J. C. (2003). Gonadotropin-inhibitory peptide in song sparrows (*Melospiza melodia*) in different reproductive conditions, and in house sparrows (*Passer domesticus*) relative to chicken-gonadotropin-releasing hormone. *J. Neuroendocrinol.* 15, 794–802.

Bentley, G. E., Ubuka, T., McGuire, N. L., Chowdhury, V. S., Morita, Y., Yano, T., et al. (2008). Gonadotropin-inhibitory hormone and its receptor in the avian reproductive system. *Gen. Comp. Endocrinol.* 156, 34–43.

Bonini, J. A., Jones, K. A., Adham, N., Forray, C., Artymyshyn, R., Durkin, M. M., et al. (2000). Identification and characterization of two G protein-coupled receptors for neuropeptide FF. *J. Biol. Chem.* 275, 39324–39331.

Bronson, F. H. (1990). *Mammalian Reproductive Biology.* Chicago: University of Chicago Press.

Burgus, R., Butcher, M., Amoss, M., Ling, N., Monahan, M., Rivier, J., et al. (1972). Primary structure of the ovine hypothalamic luteinizing hormone-releasing factor (LRF) (LH-hypothalamus-LRF-gas-chromatography-mass-spectrometry-decapeptide-Edman degradation). *Proc. Natl. Acad. Sci. U.S.A.* 69, 278–282.

Calisi, R. M., Rizzo, N. O., and Bentley, G. E. (2008). Seasonal differences in hypothalamic EGR-1 and GnIH expression following capture-handling stress in house sparrows (*Passer domesticus*). *Gen. Comp. Endocrinol.* 157, 283–287.

Chowdhury, V. S., Yamamoto, K., Ubuka, T., Bentley, G. E., Hattori, A., and Tsutsui, K. (2010). Melatonin stimulates the release of gonadotropin-inhibitory hormone by the avian hypothalamus. *Endocrinology* 151, 271–280.

Ciccone, N. A., Dunn, I. C., Boswell, T., Tsutsui, K., Ubuka, T., Ukena, K., et al. (2004). Gonadotrophin inhibitory hormone depresses gonadotrophin alpha and follicle-stimulating hormone beta subunit expression in the pituitary of the domestic chicken. *J. Neuroendocrinol.* 16, 999–1006.

Clarke, I. J., Sari, I. P., Qi, Y., Smith, J. T., Parkington, H. C., Ubuka, T., et al. (2008). Potent action of RFamide-related peptide-3 on pituitary gonadotropes indicative of a hypophysiotropic role in the negative regulation of gonadotropin secretion. *Endocrinology* 149, 5811–5821.

Dardente, H., Birnie, M., Lincoln, G. A., and Hazlerigg, D. G. (2008). RFamide-related peptide and its cognate receptor in the sheep: cDNA cloning, mRNA distribution in the hypothalamus and the effect of photoperiod. *J. Neuroendocrinol.* 20, 1252–1259.

Ducret, E., Anderson, G. M., and Herbison, A. E. (2009). RFamide-related peptide-3, a mammalian gonadotropin-inhibitory hormone ortholog, regulates gonadotropin-releasing hormone neuron firing in the mouse. *Endocrinology* 150, 2799–2804.

Dockray, G. J., Reeve, J. R. Jr., Shively, J., Gayton, R. J., and Barnard, C. S. (1983). A novel active pentapeptide from chicken brain identified by antibodies to FMRFamide. *Nature* 305, 328–330.

Fukusumi, S., Habata, Y., Yoshida, H., Iijima, N., Kawamata, Y., Hosoya, M., et al. (2001). Characteristics and distribution of endogenous RFamide-related peptide-1. *Biochim. Biophys. Acta* 1540, 221–232.

Gibson, E. M., Humber, S. A., Jain, S., Williams, W. P. III, Zhao, S., Bentley, G. E., et al. (2008). Alterations in RFamide-related peptide expression are coordinated with the preovulatory luteinizing hormone surge. *Endocrinology* 149, 4958–4969.

Gingerich, S., Wang, X., Lee, P. K., Dhillon, S. S., Chalmers, J. A., Koletar, M. M., et al. (2009). The generation of an array of clonal, immortalized cell models from the rat hypothalamus: analysis of melatonin effects on kisspeptin and gonadotropin-inhibitory hormone neurons. *Neuroscience* 162, 1134–1140.

Guyomarc'h, C., Lumineau, S., Vivien-Roels, B., Richard, J., and Deregnaucourt, S. (2001). Effect of melatonin supplementation on the sexual development in European quail (*Coturnix coturnix*). *Behav. Processes* 53, 121–130.

Herbison, A. E. (1998). Multimodal influence of estrogen upon gonadotropin-releasing hormone neurons. *Endocr. Rev.* 19, 302–330.

Hinuma, S., Shintani, Y., Fukusumi, S., Iijima, N., Matsumoto, Y., Hosoya, M., et al. (2000). New neuropeptides containing carboxy-terminal RFamide and their receptor in mammals. *Nat. Cell Biol.* 2, 703–708.

Hirokawa, T., Boon-Chieng, S., and Mitaku, S. (1998). SOSUI: classification and secondary structure prediction system for membrane proteins. *Bioinformatics* 14, 378–379.

Horn, F., Weare, J., Beukers, M. W., Hörsch, S., Bairoch, A., Chen, W., et al. (1998). GPCRDB: an information system for G protein-coupled receptors. *Nucleic Acids Res.* 26, 277–281.

Johnson, M. A., Tsutsui, K., and Fraley, G. S. (2007). Rat RFamide-related peptide-3 stimulates GH secretion, inhibits LH secretion, and has variable effects on sex behavior in the adult male rat. *Horm. Behav.* 51, 171–180.

Juss, T. S., Meddle, S. L., Servant, R. S., and King V. M. (1993). Melatonin and photoperiodic time measurement in Japanese quail (*Coturnix coturnix japonica*). *Proc. Biol. Sci.* 254, 21–28.

Kaewwongse, M., Takayanagi, Y., and Onaka, T. (2011). Effects of RFamide-related peptide (RFRP)-1 and RFRP-3 on oxytocin release and anxiety-related behaviour in rats. *J. Neuroendocrinol.* 23, 20–27.

Kadokawa, H., Shibata, M., Tanaka, Y., Kojima, T., Matsumoto, K., Oshima, K., et al. (2009). Bovine C-terminal octapeptide of RFamide-related peptide-3 suppresses luteinizing hormone (LH) secretion from the pituitary as well as pulsatile LH secretion in bovines. *Domest. Anim. Endocrinol.* 36, 219–224.

King, J. A., and Millar, R. P. (1982). Structure of chicken hypothalamic luteinizing hormone-releasing hormone. I. Structural determination on partially purified material. *J. Biol. Chem.* 257, 10722–10728.

Kirby, E. D., Geraghty, A. C., Ubuka, T., Bentley, G. E., and Kaufer,

D. (2009). Stress increases putative gonadotropin inhibitory hormone and decreases luteinizing hormone in male rats. *Proc. Natl. Acad. Sci. U.S.A.* 106, 11324–11329.

Kriegsfeld, L. J., Mei, D. F., Bentley, G. E., Ubuka, T., Mason, A. O., Inoue, K., et al. (2006). Identification and characterization of a gonadotropin-inhibitory system in the brains of mammals. *Proc. Natl. Acad. Sci. U.S.A.* 103, 2410–2415.

Legagneux, K., Bernard-Franchi, G., Poncet, F., La Roche, A., Colard, C., Fellmann, D., et al. (2009). Distribution and genesis of the RFRP-producing neurons in the rat brain: comparison with melanin-concentrating hormone- and hypocretin-containing neurons. *Neuropeptides* 43, 13–19.

Li, X., Su, J., Lei, Z., Zhao, Y., Jin, M., Fang, R., et al. (2012). Gonadotropin-inhibitory hormone (GnIH) and its receptor in the female pig: cDNA cloning, expression in tissues and expression pattern in the reproductive axis during the estrous cycle. *Peptides* 36, 176–185.

Liu, Q., Guan, X. M., Martin, W. J., McDonald, T. P., Clements, M. K., Jiang, Q., et al. (2001). Identification and characterization of novel mammalian neuropeptide FF-like peptides that attenuate morphine-induced antinociception. *J. Biol. Chem.* 276, 36961–36969.

Maddineni, S. R., Ocón-Grove, O. M., Krzysik-Walker, S. M., Hendricks, G. L. III, and Ramachandran, R. (2008). Gonadotropin-inhibitory hormone (GnIH) receptor gene is expressed in the chicken ovary: potential role of GnIH in follicular maturation. *Reproduction* 135, 267–274.

Maney, D. L., Richardson, R. D., and Wingfield, J. C. (1997). Central administration of chicken gonadotropin-releasing hormone-II enhances courtship behavior in a female sparrow. *Horm. Behav.* 32, 11–18.

Mason, A. O., Duffy, S., Zhao, S., Ubuka, T., Bentley, G. E., Tsutsui, K., et al. (2010). Photoperiod and reproductive condition are associated with changes in RFamide-related peptide (RFRP) expression in Syrian hamsters (*Mesocricetus auratus*). *J. Biol. Rhythms* 25, 176–185.

Matsuo, H., Baba, Y., Nair, R. M., Arimura, A., and Schally, A. V. (1971). Structure of the porcine LH- and FSH-releasing hormone. I. The proposed amino acid sequence. *Biochem. Biophys. Res. Commun.* 43, 1334–1339.

McGuire, N. L., and Bentley, G. E. (2010). A functional neuropeptide system in vertebrate gonads: gonadotropin-inhibitory hormone and its receptor in testes of field-caught house sparrow (*Passer domesticus*). *Gen. Comp. Endocrinol.* 166, 565–572.

McGuire, N. L., Kangas, K., and Bentley, G. E. (2011). Effects of melatonin on peripheral reproductive function: regulation of testicular GnIH and testosterone. *Endocrinology* 152, 3461–3470.

Millar, R. P. (2003). GnRH II and type II GnRH receptors. *Trends Endocrinol. Metab.* 14, 35–43.

Millar, R. P. (2005). GnRHs and GnRH receptors. *Anim. Reprod. Sci.* 88, 5–28.

Miyamoto, K., Hasegawa, Y., Minegishi, T., Nomura, M., Takahashi, Y., Igarashi, M., et al. (1982). Isolation and characterization of chicken hypothalamic luteinizing hormone-releasing hormone. *Biochem. Biophys. Res. Commun.* 107, 820–827.

Miyamoto, K., Hasegawa, Y., Nomura, M., Igarashi, M., Kangawa, K., and Matsuo, H. (1984). Identification of the second gonadotropin-releasing hormone in chicken hypothalamus: evidence that gonadotropin secretion is probably controlled by two distinct gonadotropin-releasing hormones in avian species. *Proc. Natl. Acad. Sci. U.S.A.* 81, 3874–3878.

Molnár, C. S., Kalló, I., Liposits, Z., and Hrabovszky, E. (2011). Estradiol down-regulates RF-amide-related peptide (RFRP) expression in the mouse hypothalamus. *Endocrinology* 152, 1684–1690.

Moussavi, M., Wlasichuk, M., Chang, J. P., and Habibi, H. R. (2012). Seasonal effect of GnIH on gonadotrope functions in the pituitary of goldfish. *Mol. Cell. Endocrinol.* 350, 53–60.

Murakami, M., Matsuzaki, T., Iwasa, T., Yasui, T., Irahara, M., Osugi, T., et al. (2008). Hypophysiotropic role of RFamide-related peptide-3 in the inhibition of LH secretion in female rats. *J. Endocrinol.* 199, 105–112.

Ohta, M., Kadota, C., and Konishi, H. (1989). A role of melatonin in the initial stage of photoperiodism in the Japanese quail. *Biol. Reprod.* 40, 935–941.

Oishi, H., Klausen, C., Bentley, G. E., Osugi, T., Tsutsui, K., Gilks, C. B., et al. (2012). The human gonadotropin-inhibitory hormone ortholog RFamide-related peptide-3 suppresses gonadotropin-induced progesterone production in human granulosa cells. *Endocrinology* 153, 3435–3445.

Osugi, T., Ukena, K., Bentley, G. E., O'Brien, S., Moore, I. T., Wingfield, J. C., et al. (2004). Gonadotropin-inhibitory hormone in Gambel's white-crowned sparrow (*Zonotrichia leucophrys gambelii*): cDNA identification, transcript localization and functional effects in laboratory and field experiments. *J. Endocrinol.* 182, 33–42.

Papargiris, M. M., Rivalland, E. T., Clarke, I. J., Smith, J. T., Pereira, A., and Tilbrook, A. J. (2011). Evidence that RF-amide related peptide-3 is not a mediator of the inhibitory effects of psychosocial stress on gonadotrophin secretion in ovariectomised ewes. *J. Neuroendocrinol.* 23, 208–215.

Petersen, S. L., Ottem, E. N., and Carpenter, C. D. (2003). Direct and indirect regulation of gonadotropin-releasing hormone neurons by estradiol. *Biol. Reprod.* 69, 1771–1778.

Pineda, R., Garcia-Galiano, D., Sanchez-Garrido, M. A., Romero, M., Ruiz-Pino, F., Aguilar, E., et al. (2010). Characterization of the potent gonadotropin-releasing activity of RF9, a selective antagonist of RF-amide-related peptides and neuropeptide FF receptors: physiological and pharmacological implications. *Endocrinology* 151, 1902–1913.

Poling, M. C., Kim, J., Dhamija, S., and Kauffman, A. S. (2012). Development, sex steroid regulation, and phenotypic characterization of RFamide-related peptide (Rfrp) gene expression and RFamide receptors in the mouse hypothalamus. *Endocrinology* 153, 1827–1840.

Price, D. A., and Greenberg, M. J. (1977). Structure of a molluscan cardioexcitatory neuropeptide. *Science* 197, 670–671.

Qi, Y., Oldfield, B. J., and Clarke, I. J. (2009). Projections of RFamide-related peptide-3 neurones in the ovine hypothalamus, with special reference to regions regulating energy balance and reproduction. *J. Neuroendocrinol.* 21, 690–697.

Revel, F. G., Saboureau, M., Pévet, P., Simonneaux, V., and Mikkelsen, J. D. (2008). RFamide-related peptide gene is a melatonin-driven photoperiodic gene. *Endocrinology* 149, 902–912.

Rizwan, M. Z., Poling, M. C., Corr, M., Cornes, P. A., Augustine, R. A., Quennell, J. H., et al. (2012). RFamide-related peptide-3 receptor gene expression in GnRH and kisspeptin neurons and GnRH-dependent mechanism of action. *Endocrinology* 153, 3770–3779.

Rizwan, M. Z., Porteous, R., Herbison, A. E., and Anderson, G. M. (2009). Cells expressing RFamide-related peptide-1/3, the mammalian gonadotropin-inhibitory hormone orthologs, are not hypophysiotropic neuroendocrine neurons in the rat. *Endocrinology* 150, 1413–1420.

Rozenboim, I., Aharony, T., and Yahav, S. (2002). The effect of melatonin administration on circulating plasma luteinizing hormone concentration in castrated White Leghorn roosters. *Poult. Sci.* 81, 1354–1359.

Sari, I. P., Rao, A., Smith, J. T., Tilbrook, A. J., and Clarke, I. J. (2009). Effect of RF-amide-related peptide-3 on luteinizing hormone and follicle-stimulating hormone synthesis and secretion in ovine pituitary gonadotropes. *Endocrinology* 150, 5549–5556.

Satake, H., Hisada, M., Kawada, T., Minakata, H., Ukena, K., and Tsutsui, K. (2001). Characterization of a cDNA encoding a novel avian hypothalamic neuropeptide exerting an inhibitory effect on gonadotropin release. *Biochem. J.* 354, 379–385.

Sawada, K., Ukena, K., Satake, H., Iwakoshi, E., Minakata, H., and Tsutsui, K. (2002). Novel fish hypothalamic neuropeptide. *Eur. J. Biochem.* 269, 6000–6008.

Sethi, S., Tsutsui, K., and Chaturvedi, C. M. (2010a). Temporal phase relation of circadian neural oscillations alters RFamide-related peptide-3 and testicular function in the mouse. *Neuroendocrinology* 91, 189–199.

Sethi, S., Tsutsui, K., and Chaturvedi, C. M. (2010b). Age-dependent variation in the RFRP-3 neurons is inversely correlated with gonadal activity of mice. *Gen. Comp. Endocrinol.* 168, 326–332.

Shahjahan, M., Ikegami, T., Osugi, T., Ukena, K., Doi, H., Hattori, A., et al. (2011). Synchronised expressions of LPXRFamide peptide and its receptor genes: seasonal, diurnal and circadian changes during spawning period in grass puffer. *J. Neuroendocrinol.* 23, 39–51.

Sharp, P. J., Talbot, R. T., Main, G. M., Dunn, I. C., Fraser, H. M., and Huskisson, N. S. (1990). Physiological roles of chicken LHRH-I and -II in the control of gonadotrophin release in the domestic chicken. *J. Endocrinol.* 124, 291–299.

Shimizu, M., and Bédécarrats, G. Y. (2010). Activation of the chicken gonadotropin-inhibitory hormone receptor reduces gonadotropin releasing hormone receptor signaling. *Gen. Comp. Endocrinol.* 167, 331–337.

Singh, P., Krishna, A., Sridaran, R., and Tsutsui, K. (2011a). Immunohistochemical localization of GnRH and RFamide-related peptide-3 in the ovaries of mice during the estrous cycle. *J. Mol. Histol.* 42, 371–381.

Singh, P., Krishna, A., and Tsutsui, K. (2011b). Effects of gonadotropin-inhibitory hormone on folliculogenesis and steroidogenesis of cyclic mice. *Fertil. Steril.* 95, 1397–1404.

Small, T. W., Sharp, P. J., Bentley, G. E, Millar, R. P., Tsutsui, K., Mura, E., et al. (2007). Photoperiod-independent hypothalamic regulation of luteinizing hormone secretion in a free-living sonoran desert bird, the Rufous-winged sparrow (*Aimophila carpalis*). *Brain Behav. Evol.* 71, 127–142.

Smith, J. T., Shahab, M., Pereira, A., Pau, K. Y., and Clarke, I. J. (2010). Hypothalamic expression of KISS1 and gonadotropin inhibitory hormone genes during the menstrual cycle of a non-human primate. *Biol. Reprod.* 83, 568–577.

Smith, J. T., Young, I. R., Veldhuis, J. D., and Clarke, I. J. (2012). Gonadotropin-inhibitory hormone (GnIH) secretion into the ovine hypophyseal portal system. *Endocrinology* 153, 3368–3375.

Son, Y. L., Ubuka, T., Millar, R. P., Kanasaki, H., and Tsutsui, K. (2012). Gonadotropin-inhibitory hormone inhibits GnRH-induced gonadotropin subunit gene transcriptions by inhibiting AC/cAMP/PKA-dependent ERK pathway in LβT2 cells. *Endocrinology* 153, 2332–2343.

Tachibana, T., Sato, M., Takahashi, H., Ukena, K., Tsutsui, K., and Furuse, M. (2005). Gonadotropin-inhibiting hormone stimulates feeding behavior in chicks. *Brain Res.* 1050, 94–100.

Temple, J. L., Millar, R. P., and Rissman, E. F. (2003). An evolutionarily conserved form of gonadotropin-releasing hormone coordinates energy and reproductive behavior. *Endocrinology* 144, 13–19.

Tobari, Y., Iijima, N., Tsunekawa, K., Osugi, T., Okanoya, K., Tsutsui, K., et al. (2010). Identification of gonadotropin-inhibitory hormone in the zebra finch (*Taeniopygia guttata*): peptide isolation, cDNA cloning and brain distribution. *Peptides* 31, 816–826.

Tsutsui, K. (2009). A new key neurohormone controlling reproduction, gonadotropin-inhibitory hormone (GnIH): biosynthesis, mode of action and functional significance. *Prog. Neurobiol.* 88, 76–88.

Tsutsui, K., Bentley, G. E., Bedecarrats, G., Osugi, T., Ubuka, T., and Kriegsfeld, L. J. (2010a). Gonadotropin-inhibitory hormone (GnIH) and its control of central and peripheral reproductive function. *Front. Neuroendocrinol.* 31, 284–295.

Tsutsui, K., Bentley, G. E., Kriegsfeld, L. J., Osugi, T., Seong, J. Y., and Vaudry, H. (2010b). Discovery and evolutionary history of gonadotrophin-inhibitory hormone and kisspeptin: new key neuropeptides controlling reproduction. *J. Neuroendocrinol.* 22, 716–727.

Tsutsui, K., Bentley, G. E., Ubuka, T., Saigoh, E., Yin, H., Osugi, T., et al. (2007). The general and comparative biology of gonadotropin-inhibitory hormone (GnIH). *Gen. Comp. Endocrinol.* 153, 365–370.

Tsutsui, K., Saigoh, E., Ukena, K., Teranishi, H., Fujisawa, Y., Kikuchi, M., et al. (2000). A novel avian hypothalamic peptide inhibiting gonadotropin release. *Biochem. Biophys. Res. Commun.* 275, 661–667.

Tsutsui, K., and Ubuka, T. (2012). "Gonadotropin-inhibitory hormone," in *Handbook of Biologically Active Peptides. Section on Brain Peptides,* eds A. J. Kastin and H. Vaudry (London: Academic Press) (in press).

Tsutsui, K., Ubuka, T., Bentley, G. E., and Kriegsfeld, L. J. (2012). Gonadotropin-inhibitory hormone (GnIH): discovery, progress and prospect. *Gen. Comp. Endocrinol.* 177, 305–314.

Tsutsui, K., and Ukena, K. (2006). Hypothalamic LPXRF-amide peptides in vertebrates: identification, localization and hypophysiotropic activity. *Peptides* 27, 1121–1129.

Ubuka, T., and Bentley, G. E. (2009). Identification, localization, and regulation of passerine GnRH-I messenger RNA. *J. Endocrinol.* 201, 81–87.

Ubuka, T., and Bentley, G. E. (2011). "Neuroendocrine control of reproduction in birds", in *Hormones and Reproduction of Vertebrates,* Vol. 4, *Birds,* eds D. O. Norris and K. H. Lopez (London: Academic Press), 1–25.

Ubuka, T., Bentley, G. E., Ukena, K., Wingfield, J. C., and Tsutsui, K. (2005). Melatonin induces the expression of gonadotropin-inhibitory hormone in the avian brain. *Proc. Natl. Acad. Sci. U.S.A.* 102, 3052–3057.

Ubuka, T., Cadigan, P. A., Wang, A., Liu, J., and Bentley, G. E. (2009a). Identification of European starling GnRH-I precursor mRNA and its seasonal regulation. *Gen. Comp. Endocrinol.* 162, 301–306.

Ubuka, T., Lai, H., Kitani, M., Suzuuchi, A., Pham, V., Cadigan, P. A., et al. (2009b). Gonadotropin-inhibitory hormone identification, cDNA cloning, and distribution in rhesus macaque brain. *J. Comp. Neurol.* 517, 841–855.

Ubuka, T., Inoue, K., Fukuda, Y., Mizuno, T., Ukena, K., Kriegsfeld, L. J., et al. (2012a). Identification, expression, and physiological functions of Siberian hamster gonadotropin-inhibitory hormone. *Endocrinology* 153, 373–385.

Ubuka, T., Mukai, M., Wolfe, J., Beverly, R., Clegg, S., Wang, A., et al. (2012b). RNA interference of gonadotropin-inhibitory hormone gene induces arousal in songbirds. *PLoS ONE* 7, e30202. doi: 10.1371/journal.pone.0030202

Ubuka, T., Kim, S., Huang, Y. C., Reid, J., Jiang, J., Osugi, T., et al. (2008a). Gonadotropin-inhibitory hormone neurons interact directly with gonadotropin-releasing hormone-I and -II neurons in European starling brain. *Endocrinology* 149, 268–278.

Ubuka, T., McGuire, N. L., Calisi, R. M., Perfito, N., and Bentley, G. E. (2008b). The control of reproductive physiology and behavior by gonadotropin-inhibitory hormone. *Integr. Comp. Biol.* 48, 560–569.

Ubuka, T., Morgan, K., Pawson, A. J., Osugi, T., Chowdhury, V. S., Minakata, H., et al. (2009c). Identification of human GnIH homologs, RFRP-1 and RFRP-3, and the cognate receptor, GPR147 in the human hypothalamic pituitary axis. *PLoS ONE* 4, e8400. doi:10.1371/journal.pone.0008400

Ubuka, T., Ueno, M., Ukena, K., and Tsutsui, K. (2003). Developmental changes in gonadotropin-inhibitory hormone in the Japanese quail (*Coturnix japonica*) hypothalamo-hypophysial system. *J. Endocrinol.* 178, 311–318.

Ubuka, T., Ukena, K., Sharp, P. J., Bentley, G. E., and Tsutsui, K. (2006). Gonadotropin-inhibitory hormone inhibits gonadal development and maintenance by decreasing gonadotropin synthesis and release in male quail. *Endocrinology* 147, 1187–1194.

Ukena, K., Iwakoshi, E., Minakata, H., and Tsutsui, K. (2002). A novel rat hypothalamic RFamide-related peptide identified by immunoaffinity chromatography and mass spectrometry. *FEBS Lett.* 512, 255–258.

Ukena, K., Ubuka, T., and Tsutsui, K. (2003). Distribution of a novel avian gonadotropin-inhibitory hormone in the quail brain. *Cell Tissue Res.* 312, 73–79.

Underwood, H., Binkley, S., Siopes, T., and Mosher, K. (1984). Melatonin rhythms in the eyes, pineal bodies, and blood of Japanese quail (*Coturnix coturnix japonica*). *Gen. Comp. Endocrinol.* 56, 70–81.

Wilson, F. E. (1991). Neither retinal nor pineal photoreceptors mediate photoperiodic control of seasonal reproduction in American tree sparrows (*Spizella arborea*). *J. Exp. Zool.* 259, 117–127.

Wintermantel, T. M., Campbell, R. E., Porteous, R., Bock, D., Gröne, H. J., Todman, M. G., et al. (2006). Definition of estrogen receptor pathway critical for estrogen positive feedback to gonadotropin-releasing hormone neurons and fertility. *Neuron* 52, 271–280.

Wu, M., Dumalska, I., Morozova, E., van den Pol, A. N., and Alreja, M. (2009). Gonadotropin inhibitory hormone inhibits basal forebrain vGluT2-gonadotropin-releasing hormone neurons via a direct postsynaptic mechanism. *J. Physiol.* 587(Pt 7), 1401–1411.

Yin, H., Ukena, K., Ubuka, T., and Tsutsui, K. (2005). A novel G protein-coupled receptor for gonadotropin-inhibitory hormone in the Japanese quail (*Coturnix japonica*): identification, expression and binding activity. *J. Endocrinol.* 184, 257–266.

Yoshida, H., Habata, Y., Hosoya, M., Kawamata, Y., Kitada, C., and Hinuma, S. (2003). Molecular properties of endogenous RFamide-related peptide-3 and its interaction with receptors. *Biochim. Biophys. Acta* 1593, 151–157.

Zhang, Y., Li, S., Liu, Y., Lu, D., Chen, H., Huang, X., et al. (2010). Structural diversity of the GnIH/GnIH receptor system in teleost: its involvement in early development and the negative control of LH release. *Peptides* 31, 1034–1043.

Zhao, S., Zhu, E., Yang, C., Bentley G. E., Tsutsui, K., and Kriegsfeld, L. J. (2010). RFamide-related peptide and messenger ribonucleic acid expression in mammalian testis: association with the spermatogenic cycle. *Endocrinology* 151, 617–627.

5

Decoding high gonadotropin-releasing hormone pulsatility: a role for GnRH receptor coupling to the cAMP pathway

Joëlle Cohen-Tannoudji*, Charlotte Avet, Ghislaine Garrel, Raymond Counis and Violaine Simon

Equipe Physiologie de l'Axe Gonadotrope, Unité de Biologie Fonctionnelle et Adaptative, CNRS-EAC 4413, Sorbonne Paris Cité, Université Paris Diderot-Paris 7, Paris, France

Edited by:
Hubert Vaudry, University of Rouen, France

Reviewed by:
Jong-Ik Hwang, Korea University, South Korea
Yves Combarnous, Centre National de la Recherche Scientifique, France

***Correspondence:**
Joëlle Cohen-Tannoudji, Equipe Physiologie de l'Axe Gonadotrope, Unité de Biologie Fonctionnelle et Adaptative, CNRS-EAC 4413, Sorbonne Paris Cité, Université Paris Diderot-Paris 7, Case courrier 7007, 4 rue Marie-Andrée Lagroua-Weill-Hallé, 75013 Paris, France.
e-mail: joelle.cohen-tannoudji@univ-paris-diderot.fr

The gonadotropin-releasing hormone (GnRH) pulsatile pattern is critical for appropriate regulation of gonadotrope activity but only little is known about the signaling mechanisms by which gonadotrope cells decode such pulsatile pattern. Here, we review recent lines of evidence showing that the GnRH receptor (GnRH-R) activates the cyclic AMP (cAMP) pathway in gonadotrope cells, thus ending a long-lasting controversy. Interestingly, coupling of GnRH-R to the cAMP pathway as well as induction of nitric oxide synthase 1 (NOS1) or follistatin through this signaling pathway take place preferentially under high GnRH pulsatility. The preovulatory surge of GnRH *in vivo* is indeed associated with an important increase of pituitary cAMP and NOS1 expression levels, both being markedly inhibited by treatment with a GnRH antagonist. Altogether, this suggests that due to its atypical structure and desensitization properties, the GnRH-R may continue to signal through the cAMP pathway under conditions inducing desensitization for most other receptors. Such a mechanism may contribute to decode high GnRH pulsatile pattern and enable gonadotrope cell plasticity during the estrus cycle.

Keywords: pituitary, GnRH pulsatile pattern, GnRH receptor, gonadotrope cell signaling, cAMP pathway

INTRODUCTION

Reproduction success depends on the coordinated synthesis and release of several hormones from the hypothalamus–pituitary–gonadal axis. Mammalian gonadotropin-releasing hormone (known as GnRH 1) mediates brain control of reproductive activity and, as a major actor of gonadotrope axis, has received considerable attention. The neurohormone GnRH is a decapeptide produced by a small number of scattered hypothalamic neurons whose cell bodies are primarily located in the preoptic area and basal hypothalamus. GnRH neurons project to the median eminence and secrete GnRH in a pulsatile fashion into the hypophysial portal vessels through which GnRH is transported to the anterior pituitary gland. The release of GnRH by hypothalamic neurons is influenced by numerous external and internal factors acting through central nervous pathways. The pattern of pulsatile GnRH secretion thus varies widely in both males and females depending on the reproductive status. GnRH acts *via* its receptor specifically expressed in gonadotrope cells to stimulate both synthesis and exocytosis of the two gonadotropins, luteinizing hormone (LH) and follicle-stimulating hormone (FSH). LH and FSH will in turn act on the gonads in a coordinated manner to initiate sexual maturation and regulate gonadal steroidogenesis and gametogenesis in both sexes. Gonadotrope hormones are complex endocrine signals constituted of non-covalently associated glycoprotein dimers. Each gonadotropin is composed of an alpha glycoprotein subunit common to LH, FSH, thyrotropin (TSH) and placental choriogonadotropin (for a few species) and a unique beta subunit.

The GnRH pulsatile pattern is critical for appropriate regulation of LH and FSH synthesis and secretion. Indeed, intermittent stimulation *in vivo* or *in vitro* that mimics the physiological pulsatile release of GnRH efficiently stimulates the secretion of gonadotropins. In contrast, a continuous pattern leads to desensitization of gonadotrope cells and this has been exploited by clinicians to suppress gonadotropin secretion (Lahlou et al., 1987). Furthermore, pulsatility of GnRH varies throughout the ovarian cycle and accounts for the differential secretion of LH and FSH. At mid-cycle, during proestrus, an abrupt and massive increase in GnRH pulsatility is responsible for gonadotropin surge and ovulation. Only little is known about the signaling mechanisms by which the pituitary gonadotrope cells decode GnRH pulse pattern. The aim of this article is to review the current knowledge on GnRH receptor (GnRH-R) coupling to the cyclic AMP (cAMP) signaling pathway in order to highlight its potential role in decoding high GnRH pulsatility.

COUPLING OF THE GnRH RECEPTOR TO THE cAMP SIGNALING PATHWAY

GnRH binds to a receptor belonging to the G protein-coupled receptor (GPCR) family with seven transmembrane domains connected by extracellular and intracellular loops. Agonist binding is mainly associated with a rapid Gq/11-mediated increase in phospholipase Cβ (PLCβ) activity, which will in turn initiate a wide array of signaling events. Hydrolysis of phosphatidylinositol 4,5-bisphosphate (PIP2) results in the formation of diacylglycerol

(DAG) and inositol trisphosphate (IP3). Rapid formation of IP3 induces calcium release from intracellular stores and, together with GnRH-stimulated calcium influx, accounts for calcium oscillations that trigger gonadotropin exocytosis. Elevation of calcium also activates the nitric oxide synthase (NOS) cascade (NOS1/NO/soluble guanylate cyclase), resulting in a rapid increase of cyclic GMP (cGMP) levels (Naor et al., 1980; Lozach et al., 1998). GnRH-induced DAG formation activates protein kinase C (PKC) isoforms belonging to the three known families of PKC (conventional, novel, and atypical), which mediate notably activation of mitogen-activated protein kinases (MAPK) cascades. PKC and MAPK signaling are crucial for the regulation of gonadotropin subunit gene expression (Thackray et al., 2009). Following a short time lag, GnRH also activates phospholipase D (PLD) and phospholipase A2 (PLA2). PKC favors the coupling of GnRH-R to PLD leading to a sustained second wave of DAG that may contribute to maintain PKC activation during prolonged stimulation by GnRH (Zheng et al., 1994). GnRH-mediated PLA2 activation generates arachidonic acid and its lipoxygenase products that have been implicated in GnRH-induced gonadotropin synthesis and release (Naor, 2009). The GnRH-R thus activates a wide array of signaling entities to regulate gonadotropin synthesis and release.

It has been clearly established that the cAMP/protein kinase A (PKA) pathway is essential for gonadotrope function. Indeed, cAMP analogs mimic most of the effects of GnRH as they enhance the release of newly synthesized LH and the expression of several key genes including those encoding LHβ and α subunits as well as GnRH-R and NOS1 (Starzec et al., 1989; Garrel et al., 2002; Horton and Halvorson, 2004). However, the ability of GnRH to induce cAMP production in gonadotrope cells as well as the involvement of cAMP in GnRH action has long remained debated. Early observation of Borgeat et al. (1975) showed that a prolonged exposure (3 h) of rat hemipituitaries to GnRH stimulates cAMP accumulation and this observation was confirmed soon after by others (Naor et al., 1975). Since then, studies performed on dispersed rat pituitary cell cultures did not evidence any cAMP production or stimulation of adenylyl-cyclase (AC) activity in response to GnRH (Theoleyre et al., 1976; Conn et al., 1979). In 1989, the pituitary AC-activating polypeptide (PACAP) was discovered based on its ability to strongly activate AC in rat pituitary cells (Miyata et al., 1989). This probably contributed to lower the interest paid to GnRH-R signaling through the cAMP pathway. Furthermore, no GnRH-induced cAMP production could be substantiated on the first gonadotrope cell line that was established in the same period of time, the αT3-1 cell line (Horn et al., 1991). Accordingly, using photolabeling experiments, Grosse et al. (2000) argued for the exclusive coupling of GnRH-R to Gαq/11 in αT3-1 cells. Up to the early 2000s, the coupling of GnRH-R to the cAMP pathway in gonadotrope cells thus remained elusive. The ability of the mammalian GnRH-R to stimulate the cAMP pathway was however reported in several heterologous systems such as GH_3, COS-7, or HeLa cells (Arora et al., 1998; Lin et al., 1998; Oh et al., 2005), thus reinforcing the interest for such coupling. The key to moving forward was the development of novel models and technologies. The ability of GnRH to induce cAMP accumulation in gonadotrope cells was demonstrated by two different groups including ours (Liu et al., 2002; Lariviere et al., 2007) using the gonadotrope cell line LβT2, which is more fully differentiated than the αT3-1 cell line. cAMP accumulation was evidenced by biochemical and enzyme-linked immunosorbent assays (ELISAs) and was specifically induced by GnRH-R activation as shown by competition with a GnRH antagonist. Further analysis revealed that different mechanisms contribute to GnRH-R-induced cAMP accumulation. Indeed, based on photolabeling experiments and on cell-permeable peptides that uncouple the receptor from Gαs, it was shown that GnRH-R activates cAMP production *via* Gs recruitment (Liu et al., 2002). Additionally, we demonstrated, using selective pharmacological inhibitors as well as dominant negative mutants of PKC isoforms, that novel PKCδ and ε mediate GnRH-R activation of the cAMP pathway (Lariviere et al., 2007). In both studies, GnRH-induced increase in cAMP levels exhibited atypical features. Indeed, GnRH-induced maximal accumulation of cAMP levels was observed only after a lag of time of approximately 30 min and was delayed as compared to response to PACAP (Lariviere et al., 2007) or to the beta-adrenergic receptor agonist, isoproterenol (J. Cohen-Tannoudji, personal communication). Furthermore, maximal cAMP accumulation was weaker and this may explain why GnRH-R coupling to this signaling pathway has long remained controversial. This prompted us to reevaluate the coupling of GnRH-R to the cAMP signaling pathway in αT3-1 cells using a recently developed technology. As reported previously by Horn et al. (1991), we did not detect any significant increase in cAMP levels by ELISAs when cells were challenged with a GnRH agonist in contrast to response to PACAP or forskolin stimulation. We then took advantage of a sensitive technology based on the use of a cAMP biosensor (pGloSensor^{TM}-22F cAMP Plasmid). αT3-1 cells were transfected with a plasmid encoding an engineered cAMP sensitive luciferase, which becomes active upon cAMP binding. Transfected cells were challenged with a GnRH agonist and the luminescence intensity was measured in real time in living cells. This strategy allowed us to demonstrate for the first time that GnRH-R couples to the cAMP pathway in αT3-1 cells (Avet et al., 2012). Indeed, GnRH dose-dependently increased luciferase activity reflecting cAMP production with an EC_{50} in the range of 1 nM and the increase was significantly inhibited by co-incubation with the GnRH antagonist, antide. Once the ability of GnRH to stimulate cAMP production was established in both gonadotrope cell lines, our efforts turned toward trying to understand whether this could also occurred in native gonadotrope cells. A massive pituitary cAMP level increase has been reported long ago to occur during the proestrus afternoon of the rat estrus cycle, coincidently with the GnRH preovulatory surge (Kimura et al., 1980). However, despite such temporal coincidence, the precise contribution of GnRH has never been elucidated. We reevaluated this contribution *in vivo* by administrating a potent GnRH antagonist, the ganirelix, to females at the evening of the diestrus II (Garrel et al., 2010). The marked decrease in pituitary cAMP levels provided evidence for a predominant role of GnRH in mediating the proestrus-specific rise of cAMP (**Figure 1**).

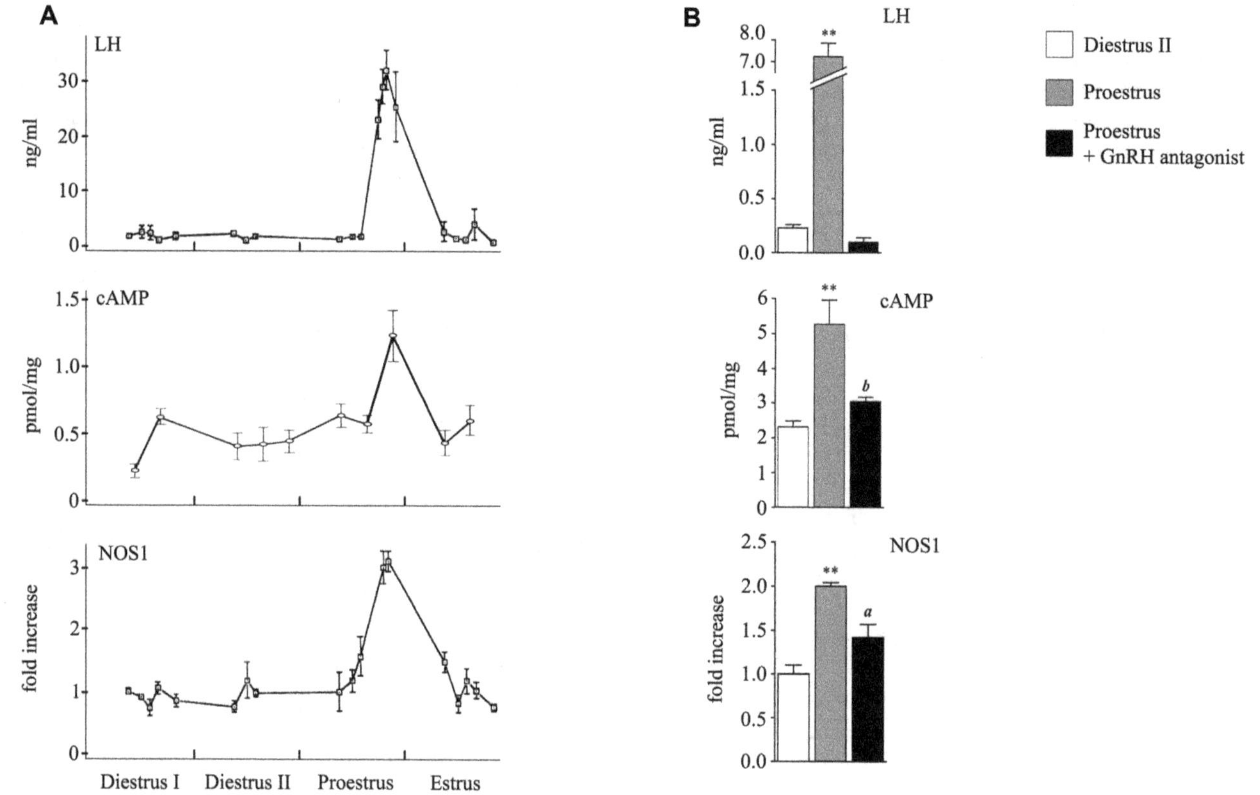

FIGURE 1 | Profiles of serum LH and pituitary cAMP and NOS1 levels during the proestrus and following administration of a GnRH antagonist. **(A)** Serum LH, pituitary cAMP, and pituitary NOS1 levels were determined by radioimmunoassay, ELISA, and western blot analysis, respectively. **(B)** Effect of an *in vivo* treatment with the GnRH antagonist, antarelix. $^{a}P < 0.05$ and $^{b}P < 0.01$ compared with proestrus, $^{**}P < 0.01$ compared with diestrus II. Modified from Kimura et al. (1980), Lozach et al. (1998), and Garrel et al. (2010).

THE ATYPICAL STRUCTURE OF GnRH RECEPTOR IS ASSOCIATED WITH RESISTANCE TO RAPID DESENSITIZATION

All mammalian pituitary GnRH-R (named type I GnRH-R) exhibit a striking structural feature, which is the lack of a cytoplasmic carboxyl-terminal tail. This carboxyl-terminal tail is present in all other GPCR including GnRH-R from non-mammalian vertebrates and is a target for kinases such as GRK (GPCR kinase). GRK-mediated phosphorylation promotes the binding of β-arrestins, which not only uncouple receptors from G proteins resulting in desensitization but also target many GPCR for internalization in clathrin-coated vesicles (Ferguson, 2001). Given the unique absence of cytoplasmic carboxyl-terminal tail, the initial rate of inositol phosphate accumulation is linear upon 10 min of GnRH stimulation showing that GnRH-R is resistance to rapid desensitization (Davidson et al., 1994). Accordingly, mammalian GnRH-R is not phosphorylated upon agonist stimulation and does not recruit β-arrestins, in contrast to non-mammalian GnRH-R (Willars et al., 1999; McArdle et al., 2002). Extensive analysis of GnRH-R internalization has been performed using biochemical approaches and fluorescent or radiolabeled GnRH in gonadotrope and heterologous cells. These studies indicated that mammalian GnRH-R is poorly internalized as compared to non-mammalian GnRH-R and that addition of a functional intracellular carboxyl-terminal tail to the receptor significantly increased internalization rates and rapid desensitization. Whereas these studies were rather measuring ligand internalization, investigations conducted by Millar's group, using an epitope-tagged receptor allowed to trace the receptor itself. These studies established that GnRH-R exhibits a low level of constitutive internalization and does not undergo rapid agonist-dependent internalization as compared to non-mammalian GnRH or the TSH-releasing hormone receptors (Pawson et al., 2008). The refractory state of gonadotrope cells under a sustained GnRH challenge is thus believed to occur through desensitization mechanism affecting downstream signaling entities such as Gαq/11, PKC isoforms, or IP3 receptors (Willars et al., 2001; Liu et al., 2003) rather than the receptor itself. Consequently, mammalian GnRH-R has the unique property amongst GPCR to face prolonged activation by its ligand.

MECHANISMS CONTRIBUTING TO GnRH-R COUPLING TO THE cAMP PATHWAY

One intriguing property of GnRH-R coupling to the cAMP pathway in LβT2 cells is that it appears to be dependent on GnRH stimulation pattern. We, indeed, observed that an intermittent stimulation of cells with GnRH, known to stimulate calcium release or MAPK activation, was ineffective in inducing cAMP accumulation (Lariviere et al., 2007). Levels of cAMP were significantly increased only under sustained stimulation of GnRH-R suggesting that this pathway may be preferentially recruited under high frequency of GnRH pulses, in agreement with the proestrus-specific elevation of pituitary cAMP levels during rat ovarian cycle (Kimura et al., 1980; Garrel et al., 2010). This shows that GnRH-R maintains cAMP pathway activation under stimulations inducing desensitization of most GPCR. This atypical feature was recently confirmed using fluorescence resonance energy transfer reporters in LβT2 cells in which high pulse frequency of GnRH desensitized DAG and calcium but not cAMP activation (Tsutsumi et al., 2010).

Only few genes regulated by GnRH through the cAMP/PKA signaling pathway have been identified so far. Among them are those encoding follistatin, Nur77, PACAP, and NOS1 (Winters et al., 2007; Hamid et al., 2008; Grafer et al., 2009; Mutiara et al., 2009; Garrel et al., 2010). Interestingly, analysis of how GnRH regulates two of these genes has revealed that they are preferentially induced under high GnRH pulse frequency. Follistatin transcript and protein are increased by GnRH administered continuously or at fast frequency pulses either *in vivo* in rat or in a perifused pituitary cells (Besecke et al., 1996) and not at slow GnRH pulse frequencies. Because follistatin binds to and neutralizes activin, stimulation of FSHβ by GnRH, which requires activin is blocked. This is believed to explain why expression of FSHβ is preferentially stimulated under low frequency of GnRH pulses. In rat anterior pituitary gland, NOS1 is expressed specifically in gonadotrope and folliculostellate cells. Our group has demonstrated from experiments performed *in vivo* in rats and *in vitro* that NOS1 expression is regulated by GnRH through the cAMP pathway (Garrel et al., 1998; Lozach et al., 1998). This was shown in particular by taking advantage of a cell-permeant PKA inhibitor (PKI) peptide delivery in primary cultures of rat pituitary cells (Garrel et al., 2010). Interestingly, we observed that NOS1 is preferentially induced by prolonged GnRH treatment. Indeed, NOS1 expression remained at high levels for at least 48 h after treatment of rats with a long-lasting GnRH agonist, whereas, at the same time, LH and FSH secretion was desensitized. Accordingly, we demonstrated in perifused rat pituitary cells that NOS1 is not induced by GnRH delivered at a frequency of one pulse per hour, although this frequency is able to trigger a massive LH release. In contrast, NOS1 was maximally induced by a continuous GnRH stimulation, which suppressed gonadotropin release. Such a result is in agreement with *in vivo* data showing a marked increase of NOS1 expression at proestrus during the preovulatory GnRH surge, which is characterized by a very high GnRH pulse frequency (Lozach et al., 1998; **Figure 1**). Interestingly, treatment with the GnRH antagonist ganirelix not only blocked the proestrus-specific cAMP increase (see above) but also significantly reduced the rise of NOS1 expression levels (Garrel et al., 2010; **Figure 1**) further supporting the physiological relevance of GnRH-R coupling to the cAMP pathway. Altogether, experiments reported here, suggest that under conditions of high GnRH pulsatility, GnRH-R, which is atypically maintained at the cell surface, still interacts with its intracellular machinery and activates the cAMP/PKA pathway. This initiates the expression of a new set of target proteins among which are NOS1 and follistatin. The role of GnRH-dependent NOS1 induction at proestrus remains to be determined. The specific increase of NOS1 expression leads to a concomitant huge increase of pituitary cGMP levels at proestrus (Lozach et al., 1998). cGMP may regulate some cyclic nucleotide-gated channels that we have characterized in pituitary gonadotrope cells (J. Cohen-Tannoudji, personal communication) and this is under investigation.

How is the preferential coupling of GnRH-R to the cAMP pathway selected? This question is still unresolved. GnRH-R is constitutively localized in low-density membrane microdomains such as rafts (Navratil et al., 2003). Intense stimulation by GnRH may alter the signaling platform associated with GnRH-R in rafts and hence favor receptor coupling to the cAMP pathway. Another potential mechanism may be related to GPCR-interacting proteins (GIP) that interact through receptor intracellular domains to regulate signaling efficacy and specificity (Bockaert et al., 2004). The idea that GIP regulate GnRH-R signaling is suggested by the fact that introduction in αT3-1 cells of synthetic peptides corresponding to intracellular domains of mammalian GnRH-R increases GnRH-R coupling to the inositol phosphate pathway (Shacham et al., 2005). We very recently identified a protein, the protein SET, as the first direct interacting partner of GnRH-R. Using cAMP and calcium biosensors in αT3-1 living cells combined with small interfering RNA directed against SET, we showed that SET significantly enhances GnRH-R coupling to the cAMP pathway. The mechanisms contributing to SET recruitment and the potential regulatory roles of SET on gonadotrope function are under current investigation.

CONCLUSION

An important question in the field of reproductive endocrinology is to understand how the GnRH pulsatile pattern is decoded by pituitary gonadotrope cells. Due to its atypical structure and desensitization properties, GnRH-R and some of its signaling mechanisms are continuing to respond under massive GnRH stimulations. Such stimulations of gonadotrope cells by GnRH thus do not lead to general cell desensitization since some genes are induced in response to GnRH at high pulse frequencies. Variation in GnRH pulse profiles may lead to preferential activation of different signaling networks and there is now evidence that the cAMP/PKA pathway contributes to the decoding of high GnRH pulsatility. This emphasizes the unique feature of gonadotrope cells, which maintain part of their functional response under conditions of stimulation inducing desensitization of most GPCR. During the ovarian cycle, the GnRH preovulatory surge lasts much longer than the LH surge (Caraty et al., 2002). Maintenance of some gonadotrope responsiveness while gonadotropins are no longer secreted may contribute to gonadotrope cell plasticity during the estrus cycle. Identifying the mechanisms directing the preferential coupling of GnRH-R to the cAMP pathway is an exciting challenge. Insight into GnRH-R interacting partners and into the dynamics of their interactions with the receptor will undoubtedly help to better understand the plasticity of gonadotrope cell signaling.

ACKNOWLEDGMENT

Authors are grateful to Richard Wargnier for his contribution to the illustration of the manuscript.

REFERENCES

Arora, K. K., Krsmanovic, L. Z., Mores, N., O'Farrell, H., and Catt, K. J. (1998). Mediation of cyclic AMP signaling by the first intracellular loop of the gonadotropin-releasing hormone receptor. *J. Biol. Chem.* 273, 25581–25586.

Avet, C., Garrel, G., Denoyelle, C., Laverrière, J. N., Counis, R., Cohen-Tannoudji, J., and Simon, V. (2012). "First identification of a direct interacting partner of the GnRH receptor, the protein SET. Differential impact on coupling to cAMP and calcium pathways," in *Keystone Symposia's Meeting*, Banff, Canada, February 17–22 (Abstract 105).

Besecke, L. M., Guendner, M. J., Schneyer, A. L., Bauer-Dantoin, A. C., Jameson, J. L., and Weiss, J. (1996). Gonadotropin-releasing hormone regulates follicle-stimulating hormone-beta gene expression through an activin/follistatin autocrine or paracrine loop. *Endocrinology* 137, 3667–3673.

Bockaert, J., Fagni, L., Dumuis, A., and Marin, P. (2004). GPCR interacting proteins (GIP). *Pharmacol. Ther.* 103, 203–221.

Borgeat, P., Garneau, P., and Labrie, F. (1975). Calcium requirement for stimulation of cyclic AMP accumulation in anterior pituitary gland by LH-RH. *Mol. Cell. Endocrinol.* 2, 117–124.

Caraty, A., Delaleu, B., Chesneau, D., and Fabre-Nys, C. (2002). Sequential role of e2 and GnRH for the expression of estrous behavior in ewes. *Endocrinology* 143, 139–145.

Conn, P. M., Morrell, D. V., Dufau, M. L., and Catt, K. J. (1979). Gonadotropin-releasing hormone action in cultured pituicytes: independence of luteinizing hormone release and adenosine 3′,5′- monophosphate production. *Endocrinology* 104, 448–453.

Davidson, J. S., Wakefield, I. K., and Millar, R. P. (1994). Absence of rapid desensitization of the mouse gonadotropin-releasing hormone receptor. *Biochem. J.* 300(Pt 2), 299–302.

Ferguson, S. S. (2001). Evolving concepts in G protein-coupled receptor endocytosis: the role in receptor desensitization and signaling. *Pharmacol. Rev.* 53, 1–24.

Garrel, G., Lerrant, Y., Siriostis, C., Berault, A., Magre, S., Bouchaud, C., and Counis, R. (1998). Evidence that gonadotropin-releasing hormone stimulates gene expression and levels of active nitric oxide synthase type I in pituitary gonadotrophs, a process altered by desensitization and, indirectly, by gonadal steroids. *Endocrinology* 139, 2163–2170.

Garrel, G., Lozach, A., Bachir, L. K., Laverriere, J. N., and Counis, R. (2002). Pituitary adenylate cyclase-activating polypeptide stimulates nitric-oxide synthase type I expression and potentiates the cGMP response to gonadotropin-releasing hormone of rat pituitary gonadotrophs. *J. Biol. Chem.* 277, 46391–46401.

Garrel, G., Simon, V., Thieulant, M. L., Cayla, X., Garcia, A., Counis, R., and Cohen-Tannoudji, J. (2010). Sustained gonadotropin-releasing hormone stimulation mobilizes the cAMP/PKA pathway to induce nitric oxide synthase type 1 expression in rat pituitary cells in vitro and in vivo at proestrus. *Biol. Reprod.* 82, 1170–1179.

Grafer, C. M., Thomas, R., Lambrakos, L., Montoya, I., White, S., and Halvorson, L. M. (2009). GnRH stimulates expression of PACAP in the pituitary gonadotropes via both the PKA and PKC signaling systems. *Mol. Endocrinol.* 23, 1022–1032.

Grosse, R., Schmid, A., Schoneberg, T., Herrlich, A., Muhn, P., Schultz, G., and Gudermann, T. (2000). Gonadotropin-releasing hormone receptor initiates multiple signaling pathways by exclusively coupling to G(q/11) proteins. *J. Biol. Chem.* 275, 9193–9200.

Hamid, T., Malik, M. T., Millar, R. P., and Kakar, S. S. (2008). Protein kinase A serves as a primary pathway in activation of Nur77 expression by gonadotropin-releasing hormone in the LbetaT2 mouse pituitary gonadotroph tumor cell line. *Int. J. Oncol.* 33, 1055–1064.

Horn, F., Bilezikjian, L. M., Perrin, M. H., Bosma, M. M., Windle, J. J., Huber, K. S., Blount, A. L., Hille, B., Vale, W., and Mellon, P. L. (1991). Intracellular responses to gonadotropin-releasing hormone in a clonal cell line of the gonadotrope lineage. *Mol. Endocrinol.* 5, 347–355.

Horton, C. D., and Halvorson, L. M. (2004). The cAMP signaling system regulates LHbeta gene expression: roles of early growth response protein-1, SP1 and steroidogenic factor-1. *J. Mol. Endocrinol.* 32, 291–306.

Kimura, F., Kawakami, M., Nakano, H., and McCann, S. M. (1980). Changes in adenosine 3′,5′-monophosphate and guanosine 3′,5′-monophosphate concentrations in the anterior pituitary and hypothalamus during the rat estrous cycle and effects of administration of sodium pentobarbital in proestrus. *Endocrinology* 106, 631–635.

Lahlou, N., Roger, M., Chaussain, J. L., Feinstein, M. C., Sultan, C., Toublanc, J. E., Schally, A. V., and Scholler, R. (1987). Gonadotropin and alpha-subunit secretion during long term pituitary suppression by D-Trp6-luteinizing hormone-releasing hormone microcapsules as treatment of precocious puberty. *J. Clin. Endocrinol. Metab.* 65, 946–953.

Lariviere, S., Garrel, G., Simon, V., Soh, J. W., Laverriere, J. N., Counis, R., and Cohen-Tannoudji, J. (2007). Gonadotropin-releasing hormone couples to 3′,5′-cyclic adenosine-5′-monophosphate pathway through novel protein kinase Cdelta and -epsilon in LbetaT2 gonadotrope cells. *Endocrinology* 148, 1099–1107.

Lin, X., Janovick, J. A., and Conn, P. M. (1998). Mutations at the consensus phosphorylation sites in the third intracellular loop of the rat gonadotropin-releasing hormone receptor: effects on receptor ligand binding and signal transduction. *Biol. Reprod.* 59, 1470–1476.

Liu, F., Austin, D. A., and Webster, N. J. (2003). Gonadotropin-releasing hormone-desensitized LbetaT2 gonadotrope cells are refractory to acute protein kinase C, cyclic AMP, and calcium-dependent signaling. *Endocrinology* 144, 4354–4365.

Liu, F., Usui, I., Evans, L. G., Austin, D. A., Mellon, P. L., Olefsky, J. M., and Webster, N. J. (2002). Involvement of both G(q/11) and G(s) proteins in gonadotropin-releasing hormone receptor-mediated signaling in L beta T2 cells. *J. Biol. Chem.* 277, 32099–32108.

Lozach, A., Garrel, G., Lerrant, Y., Berault, A., and Counis, R. (1998). GnRH-dependent up-regulation of nitric oxide synthase I level in pituitary gonadotrophs mediates cGMP elevation during rat proestrus. *Mol. Cell. Endocrinol.* 143, 43–51.

McArdle, C. A., Franklin, J., Green, L., and Hislop, J. N. (2002). Signalling, cycling and desensitisation of gonadotrophin-releasing hormone receptors. *J. Endocrinol.* 173, 1–11.

Miyata, A., Arimura, A., Dahl, R. R., Minamino, N., Uehara, A., Jiang, L., Culler, M. D., and Coy, D. H. (1989). Isolation of a novel 38 residue-hypothalamic polypeptide which stimulates adenylate cyclase in pituitary cells. *Biochem. Biophys. Res. Commun.* 164, 567–574.

Mutiara, S., Kanasaki, H., Oride, A., Purwana, I. N., Shimasaki, S., Yamamoto, H., and Miyazaki, K. (2009). Follistatin gene expression by gonadotropin-releasing hormone: a role for cyclic AMP and mitogen-activated protein kinase signaling pathways in clonal gonadotroph LbetaT2 cells. *Mol. Cell. Endocrinol.* 307, 125–132.

Naor, Z. (2009). Signaling by G-protein-coupled receptor (GPCR): studies on the GnRH receptor. *Front. Neuroendocrinol.* 30, 10–29.

Naor, Z., Koch, Y., Chobsieng, P., and Zor, U. (1975). Pituitary cyclic AMP production and mechanism of luteinizing hormone release. *FEBS Lett.* 58, 318–321.

Naor, Z., Leifer, A. M., and Catt, K. J. (1980). Calcium-dependent actions of gonadotropin-releasing hormone on pituitary guanosine 3′,5′-monophosphate production and gonadotropin release. *Endocrinology* 107, 1438–1445.

Navratil, A. M., Bliss, S. P., Berghorn, K. A., Haughian, J. M., Farmerie, T. A., Graham, J. K., Clay, C. M., and Roberson, M. S. (2003). Constitutive localization of the gonadotropin-releasing hormone (GnRH) receptor to low density membrane microdomains is necessary for GnRH signaling to ERK. *J. Biol. Chem.* 278, 31593–31602.

Oh, D. Y., Song, J. A., Moon, J. S., Moon, M. J., Kim, J. I., Kim, K., Kwon, H. B., and Seong, J. Y. (2005). Membrane-proximal region of the carboxyl terminus of the gonadotropin-releasing hormone receptor (GnRHR) confers differential signal transduction between mammalian and nonmammalian GnRHRs. *Mol. Endocrinol.* 19, 722–731.

Pawson, A. J., Faccenda, E., Maudsley, S., Lu, Z. L., Naor, Z., and Millar, R. P. (2008). Mammalian type I gonadotropin-releasing hormone receptors undergo slow, constitutive, agonist-independent internalization. *Endocrinology* 149, 1415–1422.

Shacham, S., Cheifetz, M. N., Fridkin, M., Pawson, A. J., Millar, R. P., and Naor, Z. (2005). Identification of Ser153 in ICL2 of the gonadotropin-releasing hormone (GnRH) receptor as a phosphorylation-independent site for inhibition of Gq coupling. *J. Biol. Chem.* 280, 28981–28988.

Starzec, A., Jutisz, M., and Counis, R. (1989). Cyclic adenosine monophosphate and phorbol ester, like gonadotropin-releasing hormone, stimulate the biosynthesis of luteinizing hormone polypeptide chains in a nonadditive manner. *Mol. Endocrinol.* 3, 618–624.

Thackray, V. G., Mellon, P. L., and Coss, D. (2009). Hormones in synergy: regulation of the pituitary gonadotropin genes. *Mol. Cell. Endocrinol.* 314, 192–203.

Theoleyre, M., Berault, A., Garnier, J., and Jutisz, M. (1976). Binding of gonadotropin-releasing hormone (LH-RH) to the pituitary plasma membranes and the problem of adenylate cyclase stimulation. *Mol. Cell. Endocrinol.* 5, 365–377.

Tsutsumi, R., Mistry, D., and Webster, N. J. (2010). Signaling responses to pulsatile gonadotropin-releasing hormone in LbetaT2 gonadotrope cells. *J. Biol. Chem.* 285, 20262–20272.

Willars, G. B., Heding, A., Vrecl, M., Sellar, R., Blomenrohr, M., Nahorski, S. R., and Eidne, K. A. (1999). Lack of a C-terminal tail in the mammalian gonadotropin-releasing hormone receptor confers resistance to agonist-dependent phosphorylation and rapid desensitization. *J. Biol. Chem.* 274, 30146–30153.

Willars, G. B., Royall, J. E., Nahorski, S. R., El-Gehani, F., Everest, H., and McArdle, C. A. (2001). Rapid down-regulation of the type I inositol 1,4,5-trisphosphate receptor and desensitization of gonadotropin-releasing hormone-mediated Ca2+ responses in alpha T3-1 gonadotropes. *J. Biol. Chem.* 276, 3123–3129.

Winters, S. J., Ghooray, D., Fujii, Y., Moore, J. P. Jr., Nevitt, J. R., and Kakar, S. S. (2007). Transcriptional regulation of follistatin expression by GnRH in mouse gonadotroph cell lines: evidence for a role for cAMP signaling. *Mol. Cell. Endocrinol.* 271, 45–54.

Zheng, L., Stojilkovic, S. S., Hunyady, L., Krsmanovic, L. Z., and Catt, K. J. (1994). Sequential activation of phospholipase-C and -D in agonist-stimulated gonadotrophs. *Endocrinology* 134, 1446–1454.

6

Ghrelin: central and peripheral implications in anorexia nervosa

Mathieu Méquinion[1], Fanny Langlet[1], Sara Zgheib[2], Suzanne Dickson[3,4], Bénédicte Dehouck[1,5], Christophe Chauveau[2†] and Odile Viltart[1,6*†]

[1] UMR INSERM 837, Development and Plasticity of Postnatal Brain, Lille, France
[2] Pathophysiology of inflammatory of bone diseases, Université Lille Nord de France-ULCO – Lille 2, Boulogne sur Mer, France
[3] Department of Physiology, Institute of Neuroscience and Physiology, The Sahlgrenska Academy, University of Gothenburg, Gothenburg, Sweden
[4] Department of Endocrinology, Institute of Neuroscience and Physiology, The Sahlgrenska Academy, University of Gothenburg, Gothenburg, Sweden
[5] Université Lille Nord de France – Université d'Artois, Liévin, France
[6] Université Lille Nord de France-USTL (Lille 1), Villeneuve d'Ascq, France

Edited by:
Hubert Vaudry, University of Rouen, France

Reviewed by:
Masamitsu Nakazato, University of Miyazaki, Japan
Paolo Magni, Università degli Studi di Milano, Italy

***Correspondence:**
Odile Viltart, Development and Plasticity of the Postnatal Brain, Team 2, Jean-Pierre Aubert Research Center, UMR INSERM 837, Bât Biserte, 1 place de Verdun, 59,045 Lille cedex, France.
e-mail: odile.viltart@univ-lille1.fr

† Christophe Chauveau and Odile Viltart have contributed equally to this work.

Increasing clinical and therapeutic interest in the neurobiology of eating disorders reflects their dramatic impact on health. Chronic food restriction resulting in severe weight loss is a major symptom described in restrictive anorexia nervosa (AN) patients, and they also suffer from metabolic disturbances, infertility, osteopenia, and osteoporosis. Restrictive AN, mostly observed in young women, is the third largest cause of chronic illness in teenagers of industrialized countries. From a neurobiological perspective, AN-linked behaviors can be considered an adaptation that permits the endurance of reduced energy supply, involving central and/or peripheral reprograming. The severe weight loss observed in AN patients is accompanied by significant changes in hormones involved in energy balance, feeding behavior, and bone formation, all of which can be replicated in animals models. Increasing evidence suggests that AN could be an addictive behavior disorder, potentially linking defects in the reward mechanism with suppressed food intake, heightened physical activity, and mood disorder. Surprisingly, the plasma levels of ghrelin, an orexigenic hormone that drives food-motivated behavior, are increased. This increase in plasma ghrelin levels seems paradoxical in light of the restrained eating adopted by AN patients, and may rather result from an adaptation to the disease. The aim of this review is to describe the role played by ghrelin in AN focusing on its central vs. peripheral actions. In AN patients and in rodent AN models, chronic food restriction induces profound alterations in the « ghrelin »signaling that leads to the development of inappropriate behaviors like hyperactivity or addiction to food starvation and therefore a greater depletion in energy reserves. The question of a transient insensitivity to ghrelin and/or a potential metabolic reprograming is discussed in regard of new clinical treatments currently investigated.

Keywords: ghrelin, anorexia, food intake, energy balance, central alterations, peripheral alterations, reward, animal models

INTRODUCTION

Feeding is a behavior that ensures an adequate and varied supply of nutritional substrates essential to maintain energy levels for basal metabolism, physical activity, growth, and reproduction and hence, for survival of every living organism on Earth. In the case of mammals, that must maintain a stable body temperature, the maintenance of a high metabolic rate requires constant availability of a sufficient amount of energy stores. The tight balance between energy demand and expenditure is fine-tuned by an adapted dialog between homeostatic and hedonic brain systems that are regulated by peripheral signals involved in feeding behavior and energy homeostasis. Mechanisms for feeding control remain a current and crucial scientific subject for understanding the etiology and potential therapeutic approaches for the treatment of food intake disorders that include obesity, on one hand, and severe forms of anorexia nervosa (AN) on the other.

Voluntary anorexia is a disease not unique to man and has even been described in many vertebrate species that favor migration activity (Wang et al., 2006). In this case, surviving food deprivation involves an adaptation of metabolism, such that internal energy stores available at the onset of fasting are used to maintain basal metabolism and physical activity. The biochemical and physiological adaptations that result from a lack of food help to preserve physiological function in order to maintain behaviors like food seeking or predator avoidance and also, to resume all metabolic processes necessary when food becomes available. However, absolute or long term food deprivation observed in nature or in restrictive AN proceeds in stages in which the individual/organism tries to adapt its metabolism to energy costs but that culminates in death, due to exhaustion of energy stores. As clearly described by Wang et al. (2006), the different stages progress from fasting to starvation, but "*The demarcation between these two states is rarely appreciated, perhaps owing to lack of definition. In humans, fasting often refers to abstinence from food, whereas starvation is used for a state of extreme hunger resulting from a prolonged lack of essential nutrients. In other words, starving is a state in which an animal, having depleted energy stores, normally would feed to continue normal physiological processes.*" Briefly, three metabolic phases are described during food deprivation (Wang et al., 2006) where energy metabolic adaptations occur to allow supply of fuel in the different parts of the organism, especially the brain (see **Table 1**). In regard to these metabolic stages, the transition from fasting to starvation occurs by the end of phase II or the beginning of phase III. Thus, voluntary anorexia as seen in restrictive AN should correspond to phases I and II.

Restrictive AN is a feeding behavior disorder for which severe chronic food restriction causes dramatic physiological and psychological effects that are detrimental for health. AN is most prevalent in women aged of 25 years old or younger (whose BMI reaches values largely below 18.5 kg/m^2) and is currently the third largest cause of chronic illness in teenagers (Lucas et al., 1991). The prevalence of AN has drastically increased within recent decades. It leads to central and/or peripheral reprograming that permits the individual/organism to endure a reduced energy supply. These drastic conditions not only induce severe weight loss and metabolic disturbance, but also infertility, osteopenia, and osteoporosis. Moreover, AN is increasingly recognized as an addictive behavior disorder. *-Indeed, many of its common primary characteristics – food obsession coupled with food restriction, weight loss, heightened physical activity, and the strong association with mood disorder (such as anxiety or depression), strongly suggest a potential alteration of the central (dopaminergic) reward system.

Anorexia nervosa patients exhibit significant changes in the release of key hormones involved in energy balance and feeding control (Hasan and Hasan, 2011). For example, the plasma levels of ghrelin, an orexigenic hormone mostly released from the empty stomach, are increased in AN patients along all the day (Germain et al., 2009, 2010). This hormone acts centrally to increase food intake (Wren et al., 2001a,b) and food-motivated behavior (Skibicka et al., 2012), but has also been suggested to be required for the maintenance of blood glucose homeostasis during severe calorie restriction (Zhao et al., 2010). The increases in plasma ghrelin levels in AN seem paradoxical in light of the restrained eating adopted by these patients and suggest an adaptive response to the disease. In regard to the metabolic deficiencies occurring in restrictive AN (see *infra*), the aim of this review is to highlight the impact of ghrelin in the adaptation of the organism to chronic food restriction until it falls into exhaustion and death. A better understanding of the role of this gastric hormone in dysfunctional AN like feeding behavior is important when evaluating its therapeutic potential for the treatment of AN, envisaged to be used alongside mainstay psychiatric and nutritional therapies.

Table 1 | Different metabolic phases occurring during food restriction and permitting distinction between fasting and starvation (see Wang et al., 2006).

PHASE I: FASTING
= postabsorptive phase (***Hours***)

↑ Glycogen depletion (from liver stores)
↑ Fatty acids release (from adipose tissues)

PHASE II: From FASTING to STARVATION (*Several weeks*)

=> ***End of glycogen stores***
↑ gluconeogenesis
* from adipose tissues (*rapid*)
↓
oxydation of fatty acids
↓
↗ketone bodies
* from proteolysis of muscle protein (*slow*)

PHASE III: From STARVATION to DEATH

* Dramatic depletion of adipose stores
* Degradation of muscular mass

All the metabolic changes aim to deliver sufficient amount of glucose for different organs and especially for the brain.

PHYSIOLOGICAL ALTERATIONS IN ANOREXIA NERVOSA

TYPES AND SUBTYPES OF ANOREXIA NERVOSA: NEW DSM-V CLASSIFICATION

Chronic food restriction is linked to several disorders classified in DSM-V (Diagnostic and Statistical Manuel of Mental Disorders). In the provisional version of DSM-V (of spring 2012; http://www.dsm5.org/meetus/pages/eatingdisorders.aspx), the *Feeding and Eating Disorders* category includes three disorders as manifested by persistent failure to meet appropriate nutritional and/or energy needs and significant weight loss, *AN, avoidant/restrictive food intake disorder (ARFIDO), and atypical AN.*

Diagnostic criteria for AN includes the restriction of energy intake relative to requirements, a drastic significant loss of body weight, an intense fear of gaining weight, body image disturbance, and/or a persistent lack of recognition of the seriousness of the current low body weight. In a recent review (Garcia et al., 2011), the lifetime prevalence of AN was estimated to be 1.9% in female adults to 2.6% in female adolescents in industrialized countries. In the binge eating/purging subtype, the individual engages in recurrent episodes of binge eating or purging behavior while such episodes do not occur in the restricting subtype. Patients from these two subtypes also exhibit differences in eating disorder symptom indicators (Olatunji et al., 2012). However, the subtype determination at the time of the diagnosis should be considered carefully since, over a 7-year period, the majority of women with AN were found to cross over to the restricting and binge eating/purging AN subtypes (Eddy et al., 2008). In a 21-year follow-up study, Löwe et al. (2001) showed that 16% of AN patients deceased due to consequences of their illness: about 50% died because of somatic complications leading to heart attack and the remainder committed suicide. Moreover, mortality is significantly more common among inpatients with somatic comorbidity (like renal, cardiac, bone, and digestive pathologies) than among inpatients without a somatic disease (Erdur et al., 2012). Finally, among the psychiatric comorbidities, AN is often associated with depression, anxiety, obsessive compulsive or personality disorders, and drug abuse (Erdur et al., 2012). Whether AN resembles an addiction behavior disorder remains one major question for physicians and researchers alike. The criteria proposed by Goodman (1990) to identify addictive disorder (**Table 2**) are found in AN patients. Indeed, Speranza et al. (2012) showed that 35% of the restrictive AN subtype patients, 48% of the binge eating/purging AN subtype patients and 60% of the patients have substance-use disorders and hence, exhibit an addictive disorder according to Goodman's criteria. From these criteria, an emerging hypothesis of AN implicates neurobiological mechanisms (and hence, investigation strategies for treatments and diagnostic markers) that are based on a reward deficit and on the recognition as an addictive behavior disorder (Alguacil et al., 2011). In fact, among the different theories linking AN and addiction, interestingly, the "auto-addiction opioid model" proposes that this chronic eating disorder could represent an addiction to the body's endogenous opioids, especially β-endorphins (see Davis and Claridge, 1998). Starvation and excessive exercise, that concern a high percentage of AN patients (Davis et al., 1997; Kohl et al., 2004), are associated with increased levels of β-endorphin, known to further stimulate dopamine in the mesolimbic reward centers (Bergh and Södersten, 1996; Casper, 1998). This mesolimbic pathway plays a pivotal role in addictive behaviors related to drugs and dietary behaviors (Avena and Bocarsly, 2012; Perelló and Zigman, 2012). Importantly, this mesolimbic dopamine pathway is activated by ghrelin (Abizaid et al., 2006; Jerlhag et al., 2006; see *infra*) and, since AN patients have high plasma ghrelin levels (Germain et al., 2009, 2010), it follows that there may be a dysfunctional ghrelin-(dopamine) reward signal in these patients. However, as discussed by Barbarich-Marsteller et al. (2011), there are fundamental differences between AN and addiction. Indeed, the main goal of an individual suffering from a substance abuse disorder is to pursue the immediate effects of the drug on mood and/or behavior (alleviation of anxiety, for example), whereas the goals of an AN patient are both immediate and long term. In these patients, dieting and starvation produce immediate feelings of hunger that may induce a sense of control over one's body and thereby a sense of control over one's life while, in the long term, it produces sustained weight loss and thinness that take on an irrationally important value.

In the ARFIDO, insufficient food intake is associated with significant weight loss, nutritional deficiency, dependence on enteral feeding, or nutritional supplements and/or a marked psychosocial dysfunction. In these patients, the eating disturbance does not occur exclusively during the course of AN, and is not associated with body image disturbances. ARFIDO is a new recognized eating disorder previously classified in the left over category *Eating Disorder Not Otherwise Specified* (EDNOS) corresponding to the majority of in-and-out patients treated for eating disorders. Its prevalence remains to be determined.

Table 2 | Addictive disorder criteria according to Goodman (1990).

A. Recurrent failure to resist impulses to engage in a specified behavior
B. Increasing sense of tension immediately prior the initiation of behavior
C. Pleasure or relief at the time of engaging in the behavior
D. A feeling of a lack of control while engaging in the behavior
E. At least five of the following:
  1. Frequent preoccupation with the behavior or preparatory activities
  2. Frequent engaging in the behavior to a greater extent or over a longer period than intended
  3. Repeated efforts to reduce, control, or stop the behavior
  4. A great deal of time spent in activities necessary for the behavior, engaging in the behavior, or recovering from its effects
  5. Frequent engaging in the behavior when expected to fulfill occupational, academic, domestic, or social obligations
  6. Important social, occupational, or recreational activities given up or reduced because of the behavior
  7. Continuation of the behavior despite knowledge of having a persistent or recurrent social, financial, psychological, or physical problem that is caused or exacerbated by the behavior
  8. Tolerance: need to increase the intensity or frequency of the behavior in order to achieve the desired effect or diminished effect with continued behavior of the same intensity
  9. Restlessness or irritability if unable to engage in the behavior
F. Some symptoms of the disturbance have persisted for at least 1 month or have occurred repeatedly over a longer period of time

To reach the categorical diagnosis of addictive disorder according to Goodman (1990), criteria A–D plus criterion E (five among nine symptoms) must be met for at least 1 month.

The last disorder, *atypical AN*, is in the EDNOS category. It includes all the criteria for AN diagnosis except that, despite significant weight loss, the individual's weight is within or above the normal range. The lifetime prevalence of atypical AN ranges from 2.4% in female adults to 7.7% in female adolescents (Garcia et al., 2011).

Considering this recent classification, in this review we focus on restrictive AN in which the individual is subjected to chronic food restriction that may or may not be associated with intense physical exercise. In fact, the course of AN is extremely variable, with approximately 50–60% of individuals recovering, 20–30% partially recovering, and 10–20% remain chronically ill (Löwe et al., 2001; Fisher, 2003). The unknown etiology of AN renders this complex psychiatric disease difficult to treat and current pharmacological treatments have little efficacy during the acute phase of illness or in preventing relapse (Barbarich-Marsteller, 2007). However, the physiological alterations induced by severe chronic food restriction impact on peripheral compartments (fat, bone, reproductive axis, energy balance) and on central pathways (reward, food intake, mood regulation, etc.) for which the outcome is usually similar whatever the initial cause (personal history, infancy trauma, socio-cultural pressions, personality traits, neurobiological, genetic background, etc.). Some authors even support the view that the physiological mechanisms involved in the regulation of feeding behavior in AN might, in many neurobiological effects, parallel those of obesity. As recently suggested by Jacquemont et al. (2011): "*abnormal eating behaviors, such as hyperphagia and anorexia, could represent opposite pathological manifestations of a common energy balance mechanism, although the precise relationships between these mirror phenotypes remain to be determined.*" Thus, the development of effective/new pharmacological treatments for this disease area would be enhanced if the mechanisms maintaining the abnormal behaviors characteristic of AN are better understood.

CENTRAL AND PERIPHERAL ALTERATIONS IN ANOREXIA NERVOSA

Whatever the initial and causal factors leading to AN, all patients display similar energy metabolic deficits and are unable to adapt their feeding behavior to energy demand and costs. In this state, survival requires the development of physiological changes that drive the individual/animal to adapt itself to these drastic conditions. Among all of the variations induced by chronic food restriction, the endocrine, immune, bone, and metabolic changes first allow adaptations to starvation, and are subsequently often directly involved in the complications of the disease (Estour et al., 2010). In addition, some of the feeding-regulatory factors are also involved directly (or not) in the modulation of reward-related and motivational processes, as well as in cognition and emotions associated with the disease. It should be noted that some of these endocrine changes persist after recovery and might contribute to susceptibility for AN recurrence (Lawson and Klibanski, 2008).

Among the biological factors whose levels are altered in AN patients, neurotransmitters and neuropeptides regulating appetite and feeding may contribute to some of the occurring central perturbations (**Table 3**). Overall, a high degree of heterogeneity has been observed between studies, for most of the assayed factors (plasma and cerebrospinal fluid samples). This heterogeneity could be explained by differences in the clinical characteristics of the samples (as severity and duration of the illness or subtype) and/or the increasing reliability of the methods used to ascertain factor concentrations over the last two decades. Consequentially, it is impossible to link any tendency in changes of levels and/or sensitivity to (an)orexigenic factors to AN, necessitating further investigation.

Systemic hormones directly regulating food intake have been widely studied in AN patients (**Table 4**). However, some anorexigenic hormones such as leptin decrease while others, such as peptide YY_{3-36} (PYY_{3-36}), increase. The same pattern is also observed for the orexigenic hormone, ghrelin (see *infra*). There exists sparse and contradictory data about the anorexigenic factors cholecystokinin (CKK) and glucagon-like peptide 1 (GLP1) in relation to this disease area rendering, it difficult to interpret observed

Table 3 | Compared levels of neuropeptides regulating food intake in AN patients and healthy matched population.

Neuropeptides regulating food intake*	AN/CT	Reference
Neuropeptide Y		
CSF NPY	↑	Kaye et al. (1990), Kaye (1996), Baranowska et al. (1997)
Blood NPY	→↓↑	Nedvidkova et al. (2000), Baranowska et al. (2001), Sedlackova et al. (2012)
Blood agouti-related protein	↑	Moriya et al. (2006), Merle et al. (2011)
Blood 26RFa	↑	Galusca et al. (2012)
Opioid peptides		
CSF b-endorphins	→↓	Gerner and Sharp (1982a), Baranowska (1990), Kaye (1996)
CSF dynorphins	→	Lesem et al. (1991), Kaye (1996)
Blood b-endorphins	↓↑	Baranowska (1990), Brambilla et al. (1991), Tepper et al. (1992)
Galanin		
CSF or plasma galanin	→	Berrettini et al. (1988), Baranowska et al. (1997, 2001)
Blood a-MSH	→	Moriya et al. (2006)
CSF corticotropin-releasing hormone	↑	Gerner and Gwirtsman (1981), Hotta et al. (1986), Kaye et al. (1987), Baranowska (1990)
CSF thyrotropin releasing hormone	↓	Lesem et al. (1994)
CSF neurotensin	→	Nemeroff et al. (1989)
Somatostatin (SRIF)		
CSF SRIF	↓→	Gerner and Yamada (1982b), Kaye et al. (1988)
Blood SRIF	↑↓	Pirke et al. (1994), Baranowska et al. (2000), Valevski et al. (2000)
CSF oxytocin	↓	Demitrack et al. (1990)
Blood oxytocin	→↓↑	Chiodera et al. (1991), Lawson et al. (2011a, 2012)
Brain-derived neurotrophic factor (BDNF)		
Serum BDNF	↓	Nakazato et al. (2003, 2006, 2009), Monteleone et al. (2004, 2005), Ehrlich et al. (2009), Saito et al. (2009)
Blood BDNF	↑	Mercader et al. (2007)

Adapted from Monteleone (2011).

**Neuropeptides inhibiting food intake are on a gray background.*

Table 4 | Compared levels of hormones regulating food intake in AN patients and healthy matched population.

Hormones regulating food intake*	AN/CT	Reference
Ghrelin-related		
Blood total ghrelin	↑	Otto et al. (2001, 2005), Krsek et al. (2003), Nedvidkova et al. (2003), Tanaka et al. (2003a,b,c, 2004), Tolle et al. (2003), Broglio et al. (2004a), Hotta et al. (2004), Misra et al. (2004c, 2005b, 2007, 2008), Soriano-Guillen et al. (2004), Tanaka et al. (2004), Bosy-Westphal et al. (2005), Stock et al. (2005), Troisi et al. (2005), Uehara et al. (2005), Germain et al. (2007, 2009, 2010), Janas-Kozik et al. (2007), Nakahara et al. (2007, 2008), Støving et al. (2007), Lawson et al. (2011b), Sedlackova et al. (2012)
Blood acyl ghrelin (active)	↑	Nakai et al. (2003), Hotta et al. (2004), Uehara et al. (2005), Nakahara et al. (2008), Germain et al. (2009, 2010)
Blood des-acyl ghrelin	↑	Hotta et al. (2004), Nakahara et al. (2008)
Blood obestatin	↑	Nakahara et al. (2008), Germain et al. (2009, 2010), Sedlackova et al. (2012)
Plasma insulin Leptin	(→)↓[1]	Uhe et al. (1992), Tamai et al. (1993), Støving et al. (1999), Gianotti et al. (2000), Gniuli et al. (2001), Delporte et al. (2003), Tanaka et al. (2003a), Weinbrenner et al. (2003), Misra et al. (2004a,b, 2007), Tagami et al. (2004), Bosy-Westphal et al. (2005), Housova et al. (2005), Misra et al. (2005c), Stock et al. (2005), Tomasik et al. (2005), Dolezalova et al. (2007), Dostalova et al. (2007), Kinzig et al. (2007), Nakahara et al. (2007), Støving et al. (2007), Haluzíková et al. (2009), Brick et al. (2010), Fazeli et al. (2010b), Karczewska-Kupczewska et al. (2010, 2012)
Leptin		
CSF leptin	↓	Mantzoros et al. (1997), Gendall et al. (1999)
Blood leptin	↓	Ferron et al. (1997), Hebebrand et al. (1997), Mantzoros et al. (1997), Balligand et al. (1998), Gendall et al. (1999), Støving et al. (1999), Monteleone et al. (2000, 2002a,b), Nedvidkova et al. (2000), Di Carlo et al. (2002), Krizova et al. (2002), Delporte et al. (2003), Holtkamp et al. (2003a,b, 2004), Misra et al. (2003, 2004a,b, 2005a,c, 2006, 2007, 2008), Pannacciulli et al. (2003), Tolle et al. (2003), Weinbrenner et al. (2003), Djurovic et al. (2004), Heer et al. (2004), Popovic et al. (2004), Tagami et al. (2004), Dostalova et al. (2005, 2007), Haas et al. (2005), Miljic et al. (2006), Ohwada et al. (2006, 2007), Dolezalova et al. (2007), Germain et al. (2007), Mika et al. (2007), Modan-Moses et al. (2007), Muñoz-Calvo et al. (2007), Nakahara et al. (2007), Haluzíková et al. (2009), Arimura et al. (2010), Estour et al. (2010), Fazeli et al. (2010b), Nogueira et al. (2010), Lawson et al. (2011b), Faje et al. (2012)
Total blood adiponectin	(→↓)↑[2]	Delporte et al. (2003), Iwahashi et al. (2003), Pannacciulli et al. (2003), Misra et al. (2004a), Tagami et al. (2004), Bosy-Westphal et al. (2005), Housova et al. (2005), Dolezalova et al. (2007), Dostalova et al. (2007), Modan-Moses et al. (2007), Nakahara et al. (2007), Støving et al. (2007), Haluzíková et al. (2009), Karczewska-Kupczewska et al. (2010, 2012), Nogueira et al. (2010)
Cholecystokinin (CKK)		
CSF or blood CCK	→↓	Phillipp et al. (1991), Geracioti et al. (1992), Tamai et al. (1993), Fujimoto et al. (1997), Tomasik et al. (2004, 2005)
Blood glucagon-like peptide 1	→↓	Tomasik et al. (2002, 2004, 2005)
Blood peptide YY	(→)↑[3]	Stock et al. (2005), Misra et al. (2006, 2007, 2008), Germain et al. (2007), Nakahara et al. (2007), Otto et al. (2007), Lawson et al. (2011b), Sedlackova et al. (2012)

[1] *Most of the studies found decreased insulin levels.*

[2] *Only three studies found no significant differences when compared to control group, and one found a decrease, while all the other found increased adiponectin levels.*

[3] *Most of the studies found increased PYY levels.*

**Hormones inhibiting food intake are on gray background.*

variations in the context of AN. Concerning PYY_{3-36}, most studies reported increased levels; although an anorexigenic peptide, this increase is difficult to explain as PYY_{3-36} is normally released in response to food intake. On the contrary, around 50 studies relate a very low leptin blood level in AN patients compared to a healthy matched control population (**Table 4**). This endogenous signal of energy stores is positively correlated to body mass index. Leptin is considered to be a good predictor of growth hormone (GH) burst, cortisol, estradiol, and thyroid hormone levels and its receptor is widely distributed throughout the body suggesting a pivotal role in mediating the hormonal adaptation to chronic starvation. Furthermore, AN patients display high plasma levels of adiponectin, another adipose-derived circulating cytokine. This anorexigenic hormone plays an important role in energy homeostasis and insulin sensitivity. The high levels of adiponectin in AN might contribute to the higher insulin sensitivity found in these patients. Indeed, insulin levels are usually strongly decreased that could be related to the hypoglycemia observed in AN patients.

More than 90% of adult women with AN are osteopenic, and almost 40% are osteoporotic at one or more sites (Grinspoon et al.,

2000). Osteopenia and osteoporosis are frequent consequences of AN, that very often persist after weight gain. Moreover, as synthesized by Confavreux et al. (2009), "*bone can now be considered as a true endocrine organ secreting osteocalcin, a hormone pharmacologically active on glucose and fat metabolism. Indeed osteocalcin stimulates insulin secretion and β-cell proliferation. Simultaneously, osteocalcin acts on adipocytes to induce adiponectin, which secondarily reduce insulin resistance.*" For these reasons, studies comparing bone turnover markers in AN patients with healthy control are presented in **Table 5**. Anorectic patients display increased levels of bone resorption markers and decreased bone formation markers. We may conclude that the bone mass alteration in patients with AN is dual: an increase of resorption and a decrease of bone formation. Moreover, the decrease in osteocalcin level could also contribute to the hypoinsulinemia and hypoadiponectinemia usually described.

A number of other endocrine disturbances have also been described in AN patients (**Table 6**). Hypothalamic-pituitary-adrenal axis deregulation is commonly suggested in AN. Indeed, AN is characterized by hypercortisolemia (**Table 6**) and, as mentioned by Miller (2011): "*overnight blood cortisol levels are inversely associated with bone mineral density and positively associated with severity of depression and anxiety symptoms in women with anorexia nervosa (Lawson et al., 2009). Therefore, hypercortisolemia may also contribute to the severe bone loss incurred and the highly prevalent psychiatric comorbidities in women with anorexia nervosa.*" Hypothalamic amenorrhea is another characteristic feature of AN, and has been attributed to a state of severe energy deficit from restricted energy intake, increased energy expenditure or both. Women and adolescent girls with AN have lower levels of estradiol, luteinizing hormone (LH), and for some of them follicle stimulating hormone (FSH; **Table 6**). The low levels of insulin-like growth factor-1 (IGF-1) and insulin may also contribute to this hypogonadal state and impact on bone turnover. The GH/IGF-1 axis is also altered in most of the studies (**Table 6**). Indeed, AN is associated with a nutritionally acquired hepatic resistance to GH with decreased production of IGF-1 and increased GH levels. Such an increase is due to a reduced feedback at the level of the pituitary and hypothalamus from low IGF-1 levels, and high levels of ghrelin (**Table 4**, see *infra*). Most studies report low levels of T3 and/or T4 thyroid hormones in patients with AN (**Table 6**). T3 and T4 plasma levels are enhanced by leptin administration in women with AN, and the levels of these three hormones are positively associated (Haas et al., 2005; Misra et al., 2005a). Moreover, ghrelin is known to inhibit the release of pituitary thyroid stimulating hormone (Wren et al., 2000), and studies indicate negative correlations between ghrelin and thyroid hormones plasma levels in AN (Misra et al., 2005c). These data suggest that low leptin and high ghrelin levels may contribute to lower thyroid hormone levels in AN. Finally, inflammatory cytokines were assayed in AN patients and matched healthy controls (Corcos et al., 2003). Data did not show significant variations suggesting that AN might not have an inflammatory component.

ANIMAL MODELS OF CHRONIC FOOD RESTRICTION: A WAY TO DECIPHER THE PHYSIOLOGICAL MECHANISMS OF ANOREXIA NERVOSA

The use of appropriate animal models mimicking most of the physiological changes occurring in AN might help to determine more precisely the potential mechanisms, central and/or peripheral, involved in the early adaptive state that precedes exhaustion

Table 5 | Compared levels of bone turnover markers in AN patients and healthy matched population.

Bone turnover markers*	AN/CT	Reference
Blood OC	(→)↓[1]	Calero et al. (1999), Grinspoon et al. (1999), Caillot-Augusseau et al. (2000), Gordon et al. (2002), Misra et al. (2003, 2004b, 2006, 2007, 2008), Weinbrenner et al. (2003), Galusca et al. (2006), Legroux-Gérot et al. (2007), Ohwada et al. (2007), Viapiana et al. (2007), Estour et al. (2010), Ostrowska et al. (2010, 2012a,b)
Blood procollagen type 1 N-terminal propeptide (PINP)	→↓	Calero et al. (1999), Faje et al. (2012)
Blood procollagen type 1 C-terminal propeptide (PICP)	↓	Misra et al. (2003, 2004b, 2006, 2007), Heer et al. (2004), Mika et al. (2007)
Blood bone specific alkaline phosphatase (BSAP)	(→)↓[2]	Calero et al. (1999), Gordon et al. (2002), Misra et al. (2003, 2006), Heer et al. (2004), Bolton et al. (2005), Galusca et al. (2006), Legroux-Gérot et al. (2007), Mika et al. (2007), Ohwada et al. (2007), Viapiana et al. (2007)
Blood or urinary c-terminal cross-linking telopeptide of type 1 collagen (CTX)	↑↓[3]	Caillot-Augusseau et al. (2000), Weinbrenner et al. (2003), Galusca et al. (2006), Mika et al. (2007), Estour et al. (2010), Ostrowska et al. (2010, 2012a,b), Faje et al. (2012)
Blood cross-linked N-telopeptides of type 1 collagen (NTX)	↑↓	Gordon et al. (2002), Dominguez et al. (2007)
Urinary NTX/creatinine	↑↓[4]	Grinspoon et al. (1999), Misra et al. (2003, 2006, 2007, 2008), Dominguez et al. (2007)

[1] *All but three studies found significant or non-significant decreased OC levels.*

[2] *All but three studies found significant or non-significant decreased BSAP levels*

[3] *Increased CTX found by Caillot-Augusseau et al. (2000), Weinbrenner et al. (2003), Galusca et al. (2006), Ohwada et al. (2007), and Estour et al. (2010).*

[4] *Only Grinspoon found increased urinary NTX/creatinine levels.*

**Bone resorption markers are on gray background.*

Table 6 | Compared levels of other factors altered in AN patients.

Other factors	AN/CT	Reference
Growth factors		
Blood GH	(→)↑[1]	Gianotti et al. (2000), Misra et al. (2003, 2004a,c, 2005c, 2006, 2007), Støving et al. (2003), Tolle et al. (2003), Broglio et al. (2004a), Tanaka et al. (2004), Miljic et al. (2006), Germain et al. (2007), Polli et al. (2008), Arimura et al. (2010), Estour et al. (2010)
Blood IGF-1	↓	Grinspoon et al. (1999), Støving et al. (1999, 2003, 2007), Gianotti et al. (2000), Nedvidkova et al. (2000), Di Carlo et al. (2002), Gordon et al. (2002), Misra et al. (2003, 2004a, 2005c, 2006, 2007, 2008), Tolle et al. (2003), Broglio et al. (2004a), Heer et al. (2004), Ohwada et al. (2006, 2007), Germain et al. (2007), Legroux-Gérot et al. (2007), Mika et al. (2007), Polli et al. (2008), Haas et al. (2009), Arimura et al. (2010), Brick et al. (2010), Estour et al. (2010), Fazeli et al. (2010b), Faje et al. (2012)
Steroid and sexual hormones		
Blood LH	↓	Støving et al. (1999, 2007), Di Carlo et al. (2002), Holtkamp et al. (2003b), Popovic et al. (2004), Misra et al. (2005c), Dominguez et al. (2007), Germain et al. (2007), Oswiecimska et al. (2007), Tomova et al. (2007), Nogal et al. (2008), Arimura et al. (2010), Estour et al. (2010), Ziora et al. (2011)
Blood FSH	(→)↓[2]	Støving et al. (1999, 2007), Di Carlo et al. (2002), Holtkamp et al. (2003b), Popovic et al. (2004), Dominguez et al. (2007), Germain et al. (2007), Oswiecimska et al. (2007), Tomova et al. (2007), Nogal et al. (2008), Arimura et al. (2010), Estour et al. (2010), Ziora et al. (2011)
Estrogens	(→)↑[3]	Grinspoon et al. (1999), Støving et al. (1999, 2007), Monteleone et al. (2000, 2001), Di Carlo et al. (2002), Holtkamp et al. (2003b), Misra et al. (2003, 2004a,b, 2005c, 2006, 2007, 2008), Tolle et al. (2003), Heer et al. (2004), Popovic et al. (2004), Bolton et al. (2005), Dominguez et al. (2007), Germain et al. (2007), Mika et al. (2007), Ohwada et al. (2007), Oswiecimska et al. (2007), Haas et al. (2009), Arimura et al. (2010), Brick et al. (2010), Estour et al. (2010), Buehren et al. (2011), Ziora et al. (2011), Faje et al. (2012)
Cortisol	(→)↑[4]	Grinspoon et al. (1999), Støving et al. (1999), Monteleone et al. (2000, 2001), Putignano et al. (2001), Misra et al. (2003, 2004b, 2005c, 2006, 2007, 2008), Tolle et al. (2003), Weinbrenner et al. (2003), Heer et al. (2004), Troisi et al. (2005), Miljic et al. (2006), Germain et al. (2007), Oswiecimska et al. (2007), Nogal et al. (2008), Haas et al. (2009), Arimura et al. (2010), Estour et al. (2010), Buehren et al. (2011), Ziora et al. (2011), Faje et al. (2012)
Thyroid hormones	(→)↓[5]	Nedvidkova et al. (2000), Di Carlo et al. (2002), Holtkamp et al. (2003b), Weinbrenner et al. (2003), Onur et al. (2005), Troisi et al. (2005), Brambilla et al. (2006), Ohwada et al. (2006, 2007), Oswiecimska et al. (2007), Nogal et al. (2008), Arimura et al. (2010), Estour et al. (2010), Buehren et al. (2011), Ziora et al. (2011)

[1]*All but two studies found increased GH levels.*
[2]*All but one study found decreased FSH.*
[3]*Most of the studies found decreased estrogen levels.*
[4]*Most of the studies found increased Cortisol levels.*
[5]*All but two studies found decreased T3 and/or T4 levels.*

of the individual/animal. However, developing and using animal models of psychiatric disorders is inherently difficult due to the complex nature of these illnesses. In the literature, numerous models of genetic deficient mice for one or multiple genes involved in the regulation of feeding behavior/reward/energy balance have been developed (for review, see Siegfried et al., 2003; Kim, 2012). These genetic models give essential mechanistic data related to one specific pathway but do not completely mirror the symptoms observed in human disease (Willner, 1984; Smith, 1989). Indeed, the use of more "environmental models" that mimic most of the physiological symptoms of AN are preferred as they provide insight regarding how the disease might progress toward exhaustion. Initially, the most widely used animal model, whatever the species, is the chronic food restriction model (for review, see Kim, 2012). However, it does not take into account several conditions observed in AN patients that are self-starvation, hyperactivity, and chronic stress. The rat model of self-starvation developed by Routtenberg and Kuznesof (1967) consists in housing one rat in a cage equipped with a running wheel and submitting the animal to a food restriction (1 h-feeding per day). This model later coined the term "the activity-based anorexia (ABA) model." It produces a rapid decrease in body weight and food intake, hyperactivity, hypothermia, loss of estrus, and an increase in HPA axis activity (Hall and Hanford, 1954; Routtenberg and Kuznesof, 1967; Burden et al., 1993). Moreover, in this model, the rats eat less than inactive rats fed with the same schedule, and can even starve themselves to death. In the ABA model, the long term exposure (few days) to low leptin and high ghrelin levels, induced a tissue-specific expression pattern of ghrelin and leptin receptors (Pardo et al., 2010). Furthermore, Verhagen et al. (2011) found that plasma ghrelin levels are highly associated with food anticipatory behavior, measured by running wheel activity in rats. This effect is dependent of the central ghrelin signaling system *via* growth hormone secretagogue receptor 1a (GHS-R1A). In many aspects this model mimics numerous physiological alterations observed in AN. However, as specified by Klenotich and Dulawa (2012), the ABA paradigm is strongly dependent upon factors that amplify or reduce some parts of the phenotype, i.e., the choice of rodent strain (more or less resistant to ABA, Gelegen et al., 2007), the sex of animal (female are more vulnerable to ABA), the age (younger animals are more susceptible to ABA), the temperature (increasing the temperature to 32°C strongly reduces the ABA behavior, Cerrato et al., 2012), the time of the day the animals receive food, and the hydration/dryness of the food. In fact, Boakes and Juraskova, 2001; Boakes, 2007) demonstrated that the "self-starvation" observed in ABA rats might reflect both the reduced palatability of the dry chow for a dehydrated animal and satiety signals from a stomach full of water. Thus, giving hydrated food during the 1 h-feeding schedule completely abolishes the ABA phenotype (rapid weight loss, hyperactivity, etc.). Currently, we are developing an adaptation of the ABA model in female mice that aims to follow the long term (more than 2 weeks) physiological alterations induced by a combination of physical activity and 50% food restriction. Our recent results, involving a 2-week protocol, indicate that our selected ABA model induces a rapid and stable loss of weight, changes the circadian locomotor activity, alters energy balance (corresponding to the passage from phase I to II; **Table 1**), induces hypoglycemia, hypoleptinemia, hyperghrelinemia, and a central alteration in the hypothalamic feeding centers (Méquinion, personal data). Thus, the combination of exercise (in running wheels) and food deprivation following a certain schedule might be considered as two important chronic stress factors that could reinforce the weight loss by modifying feeding behavior, as observed in our study. Other models based on chronic stress that are associated with food deprivation use tail pinching, cold swimming (Shimizu et al., 1989; Wong et al., 1993), or separation. We choose this last model, named "Separation-Based Anorexia" (SBA) to study the impact of chronic stress associated with caloric insufficiency. In our protocol, 8-week old female mice are separated and fed with a time-restricted food access for up to 10 weeks. Our recent results showed a 20–25% body weight loss with a cumulative food intake just under that of the control group. Moreover, SBA mice displayed reduced lean, fat, and bone masses associated with hypoleptinemia and alteration in GH/IGF-1 axis. Finally, an alteration of the estrous cycle was also observed (Zgheib, personal data).

To date, these described "environmental animal models" (ABA and SBA) remain the only models that enable long term studies of how chronic food restriction impacts upon physiology at different levels (energy balance, reproduction, bone/fat regulation, etc.), and of the mechanisms responsible for the sustenance of these alterations on different tissues often not available on patients (brain, bones, fat, muscle, liver, etc.). They will also facilitate determination of whether the dramatic outcome of the patients might be related to a specific dysregulation of one or many biological factors that can be considered as a marker of the disease and potentially also in its evolution. In addition, ABA and SBA models exhibit good face validity for most of the physiological symptoms of AN.

GHRELIN A KEY ENERGY BALANCE HORMONE: ROLE IN ANOREXIA NERVOSA

ORIGIN AND BIOSYNTHESIS OF GHRELIN

Ghrelin is a 28 amino acid, initially isolated from rat stomach (Kojima et al., 1999). The preproghrelin messenger RNA (mRNA) is mainly expressed in the X/A-like oxyntic gland cells of the gastric fundus mucosa equivalent to P/D1 cells in humans (Bordi et al., 2000). Ghrelin is also produced in other parts of the gastrointestinal tract, and it is expressed at lower levels in pancreas, kidney, testis, placenta, and bone (Gnanapavan et al., 2002; González et al., 2008) and hypothalamic neurons (Cowley et al., 2003). The 117 amino acid preproghrelin is processed by cleavage and results in two peptides (**Figure 1**): obestatin and proghrelin (Jeffery et al., 2005). Des-acyl ghrelin is then cleaved from the 94 amino acid proghrelin precursor by enzymes like the prohormone convertase 1/3 (Zhu et al., 2006). This 28 amino acid peptide is modified post-translationally in the active acylated form of ghrelin, capable to bind to its receptor, the GHS-R1a. The octanoylation at the third N-terminal amino acid, usually serine (Kojima et al., 1999), is catalyzed the enzyme ghrelin octanoyl-acyltransferase (GOAT, Yang et al., 2008), which is expressed predominantly in the stomach, gut, and pancreas, but also at other sites (Kang et al., 2012). Ghrelin concentrations in blood comprise principally des-acyl ghrelin (85–90%) and in lesser amounts acyl ghrelin (10–15%) and C-terminal proghrelin peptides (Pemberton and Richards, 2007).

GHRELIN RECEPTOR AND DISTRIBUTION

Ghrelin is the only known ligand to bind to GHS-R1a (Howard et al., 1996; Gutierrez et al., 2008). This receptor belongs to the G-protein coupled receptor family (GPCR; Holst and Schwartz, 2006) and has two variants, GHS-R1a and GHS-R1b, which are splice variants of the same gene. Type 1a is the full length, seven-transmembrane domain receptor, and the type 1b isoform is a C-terminally truncated, five-transmembrane domain variant (Kojima et al., 1999). Only the GHS-R1a is fully functional, binding mostly with acylated ghrelin on $G\alpha_q$-protein, whereas the 1b isoform is thought to be physiologically inactive. It should be noted that des-acyl ghrelin does not compete with acyl ghrelin for GHS-R1a to any significant extent. Indeed, supraphysiological concentrations of des-acyl ghrelin are necessary to allow binding and activation of GHS-R1a (Veldhuis and Bowers, 2010; Delhanty et al., 2012). Although derived from the same precursor, obestatin is a cognate ligand for the orphan receptor GPR39, another member of the ghrelin receptor subfamily (McKee et al., 1997; Holst et al., 2004).

Growth hormone secretagogue receptor 1a is abundantly expressed within the CNS. Notably, a large population of GHS-R1a-expressing neurons are located in the hypothalamic arcuate nucleus (ARC), which has a crucial role in energy balance control. Other hypothalamic areas expressing this receptor of relevance for feeding control include the ventromedial hypothalamus (VMH), paraventricular nucleus (PVN), anteroventral preoptic nucleus, anterior hypothalamic area, lateral hypothalamic area (LHA), suprachiasmatic nucleus, supraoptic nucleus, and the tuberomammillary nuclei (Guan et al., 1997; Gnanapavan et al., 2002; Camiña, 2006; Harrold et al., 2008). Moreover, mRNA studies also demonstrate the presence of this receptor in

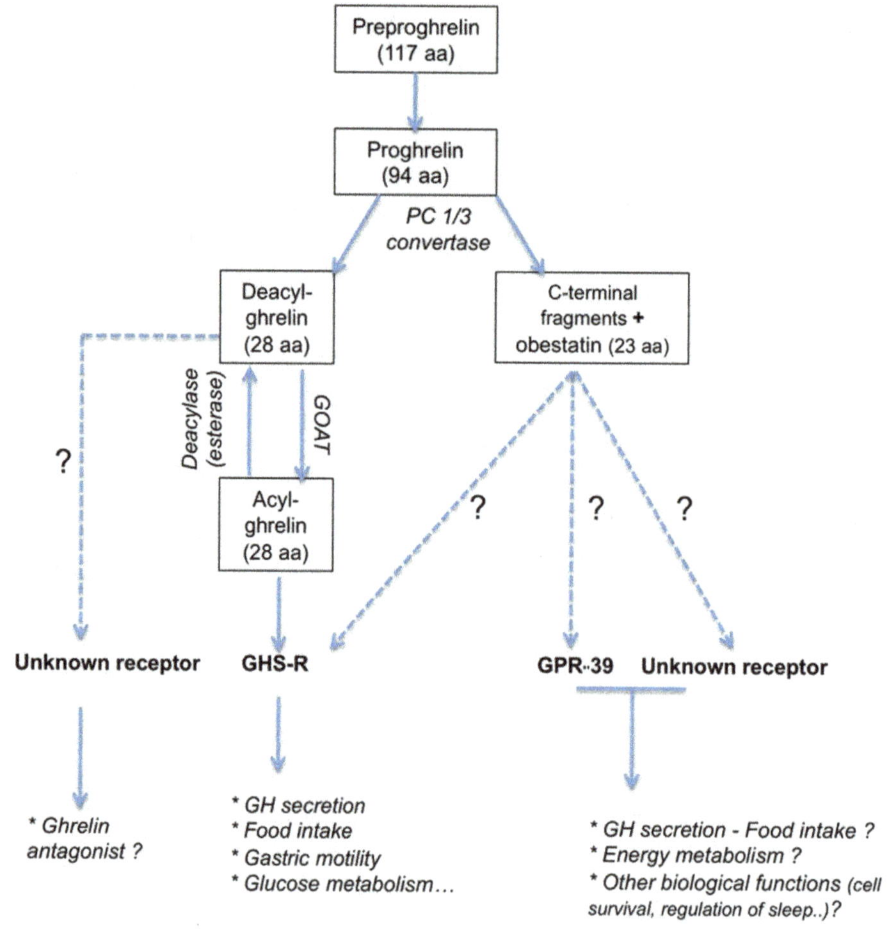

FIGURE 1 | Principal peptide products obtained by post-translational processing of preproghrelin peptide. Ghrelin and obestatin act on receptors belonging to the GPCR family. Even if the exact role of obestatin remains question of debate (see Hassouna et al., 2010), ghrelin has been first described to be a GH-secretagogue. Beside an obvious role in the regulation of food intake, ghrelin is also implicated in numerous biological function (see Veldhuis and Bowers, 2010). The active form of ghrelin, acyl ghrelin, is obtained by octanoylation of deacyl ghrelin. Its receptor is not yet identified and its function is currently unclear even if some evidences support an antagonistic effect to ghrelin (see Delhanty et al., 2012).

limbic and mesolimbic structures known to be involved in motor control, emotional reactivity and reward/motivation systems such as the hippocampus (dentate gyrus, CA2, and CA3 regions), pars compacta of the substantia nigra, ventral tegmental area (VTA), raphe nuclei, laterodorsal tegmental nucleus (Guan et al., 1997; Zigman et al., 2006), and amygdala (Alvarez-Crespo et al., 2012). In the periphery, GHS-R1a is expressed in different tissues and organs implicated in energy balance, e.g., in the anterior lobe of the pituitary on somatotroph cells (Briggs and Andrews, 2011), pancreas, spleen, stomach, intestine, heart, thyroid, gonads, adrenal, liver, skeletal muscle, and adipose tissues (Papotti et al., 2000). The truncated form is also found in various tissues but its exact role is not well known (Gnanapavan et al., 2002; Camiña, 2006). Interestingly, GHS-R1a is constitutively active even when unstimulated by the afferent ghrelin signal (Petersen et al., 2009). Finally, ghrelin receptors are able to interact with other receptors to form homo- or hetero-dimers, like GHS-R1a/GHS-R1a and GHS-R1a/GHS-R1b (Chow et al., 2012). Co-expression of the truncated variant of ghrelin receptor with the full length variant attenuated the constitutive signaling probably because the translocation of the ghrelin receptor from the plasma membrane to the cell nucleus is decreased (Mokrosinski and Holst, 2010). GHS-R1a also appears to heterodimerize with other GPCRs, at least in *in vitro* test systems, and can explain the differential ghrelin signaling (review in Schellekens et al., 2010). Heterodimerization of GHS-R1A with the dopamine receptor D2 has recently been shown to occur in mouse hypothalamic neurons that regulate appetite (Kern et al., 2012) Since GHS-R1a acts as an allosteric modulator of D1 and D2 signaling, this finding implies a functional role for the expressed GHS-R1a in brain areas that may be less accessible to peripherally produced ghrelin and where there is no local production of ghrelin (Jiang et al., 2006; Kern et al., 2012).

ROLES OF GHRELIN

In line with the broad expression of ghrelin and its receptor, this hormone is involved in multiple biological functions, many of which are linked to feeding control. Initially, this gut-brain signal was shown to have direct pituitary GH-releasing effects, reproducing the known effects of the so-called growth hormone secretagogues (GHS). This term refers a group of synthetic GHS-R1a ligands, the first group of which was derived from metenkephalin (described by Bowers et al., 1977) and included the hexapeptide GHRP-6 (Bowers et al., 1984) that is now recognized as a synthetic ghrelin mimetic. Both ghrelin and its receptor have been strongly conserved during evolution, supporting the notion that GHS-R1a and its natural ligand play a fundamentally important role in biology (Palyha et al., 2000).

Ghrelin's most characterized effects are: (i) its ability to stimulate GH secretion, likely of relevance for glucose homeostasis and energy balance; (ii) its role as an orexigenic hormone acting at key hypothalamic and midbrain circuits involved in feeding control; (iii) its involvement in various other physiological functions like gastrointestinal, cardiovascular, pulmonary and immune function, sleep duration, learning, memory, and behavior, cellular proliferation, immunomodulation, reproduction, and bone physiology. Most of these physiological functions are altered in AN indicating a potential role for ghrelin in the pathogenesis of this disease.

Role of ghrelin in the regulation of appetite, food intake, and energy balance

Ghrelin acts at different levels to stimulate GH secretion and thus modulate hepatic IGF-1 production (Peino et al., 2000). GHS-R1a is expressed by GHRH arcuate neurons but also by GH cells in the anterior pituitary gland (Kojima et al., 1999). Ghrelin and GHS activate ARC cells (Dickson et al., 1993; Hewson and Dickson, 2000) including neuroendocrine cells in this region (Dickson et al., 1996), notably a sub-population of GHRH neurons (Dickson and Luckman, 1997; Osterstock et al., 2010). Indeed, these compounds acts in synergy with GHRH to induce a greater GH release than would be induced by GHRH alone (Bowers et al., 1984; Arvat et al., 2001; Hataya et al., 2001). This ghrelin-stimulated GH release is dose-dependent and could explain why AN patients have elevated circulating GH levels (Kojima and Kangawa, 2005; Miljic et al., 2006; Misra et al., 2006; Germain et al., 2007, 2010; Estour et al., 2010). Chronic starvation is associated with GH resistance and relatively low IGF-1 levels involving a feedback mechanism, rather than body composition parameters or other circulating factors, e.g., free fatty acid or insulin levels (Støving et al., 1999; Brick et al., 2010). Besides its role in growth, GH stimulates lipolysis through a mechanism independent of IGF-1 (Fazeli et al., 2010a), for which the effects are largely anabolic. The increased GH secretion and the reduction of IGF-1 in starvation may be adaptive since they respectively serve the function of mobilizing fat stores in the setting of reduced energy availability and reduce anabolism. However, the reduction of IGF-1 levels may also have deleterious effects, contributing to bone, and muscle loss in AN women. Even if the mechanisms underlying the development of GH resistance in states of chronic undernutrition are not as well established, ghrelin might strongly participate to such endocrine dysregulation. Studies conducted in rodents support a close link between ghrelin signaling and altered GH/IGF-1 status. In rodents, fasting induced higher expression of GHS-R1a and overexpression of GHS-R1a in female mice provoked higher expression of GH and GHRH (Veldhuis and Bowers, 2010). Furthermore, suppressed ghrelin signaling (using antisense RNA knockdown against GHS-R1a or a GHS-R1a antagonist, BIM-28163), caused a decrease in GH peak pulsatility with or without a decrease in plasma levels of IGF-1 (Zizzari et al., 2005; Veldhuis and Bowers, 2010). Finally, plasma ghrelin concentration is negatively correlated with body weight and subcutaneous, visceral, and total adiposity (reviewed in Veldhuis and Bowers, 2010), probably due to a long term effect on ghrelin in driving pulsatile GH secretion, which is strongly lipolytic.

Ghrelin is perhaps best known as a circulating hunger signal necessary for meal initiation and meal anticipation with a secretion occurring in a pulsatile manner starting with a preprandial rise and postprandial fall 1 h after food intake (Ariyasu et al., 2001; Cummings et al., 2001; Tschöp et al., 2001; Zizzari et al., 2011; Merkestein et al., 2012). Moreover, whatever the route of injection, ghrelin increases food intake both in humans and animals (Wren et al., 2001a,b). In addition, prolonged food reduction or severe caloric restriction causes an increase in plasma ghrelin concentration (Wren et al., 2001b; Méquinion, personal data). In AN patients, ghrelin levels are increased up to twofold and return to normal levels after weight restoration (Otto et al., 2001, 2005; Tolle et al., 2003; Germain et al., 2009; Yi et al., 2011). However, it appears that fluctuations in ghrelin are not always influenced by food intake in AN (Germain et al., 2009) suggesting impairment in its regulation, probably due to a chronic adaptation to long term food restriction (Yi et al., 2011). Mice lacking the gene for ghrelin or its receptor have normal food intake when fed chow, probably due to compensatory adaptation during embryonic development, but show a degree of protection from obesity when fed a high-fat diet, especially from an early age (Sun et al., 2003, 2004; Wortley et al., 2004, 2005).

Ghrelin also appears to be of importance in the regulation of lipid and glucose metabolism. It has been attributed a role in the maintenance of normal blood glucose levels (Grove and Cowley, 2005). There are indications that ghrelin's effects on the GH axis may have relevance for glucose homeostasis (and even survival) during chronic food deprivation. Mice lacking acyl ghrelin (due to knockout of GOAT) lose glycemic control and become moribund by 1 week of 60% food deprivation, an effect that can be circumvented by infusion of either acyl ghrelin or GH throughout this 1-week period (Zhao et al., 2010). The work of Sun et al. (2008) on ghrelin homeostasis in ghrelin KO and GHS-R KO mice demonstrate that the ghrelin/GHS-R pathway appears to play an important role in glucose homeostasis by regulating insulin sensitivity and glucose sensing, particularly under conditions of negative energy balance. However, data indicating an action of ghrelin on plasma insulin levels are still controversial (Castañeda et al., 2010; Sangiao-Alvarellos and Cordido, 2010). Intravenous ghrelin injection leads to a decrease in plasma insulin and an increase in blood glucose (Broglio et al., 2001). This result is not found universally and it may be related to the physiological vs. pharmacological doses used (Castañeda et al., 2010). Ghrelin could potentially decrease insulin secretion by altering insulin sensitivity (Castañeda et al., 2010). This is in agreement with the results obtained during insulin and glucose tolerance tests performed in AN patients (Broglio et al., 2004a; Harada et al., 2008). Moreover, under chronic food restriction, fatty acids are mobilized and their oxidation could increase the production of octanoic acid, thereafter used to octanoylate des-acyl ghrelin, leading to a global increase of plasma ghrelin levels. Thus, the greater levels of glucose observed in ABA mice (Méquinion, personal data) or wild type mice during the early phases of the chronic food restriction might be driven by this increase in ghrelin. This might contribute to the adaptive state in the first stages of AN, before a depletion of the supply of free fatty acids and induction of ketosis. Ghrelin acts directly on the liver, to favor glycogenolysis but also on muscle and adipose tissues. Indeed, subcutaneous injection of ghrelin in rats induces an increase of hepatic triglycerides associated with an increase in the gene expression of enzymes involved in lipogenesis like acetyl-CoA carboxylase (ACC) and fatty acid synthase (FAS, Barazzoni et al., 2005) as well as increased expression of ACC and FAS mRNA in white visceral adipose tissue (Thompson et al., 2004; Barazzoni et al., 2005). By contrast, subcutaneous ghrelin injection induces a decrease of triglyceride content in muscle without modifying ACC expression and AMPK phosphorylation (Barazzoni et al., 2005). These effects are especially observed in the gastrocnemius muscle, a fast-twitch muscle that is predominantly glycolytic. Similar variations are observed in the food-restricted condition (Samec et al., 2002). Finally, Pardo et al. (2010) describe, in the ABA model, a tissue-specific expression pattern of GHS-R1a receptors in visceral and subcutaneous fat and within the muscle. Indeed, the oxidative-soleus type of muscle appears to be more susceptible to circulating ghrelin levels than the glycolytic-gastrocnemius type under exercise and food restriction situations. All of these modifications could provide a defense mechanism to maintain energy homeostasis in the unbalanced energy state that is found in AN patients.

The central orexigenic effect of ghrelin

Appetite, food intake, and energy balance are finely tuned by a complex intercommunication between neural networks and peripheral tissues (**Figure 2**). Within the CNS, various hypothalamic nuclei containing orexigenic and anorexigenic neurons regulate the different facets of food intake. The ARC cells targeted by ghrelin and its mimetics include the orexigenic neuropeptide Y (NPY) cells (Dickson and Luckman, 1997) that co-express another orexigenic peptide, agouti-related peptide (AgRP). Following administration of ghrelin, these neurons are activated, reflected by the induction of Fos-protein in discrete cell groups (Hewson and Dickson, 2000; Wang et al., 2002), by increased action potential firing (Cowley et al., 2003; Andrews et al., 2008) and by an increased expression of NPY and AgRP mRNA (Kamegai et al., 2000, 2001; Nakazato et al., 2001). Furthermore, the stimulatory effects of ghrelin on NPY/AgRP neurons are complemented by a reduction of the ARC anorexigenic pro-opiomelanocortin (POMC) neuronal activity *via* inhibitory GABA-ergic inputs from NPY/AgRP neurons (Cowley et al., 2003). Interestingly, sensitivity of the ARC cells to ghrelin appears to be nutritionally regulated as the Fos response was increased up to threefold in fasting rats relative to fed animals (Hewson and Dickson, 2000) an effect that was reversed once again upon refeeding (Luckman et al., 1999). Collectively, these data indicate that ghrelin activates a key orexigenic pathway in the hypothalamic ARC, the NPY/AgRP cells and that this response is metabolically regulated. Consistent with this, stimulation of hypothalamic GHS-R1a results in an anabolic response characterized by an increase in food intake (Wren et al., 2000) and a decrease in energy utilization (Tschöp et al., 2000). The feeding effects ghrelin appear to require normal NPY/AgRP signaling since ablation of NPY or AgRP neurons or the use of NPY receptor antagonists abolish these effects (Chen et al., 2004; Luquet et al., 2007). Conditional deletion of NPY/AgRP co-expressing neurons in the ARC of adult mice (by targeting the human diphtheria toxin to the AgRP locus) caused a rapid starvation to death (Luquet et al., 2005). Moreover, mice homozygous for the anorexia (*anx*) mutation, characterized by poor food intake and death by 3–5 weeks after birth (Maltais et al., 1984) display a lower density of hypothalamic neuropeptides. The data of Nilsson et al. (2011) support the hypothesis of degeneration of hypothalamic ARC neuron populations; the AgRP system appears to be the first system affected and the POMC system being secondary in this process. Finally, in our models of chronic food restriction (SBA and ABA), we found an alteration of the AgRP signal with an accumulation of this peptide in ARC neurons (Méquinion and Nilsson, personal data). Thus, there are numerous lines of evidence supporting the fact that in chronic food restriction (and probably in AN), a dysregulation of the AgRP system occurs that contributes to deficient ghrelin signaling at the level of the ARC. Recent neuroimaging data obtained from AN patients differing in disease duration showed a significant reduction of total white matter volume and focal gray matter atrophy in various brain areas such as the hypothalamus, especially in patients with shorter food restriction. Collectively, these studies highlight the potential role of endocrine and central (hypothalamic) dysfunction in the altered homeostatic metabolic status in AN, as described in animal models (Boghi et al., 2011).

At the hypothalamic level, ghrelin has also been reported to act directly or indirectly on other nuclei linked to feeding control such as the VMH, PVN, and LHA (López et al., 2008; Mano-Otagiri et al., 2009; Lamont et al., 2012). Although not coupled to c-fos expression, VMN cells exhibit a robust electrical response following bath application of a ghrelin agonist (Hewson et al., 1999). The elegant study of López et al. (2008) showed that, in fasted rats, an elevated ghrelin tone was associated with an increased activation of hypothalamic AMPK and a decreased mRNA expression of enzymes (like FAS) involved in the *de novo* fatty acid biosynthesis only in the VMH. They concluded that the energy peripheral signals sensed to regulate fatty acid metabolism in the hypothalamus and consequently the feeding behavior, may not be a nutrient, but ghrelin through an action at the level of the VMH.

Ghrelin's effects in the PVN are also likely linked to feeding control as direct intra-PVN injection of ghrelin induces a robust feeding response that is coupled to neuronal (c-fos) activation (Olszewski et al., 2003). Consistent with this, a reduction of GHS-R1a gene in the PVN using RNA interference in rats, significantly reduced body weight and blood ghrelin levels without affecting food intake (Shrestha et al., 2009). These data reflect a role for ghrelin in the modulation of PVN neuron activity in that is linked to energy homeostasis, but the mechanisms of action remains to be elucidated.

In the LHA, ghrelin is thought to mediate hyperphagia through orexin neurons. Indeed, central administration of ghrelin or a ghrelin mimetic induces Fos expression in orexin-containing, but not melanin-concentrating hormone-containing, neurons

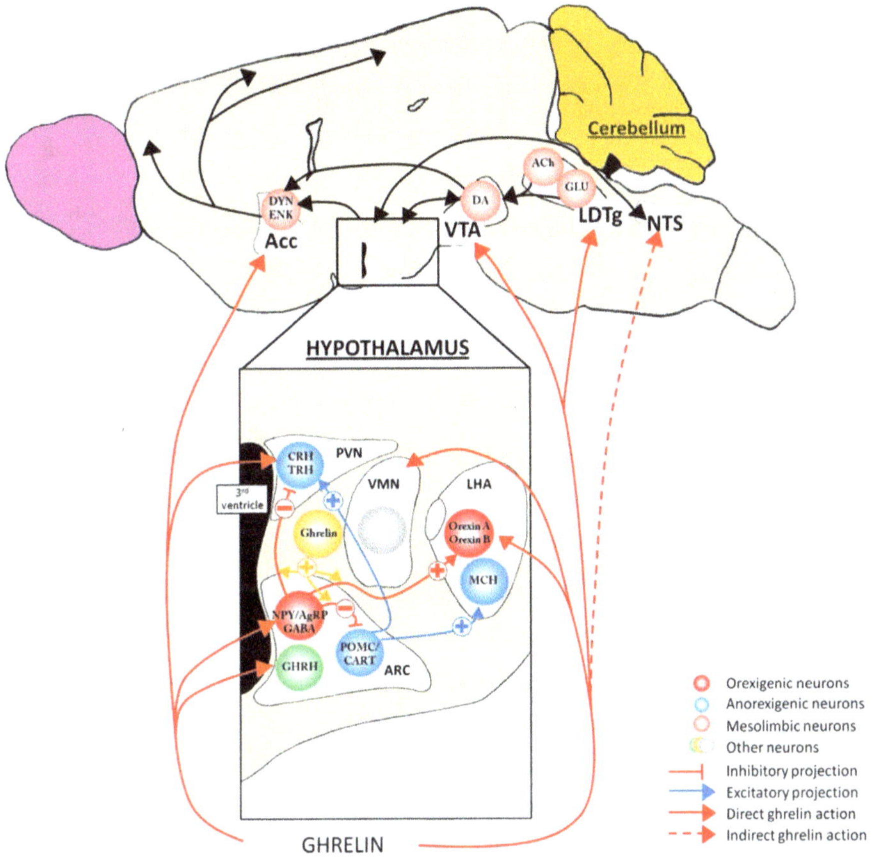

FIGURE 2 | Action of ghrelin in the brain. Ghrelin acts at different levels of the brain to stimulate food intake *via* hypothalamus and meso-cortico-limbic pathway. In the hypothalamus, ghrelin activates orexigenic neurons (AgRP/NPY), which inhibit anorexigenic neurons (POMC/CART) *via* GABA projections. They are connected to second order neurons like CRH and TRH neurons located in the PVN and/or the orexin neurons found in the LHA. POMC/CART neurons activate MCH neurons. Ghrelin acts also at different levels of meso-cortico-limbic pathway: LDTg, VTA, and Acc. Ghrelin acts directly on VTA to stimulate dopamine release in Acc. dopamine release is controlled by cholinergic LDTg neurons. Ghrelin could also act on NTS to stimulate the food intake *via* either vagal nerve or area postrema, see **Figure 4**. Acc, accumbens nucleus; ACh, acétylcholine; AgRP, agouti-related peptide; ARC, arcuate nucleus; CART, cocaine- and amphetamine-regulated transcript; CRH, corticotropin-releasing hormone; DA, dopamine; DYN, dynorphin; ENK, enkephalin; GABA, γ-aminobutyric acid; GHRH growth-hormone-releasing hormone; GLU, glutamate; LDTg, laterodorsal tegmental area; LHA, lateral hypothalamic area; MCH, melanin-concentrating hormone; NPY, neuropeptide Y; NTS, nucleus tractus solitarius; POMC, pro-opiomelanocortin; PVN, paraventricular nucleus; TRH, thyrotropin releasing hormone; VMH, ventromedial nucleus; VTA, ventral tegmental area.

(Lawrence et al., 2002; Olszewski et al., 2003), and activates glucose responding neurons (Chen et al., 2005a) in this area. Furthermore, ghrelin-induced feeding is suppressed in orexin KO mice (Toshinai et al., 2003). The role of orexin neurons to simulate feeding behavior (appetite/metabolism) is now well established although they are also especially important for sleep and wakefulness (España and Scammell, 2011; Gao, 2012) and play important roles in the stress response, in analgesia and reward/addiction (see Kukkonen, 2013). Moreover, ghrelin's effects to increase the reward value of a high-fat diet appear to involve a LHA-VTA orexin pathway (Perello et al., 2010).

The action of ghrelin to increase food intake and associated appetitive behaviors involves an integrated neurobiological response exerted at many levels, not only via the hypothalamus. For example, structures located in the caudal brainstem also express GHS-R1a. In particular, ghrelin receptors are found in all three components of the dorsal vagal complex with a highest expression within the area postrema, a moderately dense signal in the nucleus of the solitary tract and a low density signal in the dorsal motor nucleus of the vagus (Zigman et al., 2006). Peripheral injection of ghrelin and, prior to its discover, ghrelin mimetics, induces c-Fos induction in the nucleus of the solitary tract and area postrema (Bailey et al., 2000; Lawrence et al., 2002). The effects of ghrelin on food intake/behavior are similar when injected into the fourth as for the third ventricle, in terms of the amount of food eaten, the number of meals and meal size during the first few hours after treatment (Faulconbridge et al., 2003). The effects of ghrelin in the dorsal vagal complex might be more related to autonomic effects such as on the cardiovascular system. However, since the hypothalamus is strongly connected with the nucleus solitary tract, we cannot exclude an indirect effect of the ghrelin to hypothalamic structures through an activation of brainstem areas, although appears not to include a noradrenergic pathway (Bailey et al., 2000; see *infra*).

Ghrelin and the reward system

Besides the homeostatic ghrelin sensitive pathways, ghrelin also appears to target mesolimbic circuits linked to reward. Hedonic (non-homeostatic) brain pathways are also involved in feeding control and are modulated by circulating energy balance signals such as ghrelin, thereby influencing the evaluation of the pleasure derived from the taste, smell, or texture of food. Many regions of the corticolimbic and mesolimbic brain are thus involved in learning, memory, emotion, and reward processing associated with food. Among these complex feeding networks (for review, see Van Vugt, 2010; **Figure 3**), the VTA-Acc (dopaminergic) pathway plays a pivotal role in conferring reward from a wide range of reinforcers, from chemical drugs of abuse to natural rewards such as food (Nestler, 1996; Corwin et al., 2011). Using optogenetic techniques, Adamantidis et al. (2011) demonstrated that phasic activation dopaminergic VTA neurons is associated with reward-predicting cues and facilitates the development of positive reinforcement during reward-seeking and behavioral flexibility. As reviewed in Carr (2011), burst firing of VTA dopaminergic neurons may operate as a "teaching signal." For example, in the case of food intake, when rats are presented with a highly palatable food for the first time, this triggers dopamine release in the Acc (shell), whereas repeated exposure to the same palatable food blunts the dopamine response despite avid consumption. Interestingly, food restriction has been described to sustain the Acc (shell) dopamine release in this model. Moreover, simply delivering cues

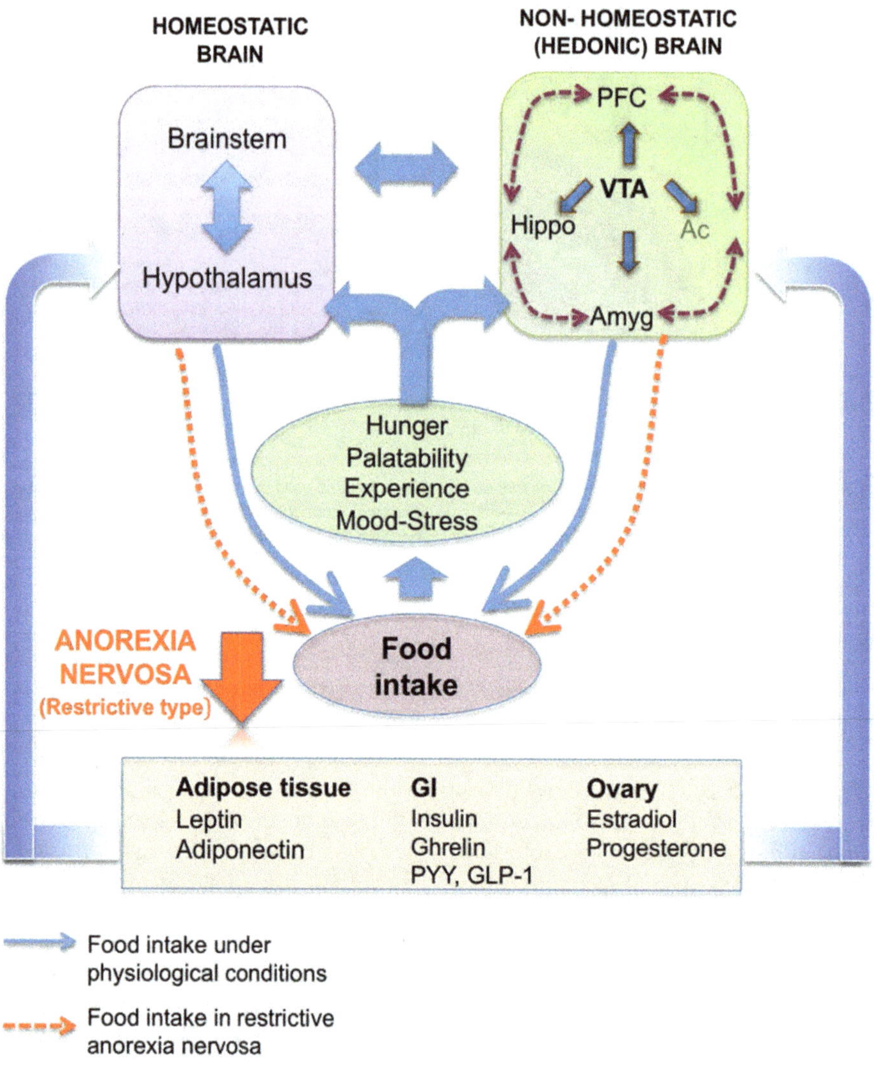

FIGURE 3 | Homeostatic brain vs. non-homeostatic (hedonic) brain. Schematic representation of the potential interaction of homeostatic hypothalamic and brainstem areas with non-homeostatic (hedonic) brain structures to control food intake. The hedonic brain comprises mainly the meso-cortico-limbic system, which includes the ventral tegmental area (VTA), nucleus accumbens (Ac), prefrontal cortex (PFC), hippocampus (Hippo), and amygdala (Amyg). Hormones from peripheral compartments like adipose tissue, gastrointestinal tract or ovary reach these areas, directly or indirectly to activate pathways controlling both energy balance (homeostatic brain) and pleasure (hedonic brain) associated with eating (hunger level, palatability of the food, past experiences, mood, level of stress). In anorexia nervosa (restrictive type), a deregulation of one or more of these pathways as well as the cross-talk between periphery and brain might be considered. Adapted from Van Vugt (2010).

linked previously to the food reward can be sufficient to reinstate the Acc (shell) dopamine response, indicating transference of the dopamine response from the reinforcer to the cue (for review, see Volkov et al. (2011). Ghrelin has emerged as one important modulator of the VTA-NAcc (dopaminergic) reward pathway (for review, see Skibicka and Dickson, 2011). More than 50% of the dopaminergic VTA neurons express GHS-R (Zigman et al., 2006), although it is also expressed on other cell types in this area (Abizaid et al., 2006). Whether administered peripherally, into the brain ventricles or into the VTA, ghrelin administration triggers a robust Acc dopamine response (Abizaid et al., 2006; Jerlhag et al., 2006, 2007) that is accompanied by an increased feeding response in rodents (Naleid et al., 2005; Egecioglu et al., 2010) and an increase in food-motivated behavior (Skibicka and Dickson, 2011; Skibicka et al., 2012). Central ghrelin signaling, *via* GHS-R1A, appears to be important not only for food reward (Egecioglu et al., 2010), but also for the reward associated with artificial rewards like alcohol, cocaine, and amphetamine (Wellman et al., 2005; Jerlhag et al., 2009, 2010). As an example, the locomotor stimulating effect of cocaine is decreased in ghrelin KO mice compared to their wild type littermates (Abizaid et al., 2010). Furthermore, in rodents, ghrelin elevates the motivation to obtain high-sugar or high-fat reward (Perello et al., 2010; Skibicka and Dickson, 2011; Skibicka et al., 2012). In particular, both peripheral and central injections of ghrelin augment the food-motivated behavior of a satiated rat to get sugar whereas blockade of ghrelin signaling reduces the operant responding of an hungry rat to the level of a satiated rat (Skibicka et al., 2012). These data strongly support the involvement of ghrelin in behaviors related to food reward. Thereby one can suggest that ghrelin could be considered as a key internal cue, available during period of energy deficit to motivate adequate food intake behavior (Skibicka and Dickson, 2011). These data reinforce the now well-documented role of ghrelin in food reward, considering that the shell region of the Acc is described to process unpredicted rewards and motivational states to reinforce food intake behaviors, but also use of drugs of abuse. However, the action of circulating ghrelin upon GHS-R1A-expressing cells in the VTA, located mostly on dopaminergic neurons, begs the question of how this hormone reaches deep brain structures that are far away from circumventricular organs (see *infra*). Finally, one study shows that presence of food is necessary to induce dopamine release (Kawahara et al., 2009). Chronic ghrelin treatment also modifies the expression of dopaminergic receptors in Acc, more specially D1 and D3 (Skibicka et al., 2012), which are described to be involved in obesity, food reward (D1 receptors) and inhibition of reward behavior (D3 receptors). Similar data were obtained from human imaging studies that emphasize the role of ghrelin in food reward. Indeed, intravenous ghrelin injection to human subjects increases activity in brain areas involved in the evaluation of the reward value attributed to food and food cues including the striatum, amygdala, insula, and orbitofrontal cortex (Malik et al., 2008).

Other functions

Almost 6000 articles have been published on ghrelin, since its discovery in Kojima et al. (1999) and it is not surprising that its biological effects extend beyond feeding and energy balance, effects that may also be relevant for AN. These include peripheral effects (e.g., gastric motility, bone homeostasis, cardiovascular system, glucose homeostasis, reproduction, immune system) as well as CNS effects (mood disorder, sleep disturbance).

There is now increasing evidence that ghrelin stimulates motor activity in the gastrointestinal tract (gastric motility and emptying). In fact, ghrelin shares high homology degree with motilin (Kojima and Kangawa, 2005), a hormone released by endocrine cells of duodenum and jejunum during fasting and which increases gastric motility after feeding (Sanger, 2008). Ghrelin has been described to use both central and local pathways to exert its effects on the gut through receptors located on vagal afferents, in the nodose ganglion and myenteric plexus. In fact in normal rodents, central pathways are operational whereas after vagotomy, ghrelin is able to exert effects *via* the myenteric plexus (see review of Peeters, 2003). Moreover, in mice, central administration of ghrelin accelerates gastric emptying (Asakawa et al., 2001) and changes the excitability of neurons located in the PVN identified as receiving ascending afferent signals from mechanoreceptors in the stomach (Zhao et al., 2003). Clinically, it has been reported that the intravenous administration of ghrelin accelerates the rate of gastric emptying and induces gastrointestinal contraction in healthy volunteers (Fujitsuka et al., 2012). Since the plasma levels of ghrelin are high in AN patients, one can hypothesize an alteration of the signaling both at central and peripheral levels that may worsen the outcome of the patients. These findings suggest that ghrelin could provide a therapeutic target for disorders related to gastrointestinal discomfort.

Surprisingly, ghrelin is also involved in sleep-wakefulness regulation. Indeed, experiments conducted in adult male rats demonstrate that repeated intravenously administrations of ghrelin stimulate wakefulness, decrease slow-wave sleep, and reduce the duration of rapid eye movement sleep (Tolle et al., 2002). This action could involve a reduction in the release of acetylcholine from the dorsal tegmental nucleus (LDTg) on neurons expressing somatotropin release-inhibiting factor known to indirectly regulate the rapid eye movement sleep periods (Tolle et al., 2002). In fact, among the various neurochemical systems involved in wakefulness (acetylcholine, norepinephrine, dopamine, serotonin, histamine), the hypothalamic orexigenic neurons are crucial promoters of wakefulness since deficiency in the orexin system leads to disorders such as narcolepsy (Modirrousta et al., 2005). The status of activity in orexin neurons is closely related with the nutritional and behavioral state of animals. Moreover, Lamont et al. (2012) observed that both GHS-R and ghrelin KO mice had fewer orexin-immunoreactive cells than their wild type littermates. Their data support the synergistic relationship between ghrelin and orexin in the coordination of metabolism, reward and arousal to adopt the adapted behavior for food seeking and restoration of energy deficiency. In humans, AN patients exhibit sleep disorders. As an example, AN adolescents have an increase in wakefulness after sleep onset, a fragmentation of sleep as well as a reduction of slow-wave sleep and slow-wave activity during their total sleep time (Lauer and Krieg, 2004; Nobili et al., 2004). Even if deepening of nocturnal sleep follows a partial weight restoration, the neurobiological mechanisms linking starvation, mood disorders, and sleep disturbance remain to be elucidated.

The impact of ghrelin on anxiety behaviors remains controversial: studies show an anxiolytic effect under caloric restriction or after subcutaneous ghrelin injection (Lutter et al., 2008) while anxiogenic effects are observed in others (acute) studies with intracerebroventricular or intraperitoneal ghrelin injection (Asakawa et al., 2001; see review Chuang and Zigman, 2010). Interestingly, chronic central ghrelin treatment was found to increase anxiety-like behavior in rats (Hansson et al., 2011). Recently, one study investigating the amygdala as a target for ghrelin found that acute ghrelin injection at this site elicits behaviors consist with a reduction in anxiety-like behavior, but only in rats that were not allowed access to food during the initial hour after injection. It was concluded that ghrelin, acting at the level of the amygdala, may provide an especially important signal to suppress anxiety-like behaviors that would otherwise prohibit the animal from finding food (Alvarez-Crespo et al., 2012). It is not yet known whether the ghrelin system regulates anxiety behavior associated with AN. One study found that a SNP in the preproghrelin gene was associated with panic disorder in a small patient group (Hansson et al., 2011).

Among the disorders described in AN, osteopenia/osteoporosis is also one major problem that cause long term outcomes with in particular a strong increase of the bone fracture incidence (Lucas et al., 1999). Ghrelin has and ghrelin mimetics have been shown to increase bone mineral density (Svensson et al., 2000; Fukushima et al., 2005; Delhanty et al., 2006) by a mechanism that appears to include the promotion of both proliferation and differentiation of osteoblasts (cells involved in bone formation), involving GHS-R1a and GHS-R1b receptors (Fukushima et al., 2005; Delhanty et al., 2006). The etiopathogenesis of bone disease in AN is complex and multifaceted. Indeed, the low bone mineral density (Legroux-Gerot et al., 2005, 2008; Legroux-Gérot et al., 2007; Estour et al., 2010) is usually linked with alteration of multiple factors (**Tables 3–6**) that are thought to contribute to the "uncoupling" of bone turnover, leading to increased bone resorption, and decreased bone formation (see Howgate et al., 2013). However, it has been demonstrated that ghrelin affects bone metabolism by operating in an autocrine/paracrine mode, independent of the GH/IGF-1 axis (see Nikolopoulos et al., 2010). Weight recovery is associated with partial recovery of bone mineral density. There is currently no approved effective therapy that completely reverses the bone mineral density deficit. The most convincing results were obtained with a treatment of recombinant human IGF-1 alone or in combination with the oral contraceptive pills (see Misra and Klibanski, 2011). The link between ghrelin and estrogen on bone metabolism is always matter of debate even if it is established that ghrelin suppresses pulsatile LH and FSH pulsatility (Meczekalski et al., 2008; Kluge et al., 2012).

Another criterion used to characterize AN patients is amenorrhea. Indeed, in negative energy balance conditions like in AN, the increase of plasma ghrelin is associated with decrease of LH secretion (**Table 6**). Evidence is mounting that ghrelin may operate as a pleitropic modulator of gonadal function and reproduction (Tena-Sempere, 2008; Muccioli et al., 2011; Repaci et al., 2011). Notably, most of the actions of ghrelin upon the reproductive axis reported to date are inhibitory. Ghrelin can suppress not only LH, but also FSH secretion in male and female rats (Fernández-Fernández et al., 2005; Martini et al., 2006). Such effects are also described in humans (Kluge et al., 2012). Centrally, ghrelin exerts a predominant action directly at the level of the GnRH pulse generator by inhibiting directly GnRH release (Fernández-Fernández et al., 2005; Muccioli et al., 2011) or by an indirect modulation of other neuronal pathways. For example, Forbes et al. (2009) recently showed the ability of ghrelin to decrease Kiss1 mRNA expression in the medial preoptic area. Given the importance of the kisspeptin system to control the reproductive axis, these data provide new hypothesis for ghrelin-induced suppression of pulsatile LH secretion. Once again, in the AN, ghrelin might dynamically mediate the suppressive effect of energy deficit on the onset of puberty, gonadal function, and fertility. Here, the effects of ghrelin on the gonadal axis might protect females in a condition of strong energy insufficiency to develop a reproductive behavior that can be deleterious for her and her progeny.

Finally, ghrelin is also involved in other physiological functions that are more or less affected in AN like cardiovascular function or immune system. Among the cardiovascular effects, this hormone improves left ventricular contractility and cardiac output in healthy humans (Enomoto et al., 2003; Tesauro et al., 2010) and lowers blood pressure in mice concomitantly with a decrease in sympathetic nerve activity that is not caused by a direct action on blood vessels (Callaghan et al., 2012). In AN, the neuroendocrine alterations are also accompanied by autonomic dysfunctions like lower blood pressure values, lack of circadian variation of blood pressure and bradycardia (Oswiecimska et al., 2007). Thus, ghrelin might participate in AN to the cardiovascular complications observed in AN (Casiero and Frishman, 2006; Jáuregui-Garrido and Jáuregui-Lobera, 2012), but no studies currently display any correlation between these cardiovascular risks and the high plasma levels of ghrelin.

The role of ghrelin on the immune system remains unclear. However, Taub (2008) describes its implication in the regulation of immune factors, by inhibiting inflammatory cytokine production, more specifically in mediating anti-inflammatory effects on IL-1, TNF-α, and IL-6 cytokine expression by T-cells and mononuclear cells *via* GHS-R, and promoting thymic function. In AN, data related to the evaluation of circulating pro-inflammatory or inflammatory cytokines or in adipocytes are still a matter of debate and, as underlined by Nova and Marcos (2006), "controversial findings have been published regarding some aspects of the immune system that are otherwise impaired in more typical types of malnutrition."

Des-acyl ghrelin and obestatin: a controversial metabolic function?

Concerning des-acyl ghrelin, its role in food intake has been much debated. The recent paper of Delhanty et al. (2012) gives numerous arguments supporting des-acyl ghrelin as an hormone that can be metabolically active, when co-administrated with acyl ghrelin, by counteracting the effects of acyl ghrelin on insulin secretion and glucose metabolism. Des-acyl ghrelin appears to be increased in AN patients (Harada et al., 2008; Germain et al., 2009). Kojima et al. (1999) showed that des-acyl ghrelin was not able to bind to GHS-R1a. Although the des-acyl ghrelin receptor remains unknown, the increasing data suggesting that des-acyl ghrelin is a biologically active molecular, indicate that a dedicated receptor may exist.

Several studies show controversial effects of des-acyl ghrelin on food intake that are either inhibitory (Asakawa et al., 2005; Chen et al., 2005b) or stimulatory (Toshinai et al., 2006) in rodents. These results can be due to the different methods used like the type of injection, the dose used, the time of injection (light or dark period), the nutritional status, fed, or fasted. However, the overexpression of des-acyl ghrelin in a transgenic mouse model results in a small phenotype, associated with a reduction of food intake and body fat mass, reduced IGF-1 plasma levels without significant changes in circulating GH and also higher des-acyl ghrelin with no change in total ghrelin plasma levels (Ariyasu et al., 2005). In these mice, no significant differences have been noticed for glycemia and insulinemia (Ariyasu et al., 2005; Asakawa et al., 2005) while studies other studies have shown that des-acyl ghrelin inhibits glucose release *in vivo* and *in vitro* (Broglio et al., 2004b; Gauna et al., 2005; Qader et al., 2008). Moreover, it appears that ghrelin and des-acyl ghrelin do not have the same blood concentration in systemic and in portal circulations suggesting that liver could be involved in ghrelin regulation (Goodyear et al., 2010).

Concerning lipid metabolism, *in vivo* studies showed that des-acyl ghrelin as well as ghrelin increase bone marrow adipogenesis in rat shinbone (Thompson et al., 2004) and both forms enhance lipid accumulation in visceral tissue in humans (Rodríguez et al., 2009). The mechanisms involved remain unclear. Similarly, acute or chronic des-acyl ghrelin injections in adult male rats cause an inhibition of LH secretion like ghrelin (Martini et al., 2006). By contrast, transgenic mice overexpressing des-acyl ghrelin do not display any changes in LH and FSH levels (Ariyasu et al., 2005).

Des-acyl ghrelin may also have a role in gastric motility. Indeed, intracerebroventricular or intravenous injections alter motor activity in the antrum with a decrease of antrum activity only in fasted rats (Chen et al., 2005b). Mice overexpressing des-acyl ghrelin exhibit a decrease in gastric emptying (Asakawa et al., 2005). Other studies are necessary to understand the mechanisms involved since vagotomy does not disrupt the (intravenous) des-acyl ghrelin effect (Chen et al., 2005b).

Studies about the effects of des-acyl ghrelin on the cardiovascular system are rare. Nevertheless, like acyl ghrelin, it promotes bradycardia and hypotension (Tsubota et al., 2005). Moreover, ghrelin and des-acyl ghrelin display vasodilator effect and no inotropic effects when they are applied on human artery *in vitro* (Kleinz et al., 2006).

Similarly, concerning obestatin, it remains again an open question whether this peptide is a physiologically relevant peptide to regulate energy homeostasis, food intake and gastric motility (Gourcerol et al., 2007). Obestatin binds to GRP 39, a receptor of the same subfamily than ghrelin receptor, to decrease food intake and body weight in an opposite manner to ghrelin (Stengel et al., 2009; Hassouna et al., 2010; Mokrosinski and Holst, 2010; Veldhuis and Bowers, 2010). Subsequent studies failed to show activation of this receptor and only few studies have reproduced the obestatin effects under specific conditions. Such results should be interpreted with caution since variations are observed according to the kits and conditions applied for obestatin assays (Hassouna et al., 2010). Due to their potential functions, it should be interesting to measure ghrelin/obestatin ratio to better understand their roles in the alteration of energy balance. It seems that AN affects obestatin blood levels with a lower ghrelin/obestatin ratio in AN patients of restrictive type compared to constitutional thin women (Germain et al., 2009, 2010). Moreover, other functions are attributed to this hormone such as the inhibition of thirst, gastric motility, cell survival, pancreatic hormone secretion, sleep, thermoregulation, memory, and anxiety (Szentirmai et al., 2009; Hassouna et al., 2010; Veldhuis and Bowers, 2010).

ACCESS OF GHRELIN TO ITS NEURONAL TARGETS

To dynamically report energy homeostasis alterations and ensure an appropriate neuronal response, blood-borne ghrelin must rapidly access the central nervous system. Intriguingly, the physiological mechanisms controlling the access of ghrelin to its neuronal target remain currently debated. Indeed, although a central origin of ghrelin has been described (Cowley et al., 2003), it is now recognized that blood-derived ghrelin is able to target neuronal networks within the central nervous system to regulate energy homeostasis. However, it remains unclear how this key energy status-signaling hormone can rapidly access sensory neurons to alter feeding responses. Ghrelin mainly targets neurons located in the ARC where different blood/brain interfaces have been described. The blood–brain barrier is one such interface and one of the best described in the hypothalamic nuclei as in all other regions of the brain. The blood–brain barrier is located on brain capillaries where endothelial cells are tightly apposed by continuous tight junctions that prevent the free passage of molecules through the paracellular pathway. For circulating factors to access to the brain through the blood–brain barrier endothelium requires transcellular transport. Many studies have investigated the transport of circulating ghrelin across the blood–brain barrier. Banks et al. (2002) demonstrated the existence of ghrelin saturable transport system in mice from the brain to the blood but transport into the brain was much less pronounced. Remarkably, human ghrelin, which differs from mouse ghrelin by 2 amino acids, can be transported in both directions in mice. So, although receptor-mediated transport of ghrelin cannot be excluded, uptake mechanisms of this peptide remain unclear. Moreover, the efficiency of this blood–brain barrier remains to be studied in a chronic caloric restriction context. Improved CNS penetration during fating is one possible mechanism to explain the threefold increase in the number of cells expressing fos after peripheral ghrelin injection in fasted vs. fed rats (Hewson and Dickson, 2000). The role of another blood/brain interface that is materialized by fenestrated vessels is also to consider. Indeed, these vessels are part of the blood-CSF barrier that is mostly described in the median eminence, the circumventricular organ adjacent to the ARC (Mullier et al., 2010). Median eminence vasculature differs from typical brain vessels as they harbor a fenestrated endothelium that lacks tight junction complexes. These structural characteristics and the presence of various blood-derived molecules in the median eminence and the other circumventricular organs parenchyma suggest high permeability of this specific vasculature (Broadwell et al., 1983; Ciofi, 2011; Morita and Miyata, 2012). Permeable vasculature can be found in the external part of the median eminence forming pituitary portal capillary plexus that displays some long intrainfundibular loops spreading into the median eminence parenchyma. Interestingly, fenestrated vessels are also found within the ARC with a higher density into the ventromedial ARC where they are bordered by NPY expressing neurons (Ciofi et al., 2009). These data give support to the access of ghrelin from the circulation to the ventromedial sensory neurons *via* median eminence/ARC fenestrated vasculature (**Figure 4**).

The action of ghrelin on food intake may not be only due to its action on hypothalamus. Indeed, an indirect role of ghrelin on hypothalamic structures through an activation of brainstem areas has been suggested. Indirect pathway may occur through the binding of ghrelin to gastric vagal afferent neurons (Date et al., 2002). However, the expression of GHS-R1a within the dorsal vagal complex supports a direct action of ghrelin to brain parenchyma. Among this complex, the area postrema is a circumventricular organ that characteristically present fenestrated vasculature. These vessels may be responsible for the diffusion of ghrelin and its delivery to the dorsal vagal complex that communicates with hypothalamic control centers (**Figure 4**).

Fenestrated vasculature could represent a direct vascular route while allowing passive diffusion of peripheral molecules into the hypothalamus and the area postrema. This route may be responsible of acute regulation and complete chronic feedback accomplished by uptake of circulating molecules *via* receptor-mediated transport across the blood–brain barrier.

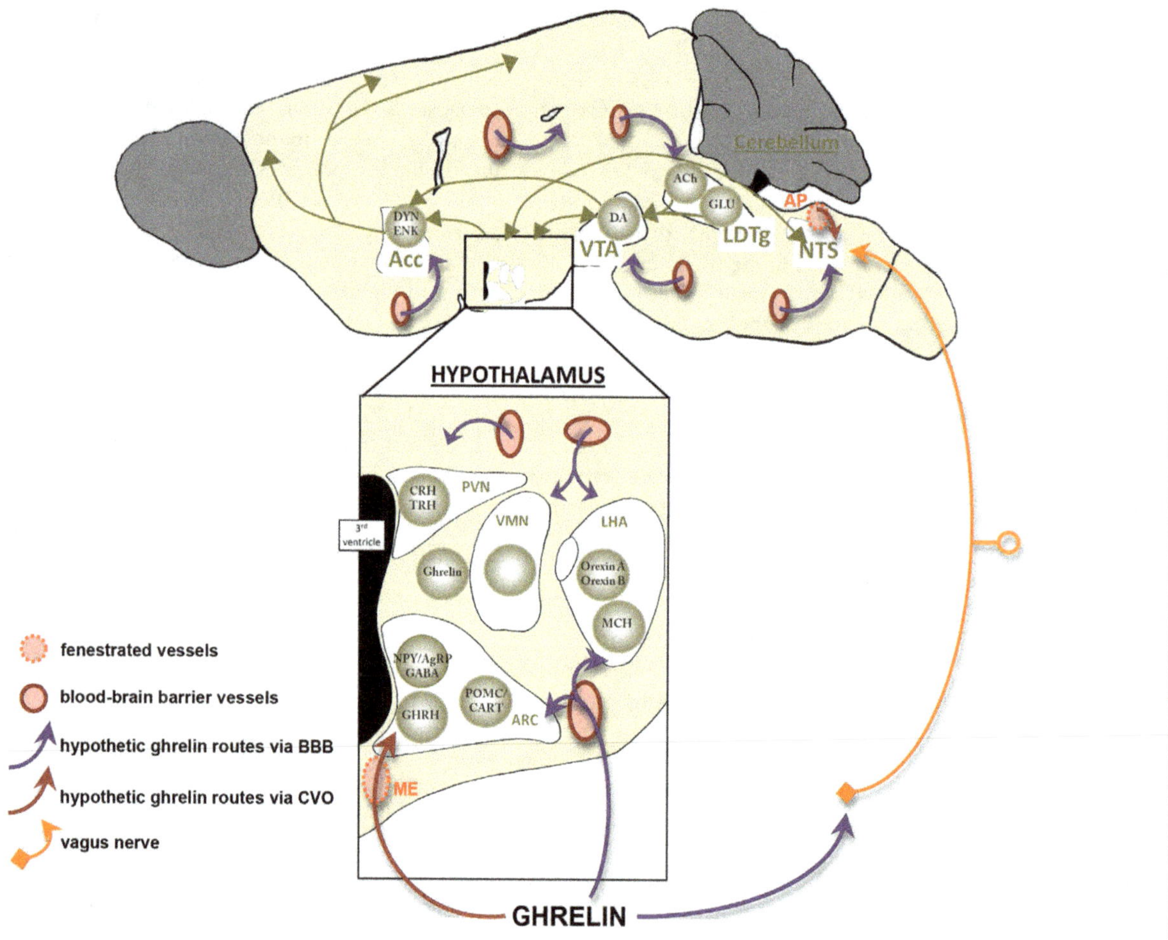

FIGURE 4 | Access of ghrelin signal to its neuronal targets. This schema summarizes the three hypothetic access routes of ghrelin toward its neuronal targets (cf **Figure 2**). First, ghrelin would be able to target neuronal networks thanks to specific transcellular transports at the level of blood–brain barrier (BBB) located on brain capillaries (purple arrows). Most ghrelin sensitive areas present blood–brain barrier vasculature and this route represent the main one described in all regions of the brain. However free-BBB regions, called the median eminence and the area postrema, are recorded in the hypothalamus and the brainstem respectively. These areas contain a rich fenestrated vasculature, which could represent a direct vascular route while allowing passive diffusion of peripheral ghrelin (red arrows). This route may be responsible of acute regulation and complete chronic feedback accomplished by uptake of circulating molecules via receptor-mediated transport across the blood–brain barrier. Finally, activation of brainstem areas by ghrelin may occur without the entrance of ghrelin in the brain, but through its binding to gastric vagal afferent neurons (orange). Acc, accumbens nucleus; ACh, acétylcholine; AgRP, agouti-related peptide; AP, area postrema; ARC, arcuate nucleus; CART, cocaine- and amphetamine-regulated transcript; CRH, corticotropin-releasing hormone; DA, dopamine; DYN, dynorphin; ENK, enkephalin; GABA, γ-aminobutyric acid; GHRH, growth-hormone-releasing hormone; GLU, glutamate; LDTg, laterodorsal tegmental area; LHA, lateral hypothalamic area; MCH, melanin-concentrating hormone; ME, median eminence; NPY, neuropeptide Y; NTS, nucleus of the solitary tract; POMC, pro-opiomelanocortin; PVN, paraventricular nucleus; TRH, thyrotropin releasing hormone; VMH, ventromedial nucleus; VTA, ventral tegmental area.

The transport of ghrelin through the blood/brain interfaces has been poorly investigated in metabolic disorders excepted in obesity where few data are available. Banks et al. (2008) showed an inverse relation between body weight and ghrelin access to the brain suggesting that physiological states influence the rate at which ghrelin is transported across the blood/brain interfaces. A better understanding of the access of ghrelin to its neuronal target may leads to novel therapeutic interventions.

CONCLUSION: GHRELIN AS A POTENTIAL TREATMENT FOR ANOREXIA NERVOSA

In restrictive AN, the high plasma levels of ghrelin, even adaptive in view of its main role in meal initiation, let us to hypothesize a potential insensitivity to this endocrine signal both peripherally and centrally in association with this disease. It should be also mentioned that AN patients often cannot increase their food intake not only because of fear of obesity, but also because of chronic or recurrent abdominal discomfort, fullness, and chronic constipation, functions in which efficient ghrelin participation is required. Injections of exogenous ghrelin have been shown to increase the adiposity and to stimulate appetite in healthy individuals and cancer patients (Peino et al., 2000; Wren et al., 2001a; Neary et al., 2004).

For AN patients, only a few preliminary studies have been performed to examine the effects of ghrelin administration (Miljic et al., 2006; Hotta et al., 2009; Ogiso et al., 2011). In these clinical studies, the mode of administration was different leading to different outcomes. In the study of Miljic et al. (2006), a single-dose continuous administration of ghrelin for 5 h failed to affect appetite in all AN patients treated. Hotta et al. (2009) report that intravenous administration of ghrelin in anorectic patients twice a day for 14 days improves epigastric discomfort or constipation and increases the hunger score, which is related to gastric emptying. An increase of the body weight was obtained, from 1.5 to 2.4 kg, and daily energy intake during ghrelin infusion increased by 12–36% compared with the pretreatment period. Nutritional parameters such as total protein and triglyceride levels improved. These findings suggest that ghrelin may have therapeutic potentials in AN patients who cannot gain weight because of gastrointestinal dysfunction. Further studies are need to elucidate the potential impact of ghrelin by itself or agonists to ameliorate the outcomes of the AN patients.

In animals, several attempts have been made (see the other chapter submitted by Hassouna et al. "Actions of agonists and antagonists of the ghrelin/GHS-R pathway on GH secretion, appetite, and c-Fos activity"). Recently, Costantini et al. (2011) detailed an unexpected effect of GSK1614343, a novel ghrelin receptor antagonist with no partial agonist properties, that induced both in rats and dogs an increase of food intake, body weight, and reduced the POMC mRNA levels in the hypothalamus of rats chronically treated with the compound. Although it may seem counterintuitive to consider the use of ghrelin antagonists in this disease area, one study in rodents suggested that suppressed ghrelin signaling reduces (food anticipatory) hyperlocomotor activity in the ABA model (Verhagen et al., 2011). Barnett et al. (2010) demonstrated that the administration of a GOAT inhibitor improved glucose tolerance and decreased weight gain in wild type mice but not in ghrelin KO mice. Such treatment also led to decreased serum levels of acyl ghrelin without any effect on serum levels of des-acyl ghrelin. Even if this GOAT inhibitor might be expected to pave the way for clinical targeting of GOAT in metabolic diseases such as obesity and diabetes mellitus, one can suggest that, a GOAT activator, which has not been reported yet, may be a potential new treatment of AN if it improves food intake and body weight gain in patients with AN.

Finally, in the future it will be possible to assess more precisely the exact contribution of ghrelin, des-acyl ghrelin, and obestatin in the evolution of the AN both in humans and adequate animal models (Cardona Cano et al., 2012). The roles played by these peptides in feeding behavior, adaptation to starvation, reward mechanisms, emotional behavior, and stress responses in animals and humans led them to be potential therapeutic targets for AN treatments. The way and the mode of administration remain to be further determined and clarified. Neuroimaging studies have reported reduced brain volumes affecting both ventral and dorsal neural circuit dysfunctions in AN patients, with altered metabolisms of serotonin and dopamine that are closely associated to ghrelin, contributing to their puzzling symptoms (Kaye et al., 2009; Brooks et al., 2011). It will be important to determine whether the ghrelin signal reaches its central targets leading, as it is observed for leptin in obesity, to a « ghrelin-resistance »or a « transient ghrelin-insensitivity ». More investigations are needed to better suppress the neuronal activity of ghrelin signaling and to identify the specific pathways that may underlie the deleterious behaviors in patients suffering from AN. Investigation of the ghrelin peptide system will open up a new window of research for tackling psychosomatic disorders beyond the gastrointestinal tract, particularly restrictive AN and obesity/metabolic syndrome, two disorders at the extreme of the body weight continuum.

AUTHOR NOTE

Cross reference with another chapter of this issue: *Actions of agonists and antagonists of the ghrelin/GHS-R pathway on GH secretion, appetite and c-Fos activity* by Rim Hassouna, Alexandra Labarthe, Philippe Zizzari, Catherine Videau, Michael Culler, Jacques Epelbaum, and Virginie Tolle (Hassouna et al., 2013).

REFERENCES

Abizaid, A., Liu, Z. W., Andrews, Z. B., Shanabrough, M., Borok, E., Elsworth, J. D., et al. (2006). Ghrelin modulates the activity and synaptic input organization of midbrain dopamine neurons while promoting appetite. *J. Clin. Invest.* 116, 3229–3239.

Abizaid, A., Mineur, Y. S., Roth, R. H., Elsworth, J. D., Sleeman, M. W., Picciotto, M. R., et al. (2010). Reduced locomotor responses to cocaine in ghrelin-deficient mice. *Neuroscience* 192, 500–506.

Adamantidis, A. R., Tsai, H. C., Boutrel, B., Zhang, F., Stuber, G. D., Budygin, E. A., et al. (2011). Optogenetic interrogation of dopaminergic modulation of the multiple phases of reward-seeking behavior. *J. Neurosci.* 31, 10829–10835.

Alguacil, L. F., Salas, E., and González-Martín, C. (2011). Identification of new drug targets and biomarkers related to obesity and eating disorders: an approach based on reward deficit and addiction. *Curr. Pharm. Des.* 17, 462–470.

Alvarez-Crespo, M., Skibicka, K. P., Farkas, I., Molnár, C. S., Egecioglu, E., Hrabovszky, E., et al. (2012). The amygdala as a neurobiological target for ghrelin in rats: neuroanatomical, electrophysiological and behavioral evidence.

PLoS ONE 7:e46321. doi:10.1371/journal.pone.0046321

Andrews, Z. B., Liu, Z. W., Walllingford, N., Erion, D. M., Borok, E., Friedman, J. M., et al. (2008). UCP2 mediates ghrelin's action on NPY/AgRP neurons by lowering free radicals. *Nature* 454, 846–851.

Arimura, C., Nozaki, T., Takakura, S., Kawai, K., Takii, M., Sudo, N., et al. (2010). Predictors of menstrual resumption by patients with anorexia nervosa. *Eat. Weight Disord.* 15, e226–e233.

Ariyasu, H., Takaya, K., Iwakura, H., Hosoda, H., Akamizu, T., Arai, Y., et al. (2005). Transgenic mice overexpressing des-acyl ghrelin show small phenotype. *Endocrinology* 146, 355–364.

Ariyasu, H., Takaya, K., Tagami, T., Ogawa, Y., Hosoda, K., Akamizu, T., et al. (2001). Stomach is a major source of circulating ghrelin, and feeding state determines plasma ghrelin-like immunoreactivity levels in humans. *J. Clin. Endocrinol. Metab.* 86, 4753–4758.

Arvat, E., Maccario, M., Di Vito, L., Broglio, F., Benso, A., Gottero, C., et al. (2001). Endocrine activities of ghrelin, a natural growth hormone secretagogue (GHS), in humans: comparison and interactions with hexarelin, a nonnatural peptidyl GHS, and GH-releasing hormone. *J. Clin. Endocrinol. Metab.* 86, 1169–1174.

Asakawa, A., Inui, A., Fujimiya, M., Sakamaki, R., Shinfuku, N., Ueta, Y., et al. (2005). Stomach regulates energy balance via acylated ghrelin and desacyl ghrelin. *Gut* 54, 18–24.

Asakawa, A., Inui, A., Kaga, T., Yuzuriha, H., Nagata, T., Ueno, N., et al. (2001). Ghrelin is an appetite-stimulatory signal from stomach with structural resemblance to motilin. *Gastroenterology* 120, 337–345.

Avena, N. M., and Bocarsly, M. E. (2012). Dysregulation of brain reward systems in eating disorders: neurochemical information from animal models of binge eating, bulimia nervosa, and anorexia nervosa. *Neuropharmacology* 63, 87–96.

Bailey, A. R., von Engelhardt, N., Leng, G., Smith, R. G., and Dickson, S. L. (2000). Growth hormone secretagogue activation of the arcuate nucleus and brainstem occurs via a non-noradrenergic pathway. *J. Neuroendocrinol.* 12, 191–197.

Balligand, J. L., Brichard, S. M., Brichard, V., Desager, J. P., and Lambert, M. (1998). Hypoleptinemia in patients with anorexia nervosa: loss of circadian rhythm and unresponsiveness to short-term refeeding. *Eur. J. Endocrinol.* 138, 415–420.

Banks, W. A., Burney, B. O., and Robinson, S. M. (2008). Effects of triglycerides, obesity, and starvation on ghrelin transport across the blood-brain barrier. *Peptides* 29, 2061–2065.

Banks, W. A., Tschop, M., Robinson, S. M., and Heiman, M. L. (2002). Extent and direction of ghrelin transport across the blood-brain barrier is determined by its unique primary structure. *J. Pharmacol. Exp. Ther.* 302, 822–827.

Baranowska, B. (1990). Are disturbances in opioid and adrenergic systems involved in the hormonal dysfunction of anorexia nervosa. *Psychoneuroendocrinology* 15, 371–379.

Baranowska, B., Radzikowska, M., Wasilewska-Dziubinska, E., Roguski, K., and Borowiec, M. (2000). The role of VIP and somatostatin in the control of GH and prolactin release in anorexia nervosa and in obesity. *Ann. N. Y. Acad. Sci.* 921, 443–455.

Baranowska, B., Wasilewska-Dziubinska, E., Radzikowska, M., Plonowski, A., and Roguski, K. (1997). Neuropeptide Y, galanin, and leptin release in obese women and in women with anorexia nervosa. *Metab. Clin. Exp.* 46, 1384–1389.

Baranowska, B., Wolinska-Witort, E., Wasilewska-Dziubinska, E., Roguski, K., and Chmielowska, M. (2001). Plasma leptin, neuropeptide Y (NPY) and galanin concentrations in bulimia nervosa and in anorexia nervosa. *Neuro Endocrinol. Lett.* 22, 356–358.

Barazzoni, R., Bosutti, A., Stebel, M., Cattin, M. R., Roder, E., Visintin, L., et al. (2005). Ghrelin regulates mitochondrial-lipid metabolism gene expression and tissue fat distribution in liver and skeletal muscle *Am. J. Physiol. Endocrinol. Metab.* 288, E228–E235.

Barbarich-Marsteller, N. C. (2007). Neurochemistry and pharmacological treatments: where is the field of anorexia nervosa heading? *Cent. Nerv. Syst. Agents Med. Chem.* 7, 35–43.

Barbarich-Marsteller, N. C., Foltin, R. W., and Walsh, B. T. (2011). Does anorexia nervosa resemble an addiction? *Curr. Drug Abuse Rev.* 4, 197–200.

Barnett, B. P., Hwang, Y., Taylor, M. S., Kirchner, H., Pfluger, P. T., Bernard, V., et al. (2010). Glucose and weight control in mice with a designed ghrelin O-acyltransferase inhibitor. *Science* 330, 1689–1692.

Bergh, C., and Södersten, P. (1996). Anorexia nervosa, self starvation and the reward of stress. *Nat. Med.* 2, 21–22.

Berrettini, W. H., Kaye, W. H., Sunderland, T., May, C., Gwirtsman, H. E., Mellow, A., et al. (1988). Galanin immunoreactivity in human CSF: studies in eating disorders and Alzheimer's disease. *Neuropsychobiology* 19, 64–68.

Boakes, R. A. (2007). Self-starvation in the rat: running versus eating. *Span. J. Psychol.* 10, 251–257.

Boakes, R. A., and Juraskova, I. (2001). The role of drinking in the suppression of food intake by recent activity. *Behav. Neurosci.* 115, 718–730.

Boghi, A., Sterpone, S., Sales, S., D'Agata, F., Bradac, G. B., Zullo, G., et al. (2011). In vivo evidence of global and focal brain alterations in anorexia nervosa. *Psychiatry Res.* 192, 154–159.

Bolton, J. G., Patel, S., Lacey, J. H., and White, S. (2005). A prospective study of changes in bone turnover and bone density associated with regaining weight in women with anorexia nervosa. *Osteoporos. Int.* 16, 1955–1962.

Bordi, C., D'Adda, T., Azzoni, C., and Ferraro, G. (2000). Classification of gastric endocrine cells at the light and electron microscopical levels. *Microsc. Res. Tech.* 48, 258–271.

Bosy-Westphal, A., Brabant, G., Haas, V., Onur, S., Paul, T., Nutzinger, D., et al. (2005). Determinants of plasma adiponectin levels in patients with anorexia nervosa examined before and after weight gain. *Eur. J. Nutr.* 44, 355–359.

Bowers, C. Y., Chang, J., Momany, F., and Folkers, K. (1977). "Effect of the enkephalins and enkephalin analogs on release of pituitary hormones in vitro," in *Molecular Endocrinology*, eds I. MacIntyre and M. Szelke (Amsterdam: Elsevier/North Holland), 287–292.

Bowers, C. Y., Momany, F. A., Reynolds, G. A., and Hong, A. (1984). On the in vitro and in vivo activity of a new synthetic hexapeptide that acts on the pituitary to specifically release growth hormone. *Endocrinology* 114, 1537–1545.

Brambilla, F., Ferrari, E., Petraglia, F., Facchinetti, F., Catalano, M., and Genazzani, A. R. (1991). Peripheral opioid secretory pattern in anorexia nervosa. *Psychiatry Res.* 39, 115–127.

Brambilla, F., Santonastaso, P., Caregaro, L., and Favaro, A. (2006). Disorders of eating behavior: correlation between hypothalamo-pituitary-thyroid function and psychopathological aspects. *Psychoneuroendocrinology* 31, 131–136.

Brick, D. J., Gerweck, A. V., Meenaghan, E., Lawson, E. A., Misra, M., Fazeli, P., et al. (2010). Determinants of IGF1 and GH across the weight spectrum: from anorexia nervosa to obesity. *Eur. J. Endocrinol.* 163, 185–191.

Briggs, D. I., and Andrews, Z. B. (2011). Metabolic status regulates ghrelin function on energy homeostasis. *Neuroendocrinology* 93, 48–57.

Broadwell, R. D., Balin, B. J., Salcman, M., and Kaplan, R. S. (1983). Brain-blood barrier? Yes and no. *Proc. Natl. Acad. Sci. U.S.A.* 80, 7352–7356.

Broglio, F., Arvat, E., Benso, A., Gottero, C., Muccioli, G., Papotti, M., et al. (2001). Ghrelin, a natural GH secretagogue produced by the stomach, induces hyperglycemia and reduces insulin secretion in humans. *J. Clin. Endocrinol. Metab.* 86, 5083–5086.

Broglio, F., Gianotti, L., Destefanis, S., Fassino, S., Abbate Daga, G., Mondelli, V., et al. (2004a). The endocrine response to acute ghrelin administration is blunted in patients with anorexia nervosa, a ghrelin hypersecretory state. *Clin. Endocrinol. (Oxf.)* 60, 592–599.

Broglio, F., Gottero, C., Prodam, F., Gauna, C., Muccioli, G., Papotti, M., et al. (2004b). Non-acylated ghrelin counteracts the metabolic but not the neuroendocrine response to acylated ghrelin in humans. *J. Clin. Endocrinol. Metab.* 89, 3062–3065.

Brooks, S. J., Barker, G. J., O'Daly, O. G., Brammer, M., Williams, S. C., Benedict, C., et al. (2011). Restraint of appetite and reduced regional brain volumes in anorexia nervosa: a voxel-based morphometric study. *BMC Psychiatry* 17:179. doi:10.1186/1471-244X-11-179

Buehren, K., Konrad, K., Schaefer, K., Kratzsch, J., Kahraman-Lanzerath, B., Lente, C., et al. (2011). Association between neuroendocrinological parameters and learning and memory functions in adolescent anorexia nervosa before and after weight recovery. *J. Neural Transm.* 118, 963–968.

Burden, V. R., White, B. D., Dean, R. G., and Martin, R. J. (1993). Activity of the hypothalamic-pituitary-adrenal axis is elevated in rats with activity-based anorexia. *J. Nutr.* 123, 1217–1225.

Caillot-Augusseau, A., Lafage-Proust, M. H., Margaillan, P., Vergely, N., Faure, S., Paillet, S., et al. (2000). Weight gain reverses bone turnover and restores circadian variation of bone resorption in anorexic patients. *Clin. Endocrinol. (Oxf.)* 52, 113–121.

Calero, J. A., Muñoz, M. T., Argente, J., Traba, M. L., Méndez-Dávila, C., García-Moreno, C., et al. (1999). A variation in Bone Alkaline Phosphatase levels that correlates positively with bone loss and normal levels of aminoterminal propeptide of collagen I in girls with anorexia nervosa. *Clin. Chim. Acta* 285, 121–129.

Callaghan, B., Hunne, B., Hirayama, H., Sartor, D. M., Nguyen, T. V., Abogafie, F. C., et al. (2012). Sites of action of ghrelin receptor ligands in cardiovascular control. *Am. J. Physiol. Heart Circ. Physiol.* 303, H1011–H1021.

Camiña, J. P. (2006). Cell biology of the ghrelin receptor. *J. Neuroendocrinol.* 18, 65–76.

Cardona Cano, S., Merkestein, M., Skibicka, K. P., Dickson, S. L., and Adan, R. A. (2012). Role of ghrelin in the pathophysiology of eating disorders: implications for pharmacotherapy. *CNS Drugs* 26, 281–296.

Carr, K. D. (2011). Food scarcity, neuroadaptations, and the pathogenic potential of dieting in an unnatural ecology: binge eating and drug abuse. *Physiol. Behav.* 104, 162–167.

Casiero, D., and Frishman, W. H. (2006). Cardiovascular complications of eating disorders. *Cardiol. Rev.* 14, 227–231.

Casper, R. C. (1998). Behavioral activation and lack of concern, core symptoms of anorexia nervosa? *Int. J. Eat. Disord.* 24, 381–393.

Castañeda, T. R., Tong, J., Datta, R., Culler, M., and Tschöp, M. H. (2010). Ghrelin in the regulation of body weight and metabolism. *Front. Neuroendocrinol.* 31, 44–60.

Cerrato, M., Carrera, O., Vazquez, R., Echevarría, E., and Gutierrez, E. (2012). Heat makes a difference in activity-based anorexia: a translational approach to treatment development in anorexia nervosa. *Int. J. Eat. Disord.* 45, 26–35.

Chen, H. Y., Trumbauer, M. E., Chen, A. S., Weingarth, D. T., Adams, J. R., Frazier, E. G., et al. (2004). Orexigenic action of peripheral ghrelin is mediated by neuropeptide Y and agouti-related protein. *Endocrinology* 145, 2607–2612.

Chen, X., Ge, Y. L., Jiang, Z. Y., Liu, C. Q., Depoortere, I., and Peeters, T. L. (2005a). Effects of ghrelin on hypothalamic glucose responding neurons in rats. *Brain Res.* 1055, 131–136.

Chen, C. Y., Inui, A., Asakawa, A., Fujino, K., Kato, I., Chen, C. C., et al. (2005b). Des-acyl ghrelin acts by CRF type 2 receptors to disrupt fasted stomach motility in conscious rats. *Gastroenterology* 129, 8–25.

Chiodera, P., Volpi, R., Capretti, L., Marchesi, C., d'Amato, L., De Ferri, A., et al. (1991). Effect of estrogen or insulin-induced hypoglycemia on plasma oxytocin levels in bulimia and anorexia nervosa. *Metab. Clin. Exp.* 40, 1226–1230.

Chow, K. B., Sun, J., Chu, K. M., Tai Cheung, W., Cheng, C. H., and Wise, H. (2012). The truncated ghrelin receptor polypeptide (GHS-R1b) is localized in the endoplasmic reticulum where it forms heterodimers with ghrelin receptors (GHS-R1a) to attenuate their cell surface expression. *Mol. Cell. Endocrinol.* 348, 247–254.

Chuang, J. C., and Zigman, J. M. (2010). Ghrelin's roles in stress, mood, and anxiety regulation. *Int. J. Pept.* 2010, pii: 460549.

Ciofi, P. (2011). The arcuate nucleus as a circumventricular organ in the mouse. *Neurosci. Lett.* 487, 187–190.

Ciofi, P., Garret, M., Lapirot, O., Lafon, P., Loyens, A., Prevot, V., et al. (2009). Brain-endocrine interactions: a microvascular route in the mediobasal hypothalamus. *Endocrinology* 150, 5509–5519.

Confavreux, C. B., Levine, R. L., and Karsenty, G. (2009). A paradigm of integrative physiology, the crosstalk between bone and energy balances. *Mol. Cell. Endocrinol.* 310, 21–29.

Corcos, M., Guilbaud, O., Paterniti, S., Moussa, M., Chambry, J., Chaouat, G., et al. (2003). Involvement of cytokines in eating disorders: a critical review of the human literature. *Psychoneuroendocrinology* 28, 229–249.

Corwin, R. L., Avena, N. M., and Boggiano, M. M. (2011). Feeding and reward: perspectives from three rat models of binge eating. *Physiol. Behav.* 104, 87–97.

Costantini, V. J., Vicentini, E., Sabbatini, F. M., Valerio, E., Lepore, S., Tessari, M., et al. (2011). GSK1614343, a novel ghrelin receptor antagonist, produces an unexpected increase of food intake and body weight in rodents and dogs. *Neuroendocrinology* 94, 158–168.

Cowley, M. A., Smith, R. G., Diano, S., Tschöp, M., Pronchuk, N., Grove, K. L., et al. (2003). The distribution and mechanism of action of ghrelin in the CNS demonstrates a novel hypothalamic circuit regulating energy homeostasis. *Neuron* 37, 649–661.

Cummings, D. E., Purnell, J. Q., Frayo, R. S., Schmidova, K., Wisse, B. E., and Weigle, D. S. (2001). A preprandial rise in plasma ghrelin levels suggests a role in meal initiation in humans. *Diabetes* 50, 1714–1719.

Date, Y., Murakami, N., Toshinai, K., Matsukura, S., Niijima, A., Matsuo, H., et al. (2002). The role of the gastric afferent vagal nerve in ghrelin-induced feeding and growth hormone secretion in rats. *Gastroenterology* 123, 1120–1128.

Davis, C., and Claridge, G. (1998). The eating disorders as addiction: a psychobiological perpspective. *Addict. Behav.* 23, 463–475.

Davis, C., Katzman, D. K., Kaptein, S., Kirsh, C., Brewer, H., Kalmbach, K., et al. (1997). The prevalence of high-level exercise in the eating disorders: etiological implications. *Compr. Psychiatry* 38, 321–326.

Delhanty, P. J., Neggers, S. J., and Van der Lely, A. J. (2012). Ghrelin: the differences between Acyl- and Desacyl Ghrelin. *Eur. J. Endocrinol.* 167, 601–608.

Delhanty, P. J., van der Eerden, B. C., van der Velde, M., Gauna, C., Pols, H. A., Jahr, H., et al. (2006). Ghrelin and unacylated ghrelin stimulate human osteoblast growth via mitogen-activated protein kinase (MAPK)/phosphoinositide 3-kinase (PI3K) pathways in the absence of GHS-R1a. *J. Endocrinol.* 188, 37–47.

Delporte, M. L., Brichard, S. M., Hermans, M. P., Beguin, C., and Lambert, M. (2003). Hyperadiponectinaemia in anorexia nervosa. *Clin. Endocrinol. (Oxf.)* 58, 22–29.

Demitrack, M. A., Lesem, M. D., Listwak, S. J., Brandt, H. A., Jimerson, D. C., and Gold, P. W. (1990). CSF oxytocin in anorexia nervosa and bulimia nervosa: clinical and pathophysiologic considerations. *Am. J. Psychiatry* 147, 882–886.

Di Carlo, C., Tommaselli, G. A., De Filippo, E., Pisano, G., Nasti, A., Bifulco, G., et al. (2002). Menstrual status and serum leptin levels in anorectic and in menstruating women with low body mass indexes. *Fertil. Steril.* 78, 376–382.

Dickson, S. L., Doutrelant-Viltart, O., Dyball, R. E., and Leng, G. (1996). Retrogradely labelled neurosecretory neurons of the rat hypothalamic arcuate nucleus express Fos protein following systemic injection of GH-releasing peptide-6. *J. Endocrinol.* 151, 323–331.

Dickson, S. L., Leng, G., and Robinson, I. C. (1993). Systemic administration of growth hormone-releasing peptide activates hypothalamic arcuate neurons. *Neuroscience* 53, 303–306.

Dickson, S. L., and Luckman, S. M. (1997). Induction of c-fos messenger ribonucleic acid in neuropeptide Y and growth hormone (GH)-releasing factor neurons in the rat arcuate nucleus following systemic injection of the GH secretagogue, GH-releasing peptide-6. *Endocrinology* 138, 771–777.

Djurovic, M., Pekic, S., Petakov, M., Damjanovic, S., Doknic, M., Dieguez, C., et al. (2004). Gonadotropin response to clomiphene and plasma leptin levels in weight recovered but amenorrhoeic patients with anorexia nervosa. *J. Endocrinol. Invest.* 27, 523–527.

Dolezalova, R., Lacinova, Z., Dolinkova, M., Kleiblova, P., Haluzikova, D., Housa, D., et al. (2007). Changes of endocrine function of adipose tissue in anorexia nervosa: comparison of circulating levels versus subcutaneous mRNA expression. *Clin. Endocrinol. (Oxf.)* 67, 674–678.

Dominguez, J., Goodman, L., Sen Gupta, S., Mayer, L., Etu, S. F., Walsh, B. T., et al. (2007). Treatment of anorexia nervosa is associated with increases in bone mineral density, and recovery is a biphasic process involving both nutrition and return of menses. *Am. J. Clin. Nutr.* 86, 92–99.

Dostalova, I., Kopsky, V., Duskova, J., Papezova, H., Pacak, K., and Nedvidkova, J. (2005). Leptin concentrations in the abdominal subcutaneous adipose tissue of patients with anorexia nervosa assessed by in vivo microdialysis. *Regul. Pept.* 128, 63–68.

Dostalova, I., Smitka, K., Papezova, H., Kvasnickova, H., and Nedvidkova, J. (2007). Increased insulin sensitivity in patients with anorexia nervosa: the role of adipocytokines. *Physiol. Res.* 56, 587–594.

Eddy, K. T., Dorer, D. J., Franko, D. L., Tahilani, K., Thompson-Brenner, H., and Herzog, D. B. (2008). Diagnostic crossover in anorexia nervosa and bulimia nervosa: implications for DSM-V. *Am. J. Psychiatry* 165, 245–250.

Egecioglu, E., Jerlhag, E., Salomé, N., Skibicka, K. P., Haage, D., Bohlooly, Y. M., et al. (2010). Ghrelin increases intake of rewarding food in rodents. *Addict. Biol.* 15, 304–311.

Ehrlich, S., Salbach-Andrae, H., Eckart, S., Merle, J. V., Burghardt, R., Pfeiffer, E., et al. (2009). Serum brain-derived neurotrophic factor and peripheral indicators of the serotonin system in underweight and weight-recovered adolescent girls and women with anorexia nervosa. *J. Psychiatry Neurosci.* 34, 323–329.

Enomoto, M., Nagaya, N., Uematsu, M., Okumura, H., Nakagawa, E., Ono, F., et al. (2003). Cardiovascular and hormonal effects of subcutaneous administration of ghrelin, a novel growth hormone-releasing peptide, in healthy humans. *Clin. Sci. (Lond.)* 105, 431–435.

Erdur, L., Kallenbach-Dermutz, B., Lehmann, V., Zimmermann-Viehoff, F., Köpp, W., Weber, C., et al. (2012). Somatic comorbidity in anorexia nervosa: first results of a 21-year follow-up study on female inpatients. *Biopsychosoc. Med.* 6, 4.

España, R. A., and Scammell, T. E. (2011). Sleep neurobiology from a clinical perspective. *Sleep* 34, 845–858.

Estour, B., Germain, N., Diconne, E., Frere, D., Cottet-Emard, J. M., Carrot, G., et al. (2010). Hormonal profile heterogeneity and short-term physical risk in restrictive anorexia nervosa. *J. Clin. Endocrinol. Metab.* 95, 2203–2210.

Faje, A. T., Fazeli, P. K., Katzman, D. K., Miller, K. K., Breggia, A., Rosen, C. J., et al. (2012). Sclerostin levels and bone turnover markers in adolescents with anorexia nervosa and healthy adolescent girls. *Bone* 51, 474–479.

Faulconbridge, L. F., Cummings, D. E., Kaplan, J. M., and Grill, H. J. (2003). Hyperphagic effects of brainstem ghrelin administration. *Diabetes* 52, 2260–2265.

Fazeli, P. K., Lawson, E. A., Prabhakaran, R., Miller, K. K., Donoho, D. A., Clemmons, D. R., et al. (2010a). Effects of recombinant human growth hormone in anorexia nervosa: a randomized, placebo-controlled study. *J. Clin. Endocrinol. Metab.* 95, 4889–4897.

Fazeli, P. K., Misra, M., Goldstein, M., Miller, K. K., and Klibanski, A. (2010b). Fibroblast growth factor-21 may mediate growth hormone resistance in anorexia nervosa. *J. Clin. Endocrinol. Metab.* 95, 369–374.

Fernández-Fernández, R., Tena-Sempere, M., Navarro, V. M., Barreiro, M. L., Castellano, J. M., Aguilar, E., et al. (2005). Effects of ghrelin upon gonadotropin-releasing hormone and gonadotropin secretion in adult female rats: in vivo and in vitro studies. *Neuroendocrinology* 82, 245–255.

Ferron, F., Considine, R. V., Peino, R., Lado, I. G., Dieguez, C., and Casanueva, F. F. (1997). Serum leptin concentrations in patients with anorexia nervosa, bulimia nervosa and nonspecific eating disorders correlate with the body mass index but are independent of the respective disease. *Clin. Endocrinol. (Oxf.)* 46, 289–293.

Fisher, M. (2003). The course and outcome of eating disorders in adults and in adolescents: a review. *Adolesc. Med.* 14, 149–158.

Forbes, S., Li, X. F., Kinsey-Jones, J., and O'Byrne, K. (2009). Effects of ghrelin on Kisspeptin mRNA expression in the hypothalamic medial preoptic area and pulsatile luteinising hormone secretion in the female rat. *Neurosci. Lett.* 460, 143–147.

Fujimoto, S., Inui, A., Kiyota, N., Seki, W., Koide, K., Takamiya, S., et al. (1997). Increased cholecystokinin and pancreatic polypeptide responses to a fat-rich meal in patients with restrictive but not bulimic anorexia nervosa. *Biol. Psychiatry* 41, 1068–1070.

Fujitsuka, N., Asakawa, A., Amitani, H., Fujimiya, M., and Inui, A. (2012). Ghrelin and gastrointestinal movement. *Meth. Enzymol.* 514, 289–301.

Fukushima, N., Hanada, R., Teranishi, H., Fukue, Y., Tachibana, T., Ishikawa, H., et al. (2005). Ghrelin directly regulates bone formation. *J. Bone Miner. Res.* 20, 790–798.

Galusca, B., Bossu, C., Germain, N., Kadem, M., Frere, D., Lafage-Proust, M. H., et al. (2006). Age-related differences in hormonal and nutritional impact on lean anorexia nervosa bone turnover uncoupling. *Osteoporos. Int.* 17, 888–896.

Galusca, B., Jeandel, L., Germain, N., Alexandre, D., Leprince, J., Anouar, Y., et al. (2012). Orexigenic neuropeptide 26RFa: new evidence for an adaptive profile of appetite regulation in anorexia nervosa. *J. Clin. Endocrinol. Metab.* 97, 2012–2018.

Gao, X. B. (2012). Plasticity in neurons synthesizing wake/arousal promoting hormone hypocretin/orexin. *Vitam. Horm.* 89, 35–59.

Garcia, F. D., Délavenne, H., and Déchelotte, P. (2011). Atypical eating disorders a review. *Nutr. Diet. Suppl.* 3, 67–75.

Gauna, C., Delhanty, P. J., Hofland, L. J., Janssen, J. A., Broglio, F., Ross, R. J., et al. (2005). Ghrelin stimulates, whereas des-octanoyl ghrelin inhibits, glucose output by primary hepatocytes. *J. Clin. Endocrinol. Metab.* 90, 1055–1060.

Gelegen, C., Collier, D. A., Campbell, I. C., Oppelaar, H., van den Heuvel, J., Adan, R. A., et al. (2007). Difference in susceptibility to activity-based anorexia in two inbred strains of mice. *Eur. Neuropsychopharmacol.* 17, 199–205.

Gendall, K. A., Kaye, W. H., Altemus, M., McConaha, C. W., and La Via, M. C. (1999). Leptin, neuropeptide Y, and peptide YY in long-term recovered eating disorder patients. *Biol. Psychiatry* 46, 292–299.

Geracioti, T. D. Jr., Liddle, R. A., Altemus, M., Demitrack, M. A., and Gold, P. W. (1992). Regulation of appetite and cholecystokinin secretion in anorexia nervosa. *Am. J. Psychiatry* 149, 958–961.

Germain, N., Galusca, B., Grouselle, D., Frere, D., Billard, S., Epelbaum, J., et al. (2010). Ghrelin and obestatin circadian levels differentiate bingeing–purging from restrictive anorexia nervosa. *J. Clin. Endocrinol. Metab.* 95, 3057–3062.

Germain, N., Galusca, B., Grouselle, D., Frere, D., Tolle, V., Zizzari, P., et al. (2009). Ghrelin/obestatin ratio in two populations with low bodyweight: constitutional thinness and anorexia nervosa. *Psychoneuroendocrinology* 34, 413–419.

Germain, N., Galusca, B., Le Roux, C. W., Bossu, C., Ghatei, M. A., Lang, F., et al. (2007). Constitutional thinness and lean anorexia nervosa display opposite concentrations of peptide YY, glucagon-like peptide 1, ghrelin, and leptin. *Am. J. Clin. Nutr.* 85, 967–971.

Gerner, R. H., and Gwirtsman, H. E. (1981). Abnormalities of dexamethasone suppression test and urinary MHPG in anorexia nervosa. *Am. J. Psychiatry* 138, 650–653.

Gerner, R. H., and Sharp, B. (1982a). CSF beta-endorphin-immunoreactivity in normal, schizophrenic, depressed, manic and anorexic subjects. *Brain Res.* 237, 244–247.

Gerner, R. H., and Yamada, T. (1982b). Altered neuropeptide concentrations in cerebrospinal fluid of psychiatric patients. *Brain Res.* 238, 298–302.

Gianotti, L., Pincelli, A. I., Scacchi, M., Rolla, M., Bellitti, D., Arvat, E., et al. (2000). Effects of recombinant human insulin-like growth factor I administration on spontaneous and growth hormone (GH)-releasing hormone-stimulated GH secretion in anorexia nervosa. *J. Clin. Endocrinol. Metab.* 85, 2805–2809.

Gnanapavan, S., Kola, B., Bustin, S. A., Morris, D. G., McGee, P., Fairclough, P., et al. (2002). The tissue distribution of the mRNA of ghrelin and subtypes of its receptor, GHS-R, in humans. *J. Clin. Endocrinol. Metab.* 87, 2988.

Gniuli, D., Liverani, E., Capristo, E., Greco, A. V., and Mingrone, G. (2001). Blunted glucose metabolism in anorexia nervosa. *Metab. Clin. Exp.* 50, 876–881.

González, C. R., Vázquez, M. J., López, M., and Diéguez, C. (2008). Influence of chronic undernutrition and leptin on GOAT mRNA levels in rat stomach mucosa. *J. Mol. Endocrinol.* 41, 415–421.

Goodman, A. (1990). Addiction: definition and implications. *Br. J. Addict.* 85, 1403–1408.

Goodyear, S., Arasaradnam, R. P., Quraishi, N., Mottershead, M., and Nwokolo, C. U. (2010). Acylated and des acyl ghrelin in human portal and systemic circulations. *Mol. Biol. Rep.* 37, 3697–3701.

Gordon, C. M., Goodman, E., Emans, S. J., Grace, E., Becker, K. A., Rosen, C. J., et al. (2002). Physiologic regulators of bone turnover in young women with anorexia nervosa. *J. Pediatr.* 141, 64–70.

Gourcerol, G., St-Pierre, D. H., and Tache, Y. (2007). Lack of obestatin effects on food intake: should obestatin be renamed ghrelin-associated peptide (GAP)? *Regul. Pept.* 141, 1–7.

Grinspoon, S., Miller, K., Coyle, C., Krempin, J., Armstrong, C., Pitts, S., et al. (1999). Severity of osteopenia in estrogen-deficient women with anorexia nervosa and hypothalamic amenorrhea. *J. Clin. Endocrinol. Metab.* 84, 2049–2055.

Grinspoon, S., Thomas, E., Pitts, S., Gross, E., Mickley, D., Miller, K., et al. (2000). Prevalence and predictive factors for regional osteopenia in women with anorexia nervosa. *Ann. Intern. Med.* 133, 790–794.

Grove, K. L., and Cowley, M. A. (2005). Is ghrelin a signal for the development of metabolic systems? *J. Clin. Invest.* 115, 3393–3397.

Guan, X. M., Yu, H., Palyha, O. C., McKee, K. K., Feighner, S. D., Sirinathsinghji, D. J., et al. (1997). Distribution of mRNA encoding the growth hormone secretagogue receptor in brain and peripheral tissues. *Brain Res. Mol. Brain Res.* 48, 23–29.

Gutierrez, J. A., Solenberg, P. J., Perkins, D. R., Willency, J. A., Knierman, M. D., Jin, Z., et al. (2008). Ghrelin octanoylation mediated by an orphan lipid transferase. *Proc. Natl. Acad. Sci. U.S.A.* 105, 6320–6325.

Haas, V., Onur, S., Paul, T., Nutzinger, D. O., Bosy-Westphal, A., Hauer, M., et al. (2005). Leptin and body weight regulation in patients with anorexia nervosa before and during weight recovery. *Am. J. Clin. Nutr.* 81, 889–896.

Haas, V. K., Kohn, M. R., Clarke, S. D., Allen, J. R., Madden, S., Müller, M. J., et al. (2009). Body composition changes in female adolescents with anorexia nervosa. *Am. J. Clin. Nutr.* 89, 1005–1010.

Hall, J. F., and Hanford, P. V. (1954). Activity as a function of a restricted feeding schedule. *J. Comp. Physiol. Psychol.* 47, 362–373.

Haluzíková, D., Dostálová, I., Kaválková, P., Roubícek, T., Mráz, M., Papezová, H., et al. (2009). Serum concentrations of adipocyte fatty acid binding protein in patients with anorexia nervosa. *Physiol. Res.* 58, 577–581.

Hansson, C., Haage, D., Taube, M., Egecioglu, E., Salomé, N., and Dickson, S. L. (2011). Central administration of ghrelin alters emotional responses in rats: behavioural, electrophysiological and molecular evidence. *Neuroscience* 180, 201–211.

Harada, T., Nakahara, T., Yasuhara, D., Kojima, S., Sagiyama, K., Amitani, H., et al. (2008). Obestatin, acyl ghrelin, and des-acyl ghrelin responses to an oral glucose tolerance test in the restricting type of anorexia nervosa. *Biol. Psychiatry* 63, 245–247.

Harrold, J. A., Dovey, T., Cai, X. J., Halford, J. C., and Pinkney, J. (2008). Autoradiographic analysis of ghrelin receptors in the rat hypothalamus. *Brain Res.* 1196, 59–64.

Hasan, T. F., and Hasan, H. (2011). Anorexia nervosa: a unified neurological perspective. *Int. J. Med. Sci.* 8, 679–703.

Hassouna, R., Labarthe, A., Zizzari, P., Videau, C., Culler, M. D., Epelbaum, J., et al. (2013). Actions of agonists and antagonists of the ghrelin/GHS-R pathway on GH secretion, appetite and cFos activity. *Front. Endocrinol.* 4:25. doi:10.3389/fendo.2013.00025

Hassouna, R., Zizzari, P., and Tolle, V. (2010). The ghrelin/obestatin balance in the physiological and pathological control of growth hormone secretion, body composition and food intake. *J. Neuroendocrinol.* 22, 793–804.

Hataya, Y., Akamizu, T., Takaya, K., Kanamoto, N., Ariyasu, H., Saijo, M., et al. (2001). A low dose of ghrelin stimulates growth hormone (GH) release synergistically with GH-releasing hormone in humans. *J. Clin. Endocrinol. Metab.* 86, 4552.

Hebebrand, J., Blum, W. F., Barth, N., Coners, H., Englaro, P., Juul, A., et al. (1997). Leptin levels in patients with anorexia nervosa are reduced in the acute stage and elevated upon short-term weight restoration. *Mol. Psychiatry* 2, 330–334.

Heer, M., Mika, C., Grzella, I., Heussen, N., and Herpertz-Dahlmann, B. (2004). Bone turnover during inpatient nutritional therapy and outpatient follow-up in patients with anorexia nervosa compared with that in healthy control subjects. *Am. J. Clin. Nutr.* 80, 774–781.

Hewson, A. K., and Dickson, S. L. (2000). Systemic administration of ghrelin induces Fos and Egr-1 proteins in the hypothalamic arcuate nucleus of fasted and fed rats. *J. Neuroendocrinol.* 12, 1047–1049.

Hewson, A. K., Viltart, O., McKenzie, D. N., Dyball, R. E., and Dickson, S. L. (1999). GHRP-6-induced changes in electrical activity of single cells in the arcuate, ventromedial and periventricular nucleus neurons [correction of nuclei] of a hypothalamic slice preparation in vitro. *J. Neuroendocrinol.* 11, 919–923. [Erratum in: *J. Neuroendocrinol.* (2000) 12, 377].

Holst, B., Holliday, N. D., Bach, A., Elling, C. E., Cox, H. M., and Schwartz, T. W. (2004). Common structural basis for constitutive activity of the ghrelin receptor family. *J. Biol. Chem.* 279, 53806–53817.

Holst, B., and Schwartz, T. W. (2006). Ghrelin receptor mutations – too little height and too much hunger. *J. Clin. Invest.* 116, 637–641.

Holtkamp, K., Hebebrand, J., Mika, C., Grzella, I., Heer, M., Heussen, N., et al. (2003a). The effect of therapeutically induced weight gain on plasma leptin levels in patients with anorexia nervosa. *J. Psychiatr. Res.* 37, 165–169.

Holtkamp, K., Mika, C., Grzella, I., Heer, M., Pak, H., Hebebrand, J., et al. (2003b). Reproductive function during weight gain in anorexia nervosa. Leptin represents a metabolic gate to gonadotropin secretion. *J. Neural Transm.* 110, 427–435.

Holtkamp, K., Hebebrand, J., Mika, C., Heer, M., Heussen, N., and Herpertz-Dahlmann, B. (2004). High serum leptin levels subsequent to weight gain predict renewed weight loss in patients with anorexia nervosa. *Psychoneuroendocrinology* 29, 791–797.

Hotta, M., Ohwada, R., Akamizu, T., Shibasaki, T., Takano, K., and Kangawa, K. (2009). Ghrelin increases hunger and food intake in patients with restricting-type anorexia nervosa: a pilot study. *Endocr. J.* 56, 1119–1128.

Hotta, M., Ohwada, R., Katakami, H., Shibasaki, T., Hizuka, N., and Takano, K. (2004). Plasma levels of intact and degraded ghrelin and their responses to glucose infusion in anorexia nervosa. *J. Clin. Endocrinol. Metab.* 89, 5707–5712.

Hotta, M., Shibasaki, T., Masuda, A., Imaki, T., Demura, H., Ling, N., et al. (1986). The responses of plasma adrenocorticotropin and cortisol to corticotropin-releasing hormone (CRH) and cerebrospinal fluid immunoreactive CRH in anorexia nervosa patients. *J. Clin. Endocrinol. Metab.* 62, 319–324.

Housova, J., Anderlova, K., Krizova, J., Haluzikova, D., Kremen, J., Kumstyrova, T., et al. (2005). Serum adiponectin and resistin concentrations in patients with restrictive and binge/purge form of anorexia nervosa and bulimia nervosa. *J. Clin. Endocrinol. Metab.* 90, 1366–1370.

Howard, A. D., Feighner, S. D., Cully, D. F., Arena, J. P., Liberator, P. A., Rosenblum, C. I., et al. (1996). A receptor in pituitary and hypothalamus that functions in growth hormone release. *Science* 273, 974–977.

Howgate, D. J., Graham, S. M., Leonidou, A., Korres, N., Tsiridis, E., and Tsapakis, E. (2013). Bone metabolism in anorexia nervosa: molecular pathways and current treatment modalities. *Osteoporos. Int.* 24, 407–421.

Iwahashi, H., Funahashi, T., Kurokawa, N., Sayama, K., Fukuda, E., Okita, K., et al. (2003). Plasma adiponectin levels in women with anorexia nervosa. *Horm. Metab. Res.* 35, 537–540.

Jacquemont, S., Reymond, A., Zufferey, F., Harewood, L., Walters, R. G., Kutalik, Z., et al. (2011). Mirror extreme BMI phenotypes associated with gene dosage at the chromosome 16p11.2 locus. *Nature* 478, 97–102.

Janas-Kozik, M., Krupka-Matuszczyk, I., Malinowska-Kolodziej, I., and Lewin-Kowalik, J. (2007). Total ghrelin plasma level in patients with the restrictive type of anorexia nervosa. *Regul. Pept.* 140, 43–46.

Jáuregui-Garrido, B., and Jáuregui-Lobera, I. (2012). Sudden death in eating disorders. *Vasc. Health Risk Manag.* 8, 91–98.

Jeffery, P. L., Duncan, R. P., Yeh, A. H., Jaskolski, R. A., Hammond, D. S., Herington, A. C., et al. (2005). Expression of the ghrelin axis in the mouse: an exon 4-deleted mouse proghrelin variant encodes a novel C terminal peptide. *Endocrinology* 146, 432–440.

Jerlhag, E., Egecioglu, E., Dickson, S. L., Andersson, M., Svensson, L., and Engel, J. A. (2006). Ghrelin stimulates locomotor activity and accumbal dopamine-overflow via central cholinergic systems in mice: implications for its involvement in brain reward. *Addict. Biol.* 11, 45–54.

Jerlhag, E., Egecioglu, E., Dickson, S. L., Douhan, A., Svensson, L., and Engel, J. A. (2007). Ghrelin administration into tegmental areas stimulates locomotor activity and increases extracellular concentration of dopamine in the nucleus accumbens. *Addict. Biol.* 12, 6–16.

Jerlhag, E., Egecioglu, E., Dickson, S. L., and Engel, J. A. (2010). Ghrelin receptor antagonism attenuates cocaine- and amphetamine-induced locomotor stimulation, accumbal dopamine release, and conditioned place preference. *Psychopharmacology (Berl.)* 211, 415–422.

Jerlhag, E., Egecioglu, E., Landgren, S., Salomé, N., Heilig, M., Moechars, D., et al. (2009). Requirement of central ghrelin signaling for alcohol reward. *Proc. Natl. Acad. Sci. U.S.A.* 106, 11318–11323.

Jiang, H., Betancourt, L., and Smith, R. G. (2006). Ghrelin amplifies dopamine signaling by cross talk involving formation of growth hormone secretagogue receptor/dopamine receptor subtype 1 heterodimers. *Mol. Endocrinol.* 20, 1772–1785.

Kamegai, J., Tamura, H., Shimizu, T., Ishii, S., Sugihara, H., and Wakabayashi, I. (2000). Central effect of ghrelin, an endogenous growth hormone secretagogue, on hypothalamic peptide gene expression. *Endocrinology* 141, 4797–4780.

Kamegai, J., Tamura, H., Shimizu, T., Ishii, S., Sugihara, H., and Wakabayashi, I. (2001). Chronic central infusion of ghrelin increases hypothalamic neuropeptide Y and agouti-related protein mRNA levels and body weight in rats. *Diabetes* 50, 2438–2443.

Kang, K., Schmahl, J., Lee, J. M., Garcia, K., Patil, K., Chen, A., et al. (2012). Mouse ghrelin-O-acyltransferase (GOAT) plays a critical role in bile acid reabsorption. *FASEB J.* 26, 259–271.

Karczewska-Kupczewska, M., Kowalska, I., Nikolajuk, A., Adamska, A., Otziomek, E., Gorska, M., et al. (2012). Hyperinsulinemia acutely increases serum macrophage inhibitory cytokine-1 concentration in anorexia nervosa and obesity. *Clin. Endocrinol. (Oxf.)* 76, 46–50.

Karczewska-Kupczewska, M., Straczkowski, M., Adamska, A., Nikolajuk, A., Otziomek, E., Górska, M., et al. (2010). Insulin sensitivity, metabolic flexibility, and serum adiponectin concentration in women with anorexia nervosa. *Metab. Clin. Exp.* 59, 473–477.

Kawahara, Y., Kawahara, H., Kaneko, F., Yamada, M., Nishi, Y., Tanaka, E., et al. (2009). Peripherally administered ghrelin induces bimodal effects on the mesolimbic dopamine system depending on food-consumptive states. *Neuroscience* 161, 855–864.

Kaye, W. H. (1996). Neuropeptide abnormalities in anorexia nervosa. *Psychiatry Res.* 62, 65–74.

Kaye, W. H., Berrettini, W., Gwirtsman, H., and George, D. T. (1990). Altered cerebrospinal fluid neuropeptide Y and peptide YY immunoreactivity in anorexia and bulimia nervosa. *Arch. Gen. Psychiatry* 47, 548–556.

Kaye, W. H., Fudge, J. L., and Paulus, M. (2009). New insights into symptoms and neuro-circuit function of anorexia nervosa. *Nat. Rev. Neurosci.* 10, 573–584.

Kaye, W. H., Gwirtsman, H. E., George, D. T., Ebert, M. H., Jimerson, D. C., Tomai, T. P., et al. (1987). Elevated cerebrospinal fluid levels of immunoreactive corticotrophin-releasing hormone in anorexia nervosa: relation to state of nutrition, adrenal function and intensity of depression. *J. Clin. Endocrinol. Metab.* 64, 203–208.

Kaye, W. H., Rubinow, D., Gwirtsman, H. E., George, D. T., Jimerson, D. C., and Gold, P. W. (1988). CSF somatostatin in anorexia nervosa and bulimia: relationship to the hypothalamic pituitary-adrenal cortical axis. *Psychoneuroendocrinology* 13, 265–272.

Kern, A., Albarran-Zeckler, R., Walsh, H. E., and Smith, R. G. (2012). Apo-ghrelin receptor forms heteromers with DRD2 in hypothalamic neurons and is essential for anorexigenic effects of DRD2 agonism. *Neuron* 73, 317–332.

Kim, S. F. (2012). Animal models of eating disorders. *Neuroscience* 211, 2–12.

Kinzig, K. P., Coughlin, J. W., Redgrave, G. W., Moran, T. H., and Guarda, A. S. (2007). Insulin, glucose, and pancreatic polypeptide responses to a test meal in restricting type anorexia nervosa before and after weight restoration. *Am. J. Physiol. Endocrinol. Metab.* 292, E1441–E1446.

Kleinz, M. J., Maguire, J. J., Skepper, J. N., and Davenport, A. P. (2006). Functional and immunocytochemical evidence for a role of ghrelin and des-octanoyl ghrelin in the regulation of vascular tone in man. *Cardiovasc. Res.* 69, 227–235.

Klenotich, S. J., and Dulawa, S. C. (2012). The activity-based anorexia mouse model. *Methods Mol. Biol.* 829, 377–393.

Kluge, M., Schüssler, P., Schmidt, D., Uhr, M., and Steiger, A. (2012). Ghrelin suppresses secretion of luteinizing hormone (LH) and follicle-stimulating hormone (FSH) in women. *J. Clin. Endocrinol. Metab.* 97, E448–E451.

Kohl, M., Foulon, C., and Guelfi, J. D. (2004). Hyperactivity and anorexia nervosa: behavioural and biological perspective. *Encephale* 30, 492–499.

Kojima, M., Hosoda, H., Date, Y., Nakazato, M., Matsuo, H., and Kangawa, K. (1999). Ghrelin is a growth-hormone-releasing acylated peptide from stomach. *Nature* 402, 656–660.

Kojima, M., and Kangawa, K. (2005). Ghrelin: structure and function. *Physiol. Rev.* 85, 495–522.

Krizova, J., Papezova, H., Haluzikova, D., Parizkova, J., Jiskra, J., Kotrlikova, E., et al. (2002). Soluble leptin receptor levels in patients with anorexia nervosa. *Endocr. Res.* 28, 199–205.

Krsek, M., Rosicka, M., Papezova, H., Krizova, J., Kotrikova, E., Haluzk, M., et al. (2003). Plasma ghrelin levels and malnutrition: a comparison of two etiologies. *Eat. Weight Disord.* 8, 207–211.

Kukkonen, J. P. (2013). Physiology of the orexinergic/hypocretinergic system: a revisit in 2012. *Am. J. Physiol. Cell Physiol.* 304, C2–C32.

Lamont, E. W., Patterson, Z., Rodrigues, T., Vallejos, O., Blum, I. D., and Abizaid, A. (2012). Ghrelin-deficient mice have fewer orexin cells and reduced cFOS expression in the mesolimbic dopamine pathway under a restricted feeding paradigm. *Neuroscience* 218, 12–19.

Lauer, C. J., and Krieg, J. C. (2004). Sleep in eating disorders. *Sleep Med. Rev.* 8, 109–118.

Lawrence, C. B., Snape, A. C., Baudoin, F. M., and Luckman, S. M. (2002). Acute central ghrelin and GH secretagogues induce feeding and activate brain appetite centers. *Endocrinology* 143, 155–162.

Lawson, E. A., Donoho, D., Miller, K. K., Misra, M., Meenaghan, E., Lydecker, J., et al. (2009). Hypercortisolemia is associated with severity of bone loss and depression in hypothalamic amenorrhea and anorexia nervosa. *J. Clin. Endocrinol. Metab.* 94, 4710–4716.

Lawson, E. A., Donoho, D. A., Blum, J. I., Meenaghan, E. M., Misra, M., Herzog, D. B., et al. (2011a). Decreased nocturnal oxytocin levels in anorexia nervosa are associated with low bone mineral density and fat mass. *J. Clin. Psychiatry* 72, 1546–1551.

Lawson, E. A., Eddy, K. T., Donoho, D., Misra, M., Miller, K. K., Meenaghan, E., et al. (2011b). Appetite-regulating hormones cortisol and peptide YY are associated with disordered eating psychopathology, independent of body mass index. *Eur. J. Endocrinol.* 164, 253–261.

Lawson, E. A., Holsen, L. M., Santin, M., Meenaghan, E., Eddy, K. T., Becker, A. E., et al. (2012). Oxytocin secretion is associated with severity of disordered eating psychopathology and insular cortex hypoactivation in anorexia nervosa. *J. Clin. Endocrinol. Metab.* 97, E1898–E1908.

Lawson, E. A., and Klibanski, A. (2008). Endocrine abnormalities in anorexia nervosa. *Nat. Clin. Pract. Endocrinol. Metab.* 4, 407–414.

Legroux-Gerot, I., Vignau, J., Collier, F., and Cortet, B. (2005). Bone loss associated with anorexia nervosa. *Joint Bone Spine* 72, 489–495.

Legroux-Gerot, I., Vignau, J., Collier, F., and Cortet, B. (2008). Factors influencing changes in bone mineral density in patients with anorexia nervosa-related osteoporosis: the effect of hormone replacement therapy. *Calcif. Tissue Int.* 83, 315–323.

Legroux-Gérot, I., Vignau, J., D'Herbomez, M., Collier, F., Marchandise, X., Duquesnoy, B., et al. (2007). Evaluation of bone loss and its mechanisms in anorexia nervosa. *Calcif. Tissue Int.* 81, 174–182.

Lesem, M. D., Berrettini, W. H., Kaye, W. H., and Jimerson, D. C. (1991). Measurement of CSF dynorphin A 1-8 immunoreactivity in anorexia nervosa and normal-weight bulimia. *Biol. Psychiatry* 29, 244–252.

Lesem, M. D., Kaye, W. H., Bissette, G., Jimerson, D. C., and Nemeroff, C. B. (1994). Cerebrospinal fluid TRH immunoreactivity in anorexia nervosa. *Biol. Psychiatry* 35, 48–53.

López, M., Lage, R., Saha, A. K., Pérez-Tilve, D., Vázquez, M. J., Varela, L., et al. (2008). Hypothalamic fatty acid metabolism mediates the orexigenic action of ghrelin. *Cell Metab.* 7, 389–399.

Löwe, B., Zipfel, S., Buchholz, C., Dupont, Y., Reas, D. L., and Herzog, W. (2001). Long-term outcome of anorexia nervosa in a prospective 21-year follow-up study. *Psychol. Med.* 31, 881–890.

Lucas, A. R., Beard, C. M., O'Fallon, W. M., and Kurland, L. T. (1991). 50-Year trends in the incidence of anorexia nervosa in Rochester, Minn.: a population-based study. *Am. J. Psychiatry* 148, 917–922.

Lucas, A. R., Melton, L. J. III, Crowson, C. S., and O'Fallon, W. M. (1999). Long-term frac-ture risk among women with anorexia nervosa: a population-based co-hort study. *Mayo Clin. Proc.* 74, 972–977.

Luckman, S. M., Rosenzweig, I., and Dickson, S. L. (1999). Activation of arcuate nucleus neurons by systemic administration of leptin and growth hormone-releasing peptide-6 in normal and fasted rats. *Neuroendocrinology* 70, 93–100.

Luquet, S., Perez, F. A., Hnasko, T. S., and Palmiter, R. D. (2005). NPY/AgRP neurons are essential for feeding in adult mice but can be ablated in neonates. *Science* 310, 683–685.

Luquet, S., Phillips, C. T., and Palmiter, R. D. (2007). NPY/AgRP neurons are not essential for feeding responses to glucoprivation. *Peptides* 28, 214–225.

Lutter, M., Sakata, I., Osborne-Lawrence, S., Rovinsky, S. A., Anderson, J. G., Jung, S., et al. (2008). The orexigenic hormone ghrelin defends against depressive symptoms of chronic stress. *Nat. Neurosci.* 11, 752–763.

Malik, S., McGlone, F., Bedrossian, D., and Dagher, A. (2008). Ghrelin modulates brain activity in areas that control appetitive behavior. *Cell Metab.* 7, 400–509.

Maltais, L. J., Lane, P. W., and Beamer, W. G. (1984). Anorexia, a recessive mutation causing starvation in preweanling mice. *J. Hered.* 75, 468–472.

Mano-Otagiri, A., Ohata, H., Iwasaki-Sekino, A., Nemoto, T., and Shibasaki, T. (2009). Ghrelin suppresses noradrenaline release in the brown adipose tissue of rats. *J. Endocrinol.* 201, 341–349.

Mantzoros, C., Flier, J. S., Lesem, M. D., Brewerton, T. D., and Jimerson, D. C. (1997). Cerebrospinal fluid leptin in anorexia nervosa: correlation with nutritional status and potential role in resistance to weight gain. *J. Clin. Endocrinol. Metab.* 82, 1845–1851.

Martini, A. C., Fernández-Fernández, R., Tovar, S., Navarro, V. M., Vigo, E., Vazquez, M. J., et al. (2006). Comparative analysis of the effects of ghrelin and unacylated ghrelin on luteinizing hormone secretion in male rats. *Endocrinology* 147, 2374–2382.

McKee, K. K., Tan, C. P., Palyha, O. C., Liu, J., Feighner, S. D., Hreniuk, D. L., et al. (1997). Cloning and characterization of two human G protein-coupled receptor genes

(GPR38 and GPR39) related to the growth hormone secretagogue and neurotensin receptors. *Genomics* 46, 426–434.

Meczekalski, B., Podfigurna-Stopa, A., Warenik-Szymankiewicz, A., and Genazzani, A. R. (2008). Functional hypothalamic amenorrhea: current view on neuroendocrine aberrations. *Gynecol. Endocrinol.* 24, 4–11.

Mercader, J. M., Ribasés, M., Gratacòs, M., González, J. R., Bayés, M., de Cid, R., et al. (2007). Altered brain-derived neurotrophic factor blood levels and gene variability are associated with anorexia and bulimia. *Genes Brain Behav.* 6, 706–716.

Merkestein, M., Brans, M. A., Luijendijk, M. C., de Jong, J. W., Egecioglu, E., Dickson, S. L., et al. (2012). Ghrelin mediates anticipation to a palatable meal in rats. *Obesity (Silver Spring)* 20, 963–971.

Merle, J. V., Haas, V., Burghardt, R., Döhler, N., Schneider, N., Lehmkuhl, U., et al. (2011). Agouti-related protein in patients with acute and weight-restored anorexia nervosa. *Psychol. Med.* 41, 2183–2192.

Mika, C., Holtkamp, K., Heer, M., Günther, R. W., and Herpertz-Dahlmann, B. (2007). A 2-year prospective study of bone metabolism and bone mineral density in adolescents with anorexia nervosa. *J. Neural Transm.* 114, 1611–1618.

Miljic, D., Pekic, S., Djurovic, M., Doknic, M., Milic, N., Casanueva, F. F., et al. (2006). Ghrelin has partial or no effect on appetite, growth hormone, prolactin, and cortisol release in patients with anorexia nervosa. *J. Clin. Endocrinol. Metab.* 91, 1491–1495.

Miller, K. K. (2011). Endocrine dysregulation in anorexia nervosa update. *J. Clin. Endocrinol. Metab.* 96, 2939–2949.

Misra, M., and Klibanski, A. (2011). The neuroendocrine basis of anorexia nervosa and its impact on bone metabolism. *Neuroendocrinology* 93, 65–73.

Misra, M., Miller, K. K., Almazan, C., Ramaswamy, K., Aggarwal, A., Herzog, D. B., et al. (2004a). Hormonal and body composition predictors of soluble leptin receptor, leptin, and free leptin index in adolescent girls with anorexia nervosa and controls and relation to insulin sensitivity. *J. Clin. Endocrinol. Metab.* 89, 3486–3495.

Misra, M., Miller, K. K., Almazan, C., Ramaswamy, K., Lapcharoensap, W., Worley, M., et al. (2004b). Alterations in cortisol secretory dynamics in adolescent girls with anorexia nervosa and effects on bone metabolism. *J. Clin. Endocrinol. Metab.* 89, 4972–4980.

Misra, M., Miller, K., Herzog, D., Ramaswamy, K., Aggarwal, A., Almzan, C., et al. (2004c). Growth hormone and ghrelin responses to an oral glucose load in adolescent girls with anorexia nervosa and controls. *J. Clin. Endocrinol. Metab.* 89, 1605–1612.

Misra, M., Miller, K. K., Bjornson, J., Hackman, A., Aggarwal, A., Chung, J., et al. (2003). Alterations in growth hormone secretory dynamics in adolescent girls with anorexia nervosa and effects on bone metabolism. *J. Clin. Endocrinol. Metab.* 88, 5615–5623.

Misra, M., Miller, K. K., Cord, J., Prabhakaran, R., Herzog, D. B., Goldstein, M., et al. (2007). Relationships between serum adipokines, insulin levels, and bone density in girls with anorexia nervosa. *J. Clin. Endocrinol. Metab.* 92, 2046–2052.

Misra, M., Miller, K. K., Kuo, K., Griffin, K., Stewart, V., Hunter, E., et al. (2005a). Secretory dynamics of leptin in adolescent girls with anorexia nervosa and healthy adolescents. *Am. J. Physiol. Endocrinol. Metab.* 289, E373–E381.

Misra, M., Miller, K. K., Stewart, V., Hunter, E., Kuo, K., Herzog, D. B., et al. (2005b). Ghrelin and bone metabolism in adolescent girls with anorexia nervosa and healthy adolescents. *J. Clin. Endocrinol. Metab.* 90, 5082–5087.

Misra, M., Miller, K. K., Kuo, K., Griffin, K., Stewart, V., Hunter, E., et al. (2005c). Secretory dynamics of ghrelin in adolescent girls with anorexia nervosa and healthy adolescents. *Am. J. Physiol. Endocrinol. Metab.* 289, E347–E356.

Misra, M., Miller, K. K., Tsai, P., Gallagher, K., Lin, A., Lee, N., et al. (2006). Elevated peptide YY levels in adolescent girls with anorexia nervosa. *J. Clin. Endocrinol. Metab.* 91, 1027–1033.

Misra, M., Prabhakaran, R., Miller, K. K., Goldstein, M. A., Mickley, D., Clauss, L., et al. (2008). Prognostic indicators of changes in bone density measures in adolescent girls with anorexia nervosa-II. *J. Clin. Endocrinol. Metab.* 93, 1292–1297.

Modan-Moses, D., Stein, D., Pariente, C., Yaroslavsky, A., Ram, A., Faigin, M., et al. (2007). Modulation of adiponectin and leptin during refeeding of female anorexia nervosa patients. *J. Clin. Endocrinol. Metab.* 92, 1843–1847.

Modirrousta, M., Mainville, L., and Jones, B. E. (2005). Orexin and MCH neurons express c-Fos differently after sleep deprivation vs. recovery and bear different adrenergic receptors. *Eur. J. Neurosci.* 21, 2807–2816.

Mokrosinski, J., and Holst, B. (2010). Modulation of the constitutive activity of the ghrelin receptor by use of pharmacological tools and mutagenesis. *Meth. Enzymol.* 484, 53–73.

Monteleone, P. (2011). New frontiers in endocrinology of eating disorders. *Curr. Top. Behav. Neurosci.* 6, 189–208.

Monteleone, P., Di Lieto, A., Tortorella, A., Longobardi, N., and Maj, M. (2000). Circulating leptin in patients with anorexia nervosa, bulimia nervosa or binge-eating disorder: relationship to body weight, eating patterns, psychopathology and endocrine changes. *Psychiatry Res.* 94, 121–129.

Monteleone, P., Fabrazzo, M., Martiadis, V., Serritella, C., Pannuto, M., and Maj, M. (2005). Circulating brain-derived neurotrophic factor is decreased in women with anorexia and bulimia nervosa but not in women with binge-eating disorder: relationships to co-morbid depression, psychopathology and hormonal variables. *Psychol. Med.* 35, 897–905.

Monteleone, P., Fabrazzo, M., Tortorella, A., Fuschino, A., and Maj, M. (2002a). Opposite modifications in circulating leptin and soluble leptin receptor across the eating disorder spectrum. *Mol. Psychiatry* 7, 641–646.

Monteleone, P., Martiadis, V., Colurcio, B., and Maj, M. (2002b). Leptin secretion is related to chronicity and severity of the illness in bulimia nervosa. *Psychosom. Med.* 64, 874–879.

Monteleone, P., Luisi, M., Colurcio, B., Casarosa, E., Monteleone, P., Ioime, R., et al. (2001). Plasma levels of neuroactive steroids are increased in untreated women with anorexia nervosa or bulimia nervosa. *Psychosom. Med.* 63, 62–68.

Monteleone, P., Tortorella, A., Martiadis, V., Serritella, C., Fuschino, A., and Maj, M. (2004). Opposite changes in the serum brain-derived neurotrophic factor in anorexia nervosa and obesity. *Psychosom. Med.* 66, 744–748.

Morita, S., and Miyata, S. (2012). Different vascular permeability between the sensory and secretory circumventricular organs of adult mouse brain. *Cell Tissue Res.* 349, 589–603.

Moriya, J., Takimoto, Y., Yoshiuchi, K., Shimosawa, T., and Akabayashi, A. (2006). Plasma agouti-related protein levels in women with anorexia nervosa. *Psychoneuroendocrinology* 31, 1057–1061.

Muccioli, G., Lorenzi, T., Lorenzi, M., Ghè, C., Arnoletti, E., Raso, G. M., et al. (2011). Beyond the metabolic role of ghrelin: a new player in the regulation of reproductive function. *Peptides* 32, 2514–2521.

Mullier, A., Bouret, S. G., Prevot, V., and Dehouck, B. (2010). Differential distribution of tight junction proteins suggests a role for tanycytes in blood-hypothalamus barrier regulation in the adult mouse brain. *J. Comp. Neurol.* 518, 943–962.

Muñoz-Calvo, M. T., Barrios, V., García de Alvaro, M. T., Lefort, M., Méndez-Dávila, C., Argente, J., et al. (2007). Maintained malnutrition produces a progressive decrease in (OPG)/RANKL ratio and leptin levels in patients with anorexia nervosa. *Scand. J. Clin. Lab. Invest.* 67, 387–393.

Nakahara, T., Harada, T., Yasuhara, D., Shimada, N., Amitani, H., Sakoguchi, T., et al. (2008). Plasma obestatin concentrations are negatively correlated with body mass index, insulin resistance index, and plasma leptin concentrations in obesity and anorexia nervosa. *Biol. Psychiatry* 64, 252–255.

Nakahara, T., Kojima, S., Tanaka, M., Yasuhara, D., Harada, T., Sagiyama, K., et al. (2007). Incomplete restoration of the secretion of ghrelin and PYY compared to insulin after food ingestion following weight gain in anorexia nervosa. *J. Psychiatr. Res.* 41, 814–820.

Nakai, Y., Hosoda, H., Nin, K., Ooya, C., Hayashi, H., Akamizu, T., et al. (2003). Plasma levels of active form of ghrelin during oral glucose tolerance test in patients with anorexia nervosa. *Eur. J. Endocrinol.* 149, R1–R3.

Nakazato, M., Hashimoto, K., Shimizu, E., Kumakiri, C., Koizumi, H., Okamura, N., et al. (2003). Decreased levels of serum brain-derived neurotrophic factor in female patients with eating disorders. *Biol. Psychiatry* 54, 485–490.

Nakazato, M., Hashimoto, K., Yoshimura, K., Hashimoto, T., Shimizu, E., and Iyo, M. (2006). No change between the serum brain-derived neurotrophic factor in female patients with anorexia nervosa before and after partial weight recovery.

Prog. Neuropsychopharmacol. Biol. Psychiatry 30, 1117–1121.

Nakazato, M., Murakami, N., Date, Y., Kojima, M., Matsuo, H., Kangawa, K., et al. (2001). A role for ghrelin in the central regulation of feeding. *Nature* 409, 194–198.

Nakazato, M., Tchanturia, K., Schmidt, U., Campbell, I. C., Treasure, J., Collier, D. A., et al. (2009). Brain-derived neurotrophic factor (BDNF) and set-shifting in currently ill and recovered anorexia nervosa (AN) patients. *Psychol. Med.* 39, 1029–1035.

Naleid, A. M., Grace, M. K., Cummings, D. E., and Levine, A. S. (2005). Ghrelin induces feeding in the mesolimbic reward pathway between the ventral tegmental area and the nucleus accumbens. *Peptides* 26, 2274–2279.

Neary, N. M., Small, C. J., Wren, A. M., Lee, J. L., Druce, M. R., Palmieri, C., et al. (2004). Ghrelin increases energy intake in cancer patients with impaired appetite: acute, randomized, placebo controlled trial. *J. Clin. Endocrinol. Metab.* 89, 2832–2836.

Nedvidkova, J., Krykorkova, I., Bartak, V., Papezova, H., Gold, P. W., Alesci, S., et al. (2003). Loss of meal-induced decrease in plasma ghrelin levels in patients with anorexia nervosa. *J. Clin. Endocrinol. Metab.* 88, 1678–1682.

Nedvidkova, J., Papezova, H., Haluzik, M., and Schreiber, V. (2000). Interaction between serum leptin levels and hypothalamo-hypophyseal-thyroid axis in patients with anorexia nervosa. *Endocr. Res.* 26, 219–230.

Nemeroff, C. B., Bissette, G., Widerlov, E., Beckmann, H., Gerner, R., Manberg, P. J., et al. (1989). Neurotensin-like immunoreactivity in cerebrospinal fluid of patients with schizophrenia, depression, anorexia nervosa-bulimia, and premenstrual syndrome. *J. Neuropsychiatry Clin. Neurosci.* 1, 16–20.

Nestler, E. J. (1996). Under siege: the brain on opiates. *Neuron* 16, 897–900.

Nikolopoulos, D., Theocharis, S., and Kouraklis, G. (2010). Ghrelin, another factor affecting bone metabolism. *Med. Sci. Monit.* 16, RA147–RA162.

Nilsson, I. A., Thams, S., Lindfors, C., Bergstrand, A., Cullheim, S., Hökfelt, T., et al. (2011). Evidence of hypothalamic degeneration in the anorectic anx/anx mouse. *Glia* 59, 45–57.

Nobili, L., Baglietto, M. G., Beelke, M., De Carli, F., Di Comite, R., Fiocchi, I., et al. (2004). Impairment of the production of delta sleep in anorectic adolescents. *Sleep* 27, 1553–1559.

Nogal, P., Pniewska-Siark, B., and Lewinski, A. (2008). Evaluation of selected clinical and diagnostic parameters in girls with anorexia nervosa (I). *Neuro Endocrinol. Lett.* 29, 421–427.

Nogueira, J. P., Maraninchi, M., Lorec, A. M., Corroller, A. B., Nicolay, A., Gaudart, J., et al. (2010). Specific adipocytokines profiles in patients with hyperactive and/or binge/purge form of anorexia nervosa. *Eur. J. Clin. Nutr.* 64, 840–844.

Nova, E., and Marcos, A. (2006). Immunocompetence to assess nutritional status in eating disorders. *Expert Rev. Clin. Immunol.* 2, 433–444.

Ogiso, K., Asakawa, A., Amitani, H., and Inui, A. (2011). Ghrelin and anorexia nervosa: a psychosomatic perspective. *Nutrition* 27, 988–993.

Ohwada, R., Hotta, M., Oikawa, S., and Takano, K. (2006). Etiology of hypercholesterolemia in patients with anorexia nervosa. *Int. J. Eat. Disord.* 39, 598–601.

Ohwada, R., Hotta, M., Sato, K., Shibasaki, T., and Takano, K. (2007). The relationship between serum levels of estradiol and osteoprotegerin in patients with anorexia nervosa. *Endocr. J.* 54, 953–959.

Olatunji, B. O., Broman-Fulks, J. J., Ciesielski, B. G., Zawilinski, L. L., Shewmaker, S., and Wall, D. (2012). A taxometric investigation of the latent structure of eating disorders. *Psychiatry Res.* 197, 97–102.

Olszewski, P. K., Li, D., Grace, M. K., Billington, C. J., Kotz, C. M., and Levine, A. S. (2003). Neural basis of orexigenic effects of ghrelin acting within lateral hypothalamus. *Peptides* 24, 597–602.

Onur, S., Haas, V., Bosy-Westphal, A., Hauer, M., Paul, T., Nutzinger, D., et al. (2005). L-tri-iodothyronine is a major determinant of resting energy expenditure in underweight patients with anorexia nervosa and during weight gain. *Eur. J. Endocrinol.* 152, 179–184.

Osterstock, G., Escobar, P., Mitutsova, V., Gouty-Colomer, L. A., Fontanaud, P., Molino, F., et al. (2010). Ghrelin stimulation of growth hormone-releasing hormone neurons is direct in the arcuate nucleus. *PLoS ONE* 5:e9159. doi:10.1371/journal.pone.0009159

Ostrowska, Z., Ziora, K., Kos-Kudla, B., Swietochowska, E., Oswiecimska, J., Dyduch, A., et al. (2010). Melatonin, the RANKL/RANK/OPG system, and bone metabolism in girls with anorexia nervosa. *Endokrynol. Pol.* 61, 117–123.

Ostrowska, Z., Ziora, K., Oswiecimska, J., Swietochowska, E., and Wolkowska-Pokrywa, K. (2012a). Dehydroepiandrosterone sulfate, osteoprotegerin and its soluble ligand sRANKL and bone metabolism in girls with anorexia nervosa. *Postepy Hig. Med. Dosw. (Online)* 66, 655–662.

Ostrowska, Z., Ziora, K., Oswiecimska, J., Swietochowska, E., Szapska, B., Wolkowska-Pokrywa, K., et al. (2012b). RANKL/RANK/OPG system and bone status in females with anorexia nervosa. *Bone* 50, 156–160.

Oswiecimska, J., Ziora, K., Adamczyk, P., Roczniak, W., Pikiewicz-Koch, A., Stojewska, M., et al. (2007). Effects of neuroendocrine changes on results of ambulatory blood pressure monitoring (ABPM) in adolescent girls with anorexia nervosa. *Neuro Endocrinol. Lett.* 28, 410–416.

Otto, B., Cuntz, U., Fruehauf, E., Wawarta, R., Folwaczny, C., Riepl, R. L., et al. (2001). Weight gain decreases elevated plasma ghrelin concentrations of patients with anorexia nervosa. *Eur. J. Endocrinol.* 145, 669–673.

Otto, B., Cuntz, U., Otto, C., Heldwein, W., Riepl, R. L., and Tschop, M. H. (2007). Peptide YY release in anorectic patients after liquid meal. *Appetite* 48, 301–304.

Otto, B., Tschop, M., Frühauf, E., Heldwein, W., Fichter, M., Otto, C., et al. (2005). Postprandial ghrelin release in anorectic patients before and after weight gain. *Psychoneuroendocrinology* 30, 577–581.

Palyha, O. C., Feighner, S. D., Tan, C. P., McKee, K. K., Hreniuk, D. L., Gao, Y. D., et al. (2000). Ligand activation domain of human orphan growth hormone (GH) secretagogue receptor (GHS-R) conserved from Pufferfish to humans. *Mol. Endocrinol.* 14, 160–169.

Pannacciulli, N., Vettor, R., Milan, G., Granzotto, M., Catucci, A., and Federspil, G. (2003). Anorexia nervosa is characterized by increased adiponectin plasma levels and reduced nonoxidative glucose metabolism. *J. Clin. Endocrinol. Metab.* 88, 1748–1752.

Papotti, M., Ghè, C., Cassoni, P., Catapano, F., Deghenghi, R., Ghigo, E., et al. (2000). Growth hormone secretagogue binding sites in peripheral human tissues. *Clin. Endocrinol. Metab.* 85, 3803–3807.

Pardo, M., Roca-Rivada, A., Al-Massadi, O., Seoane, L. M., Camiña, J. P., and Casanueva, F. F. (2010). Peripheral leptin and ghrelin receptors are regulated in a tissue-specific manner in activity-based anorexia. *Peptides* 31, 1912–1919.

Peeters, T. L. (2003). Central and peripheral mechanisms by which ghrelin regulates gut motility. *J. Physiol. Pharmacol.* 54(Suppl. 4), 95–103.

Peino, R., Baldelli, R., Rodriguez-Garcia, J., Rodriguez-Segade, S., Kojima, M., Kangawa, K., et al. (2000). Ghrelin – induced growth hormone secretion in humans. *Eur. J. Endocrinol.* 143, R11–R14.

Pemberton, C. J., and Richards, A. M. (2007). Biochemistry of ghrelin precursor peptides. *Vitam. Horm.* 77, 13–30.

Perello, M., Sakata, I., Birnbaum, S., Chuang, J. C., Osborne-Lawrence, S., Rovinsky, S. A., et al. (2010). Ghrelin increases the rewarding value of high-fat diet in an orexin-dependent manner. *Biol. Psychiatry* 67, 880–886.

Perelló, M., and Zigman, J. M. (2012). The role of ghrelin in reward-based eating. *Biol. Psychiatry* 72, 347–353.

Petersen, P. S., Woldbye, D. P., Madsen, A. N., Egerod, K. L., Jin, C., Lang, M., et al. (2009). In vivo characterization of high Basal signaling from the ghrelin receptor. *Endocrinology* 150, 4920–4930.

Phillipp, E., Pirke, K. M., Kellner, M. B., and Krieg, J. C. (1991). Disturbed cholecystokinin secretion in patients with eating disorders. *Life Sci.* 48, 2443–2450.

Pirke, K. M., Friess, E., Kellner, M. B., Krieg, J. C., and Fichter, M. M. (1994). Somatostatin in eating disorders. *Int. J. Eat. Disord.* 15, 99–102.

Polli, N., Scacchi, M., Pecori Giraldi, F., Sormani, M., Zappulli, D., and Cavagnini, F. (2008). Low insulin-like growth factor I and leukopenia in anorexia nervosa. *Int. J. Eat. Disord.* 41, 355–359.

Popovic, V., Djurovic, M., Cetkovic, A., Vojvodic, D., Pekic, S., Spremovic, S., et al. (2004). Inhibin B: a potential marker of gonadal activity in patients with anorexia nervosa during weight recovery. *J. Clin. Endocrinol. Metab.* 89, 1838–1843.

Putignano, P., Dubini, A., Toja, P., Invitti, C., Bonfanti, S., Redaelli, G., et al. (2001). Salivary cortisol measurement in normal-weight, obese and anorexic women: comparison with plasma cortisol. *Eur. J. Endocrinol.* 145, 165–171.

Qader, S. S., Håkanson, R., Rehfeld, J. F., Lundquist, I., and Salehi, A.

(2008). Proghrelin-derived peptides influence the secretion of insulin, glucagon, pancreatic polypeptide and somatostatin: a study on isolated islets from mouse and rat pancreas. *Regul. Pept.* 146, 230–237.

Repaci, A., Gambineri, A., Pagotto, U., and Pasquali, R. (2011). Ghrelin and reproductive disorders. *Mol. Cell. Endocrinol.* 340, 70–79.

Rodríguez, A., Gómez-Ambrosi, J., Catalán, V., Gil, M. J., Becerril, S., Sáinz, N., et al. (2009). Acylated and desacyl ghrelin stimulate lipid accumulation in human visceral adipocytes. *Int. J. Obes. (Lond.)* 33, 541–552.

Routtenberg, A., and Kuznesof, A. W. (1967). Self-starvation of rats living in activity wheels on a restricted feeding schedule. *J. Comp. Physiol. Psychol.* 64, 414–421.

Saito, S., Watanabe, K., Hashimoto, E., and Saito, T. (2009). Low serum BDNF and food intake regulation: a possible new explanation of the pathophysiology of eating disorders. *Prog. Neuropsychopharmacol. Biol. Psychiatry* 33, 312–316.

Samec, S., Seydoux, J., Russell, A. P., Montani, J. P., and Dulloo, A. G. (2002). Skeletal muscle heterogeneity in fasting-induced upregulation of genes encoding UCP2, UCP3, PPARgamma and key enzymes of lipid oxidation. *Pflugers Arch.* 445, 80–86.

Sanger, G. J. (2008). Motilin, ghrelin and related neuropeptides as targets for the treatment of GI diseases. *Drug Discov. Today* 13, 234–239.

Sangiao-Alvarellos, S., and Cordido, F. (2010). Effect of ghrelin on glucose-insulin homeostasis: therapeutic implications. *Int. J. Pept.* 2010, pii: 234709.

Schellekens, H., Dinan, T. G., and Cryan, J. F. (2010). Lean mean fat reducing "ghrelin" machine: hypothalamic ghrelin and ghrelin receptors as therapeutic targets in obesity. *Neuropharmacology* 58, 2–16.

Sedlackova, D., Kopeckova, J., Papezova, H., Hainer, V., Kvasnickova, H., Hill, M., et al. (2012). Comparison of a high-carbohydrate and highprotein breakfast effect on plasma ghrelin, obestatin, NPY and PYY levels in women with anorexia and bulimia nervosa. *Nutr. Metab. (Lond.)* 9, 52.

Shimizu, N., Oomura, Y., and Kai, Y. (1989). Stress-induced anorexia in rats mediated by serotonergic mechanisms in the hypothalamus. *Physiol. Behav.* 46, 835–841.

Shrestha, Y. B., Wickwire, K., and Giraudo, S. (2009). Effect of reducing hypothalamic ghrelin receptor gene expression on energy balance. *Peptides* 30, 1336–1341.

Siegfried, Z., Berry, E. M., Hao, S., and Avraham, Y. (2003). Animal models in the investigation of anorexia. *Physiol. Behav.* 79, 39–45.

Skibicka, K. P., and Dickson, S. L. (2011). Ghrelin and food reward: the story of potential underlying substrates. *Peptides* 32, 2265–2273.

Skibicka, K. P., Hansson, C., Egecioglu, E., and Dickson, S. L. (2012). Role of ghrelin in food reward: impact of ghrelin on sucrose self-administration and mesolimbic dopamine and acetylcholine receptor gene expression. *Addict. Biol.* 17, 95–107.

Smith, G. P. (1989). Animal models of human eating disorders. *Ann. N. Y. Acad. Sci.* 575, 63–72.

Soriano-Guillen, L., Barrios, V., Campos-Barros, A., and Argente, J. (2004). Ghrelin levels inobesityand anorexia nervosa: effect of weight reduction or recuperation. *J. Pediatr.* 144, 36–42.

Speranza, M., Revah-Levy, A., Giquel, L., Loas, G., Venisse, J. L., Jeammet, P., et al. (2012). An investigation of Goodman's addictive disorder criteria in eating disorders. *Eur. Eat. Disord. Rev.* 20, 182–189.

Stengel, A., Keire, D., Goebel, M., Evilevitch, L., Wiggins, B., Taché, Y., et al. (2009). The RAPID method for blood processing yields new insight in plasma concentrations and molecular forms of circulating gut peptides. *Endocrinology* 150, 5113–5118.

Stock, S., Leichner, P., Wong, A. C., Ghatei, M. A., Kieffer, T. J., Bloom, S. R., et al. (2005). Ghrelin, peptide YY, glucose-dependent insulinotropic polypeptide, and hunger responses to a mixed meal in anorexic, obese, and control female adolescents. *J. Clin. Endocrinol. Metab.* 90, 2161–2168.

Støving, R. K., Chen, J. W., Glintborg, D., Brixen, K., Flyvbjerg, A., Hørder, K., et al. (2007). Bioactive insulin-like growth factor (IGF) I and IGF-binding protein-1 in anorexia nervosa. *J. Clin. Endocrinol. Metab.* 92, 2323–2329.

Støving, R. K., Hangaard, J., Hagen, C., and Flyvbjerg, A. (2003). Low levels of the 150-kD insulin-like growth factor binding protein 3 ternary complex in patients with anorexia nervosa: effect of partial weight recovery. *Horm. Res.* 60, 43–48.

Støving, R. K., Veldhuis, J. D., Flyvbjerg, A., Vinten, J., Hangaard, J., Koldkjaer, O. G., et al. (1999). Jointly amplified basal and pulsatile growth hormone (GH) secretion and increased process irregularity in women with anorexia nervosa: indirect evidence for disruption of feedback regulation within the GH-insulin-like growth factor I axis. *J. Clin. Endocrinol. Metab.* 84, 2056–2063.

Sun, Y., Ahmed, S., and Smith, R. G. (2003). Deletion of ghrelin impairs neither growth nor appetite. *Mol. Cell. Biol.* 23, 7973–7981.

Sun, Y., Butte, N. F., Garcia, J. M., and Smith, R. G. (2008). Characterization of adult ghrelin and ghrelin receptor knockout mice under positive and negative energy balance. *Endocrinology* 149, 843–850.

Sun, Y., Wang, P., Zheng, H., and Smith, R. G. (2004). Ghrelin stimulation of growth hormone release and appetite is mediated through the growth hormone secretagogue receptor. *Proc. Natl. Acad. Sci. U.S.A.* 101, 4679–4684.

Svensson, J., Lall, S., Dickson, S. L., Bengtsson, B. A., Rømer, J., Ahnfelt-Rønne, I., et al. (2000). The GH secretagogues ipamorelin and GH-releasing peptide-6 increase bone mineral content in adult female rats. *J. Endocrinol.* 165, 569–577.

Szentirmai, E., Kapás, L., Sun, Y., Smith, R. G., and Krueger, J. M. (2009). The preproghrelin gene is required for the normal integration of thermoregulation and sleep in mice. *Proc. Natl. Acad. Sci. U.S.A.* 106, 14069–14074.

Tagami, T., Satoh, N., Usui, T., Yamada, K., Shimatsu, A., and Kuzuya, H. (2004). Adiponectin in anorexia nervosa and bulimia nervosa. *J. Clin. Endocrinol. Metab.* 89, 1833–1837.

Tamai, H., Takemura, J., Kobayashi, N., Matsubayashi, S., Matsukura, S., and Nakagawa, T. (1993). Changes in plasma cholecystokinin concentrations after oral glucose tolerance test in anorexia nervosa before and after therapy. *Metab. Clin. Exp.* 42, 581–584.

Tanaka, M., Nakahara, T., Kojima, S., Nakano, T., Muranaga, T., Nagai, N., et al. (2004). Effect of nutritional rehabilitation on circulating ghrelin and growth hormone levels in patients with anorexia nervosa. *Regul. Pept.* 122, 163–168.

Tanaka, M., Tatebe, Y., Nakahara, T., Yasuhara, D., Sagiyama, K., Muranaga, T., et al. (2003a). Eating pattern and the effect of oral glucose on ghrelin and insulin secretion in patients with anorexia nervosa. *Clin. Endocrinol. (Oxf.)* 59, 574–549.

Tanaka, M., Naruo, T., Yasuhara, D., Tatebe, Y., Nagai, N., Shiiya, T., et al. (2003b). Fasting plasma ghrelin levels in subtypes of anorexia nervosa. *Psychoneuroendocrinology* 28, 829–835.

Tanaka, M., Narau, T., Nagai, N., Kuroki, N., Shiiya, T., Nakazato, M., et al. (2003c). Habitual binge/purge behavior influences circulating ghrelin levels in eating disorders. *J. Psychiatr. Res.* 37, 17–22.

Taub, D. D. (2008). Novel connections between the neuroendocrine and immune systems: the ghrelin immunoregulatory network. *Vitam. Horm.* 77, 325–346.

Tena-Sempere, M. (2008). Ghrelin as a pleotrophic modulator of gonadal function and reproduction. *Nat. Clin. Pract. Endocrinol. Metab.* 4, 666–674.

Tepper, R., Weizman, A., Apter, A., Tyano, S., and Beyth, Y. (1992). Elevated plasma immunoreactive b-endorphin in anorexia nervosa. *Clin. Neuropharmacol.* 15, 387–391.

Tesauro, M., Schinzari, F., Caramanti, M., Lauro, R., and Cardillo, C. (2010). Metabolic and cardiovascular effects of ghrelin. *Int. J. Pept.* 2010, 1–7.

Thompson, N. M., Gill, D. A., Davies, R., Loveridge, N., Houston, P. A., Robinson, I. C., et al. (2004). Ghrelin and des-octanoyl ghrelin promote adipogenesis directly in vivo by a mechanism independent of the type 1a growth hormone secretagogue receptor. *Endocrinology* 145, 234–242.

Tolle, V., Bassant, M. H., Zizzari, P., Poindessous-Jazat, F., Tomasetto, C., Epelbaum, J., et al. (2002). Ultradian rhythmicity of ghrelin secretion in relation with GH, feeding behavior, and sleep-wake patterns in rats. *Endocrinology* 143, 1353–1361.

Tolle, V., Kadem, M., Bluet-Pajot, M. T., Frere, D., Foulon, C., Bossu, C., et al. (2003). Balance in ghrelin and leptin plasma levels in anorexia nervosa patients and constitutionally thin women. *J. Clin. Endocrinol. Metab.* 88, 109–116.

Tomasik, P. J., Sztefko, K., and Malek, A. (2002). GLP-1 as a satiety factor in children with eating disorders. *Horm. Metab. Res.* 34, 77–80.

Tomasik, P. J., Sztefko, K., and Starzyk, J. (2004). Cholecystokinin, glucose dependent insulinotropic peptide and glucagon-like peptide 1 secretion in childrenwith anorexia nervosa and simple obesity. *J. Pediatr. Endocrinol. Metab.* 17, 1623–1631.

Tomasik, P. J., Sztefko, K., Starzyk, J., Rogatko, I., and Szafran, Z. (2005). Entero-insular axis in children with anorexia nervosa. *Psychoneuroendocrinology* 30, 364–372.

Tomova, A., Makker, K., Kirilov, G., Agarwal, A., and Kumanov, P. (2007). Disturbances in gonadal axis in women with anorexia nervosa. *Eat. Weight Disord.* 12, e92–e97.

Toshinai, K., Date, Y., Murakami, N., Shimada, M., Mondal, M. S., Shimbara, T., et al. (2003). Ghrelin-induced food intake is mediated via the orexin pathway. *Endocrinology* 144, 1506–1512.

Toshinai, K., Yamaguchi, H., Sun, Y., Smith, R. G., Yamanaka, A., Sakurai, T., et al. (2006). Des-acyl ghrelin induces food intake by a mechanism independent of the growth hormone secretagogue receptor. *Endocrinology* 147, 2306–2314.

Troisi, A., Di Lorenzo, G., Lega, I., Tesauro, M., Bertoli, A., Leo, R., et al. (2005). Plasma ghrelin in anorexia, bulimia, and binge-eating disorder: relations with eating patterns and circulating concentrations of cortisol and thyroid hormones. *Neuroendocrinology* 81, 259–266.

Tschöp, M., Smiley, D. L., and Heiman, M. L. (2000). Ghrelin induces adiposity in rodents. *Nature* 407, 908–910.

Tschöp, M., Wawarta, R., Riepl, R. L., Friedrich, S., Bidlingmaier, M., Landgraf, R., et al. (2001). Postprandial decrease of circulating human ghrelin levels. *J. Endocrinol. Invest.* 24, RC19–RC21.

Tsubota, Y., Owada-Makabe, K., Yukawa, K., and Maeda, M. (2005). Hypotensive effect of des-acyl ghrelin at nucleus tractus solitarii of rat. *Neuroreport* 16, 163–166.

Uehara, T., Omori, I., Nakamura, K., Suda, M., Hosoda, Y., Minegishi, T., et al. (2005). Plasma des-acyl and acyl ghrelin in patients with eating disorders. *Eat. Weight Disord.* 10, 264–266.

Uhe, A. M., Szmukler, G. I., Collier, G. R., Hansky, J., O'Dea, K., and Young, G. P. (1992). Potential regulators of feeding behavior in anorexia nervosa. *Am. J. Clin. Nutr.* 55, 28–32.

Valevski, A., Fridberg, G., Gil-Ad, I., Laron, Z., and Weizman, A. (2000). Neuroendocrinological response to standardized mixed meal in female anorectic patients during active and refeeding phases. *J. Pediatr. Endocrinol. Metab.* 13, 195–199.

Van Vugt, D. A. (2010). Brain imaging studies of appetite in the context of obesity and the menstrual cycle. *Hum. Reprod. Update* 16, 276–292.

Veldhuis, J. D., and Bowers, C. Y. (2010). Integrating GHS into the ghrelin system. *Int. J. Pept.* 2010, 1–40.

Verhagen, L. A., Egecioglu, E., Luijendijk, M. C., Hillebrand, J. J., Adan, R. A., and Dickson, S. L. (2011). Acute and chronic suppression of the central ghrelin signaling system reveals a role in food anticipatory activity. *Eur. Neuropsychopharmacol.* 21, 384–392.

Viapiana, O., Gatti, D., Dalle Grave, R., Todesco, T., Rossini, M., Braga, V., et al. (2007). Marked increases in bone mineral density and biochemical markers of bone turnover in patients with anorexia nervosa gaining weight. *Bone* 40, 1073–1077.

Volkov, N. D., Wang, G. J., and Baler, R. D. (2011). Reward, dopamine and the control of food intake: implications for obesity. *Trends Cogn. Sci. (Regul. Ed.)* 15, 37–46.

Wang, L., Saint-Pierre, D. H., and Tache, Y. (2002). Peripheral ghrelin selectively increases Fos expression in neuropeptide Y-synthesizing neurons in mouse hypothalamic arcuate nucleus. *Neurosci. Lett.* 325, 47–51.

Wang, T., Hung, C. C., and Randall, D. J. (2006). The comparative physiology of food deprivation: from feast to famine. *Annu. Rev. Physiol.* 68, 223–251.

Weinbrenner, T., Zittermann, A., Gouni-Berthold, I., Stehle, P., and Berthold, H. K. (2003). Body mass index and disease duration are predictors of disturbed bone turnover in anorexia nervosa. A case-control study. *Eur. J. Clin. Nutr.* 57, 1262–1267.

Wellman, P. J., Davis, K. W., and Nation, J. R. (2005). Augmentation of cocaine hyperactivity in rats by systemic ghrelin. *Regul. Pept.* 125, 151–154.

Willner, P. (1984). The validity of animal models of depression. *Psychopharmacology (Berl.)* 83, 1–16.

Wong, M. L., Licinio, J., Gold, P. W., and Glowa, J. (1993). Activity-induced anorexia in rats does not affect hypothalamic neuropeptide gene expression chronically. *Int. J. Eat. Disord.* 13, 399–405.

Wortley, K. E., Anderson, K. D., Garcia, K., Murray, J. D., Malinova, L., Liu, R., et al. (2004). Genetic deletion of ghrelin does not decrease food intake but influences metabolic fuel preference. *Proc. Natl. Acad. Sci. U.S.A.* 101, 8227–8232.

Wortley, K. E., del Rincon, J. P., Murray, J. D., Garcia, K., Iida, K., Thorner, M. O., et al. (2005). Absence of ghrelin protects against early-onset obesity. *J. Clin. Invest.* 115, 3573–3578.

Wren, A. M., Seal, L. J., Cohen, M. A., Brynes, A. E., Frost, G. S., Murphy, K. G., et al. (2001a). Ghrelin enhances appetite and increases food intake in humans. *J. Clin. Endocrinol. Metab.* 86, 5992.

Wren, A. M., Small, C. J., Abbott, C. R., Dhillo, W. S., Seal, L. J., Cohen, M. A., et al. (2001b). Ghrelin causes hyperphagia and obesity in rats. *Diabetes* 50, 2540–2547.

Wren, A. M., Small, C. J., Ward, H. L., Murphy, K. G., Dakin, C. L., Taheri, S., et al. (2000). The novel hypothalamic peptide ghrelin stimulates food intake and growth hormone secretion. *Endocrinology* 141, 4325–4328.

Yang, J., Brown, M. S., Liang, G., Grishin, N. V., and Goldstein, J. L. (2008). Identification of the acyltransferase that octanoylates ghrelin, an appetite-stimulating peptide hormone. *Cell* 132, 387–396.

Yi, C. X., Heppner, K., and Tschöp, M. H. (2011). Ghrelin in eating disorders. *Mol. Cell. Endocrinol.* 340, 29–34.

Zhao, C. P., Tang, M., Peeters, T. L., and Depoortere, I. (2003). In the rat ghrelin changes the excitability of neurons in the paraventricular nucleus of the hypothalamus. *Neurogastroent. Mot.* 15, 571–590.

Zhao, T. J., Liang, G., Li, R. L., Xie, X., Sleeman, M. W., Murphy, A. J., et al. (2010). Ghrelin O-acyltransferase (GOAT) is essential for growth hormone-mediated survival of calorie-restricted mice. *Proc. Natl. Acad. Sci. U.S.A.* 107, 7467–7472.

Zhu, X., Cao, Y., Voogd, K., and Steiner, D. F. (2006). On the processing of proghrelin to ghrelin. *J. Biol. Chem.* 281, 38867–38870.

Zigman, J. M., Jones, J. E., Lee, C. E., Saper, C. B., and Elmquist, J. K. (2006). Expression of ghrelin receptor mRNA in the rat and the mouse brain. *J. Comp. Neurol.* 494, 528–548.

Ziora, K. T., Oswiecimska, J. M., Swietochowska, E., Ostrowska, Z., Stojewska, M., Gorczyca, P., et al. (2011). Assessment of serum levels resistin in girls with anorexia nervosa. Part II. Relationships between serum levels of resistin and thyroid, adrenal and gonadal hormones. *Neuro Endocrinol. Lett.* 32, 697–703.

Zizzari, P., Halem, H., Taylor, J., Dong, J. Z., Datta, R., Culler, M. D., et al. (2005). Endogenous ghrelin regulates episodic growth hormone (GH) secretion by amplifying GH Pulse amplitude: evidence from antagonism of the GH secretagogue-R1a receptor. *Endocrinology* 146, 3836–3842.

Zizzari, P., Hassouna, R., Longchamps, R., Epelbaum, J., and Tolle, V. (2011). Meal anticipatory rise in acylated ghrelin at dark onset is blunted after long-term fasting in rats. *J. Neuroendocrinol.* 23, 804–814.

7

Actions of agonists and antagonists of the ghrelin/GHS-R pathway on GH secretion, appetite, and cFos activity

Rim Hassouna[1], Alexandra Labarthe[1], Philippe Zizzari[1], Catherine Videau[1], Michael Culler[2], Jacques Epelbaum[1] and Virginie Tolle[1]*

[1] *UMR-S 894 INSERM, Centre de Psychiatrie et Neurosciences, Université Paris Descartes, Sorbonne Paris Cité, Paris, France*
[2] *IPSEN, Milford, MA, USA*

Edited by:
Hubert Vaudry, University of Rouen, France

Reviewed by:
Rhonda D. Kineman, University of Illinois at Chicago, USA
Vivian J. Costantini, Aptuit s.r.l., Italy

****Correspondence:***
Virginie Tolle, UMR894 INSERM, Centre de Psychiatrie et Neurosciences, 2 ter rue d'Alésia, 75014 Paris, France.
e-mail: virginie.tolle@inserm.fr

The stimulatory effects of ghrelin, a 28-AA acylated peptide originally isolated from stomach, on growth hormone (GH) secretion and feeding are exclusively mediated through the growth hormone secretagogue 1a receptor (GHS-R1a), the only ghrelin receptor described so far. Several GHS-R1a agonists and antagonists have been developed to treat metabolic or nutritional disorders but their mechanisms of action in the central nervous system remain poorly understood. In the present study, we compared the activity of BIM-28163, a GHS-R1a antagonist, and of several agonists, including native ghrelin and the potent synthetic agonist, BIM-28131, to modulate food intake, GH secretion, and cFos activity in arcuate nucleus (ArcN), nucleus tractus solitarius (NTS), and area postrema (AP) in wild-type and NPY-GFP mice. BIM-28131 was as effective as ghrelin in stimulating GH secretion, but more active than ghrelin in inducing feeding. It stimulated cFos activity similarly to ghrelin in the NTS and AP but was more powerful in the ArcN, suggesting that the super-agonist activity of BIM-28131 is mostly mediated in the ArcN. BIM-28163 antagonized ghrelin-induced GH secretion but not ghrelin-induced food consumption and cFos activation, rather it stimulated food intake and cFos activity without affecting GH secretion. The level of cFos activation was dependent on the region considered: BIM-28163 was as active as ghrelin in the NTS, but less active in the ArcN and AP. All compounds also induced cFos immunoreactivity in ArcN NPY neurons but BIM-28131 was the most active. In conclusion, these data demonstrate that two peptide analogs of ghrelin, BIM-28163, and BIM-28131, are powerful stimulators of appetite in mice, acting through pathways and key brain regions involved in the control of appetite that are only partially superimposable from those activated by ghrelin. A better understanding of the molecular pathways activated by these compounds could be useful in devising future therapeutic applications, such as for cachexia and anorexia.

Keywords: ghrelin, GHS-R, BIM-28163, BIM-28131, antagonist, food intake, GH secretion, cFos

INTRODUCTION

Ghrelin is a 28 amino acid acylated peptide originally discovered in stomach tissues by inverse pharmacology (Kojima et al., 1999) as the endogenous ligand for the growth hormone (GH) Secretagogue-1a Receptor (GHS-R1a), an orphan receptor cloned a few years earlier from pig pituitaries (Howard et al., 1996). GH secretagogues are a family of synthetic peptidic or non-peptidic compounds developed from the early 1980s to stimulate GH secretion (Bluet-Pajot et al., 2001). As anticipated, ghrelin was initially described for its ability to stimulate GH secretion in several species including rodents and humans (Kojima et al., 1999; Tolle et al., 2001) but it is still to date the only orexigenic hormone produced in the gastrointestinal tract (Tschop et al., 2000).

The actions of ghrelin on GH secretion and feeding require the addition of an eight-carbon fatty acid that is attached on a serine in position 3 by the enzyme ghrelin-*O*-acyl-transferase (GOAT) (Gutierrez et al., 2008; Yang et al., 2008). They are exclusively mediated through the GHS-R1a (Sun et al., 2004), the only ghrelin receptor described so far. GHS-R1a is highly expressed in the hypothalamus, a region involved in the control of GH secretion and appetite, and also in the brainstem that receives informations from gut vagal afferents (Guan et al., 1997; Katayama et al., 2000). Within the hypothalamus, NPY neurons in the arcuate nucleus (ArcN) express the GHS-R1a (Willesen et al., 1999; Tannenbaum et al., 2003), and are a well-characterized target for ghrelin actions (Tannenbaum et al., 2003; Chen et al., 2004). Nevertheless, several studies have suggested that certain ghrelin actions may be mediated through a receptor that has yet to be identified.

Several GHS-R1a antagonists have been developed to decipher the function of the ghrelin/GHS-R pathway in the regulation of feeding behavior and GH secretion (Asakawa et al., 2003; Okimura et al., 2003; Beck et al., 2004; Halem et al., 2004; Demange et al., 2007; Esler et al., 2007; Petersen et al., 2009; Costantini et al., 2011; Moulin et al., 2013). Although they have all been clearly shown to antagonize exogenous ghrelin actions on GH secretion both in *in vitro* systems and *in vivo*, their biological effects *per se* on several biological parameters are contradictory and their mechanisms of action in the central nervous system remain poorly understood.

Indeed, intracerebroventricular injections of two antagonists [D-Lys3]-GHRP6, an analog of one of the synthetic GHS (Asakawa et al., 2003) or [D-Arg-1, D-Phe-5, D-Trp-7,9,Leu-11]-substance P, an analog of substance P (Petersen et al., 2009) induces suppression of feeding in mice. In contrast [D-Lys3]-GHRP6 has no action on spontaneous ultradian GH secretion (Okimura et al., 2003). But results are biased by the fact that [D-Lys3]-GHRP6 also binds to all melanocortin receptors (Schioth et al., 1997) and [D-Arg-1, D-Phe-5, D-Trp-7,9,Leu-11]-substance P also has full inverse agonist action *in vitro* and *in vivo* (Holst et al., 2003; Petersen et al., 2009). To date, the effects of JMV2810, another recently developed GHS-R1a antagonist, on spontaneous feeding or GH secretion have not been reported (Demange et al., 2007).

Only the full-length ghrelin analog, BIM-28163 (now called RM-28163), has been tested on both spontaneous GH secretion and food intake. Treatment with this selective GHS-R1a antagonist over 48 h in rats reduces pulsatile GH secretion (Zizzari et al., 2005). In contrast, it increases food intake and weight gain as effectively as ghrelin when administered at 5- to 10-fold higher doses than ghrelin (Halem et al., 2004, 2005). Interestingly, BIM-28163 induces cFos activation in the dorsomedial nucleus of the hypothalamus (DMH) while it acts as an antagonist in the ArcN of the hypothalamus. These data are corroborated by a more recent study also describing a stimulatory effect of another GHS-R1a antagonist, GSK1614343, on feeding in rats and dogs (Costantini et al., 2011). Altogether these data are intriguing and suggest the existence of an unknown pathway mediating the effects of these ghrelin antagonists on feeding through either the GHS-R1a or another unknown receptor. Understanding the mechanisms of action of this compound that differentially affect feeding and GH secretion can be of clinical interest.

In the present study, we compared the effect of BIM-28163, BIM-28131(Strassburg et al., 2008; Palus et al., 2011), native ghrelin, and the combination of BIM-28163 + ghrelin in the modulation of food intake, GH secretion, and cFos activity in fed mice. Our aim was to map changes in cFos activation in several key brain regions controlling appetite and/or GH secretion, including the hypothalamic ArcN, ventromedial nucleus of the hypothalamus (VMH), nucleus tractus solitarius (NTS), and area postrema (AP) of the brainstem. In addition, we used NPY-GFP mice to test whether the feeding effects of the analogs were mediated, like ghrelin, through the orexigenic NPY neurons.

MATERIALS AND METHODS

ANIMALS

About 18–25-week-old C57BL6/J male and female mice, obtained either from Charles River or from our own colony, were used for feeding experiments. About 18–25-week-old C57BL6/J or NPY-Renilla GFP transgenic male and female mice backcrossed on the C57BL6/J background and expressing Renilla GFP under the transcriptional control of the NPY genomic sequence (Van Den Pol et al., 2009) were used for cFos experiments. Mice were housed at constant temperature and humidity, with a fixed 12-h light/dark cycle (lights-on at 7.00 a.m.) and free access to food and water. In addition, the animals were handled weekly to minimize stress. All experiments were carried out in accordance with the European Communities Council Directive (86/609/EEC) and were approved by the animal experimentation committee of Paris Descartes University.

PEPTIDES

Native ghrelin, BIM-28131 (a small peptide ghrelin agonist), and BIM-28163 (a full-length ghrelin analog antagonist) were obtained from IPSEN (Milford, MA, USA). Peptides were dissolved in a vehicle containing 0.9% saline +0.25% of bovin serum albumin (BSA).

AUTOMATED FOOD INTAKE MONITORING

One week prior to the experiments, 18–25-week-old C57BL6/J male mice were individually housed and acclimatized to the automated drinking/feeding stations (TSE Systems, GmbH, Germany). Feeding behavior was recorded continuously by means of high precision sensors, attached to the top of the cage lids. Meal patterns were analyzed using the following definition: a meal consists of the consumption of 0.03 g of food separated from the next feeding episode by at least 10 min as previously described (Yu et al., 2009; Stengel et al., 2010; Wang et al., 2011). For each mouse, the meal number, the total meal size (g), and the total meal duration (min) were measured within 4 h following peptide injections.

Experiments were performed during the light phase (10.00 a.m.–11.00 a.m.) and carried out in a cross-over designed manner so that each mouse received all treatments randomly separated by two washout days. On each experimental day, mice were injected intraperitoneally (ip) with either vehicle (0.9% saline containing 0.25% BSA), native ghrelin (30 nmol), BIM-28131 (30 nmol), BIM-28163 (150 nmol), or native ghrelin (30 nmol) combined with BIM-28163 (150 nmol).

cFos IMMUNOHISTOCHEMISTRY, FEEDING, AND GH MEASUREMENTS

About 18–25-week-old male and female C57BL6/J and NPY-GFP mice were individually housed and had free access to food and water at the time of injections. Vehicle, native ghrelin (30 nmol), BIM-28131 (30 nmol), BIM-28163 (150 nmol), or native ghrelin (30 nmol) combined with BIM-28163 (150 nmol) were injected ip in the early light phase (9.00 a.m.–11.00 a.m.).

A pre-weighed amount of food was distributed in each cage at the time of injections and weighed 90 min later in order to confirm the effects of the treatments on food consumption and to correlate food intake to the number of activated cFos nuclei. 15 min following the injection, 4 μl of whole blood was withdrawn from the tail vein, homogenized in 116 μl of GH buffer (PBS, 0.05% Tween) for GH measurements. Whole blood GH concentrations were evaluated by EIA as previously described (Steyn et al., 2011).

The number of nuclei immunoreactive for cFos protein were quantified 90 min after ip injection of peptides to determine which brain regions were activated by the compounds. Mice were deeply anesthetized with pentobarbital (5.5 mg/30 g BW) and perfused through the ascending aorta with saline 0.9% for 1 min followed by 4% paraformaldehyde (PFA) in phosphate buffer 0.1 M (PB) for an additional 9 min. The brains were removed, post-fixed for 2 h in 4% PFA and cryoprotected in 30% sucrose for 2 days at 4°C. Brains were then frozen in 2-methyl-butane and sectioned in the coronal plane at a thickness of 25 μm using a freezing microtome (Frigomobile, Leica, Wetzlar, Germany).

For the detection of cFos protein expression, free-floating sections were processed for immunohistochemistry. Sections were incubated in blocking buffer (10% Normal Donkey Serum, 0.3% Triton X-100 in 0.1 M TBS) for 1 h at room temperature then incubated with rabbit cFos antibody (1:20000, Ab-5, Jackson Laboratories, West Grove, PA, USA) in 1% NDS, 0.3% Triton X-100 in 0.1 M TBS overnight at room temperature. Sections were then rinsed 4 × 10 min in 0.1 M TBS and incubated with Cy3 conjugated Donkey Anti-Rabbit antibody (1:800 DAR-Cy3, Jackson Laboratories, West Grove, PA, USA) 1 h at room temperature and then rinsed 4 × 10 min in 0.1 M TBS. Sections were mounted with fluoromount and quantified using a Zeiss Axioplan epifluorescence microscope (Carl Zeiss, Le Pecq, France) under 40× magnification. Quantifications were performed bilaterally every 100 μm sections through the ArcN (2.3–1.6 mm anterior to the interaural line) and ventromedial nucleus (VMH, 2.5–2.3 mm anterior to the interaural line) of the hypothalamus and in the NTS (3.7 mm posterior to the interaural line) and AP (3.7 mm posterior to the interaural line) of the brainstem (Franklin and Paxinos, 1997).

NPY neurons were visualized using GFP fluorescence. GFP-positive cell bodies expressing cFos were quantified unilaterally under 40× magnification using a confocal SP5 microscope (Leica, Wetzlar, Germany). Co-localizations were determined with the Image-J software (http://rsbweb.nih.gov/ij/) on series of continuous optical sections with 0.5 μm increment along the z-axis of the section.

STATISTICAL ANALYSES

Values are given as mean ± SEM. Statistical analyses were performed using ANOVA, repeated measures ANOVA followed by Fisher PLSD *post hoc* test using the Statview software (SAS Institute Inc., Cary, NC, USA).

RESULTS

EFFECT OF GHS-R1a AGONISTS AND ANTAGONISTS ON FEEDING BEHAVIOR

Feeding was monitored after intraperitoneal injections of native ghrelin (30 nmol), BIM-28163 (150 nmol), BIM-28131 (30 nmol), or after co-administration of native ghrelin + BIM-28163 in the early light phase. In a first subset of mice, feeding was monitored manually after injection of the treatments in randomly assigned groups of animals. Ninety minutes after the injections, a significant effect of treatment on food consumption was observed (**Figure 1A**). Although native ghrelin increased food intake by twofold, the effect of this compound was not significant. Only BIM-28131 and BIM-28163 increased food consumption significantly with BIM-28131 being three times more effective and BIM-28163 two times more effective than ghrelin, respectively. Food intake was identical after co-administration of BIM-28163 and native ghrelin or after administration of ghrelin alone. Automated feeding stations were also used to monitor cumulative food intake and meal pattern during 7 h following the injection in a second set of mice: animals received each treatment randomly in a cross-over designed manner (**Figure 2** and **Table 1**). When data were analyzed as repeated measures in the same mouse and over time, there was a significant interaction between time and treatment. BIM-28131 was the only compound to stimulate appetite even in mice that did not respond well to ghrelin. Increased food consumption in this group was associated with a tendency to increased meal number, total meal size, and total meal duration (**Table 1**).

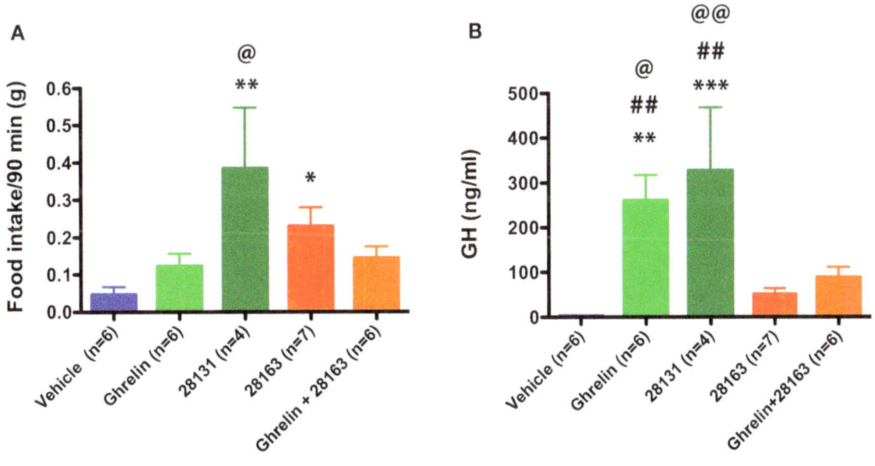

FIGURE 1 | Effect of native ghrelin and BIM compounds on cumulative food intake and GH secretion measured during the light cycle in mice. Data represent mean ± SEM. **(A)** Mean cumulative food intake (90 min) after ip injection of native ghrelin (30 nmol), BIM-28131 (30 nmol), BIM-28163 (150 nmol), and native ghrelin (30 nmol) co-administered with BIM-28163 (150 nmol). ANOVA shows an effect of treatment on 90 min food intake: $*p < 0.05$ BIM-28163 vs. vehicle, $**P < 0.01$ BIM-28131 vs. vehicle, and native ghrelin, $^{@}P < 0.05$ BIM-28131 vs. native ghrelin + BIM-28163, Fisher PLSD *post hoc* test. **(B)** GH secretion measured by tail bleeding 15 min after ip injection of BIM compounds in the same animals. ANOVA shows an effect of treatment on GH levels: $**p < 0.01$ native ghrelin vs. vehicle, $***P < 0.001$ BIM-28131 vs. vehicle, $^{@}P < 0.05$ native ghrelin vs. native ghrelin + BIM-28163, $^{@@}P < 0.01$ BIM-28131 vs. native ghrelin + BIM-28163, $^{\#\#}P < 0.01$ native ghrelin or BIM-28131 vs. BIM-28163, Fisher PLSD *post hoc* test.

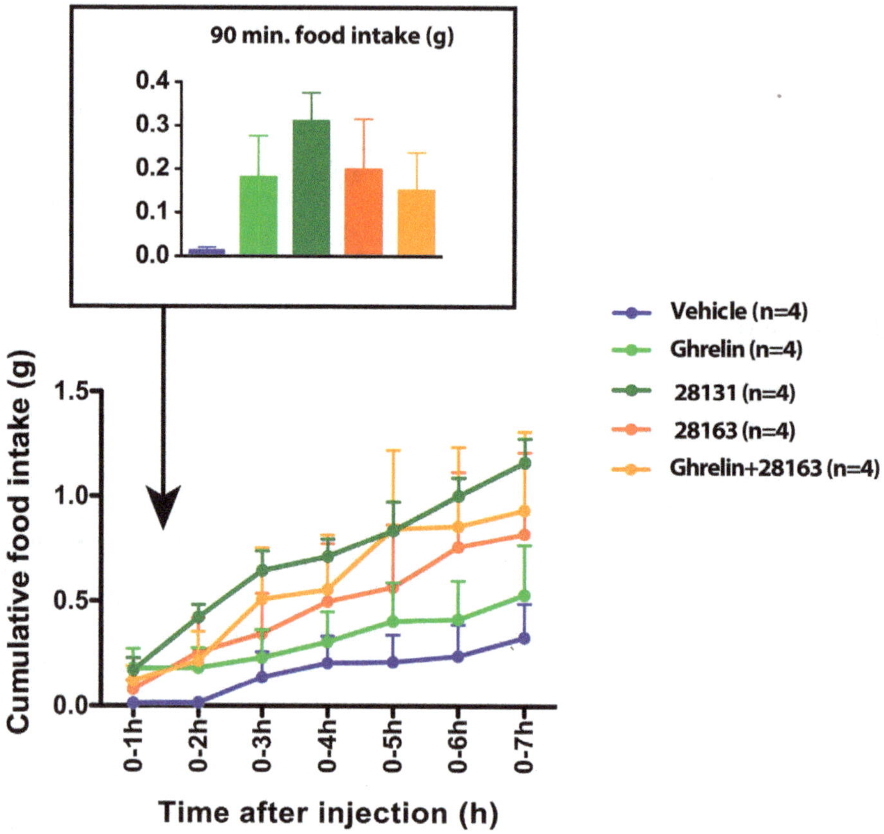

FIGURE 2 | Effect of native ghrelin and BIM compounds on cumulative food intake measured with the automated feeding station in mice. Mean cumulative food intake (0–7 h) after ip injection of native ghrelin (30 nmol), BIM-28131 (30 nmol), BIM-28163 (150 nmol), and native ghrelin (30 nmol) co-administered with BIM-28163 (150 nmol). Data represent mean ± SEM. Repeated measures ANOVA over time (7 h) and across treatments shows an interaction between time and treatment on cumulative food intake. $P = 0.06$ BIM-28131 vs. vehicle, Fisher PLSD *post-hoc* test.

Table 1 | Effect of native ghrelin and BIM compounds on meal pattern measured with the automated feeding station in mice.

	Meal number $n = 3$	Total meal size (g) $n = 4$	Total meal duration (min) $n = 4$
Vehicle	1.25 ± 0.75	0.23 ± 0.15	7.50 ± 4.97
Ghrelin	3.00 ± 1.08	0.41 ± 0.17	15.50 ± 9.90
BIM-28131	4.00 ± 0.41	0.82 ± 0.10	31.50 ± 4.99
BIM-28163	3.50 ± 2.02	0.92 ± 0.57	26.75 ± 14.73
Ghrelin + BIM-28163	3.50 ± 1.04	0.76 ± 0.29	27.75 ± 12.37

Meal number, total meal size, and total meal duration measured (0–7 h) after ip injection of native ghrelin (30 nmol), BIM-28131 (30 nmol), BIM-28163 (150 nmol), and native ghrelin (30 nmol) co-administered with BIM-28163 (150 nmol). Data represent mean ± SEM.

EFFECT OF GHS-R1a AGONISTS AND ANTAGONISTS ON GH SECRETION

GH plasma levels were monitored 15 min following the injections in the same animals used to monitor food intake manually (**Figure 1B**). Native ghrelin and BIM-28131 equally stimulated GH secretion whereas GH secretion was not increased after injection of BIM-28163 alone. In contrast to feeding data, BIM-28163 antagonized ghrelin-induced GH secretion.

EFFECT OF GHS-R1a AGONISTS AND ANTAGONISTS ON cFos ACTIVATION IN THE HYPOTHALAMIC ArcN

cFos activation was monitored after intraperitoneal injections of native ghrelin (30 nmol), BIM-28163 (150 nmol), BIM-28131 (30 nmol), or after co-administration of native ghrelin + BIM-28163 in the early light phase. Repeated measures ANOVA over the rostro-caudal extent of the ArcN showed an effect of treatment on cFos immunoreactive nuclei (**Figure 3A**). All treatment groups were significantly elevated compared to the vehicle-treated group, except BIM-28163 which had a modest effect (**Figure 3B**). Injection of native ghrelin induced cFos activation and this was not antagonized by co-administration of BIM-28163. Administration of BIM-28131 induced a more pronounced activation than all other treatments. Thus the efficiency of activation in the ArcN was BIM-28131 > native ghrelin > native ghrelin + BIM-28163 > BIM-28163. Differences were greater around 2.1–2.0 mm anterior to the interaural line where most NPY neurons are localized.

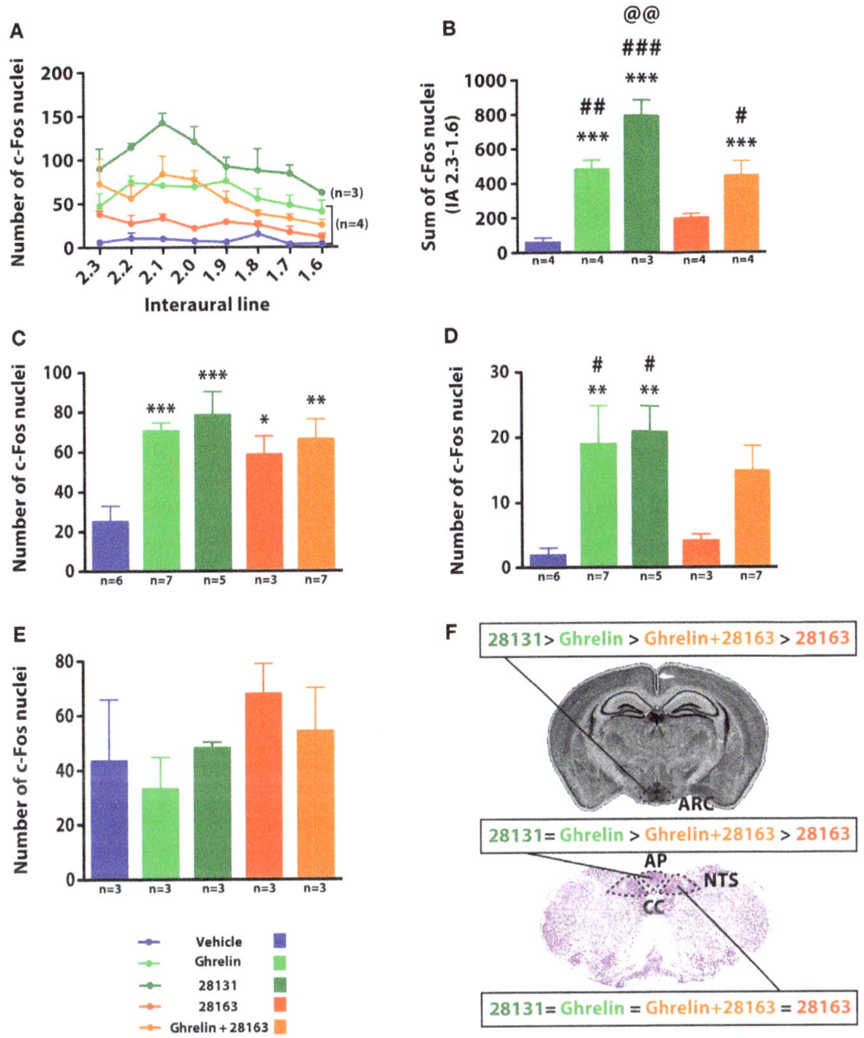

FIGURE 3 | Effect of native ghrelin and BIM compounds on cFos immunoreactivity in mice in the ArcN, AP, NTS, and VMH. (A) Number of cFos immunoreactive nuclei and **(B)** sum of cFos immunoreactive nuclei along the rostro-caudal extent of the ArcN (2.3–1.6 mm anterior to the interaural line). Data represent mean ± SEM. **(A)** Repeated measures ANOVA over the rostro-caudal extent of the ArcN shows an effect of treatment on the number of cFos-positive nuclei: $P < 0.0001$ native ghrelin vs. Vehicle, BIM-28163, and BIM-28131, $P < 0.0001$ BIM-28131 vs. all other treatments, $P < 0.0001$ BIM-28163 vs. all other treatments except vehicle, $P < 0.01$ BIM-28163 vs. vehicle, $P < 0.0001$ native ghrelin + BIM-28163 vs. vehicle, BIM-28163, and BIM-28131, Fisher PLSD *post hoc* test. **(B)** $^{***}P < 0.001$ vs. vehicle, $^{\#}P < 0.05$ vs. BIM-28163, $^{\#\#}P < 0.01$ vs. BIM-28163, $^{\#\#\#}P < 0.001$ vs. BIM-28163, $^{@@}P < 0.01$ vs. ghrelin + BIM-28163, Fisher PLSD *post hoc* test. **(C,D)** Number of cFos immunoreactive nuclei in the NTS and AP (3.7 mm posterior to the interaural line). Data represent mean ± SEM. ANOVA shows an effect of treatment on the number of cFos nuclei in the NTS and AP. $^{*}P < 0.05$, $^{**}P < 0.01$ and $^{***}P < 0.001$ vs. vehicle, $^{\#}P < 0.05$ vs. 28163, Fisher PLSD *post hoc* test. **(E)** Number of cFos immunoreactive nuclei in the VMH (2.5–2.3 mm anterior to the interaural line). Data represent mean ± SEM. No significant effect of treatments is observed in the VMH. **(F)** Summary of the effect of the different BIM compounds on cFos activation in the ArcN, NTS, and AP. Cc, central canal.

EFFECT OF GHS-R1a AGONISTS AND ANTAGONISTS ON cFos ACTIVATION IN THE NTS AND AP OF THE BRAINSTEM

cFos activation was also observed in the AP and nucleus tractus solitarius (NTS) (**Figures 3C,D**). In the NTS, in contrast to the ArcN, all treatments significantly increased the number of cFos-immunoreactive cells. BIM-28131 stimulated cFos as efficiently as native ghrelin. BIM-28163 had an activity *per se* but was inefficient in antagonizing ghrelin-induced cFos. In the AP, the compounds had different activities. Native ghrelin and BIM-28131 had the same efficiency in activating cFos, but BIM-28163 was ineffective.

EFFECT OF GHS-R1a AGONISTS AND ANTAGONISTS ON cFos ACTIVATION IN THE HYPOTHALAMIC VMH

In a separate group of animals, cFos activation was quantified in the VMH (Interaural line: −2.5, −2.3). Due to the high level of cFos activation and high variability in vehicle-treated animals, statistical differences were not observed between treatments (**Figure 3E**). The number of cFos nuclei in vehicle, ghrelin, and BIM-28131-treated animals were identical; however, in mice treated with BIM-28163, the number of cFos nuclei was twice as elevated as in ghrelin-treated mice.

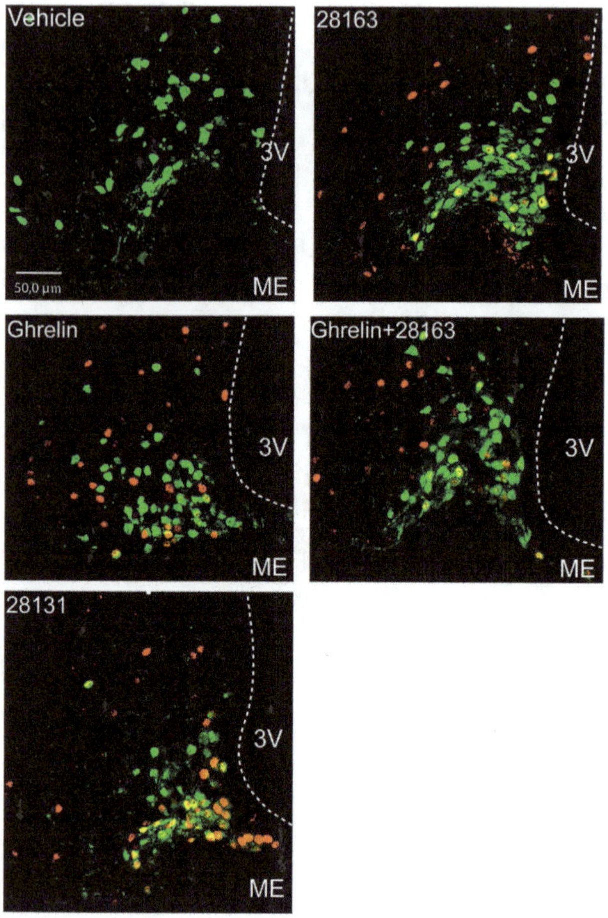

FIGURE 4 | Effect of native ghrelin and BIM compounds on cFos immunoreactivity in ArcN NPY neurons in NPY-Renilla GFP mice. Representative confocal microphotographs showing GFP neurons (green), cFos nuclei (red), and the merge of both signals (yellow/orange) in coronal sections of the ArcN at approximately 2.1–1.9 mm anterior to the interaural line. Data represent mean ± SEM. Scale bar represents 50 µm in the ArcN. 3V, third ventricle; ME, median eminence.

EFFECT OF GHS-R1a AGONISTS AND ANTAGONISTS ON cFos ACTIVATION IN NPY NEURONS

To measure cFos immunoreactivity in NPY neurons, we used NPY-GFP mice. All treatments induced cFos activation in NPY neurons as compared with vehicle-treated mice (**Figure 4** and **Table 2**). Treatments did not modify the number of GFP-positive neurons. BIM-28131 and native ghrelin co-administered with BIM-28163 induced the greatest activation of NPY neurons with more than 20% of NPY cells activated, whereas native ghrelin and BIM-28163 alone induced cFos in less than 15% of NPY neurons (**Table 2**).

DISCUSSION

The present study demonstrates that two GHS-R1a synthetic ligands, BIM-28163 and BIM-28131, are powerful stimulators of appetite in mice, acting through pathways and brain regions that are distinct from the ones activated by ghrelin (**Figure 3F** and **Table 3**).

BIM-28163 is a full GHS-R1a antagonist as it has no intrinsic activity at the GHS-R1a, and can fully block the ability of ghrelin to activate the GHS-R1a, as well as block ghrelin-induced GH release, both *in vitro* and *in vivo* (Halem et al., 2004). It is thus a pharmacological tool to dissect the role of endogenous ghrelin. However, whereas previous investigations in rats with this GHS-R1a antagonist revealed a role of the endogenous ligand in amplifying GH pulsatile pattern, blocking GHS-R1a fails to inhibit food intake (Zizzari et al., 2005), and BIM-28163 even stimulates appetite and weight gain after daily treatment in rats (Halem et al., 2004, 2005). In the current study performed in mice, we also demonstrate that acute injection of BIM-28163 increases food consumption and show for the first time that the compound induces cFos in two brain regions involved in the control of appetite, the hypothalamus and brainstem. The feeding effect of BIM-28163 is observed as early as 15–30 min after its injection (i.e., same time-course as native ghrelin) (data not shown).

It was previously described in the rat that intraperitoneal (ip) injection of native ghrelin in the early light phase induces feeding and cFos activation in the ArcN, NTS, and AP (Hewson and Dickson, 2000; Lawrence et al., 2002; Takayama et al., 2007). A dose of 30 nmol/30 g body weight was chosen here based on a published study showing that this dose stimulates food intake in mice (Zizzari et al., 2007). Although ghrelin was very potent in activating cFos in the ArcN, NTS, and AP in the present study, its effects on feeding did not reach statistical significance. It may be due to the fact that different sets of animals were used for feeding experiments and cFos experiments. Another possible interpretation is that cFos activation in these nuclei is required but not alone sufficient to induce an effect on appetite. We indeed recently observed that after ip injection of ghrelin, animals can be subdivided into two groups: high and low responders, suggesting an interindividual variability in the feeding effects of ghrelin (Hassouna et al., 2012b).

BIM-28131 is a super-agonist with regard to food intake in rats (Strassburg et al., 2008; Palus et al., 2011). It is also very potent to stimulate both appetite and cFos in the current study even in mice that were not responsive to ghrelin in the cross-over designed study. Differences in stability between native ghrelin and BIM-28131 would partly explain the differential activities of these two compounds. Indeed, in addition to a fivefold higher affinity than native ghrelin in binding to the GHS-R1a and a 10-fold increased potency in activating the receptor, BIM-28131 has a 10-fold greater circulating half-life. However, BIM-28131 is comparable to ghrelin with regard to stimulating GH secretion. The equal effect on GH release may be possible because the action of the compounds may be partly relayed at the pituitary level and the time of blood sampling occurred after a relatively short time (15 min) whereas the food intake was measured over 90 min or greater. By analyzing the feeding response every 15 min following the injection, BIM-28131 did not have a stronger feeding effect over native ghrelin at 15–30 min post-injection (data not shown) but from 60 min following the injection. Thus, BIM-28131 is more powerful than ghrelin in stimulating appetite at equimolar doses, and is also more powerful in activating cFos in the ArcN, but not in the NTS and AP, suggesting that the activity of this super-agonist is mostly mediated in the ArcN. This is further substantiated by cFos activation

Table 2 | Effect of native ghrelin and BIM compounds on the number of GFP-positive cells, number of cFos-positive nuclei, number, and percentage of GFP-positive cells expressing cFos protein in the ArcN in NPY-Renilla GFP mice.

	GFP-positive cells	cFos-positive nuclei	GFP-positive cells expressing cFos	% GFP-positive cells expressing cFos
Vehicle ($n=5$)	78.2 ± 10.5	6.0 ± 2.1	1.0 ± 0.4	1.5 ± 0.7
Ghrelin ($n=4$)	106.0 ± 9.5	35.7 ± 11.4*	14.8 ± 5.8	13.9 ± 4.9
BIM-28131 ($n=4$)	84.5 ± 9.4	43.5 ± 7.6**	18.0 ± 4.9*	20.7 ± 3.9**
BIM-28163 ($n=4$)	102.5 ± 14.9	24.2 ± 7.5	11.5 ± 4.1	11.9 ± 3.7
Ghrelin + BIM-28163 ($n=4$)	81.2 ± 23.1	30.2 ± 8.6*	16.0 ± 7.7*	23.4 ± 7.5**

Coronal sections of the ArcN at approximately 2.0–1.9 mm anterior to the interaural line were quantified unilaterally. Data represent mean ± SEM.
$^*P < 0.05$ and $^{**}P < 0.01$ vs. vehicle.

Table 3 | Summary of the effects of the different BIM compounds on GH secretion, food intake, and cFos activity in the ArcN, NTS, and AP after intraperitoneal administration in the mouse.

	Food intake	GH secretion	cfos ArcN	cfos AP	cfos NTS	cfos VMH
Ghrelin	±	+++	++	+++	+++	=
28131	+++	+++	+++	+++	+++	=
28163	++	=	±	±	+++	=
Ghrelin + 28163	No antagonistic action	Antagonistic action	No antagonistic action	No antagonistic action	No antagonistic action	=

Food intake and cFos measured 90 min and GH 15 min post-injection.

in orexigenic NPY ArcN neurons in BIM-28131-treated mice as compared with ghrelin-treated ones. NPY neurons are well-known targets for ghrelin actions (Tannenbaum et al., 2003; Chen et al., 2004) and induction of cFos in NPY neurons in rats was previously demonstrated with other ghrelin agonists (Dickson and Luckman, 1997).

In the current study, BIM-28163 activates several brain nuclei. The intensity of activation seems to be different depending on the region and relative to that of native ghrelin. BIM-28163 appears to have greater activity in the NTS than in the ArcN and AP, two structures outside the blood brain barrier (BBB). Indeed, in the NTS, BIM-28163 is as potent as both native ghrelin and BIM-28131 in inducing cFos with more than a twofold increase as compared with saline treated animals although the effect does not reach statistical significance. In the ArcN, however, BIM-28163 is not as effective as ghrelin in stimulating cFos, and is much less active than BIM-28131. This suggests that BIM-28163 uses alternative pathways other than through these BBB free structures to relay its orexigenic actions. These data are consistent with previous reports in rats showing that BIM-28163 selectively activates cFos in the DMH after icv injections, whereas, in the ArcN, it acts exclusively as an antagonist by blocking ghrelin-induced cFos activation without any intrinsic effect (Halem et al., 2004, 2005). Our data here slightly differ from the above studies in rats because BIM-28163 still activates cFos in the ArcN, although to a much lesser extent than ghrelin. In addition, we were not able to observe any antagonistic actions of BIM-28163 either on food intake or cFos activity when co-administered with ghrelin. Differences may be due to the species studied (mouse vs. rat), to the mode of administration (ip vs. icv), as well as the dose injected (5 nmol/g ip vs. 1.5 nmol/rat icv).

Differences in antagonizing ghrelin-induced food consumption or cFos may be due to the fact that BIM-28163 was injected at a fivefold higher dose than ghrelin instead of a 10-fold higher dose (IC50 for BIM-28163 at GHS-R1a is 10-fold higher than for native ghrelin). However, the antagonistic effect of BIM-28163 on ghrelin-induced cFos activity in rats was still observed when BIM-28163 was administered at a fivefold dose (Halem et al., 2005). The recent report by Costantini et al. (2011) shows that another novel and selective GHS-R1a antagonist with no partial agonist activity, GSK1614343 was also not able to antagonize ghrelin-induced food intake at a dose of 10 mg/kg.

Concerning the VMH, a high level of activation and high interindividual variability in vehicle-treated animals are observed. Consequently, ghrelin seems to have no stimulatory action in this nucleus. This is consistent with other data in rats showing that ghrelin does not activate cFos in the VMH (Lawrence et al., 2002). In contrast, the number of cFos-positive nuclei after treatment with BIM-28163 is almost twofold higher than in the ghrelin-treated group.

Within the hypothalamus, the ArcN is one of the main targets of peripheral signals, such as leptin and ghrelin, which relay information about energy stores and/or nutritional status. The efficiency of the compounds used in this study in activating the ArcN is BIM-28131 > native ghrelin > native ghrelin + BIM-28163 > BIM-28163. The GHS-R1a has been shown to be co-expressed with several neuropeptides in the ArcN. It is expressed on the orexigenic NPY and GHRH neurons (Willesen et al., 1999; Tannenbaum et al., 2003) and these populations of neurons relay ghrelin orexigenic and GH-releasing actions in rats (Tannenbaum et al., 2003; Chen et al., 2004). In mice, ghrelin also induces cFos in NPY-expressing neurons (Wang et al., 2002). To determine whether BIM-28163 and BIM-28131 orexigenic actions could be partly mediated through NPY neurons as is the case for ghrelin, we investigated the effect of these compounds in NPY-GFP mice. Indeed, ip administration of 30 nmol ghrelin during the light cycle induced cFos activation in approximately 26% of NPY neurons (Hassouna et al., 2012a,b). Here we observed that about 15% of NPY-positive cells were activated after BIM-28163 or native ghrelin administration whereas about 20% were activated after BIM-28131 treatment. The orexigenic action of BIM-28163 could be partly mediated through an activation of ArcN NPY neurons. Orexigenic actions of ghrelin may also be mediated by a reduced activity in POMC cells (Cowley et al., 2003). Modified activity of the anorexigenic POMC neurons after treatment with GHS-R1a compounds can thus not be excluded. Orexigenic actions of GSK1614343, another GHS-R1a antagonist, was accompanied by a reduced expression of POMC in the ArcN after chronic treatment with the compound (Costantini et al., 2011).

Although the majority of studies demonstrated that acylation is essential for ghrelin feeding activities (Inhoff et al., 2009), one study showed that desacyl ghrelin was able to stimulate food intake after intracerebroventricular administration by a mechanisms independent of the GHS-R1a (Toshinai et al., 2006). Interestingly, feeding effects of desacyl ghrelin was more pronounced in GHS-R1a deficient mice. Thus it can be postulated that blocking the GHS-R1a with the antagonist may allow desacyl to stimulate feeding through a GHS-R1a independent pathway. Whereas a distinct receptor from the known GHS-R1a would possibly mediate the orexigenic actions of BIM-28163, we can not exclude that these effects are also dependent on the GHS-R1a. Indeed, a recent study using the antagonist, GSK1614343, showed that the appetite-mediated action of this compound was abolished in GHS-R null mice (Costantini et al., 2011), suggesting that the orexigenic effects of GSK1614343 is relayed by GHS-R1a or that the ghrelin receptor may be needed. GHS-R1a is associated with multiple signal transduction pathways (Carreira et al., 2004; Holst et al., 2005) and it is possible that BIM-28163 could activate a specific pathway on the GHS-R1a that is independent from the one mediating GH-releasing activities. In addition, the formation of heterodimers between the GHS-R1a and other receptors has been evidenced (Kern et al., 2012), and raises the question as to whether the orexigenic actions of BIM-28163 could be mediated through interaction with a GHS-R1a dimer that differs from the GHS-R1a receptor form that regulates GH secretion. BIM-28163 could possibly interact with a receptor that needs to dimerize with the GHS-R1a.

The present study demonstrates that two GHS-R1a synthetic ligands, BIM-28163, and BIM-28131, are powerful stimulators of appetite in mice, acting through pathways and brain regions that are distinct from those activated by ghrelin.

In conclusion, utilization of synthetic GHS-R1a ligands, such as BIM-28163 and BIM-28131 that are powerful stimulators of appetite and act through pathways that are distinct from those activated by ghrelin, even in situations when ghrelin seems modestly effective, can have important clinical implications, in conditions such as cachexia or anorexia [*see other chapter in the same issue: Ghrelin: Central and Peripheral Implications in Anorexia Nervosa* (Mequinion et al., 2012)]. BIM-28131 was previously demonstrated to be very efficient in a rat heart failure model of cachexia (Strassburg et al., 2008; Palus et al., 2011). In addition, observations that BIM-28163 is able to selectively stimulate feeding and increase weight gain without altering GH secretion may suggest the possibility of treating pathologies in which hyper-activity of the GH/IGF-1 axis may be deleterious. A better understanding of the molecular pathways activated by these compounds will be useful for devising future therapeutic applications.

ACKNOWLEDGMENTS

This work was supported by an IPSEN grant to Virginie Tolle and Jacques Epelbaum. We are grateful to Alice Cougnon for the care of the animals and to Julie Cognet for technical assistance. The compounds utilized in this study, BIM-28131 and BIM-28163, are now known as RM131 and RM163. RM131 is currently in clinical development by Rhythm, Boston, MA, USA.

REFERENCES

Asakawa, A., Inui, A., Kaga, T., Katsuura, G., Fujimiya, M., Fujino, M. A., et al. (2003). Antagonism of ghrelin receptor reduces food intake and body weight gain in mice. *Gut* 52, 947–952.

Beck, B., Richy, S., and Stricker-Krongrad, A. (2004). Feeding response to ghrelin agonist and antagonist in lean and obese Zucker rats. *Life Sci.* 76, 473–478.

Bluet-Pajot, M. T., Tolle, V., Zizzari, P., Robert, C., Hammond, C., Mitchell, V., et al. (2001). Growth hormone secretagogues and hypothalamic networks. *Endocrine* 14, 1–8.

Carreira, M. C., Camiña, J. P., Smith, R. G., and Casanueva, F. F. (2004). Agonist-specific coupling of growth hormone secretagogue receptor type 1a to different intracellular signaling systems. Role of adenosine. *Neuroendocrinology* 79, 13–25.

Chen, H. Y., Trumbauer, M. E., Chen, A. S., Weingarth, D. T., Adams, J. R., Frazier, E. G., et al. (2004). Orexigenic action of peripheral ghrelin is mediated by neuropeptide Y and agouti-related protein. *Endocrinology* 145, 2607–2612.

Costantini, V. J., Vicentini, E., Sabbatini, F. M., Valerio, E., Lepore, S., Tessari, M., et al. (2011). GSK1614343, a novel ghrelin receptor antagonist, produces an unexpected increase of food intake and body weight in rodents and dogs. *Neuroendocrinology* 94, 158–168.

Cowley, M. A., Smith, R. G., Diano, S., Tschöp, M., Pronchuk, N., Grove, K. L., et al. (2003). The distribution and mechanism of action of ghrelin in the CNS demonstrates a novel hypothalamic circuit regulating energy homeostasis. *Neuron* 37, 649–661.

Demange, L., Boeglin, D., Moulin, A., Mousseaux, D., Ryan, J., Bergé, G., et al. (2007). Synthesis and pharmacological in vitro and in vivo evaluations of novel triazole derivatives as ligands of the ghrelin receptor. 1. *J. Med. Chem.* 50, 1939–1957.

Dickson, S. L., and Luckman, S. M. (1997). Induction of c-fos messenger ribonucleic acid in neuropeptide Y and growth hormone (GH)-releasing factor neurons in the rat arcuate nucleus following systemic injection of the GH secretagogue, GH-releasing peptide-6. *Endocrinology* 138, 771–777.

Esler, W. P., Rudolph, J., Claus, T. H., Tang, W., Barucci, N., Brown, S. E., et al. (2007). Small-molecule ghrelin receptor antagonists improve glucose tolerance, suppress appetite, and promote weight loss. *Endocrinology* 148, 5175–5185.

Franklin, K. B. J., and Paxinos, G. (1997). *The Mouse Brain in Stereotaxic Coordinates.* San Diego: Academic Press.

Guan, X. M., Yu, H., Palyha, O. C., Mckee, K. K., Feighner, S. D., Sirinathsinghji, D. J., et al. (1997). Distribution of mRNA encoding the growth hormone secretagogue receptor in brain and peripheral tissues. *Brain Res. Mol. Brain Res.* 48, 23–29.

Gutierrez, J. A., Solenberg, P. J., Perkins, D. R., Willency, J. A., Knierman, M. D., Jin, Z., et al. (2008). Ghrelin octanoylation mediated by an orphan lipid transferase. *Proc. Natl. Acad. Sci. U.S.A.* 105, 6320–6325.

Halem, H. A., Taylor, J. E., Dong, J. Z., Shen, Y., Datta, R., Abizaid, A., et al. (2004). Novel analogs of ghrelin: physiological and clinical implications. *Eur. J. Endocrinol.* 151(Suppl. 1), S71–S75.

Halem, H. A., Taylor, J. E., Dong, J. Z., Shen, Y., Datta, R., Abizaid, A., et al. (2005). A novel growth hormone secretagogue-1a receptor antagonist that blocks ghrelin-induced growth hormone secretion but induces increased body weight gain. *Neuroendocrinology* 81, 339–349.

Hassouna, R., Viltart, O., Tallot, L., Bouyer, K., Videau, C., Epelbaum, J., et al. (2012a). "Visualization techniques: from immunohistochemistry to magnetic resonance imaging," in *Visualization Techniques: From Immunohistochemistry to Magnetic Resonance Imaging*, ed. E. Badoer (Australia: Humana Press), 207–223.

Hassouna, R., Zizzari, P., Viltart, O., Yang, S.-K., Gardette, R., Videau, C., et al. (2012b). A natural variant of obestatin, Q90L, inhibits ghrelin's action on food intake and GH secretion and targets NPY and GHRH neurons in mice. *PLoS ONE* 7:e51135. doi:10.1371/journal.pone.0051135

Hewson, A. K., and Dickson, S. L. (2000). Systemic administration of ghrelin induces Fos and Egr-1 proteins in the hypothalamic arcuate nucleus of fasted and fed rats. *J. Neuroendocrinol.* 12, 1047–1049.

Holst, B., Brandt, E., Bach, A., Heding, A., and Schwartz, T. W. (2005). Nonpeptide and peptide growth hormone secretagogues act both as ghrelin receptor agonist and as positive or negative allosteric modulators of ghrelin signaling. *Mol. Endocrinol.* 19, 2400–2411.

Holst, B., Cygankiewicz, A., Jensen, T. H., Ankersen, M., and Schwartz, T. W. (2003). High constitutive signaling of the ghrelin receptor – identification of a potent inverse agonist. *Mol. Endocrinol.* 17, 2201–2210.

Howard, A. D., Feighner, S. D., Cully, D. F., Arena, J. P., Liberator, P. A., Rosenblum, C. I., et al. (1996). A receptor in pituitary and hypothalamus that functions in growth hormone release. *Science* 273, 974–977.

Inhoff, T., Wiedenmann, B., Klapp, B. F., Mönnikes, H., and Kobelt, P. (2009). Is desacyl ghrelin a modulator of food intake? *Peptides* 30, 991–994.

Katayama, M., Nogami, H., Nishiyama, J., Kawase, T., and Kawamura, K. (2000). Developmentally and regionally regulated expression of growth hormone secretagogue receptor mRNA in rat brain and pituitary gland. *Neuroendocrinology* 72, 333–340.

Kern, A., Albarran-Zeckler, R., Walsh, H. E., and Smith, R. G. (2012). Apo-ghrelin receptor forms heteromers with DRD2 in hypothalamic neurons and is essential for anorexigenic effects of DRD2 agonism. *Neuron* 73, 317–332.

Kojima, M., Hosoda, H., Date, Y., Nakazato, M., Matsuo, H., and Kangawa, K. (1999). Ghrelin is a growth-hormone-releasing acylated peptide from stomach. *Nature* 402, 656–660.

Lawrence, C. B., Snape, A. C., Baudoin, F. M.-H., and Luckman, S. M. (2002). Acute central ghrelin and GH secretagogues induce feeding and activate brain appetite centers. *Endocrinology* 143, 155–162.

Mequinion, M., Langlet, F., Zgheib, S., Dehouck, B., Chauveau, C., and Viltart, O. (2012). Ghrelin: central and peripheral implications in anorexia nervosa. *Front. Endocrinol.* 4:15. doi:10.3389/fendo.2013.00015

Moulin, A., Brunel, L., Boeglin, D., Demange, L., Ryan, J., M'kadmi, C., et al. (2013). The 1,2,4-triazole as a scaffold for the design of ghrelin receptor ligands: development of JMV 2959, a potent antagonist. *Amino Acids* 44, 301–314.

Okimura, Y., Ukai, K., Hosoda, H., Murata, M., Iguchi, G., Iida, K., et al. (2003). The role of circulating ghrelin in growth hormone (GH) secretion in freely moving male rats. *Life Sci.* 72, 2517–2524.

Palus, S., Schur, R., Akashi, Y. J., Bockmeyer, B., Datta, R., Halem, H., et al. (2011). Ghrelin and its analogues, BIM-28131 and BIM-28125, improve body weight and regulate the expression of MuRF-1 and MAFbx in a rat heart failure model. *PLoS ONE* 6:e26865. doi:10.1371/journal.pone.0026865

Petersen, P. S., Woldbye, D. P. D., Madsen, A. N., Egerod, K. L., Jin, C., Lang, M., et al. (2009). In vivo characterization of high basal signaling from the ghrelin receptor. *Endocrinology* 150, 4920–4930.

Schioth, H. B., Muceniece, R., and Wikberg, J. E. (1997). Characterization of the binding of MSH-B, HB-228, GHRP-6 and 153N-6 to the human melanocortin receptor subtypes. *Neuropeptides* 31, 565–571.

Stengel, A., Goebel, M., Wang, L., Rivier, J., Kobelt, P., Monnikes, H., et al. (2010). Activation of brain somatostatin 2 receptors stimulates feeding in mice: analysis of food intake microstructure. *Physiol. Behav.* 101, 614–622.

Steyn, F. J., Huang, L., Ngo, S. T., Leong, J. W., Tan, H. Y., Xie, T. Y., et al. (2011). Development of a method for the determination of pulsatile growth hormone secretion in mice. *Endocrinology* 152, 3165–3171.

Strassburg, S., Anker, S. D., Castaneda, T. R., Burget, L., Perez-Tilve, D., Pfluger, P. T., et al. (2008). Long-term effects of ghrelin and ghrelin receptor agonists on energy balance in rats. *Am. J. Physiol. Endocrinol. Metab.* 295, E78–E84.

Sun, Y., Wang, P., Zheng, H., and Smith, R. G. (2004). Ghrelin stimulation of growth hormone release and appetite is mediated through the growth hormone secretagogue receptor. *Proc. Natl. Acad. Sci. U.S.A.* 101, 4679–4684.

Takayama, K., Johno, Y., Hayashi, K., Yakabi, K., Tanaka, T., and Ro, S. (2007). Expression of c-Fos protein in the brain after intravenous injection of ghrelin in rats. *Neurosci. Lett.* 417, 292–296.

Tannenbaum, G. S., Epelbaum, J., and Bowers, C. Y. (2003). Interrelationship between the novel peptide ghrelin and somatostatin/growth hormone-releasing hormone in regulation of pulsatile growth hormone secretion. *Endocrinology* 144, 967–974.

Tolle, V., Zizzari, P., Tomasetto, C., Rio, M. C., Epelbaum, J., and Bluet-Pajot, M. T. (2001). In vivo and in vitro effects of ghrelin/motilin-related peptide on growth hormone secretion in the rat. *Neuroendocrinology* 73, 54–61.

Toshinai, K., Yamaguchi, H., Sun, Y., Smith, R. G., Yamanaka, A., Sakurai, T., et al. (2006). Des-acyl ghrelin induces food intake by a mechanism independent of the growth hormone secretagogue receptor. *Endocrinology* 147, 2306–2314.

Tschop, M., Smiley, D. L., and Heiman, M. L. (2000). Ghrelin induces adiposity in rodents. *Nature* 407, 908–913.

Van Den Pol, A. N., Yao, Y., Fu, L.-Y., Foo, K., Huang, H., and Coppari, R. (2009). Neuromedin B and gastrin-releasing peptide excite arcuate nucleus neuropeptide Y neurons in a novel transgenic mouse expressing strong renilla green fluorescent protein in NPY neurons. *J. Neurosci.* 29, 4622–4639.

Wang, L., Saint-Pierre, D. H., and Tache, Y. (2002). Peripheral ghrelin selectively increases Fos expression in neuropeptide Y – synthesizing neurons in mouse hypothalamic arcuate nucleus. *Neurosci. Lett.* 325, 47–51.

Wang, L., Stengel, A., Goebel, M., Martinez, V., Gourcerol, G., Rivier, J., et al. (2011). Peripheral activation of corticotropin-releasing factor receptor 2 inhibits food intake and alters meal structures in mice. *Peptides* 32, 51–59.

Willesen, M. G., Kristensen, P., and Rømer, J. (1999). Co-localization of growth hormone secretagogue receptor and NPY mRNA in the arcuate nucleus of the rat. *Neuroendocrinology* 70, 306–316.

Yang, J., Brown, M. S., Liang, G., Grishin, N. V., and Goldstein, J. L. (2008). Identification of the acyltransferase that octanoylates ghrelin, an appetite-stimulating peptide hormone. *Cell* 132, 387–396.

Yu, Y., South, T., and Huang, X. F. (2009). Inter-meal interval is increased in mice fed a high whey, as opposed to soy and gluten, protein diets. *Appetite* 52, 372–379.

Zizzari, P., Halem, H., Taylor, J., Dong, J. Z., Datta, R., Culler, M. D., et al. (2005). Endogenous ghrelin regulates episodic growth hormone (GH) secretion by amplifying GH Pulse amplitude: evidence from antagonism of the GH secretagogue-R1a receptor. *Endocrinology* 146, 3836–3842.

Zizzari, P., Longchamps, R., Epelbaum, J., and Bluet-Pajot, M. T. (2007). Obestatin partially affects ghrelin stimulation of food intake and growth hormone secretion in rodents. *Endocrinology* 148, 1648–1653.

8

Oxytocin, feeding, and satiety

Nancy Sabatier, Gareth Leng and John Menzies*

Centre for Integrative Physiology, School of Biomedical Sciences, The University of Edinburgh, Edinburgh, UK

Edited by:
Hubert Vaudry, University of Rouen, France

Reviewed by:
Aldo Lucion, Universidade Federal do Rio Grande do Sul, Brazil
Ruud Buijs, Universidad Autónoma de México, Mexico

****Correspondence:***
John Menzies, Centre for Integrative Physiology, University of Edinburgh, George Square, Edinburgh, EH8 9XD, UK.
e-mail: john.menzies@ed.ac.uk

Oxytocin neurons have a physiological role in food intake and energy balance. Central administration of oxytocin is powerfully anorexigenic, reducing food intake and meal duration. The central mechanisms underlying this effect of oxytocin have become better understood in the past few years. Parvocellular neurons of the paraventricular nucleus project to the caudal brainstem to regulate feeding via autonomic functions including the gastrointestinal vago-vagal reflex. In contrast, magnocellular neurons of the supraoptic and paraventricular nuclei release oxytocin from their dendrites to diffuse to distant hypothalamic targets involved in satiety. The ventromedial hypothalamus, for example, expresses a high density of oxytocin receptors but does not contain detectable oxytocin nerve fibers. Magnocellular neurons represent targets for the anorexigenic neuropeptide α-melanocyte stimulating hormone. In addition to homeostatic control, oxytocin may also have a role in reward-related feeding. Evidence suggests that oxytocin can selectively suppress sugar intake and that it may have a role in limiting the intake of palatable food by inhibiting the reward pathway.

Keywords: oxytocin, food, appetite, satiety, reward

INTRODUCTION

Unlike Roald Dahl's "enormously fat" Augustus Gloop – a boy who pursued eating as a hobby – humans usually eat much less than they could. Obesity is typically the result of a modest excess of energy intake over expenditure, but one that is sustained over a prolonged period. In fact, humans, like other animals, are very efficient at balancing energy intake and expenditure. If rats are allowed unlimited access to a high-energy palatable diet, their energy intake diverges quickly from control animals fed a bland diet, but the difference in energy intake stabilizes within days (Archer and Mercer, 2007). Thus rats, which presumably do not feel societal pressure to be slim, will overeat palatable food, but only to a certain extent. When their access to palatable food ends, rats typically *undereat*, failing to defend the extra body weight they have accumulated.

A variety of peripheral signals convey information to control meal size and, in the longer term, these signals are modified according to physiological state and the size of energy reserves. Several "satiety" peptides are secreted from the gastrointestinal tract, including cholecystokinin (CCK), glucagon-like-peptide-1 (GLP-1), and peptide YY (PYY) (Strader and Woods, 2005); some of these act on the brain at sites that lack a blood-brain barrier, others are transported across the blood-brain barrier, and others act via vagal neuronal afferents (Verbalis et al., 1986). Leptin, which is secreted from adipose tissue in proportion to the size of fat stores, is not itself a satiety signal, but by signaling the size of peripheral fat reserves it has a long term anorectic influence, and in part it may act by moderating acute satiety signals arising from the gastrointestinal tract. Whether these satiety signals and leptin all converge at a discrete "satiety center" in the brain is unclear but several neuronal populations have been identified as likely candidates for mediating satiety. In part, these have been identified because they synthesize peptides that have marked anorexic actions when administered centrally.

One of those potently anorectic neuropeptides is oxytocin – a peptide classically thought to be involved mainly in reproductive functions. However, as we review here, there is now considerable evidence that oxytocin also plays an important role in satiety.

PHYSIOLOGICAL ROLES OF OXYTOCIN

Oxytocin is produced in two hypothalamic regions: the supraoptic nucleus (SON) and paraventricular nucleus (PVN). Magnocellular neuroendocrine neurons in these nuclei project to the posterior pituitary gland, from where oxytocin is secreted into the blood. Classically, oxytocin secreted from the pituitary gland is involved in efficient and timely fetal expulsion, and is indispensable for the milk-ejection reflex and successful lactation (Nishimori et al., 1996); in some species, including rodents but not humans, it also regulates sodium excretion (natriuresis) (Verbalis et al., 1991), both by direct actions at the kidneys and indirectly be regulating the secretion of natriuretic peptides from the heart (McCann et al., 2003); in these species it is secreted in response to raised plasma osmotic pressure (Huang et al., 1996). All of the oxytocin neurons in the SON are magnocellular neuroendocrine neurons, but the PVN also contains parvocellular oxytocin neurons that project within the brain – to the spinal cord, caudal brainstem, amygdala, and substantia nigra (Sofroniew, 1980). These neurons are important in sexual behavior in males (Melis et al., 1986), and, as we discuss below, in the regulation of gastric reflexes.

Recently it has become apparent that oxytocin has an important "pro-social" role. In rodents, it has been implicated in recognition and positive social behavior between rodent mothers and their offspring and between adult members of the same social group (Neumann, 2009). However, behaviors linked to oxytocin are not all positive. In the rat, for example, patterns of central oxytocin release correlate with maternal aggression against unfamiliar intruders (Bosch et al., 2005). Various "social" effects of oxytocin in humans have also been reported, but mainly following the intranasal administration of doses of oxytocin so large that it is hard to be confident of where or how they are acting.

It is unclear to what extent these "behavioral" roles of oxytocin are attributable to the parvocellular oxytocin system or the magnocellular system, because many of the sites of action of oxytocin in this regard lack conspicuous innervation by oxytocin-containing fibers. Accordingly, it seems likely that oxytocin reaches these sites by volume transmission following release from possibly quite distant sites. Large amounts of oxytocin are released in some circumstances from the dendrites of magnocellular neurons (Ludwig and Leng, 2006), and interestingly, such dendritic released is regulated independently of axonal secretion – thus magnocellular neurons can release oxytocin either centrally or peripherally depending upon the stimulus (Sabatier et al., 2003).

OXYTOCIN AND FOOD INTAKE

In early studies of hypothalamic function, lesions of oxytocin-containing hypothalamic nuclei were shown to result in an increase in food intake and body weight (Leibowitz et al., 1981; Shor-Posner et al., 1985; Sims and Lorden, 1986; Kirchgessner et al., 1988). Then, in the 1990s, several studies reported anorexigenic effects of central oxytocin: low doses of oxytocin given icv dose-dependently inhibited food intake in rats, increased the latency to begin feeding and reduced meal duration in both hungry and satiated animals, and these actions could be blocked by oxytocin receptor antagonists (Arletti et al., 1990; Olson et al., 1991a). Longer term central infusions of oxytocin were also reported to reduce body weight gain in rats given a high-fat diet, but in contrast to oxytocin's acute effects, chronic oxytocin infusions did not alter total food intake or meal patterning, but instead appeared to stimulate lipid metabolism in adipose tissue (Deblon et al., 2011). It was noted that, in rats, dehydration or sodium loading potently increased oxytocin secretion and at the same time suppressed appetite (Flanagan et al., 1992a); given that (in rats) oxytocin promotes natriuresis (Verbalis et al., 1991), the suppression of appetite by oxytocin appeared to be part of a general homeostatic role in sodium balance. As oxytocin secretion is not stimulated by hyperosmolarity in humans (Williams et al., 1986) it seemed that this role of oxytocin might be one peculiar to rodents. However, recent findings in humans with rare genetic mutations linked to monogenic obesity indicate that oxytocin may also have a role in appetite regulation in humans.

Male (but not female) oxytocin receptor-deficient mice express an obese phenotype in later adulthood despite no difference in food intake or motor activity (Takayanagi et al., 2008). Male and female oxytocin-knockout mice show an elevation in body weight and fat stores in adulthood but as with oxytocin receptor-deficient mice this is not due to an increase in food intake (Nishimori et al., 1996). There have been no published reports of humans completely lacking either oxytocin or its receptor, probably because the absence of oxytocin or its receptor is incompatible with successful reproduction, but a partial deficiency in central oxytocin production has been associated with the development of obesity in humans in two documented conditions.

The transcription factor Single-minded 1 (Sim1) is one of the few genes associated with human monogenic obesity (Holder et al., 2000; Farooqi and O'Rahilly, 2005). In mice, Sim1 is expressed in the SON and PVN and is essential for the development of these nuclei (Michaud et al., 1998). Homozygous Sim1 knockout mice do not survive gestation; but heterozygous mice are viable and are hyperphagic and become obese early in life (Michaud et al., 2001). These mice have much-reduced levels of oxytocin mRNA and immunoreactive oxytocin in both the SON and PVN (Michaud et al., 2001), and their hyperphagia can be reversed by oxytocin given icv (Kublaoui et al., 2008). Conditional deletion of Sim1 after gestational development of the PVN also results in both a reduction in oxytocin mRNA expression, and in hyperphagia and obesity (Tolson et al., 2010). In contrast, mice overexpressing Sim1 do not increase their food intake when given a high-fat diet, and are resistant to diet-induced obesity (Kublaoui et al., 2006b).

Patients affected by Prader–Willi syndrome (PWS) caused by the lack of a segment in the paternal chromosome 15 suffer from morbid obesity due to extreme hyperphagia. The PVN of these patients contains fewer oxytocin neurons than controls (Swaab et al., 1995), leading to speculation that a deficiency in oxytocin may be instrumental in the development of obesity in this condition. Mice in which specific genes associated with the PWS syndrome have been knocked out similarly develop late-onset obesity due to hyperphagia, and this can be partly explained by a deficient production of oxytocin in the hypothalamus (Dombret et al., 2012) or by a reduction in the number of oxytocin neurons (Muscatelli et al., 2000).

WHERE DOES APPETITE-INHIBITORY OXYTOCIN COME FROM?

In the last 20 years it has become apparent that oxytocin neurons in both the SON and PVN are powerfully regulated by appetite-related signals (Renaud et al., 1987; Olson et al., 1991a,b). The role of central oxytocin in the regulation of energy homeostasis appears to involve both the magnocellular neurons and centrally projecting parvocellular neurons.

PARVOCELLULAR NEURONS OF THE PVN

The PVN has a major role in the regulation of appetite and metabolism, and is an important direct target of projections from the primary leptin- and ghrelin-receptive neurons of the arcuate nucleus – from orexigenic neurons that co-express neuropeptide Y (NPY) and agouti-related peptide (AgRP) and the inhibitory neurotransmitter GABA, and from pro-opiomelanocortin (POMC)-containing neurons, which express the potent satiety peptides α-melanocyte stimulating hormone (α-MSH) and cocaine-and amphetamine regulating transcript (CART) (Valassi et al., 2008). The PVN regulates metabolism via neuroendocrine neurons that release thyrotropin releasing hormone to regulate the thyroid gland (Alkemade, 2010; Nillni, 2010), it regulates glucocorticoid production via its regulation of pituitary adrenocorticotropin secretion (Herman et al., 2003), and it regulates the sympathetic nervous system via a large population of pre-autonomic neurons (Ferguson et al., 2008; Kc and Dick, 2010). However, the oxytocin neurons in the PVN, like those in the SON, are also conspicuous targets for α-MSH (Kim et al., 2000), and are particularly powerfully influenced by food intake and a variety of nutritionally related signals.

In rats, the expression of oxytocin mRNA in the PVN is markedly reduced by fasting; this reduction can be reversed by leptin administration (Kublaoui et al., 2008) and these effects apparently involve both magnocellular neurons and parvocellular neurons. Oxytocin neurons in the PVN are also contacted by fibers arising from the NPY/AgRP/GABA neurons of the arcuate nucleus. The PVN expresses abundant GABA receptors (Kalsbeek et al., 2004) and NPY Y1 receptors (Yokosuka et al., 1999). Optogenetic activation of the GABAergic axons in the PVN that arise from the arcuate nucleus increases food intake. Similarly, direct optogenetic activation of PVN oxytocin neurons increases c-Fos expression in these neurons and suppresses food intake. In the same study, a pharmacogenetic approach showed that while acute silencing of arcuate POMC neurons has surprisingly little effect, silencing Sim1-expressing PVN neurons markedly increases food intake (Atasoy et al., 2012).

Many parvocellular oxytocin neurons project to the nucleus tractus solitarii (NTS) in the caudal brainstem (Rinaman, 1998) where oxytocin modulates vagal efferent pathways that regulate gastric motility (McCann and Rogers, 1990). These neurons are critically involved in a reflex that is triggered by food intake, and mediated in part by gastric distension and in part by the secretion of CCK from the duodenum. Peripheral administration of CCK leads to activation of gastric vagal afferent neurons and thence to activation of brainstem structures, notably the NTS and ventrolateral medulla (Simpson et al., 2012). These in turn project to, and activate, centrally projecting oxytocin neurons of the PVN. As the CCK-stimulated NTS neurons are densely innervated by oxytocin-containing fibers from the PVN (Blevins et al., 2003), it appears that there is a recurrent circuit involving parvocellular oxytocin neurons that modulates the gastrointestinal vago-vagal reflex.

The gastrointestinal vago-vagal reflex involves main three-components: the gastrointestinal tract, the NTS, and the dorsal motor nucleus of the vagus (DMV). Visceral afferent fibers carrying digestion-related information ascend the vagus nerve and terminate in the medial NTS. NTS neurons integrate the information and send afferent projections to the DMV, and DMV neurons in turn project back down to the intrinsic ganglia in the gastrointestinal tract. In addition to this main loop, catecholaminergic and peptidergic neurons of the NTS also send ascending projections to structures in the forebrain including the PVN and the SON, and parvocellular PVN neurons project back to both the NTS and the DMN (Saper et al., 1976; Swanson and Kuypers, 1980). There is clear evidence that oxytocin acts in the DMN to inhibit gastric motility: the DMN contains oxytocin receptors (Dubois-Dauphin et al., 1992) and injection of oxytocin into the DMN decreases gastric motility, while oxytocin antagonists have the opposite effect (Rogers and Hermann, 1987). Electrical stimulation of the PVN inhibits gastric motility, and this effect can be attenuated by injection of an oxytocin antagonist in the DMN (Rogers and Hermann, 1987). Similar results were observed in conscious, freely moving animals, in which gastric motility was reduced by icv injection of oxytocin and by stimulation of the PVN, and in both cases the inhibition was prevented by icv injection of an oxytocin antagonist (Flanagan et al., 1992b). Finally, icv administration of an oxytocin antagonist alone increased baseline gastric motility, suggesting a tonic inhibitory effect of oxytocin on gastric motility. However, it seems unlikely that the inhibitory action of CCK on gastric motility is mediated by oxytocin, as icv injection of an oxytocin antagonist did not prevent CCK-induced inhibition of gastric motility (Flanagan et al., 1992b).

Thus there is a well-established role of parvocellular oxytocin neurons in the regulation of the gastrointestinal tract. Moreover, the magnocellular oxytocin neurons of the SON and PVN also appear to be involved in regulating appetite, possibly by the actions of dendritically released oxytocin on the ventromedial nucleus of the hypothalamus (VMN). This large nucleus is known to have an important role in both energy balance and sexual behavior, and is a site at which oxytocin receptors are expressed at an exceptionally high density (Tribollet et al., 1988) as well as insulin-regulated aminopeptidase (IRAP), an enzyme involved in the inactivation of oxytocin (Fernando et al., 2005).

MAGNOCELLULAR NEURONS OF THE SON AND PVN

As we discuss further below, there is powerful evidence that magnocellular oxytocin neurons have an important role in the regulation of appetite – but it is important to note that this role is not necessarily mediated by oxytocin alone. In magnocellular neurons of the SON and PVN, oxytocin is co-localized with a number of anorexigenic factors, including the neuropeptides CART (Vrang et al., 1999), pituitary adenylate cyclase activating polypeptide (PACAP) (Koves et al., 1994), corticotropin-releasing factor (CRF) (Sawchenko et al., 1984), CCK (Vanderhaeghen et al., 1981), and nesfatin-1 (Foo et al., 2008). Indeed, it has been suggested that oxytocin actually mediates the inhibitory action of nesfatin-1 on food intake, as nesfatin-1 induces the release of oxytocin in the PVN (Maejima et al., 2009) and as the anorexigenic effect of nesfatin-1 can be blocked by an oxytocin antagonist (Yosten and Samson, 2010). The fat mass and obesity-associated (FTO) gene that has been associated with obesity in humans is also co-localized with oxytocin in both the PVN and SON. This gene encodes a transcription co-factor (Fto) that is believed to regulate the expression of appetite-related genes (Jia et al., 2008), and Fto over-expression increases oxytocin mRNA levels in cell cultures (Olszewski et al., 2011).

Magnocellular oxytocin neurons are activated during feeding: thus, in schedule-fed rats trained to expect to receive food for just 2 h each day, magnocellular oxytocin neurons in both the SON and PVN densely express Fos protein soon after the initiation of food intake (Johnstone et al., 2006). These neurons are also activated by gastric distension, and by systemic application of the satiety peptides CCK (Renaud et al., 1987) and GLP-1 (Bojanowska and Stempniak, 2000). Moreover, the intestinal lipid amide oleoylethanolamide (OEA), which suppresses feeding via activation of the vagus nerve (Lo Verme et al., 2005), stimulates oxytocin mRNA expression in the PVN and SON, this anorexic effect is prevented by blockade of central oxytocin receptors (Gaetani et al., 2010).

The best understood pathway involving feeding-evoked activation of magnocellular oxytocin neurons is that where peripheral injections of CCK leads to secretion of oxytocin from the posterior pituitary gland in rats. In brief, CCK is released from the duodenum in response to food intake and peripheral administration of CCK can inhibit food intake via stimulation of vagal afferent neurons and activation of brainstem structures, notably the NTS and ventrolateral medulla. CCK given intraperitoneally or intravenously increases Fos expression in oxytocin neurons in the PVN and SON (Caquineau et al., 2010), increases the electrical activity of oxytocin neurons in the SON (Renaud et al., 1987; Leng et al., 1991) and increases plasma oxytocin secretion (Kutlu et al., 2010). These actions are mediated by a direct projection from noradrenergic neurons of the A2 cell group, which co-express the potent appetite-inhibiting peptide prolactin-releasing peptide (PrRP). The activation of oxytocin neurons can be blocked by selective lesioning of the noradrenergic afferents or by blocking the actions at the SON of noradrenaline itself or those of PrRP (Onaka et al., 2012). Interestingly, central pretreatment with an oxytocin receptor antagonist reduces the anorexigenic effect of CCK (Olson et al., 1991b; Blevins et al., 2003) suggesting that CCK-evoked satiety may be mediated in part by oxytocin.

INTERACTIONS BETWEEN MAGNOCELLULAR OXYTOCIN NEURONS AND THE MELANOCORTINS

Like parvocellular oxytocin neurons, magnocellular oxytocin neurons abundantly express leptin receptors and are a target for this important hormone (Hakansson et al., 1998; Yarnell et al., 1998; Brogan et al., 2000). Leptin activates Fos expression in the PVN (Yokosuka et al., 1998; Caquineau et al., 2010; Qi et al., 2010), particularly in parvocellular PVN neurons projecting to CCK-sensitive neurons in the NTS. In the SON, however, central administration of leptin does not induce Fos expression (Caquineau et al., 2010) or nuclear translocation of STAT3 (Hakansson and Meister, 1998), but it does increase nuclear STAT5 expression (Mutze et al., 2007).

In addition to this direct modulation by leptin, magnocellular oxytocin neurons are regulated indirectly via the effects of leptin on POMC neurons of the arcuate nucleus. Like the PVN, the SON receives a strong projection from POMC neurons. Oxytocin neurons in the SON, like those in the PVN, densely express α-MSH receptors (MC4) (Garza et al., 2008). α-MSH is a powerful anorexigenic peptide: centrally administered α-MSH reduces food intake and body weight, and mice lacking MC4 receptors are hyperphagic and obese (Adan et al., 2006). As mentioned above, magnocellular oxytocin neurons can secrete a large amount of peptide from their dendrites in response to certain stimuli, and notably they do so in response to α-MSH. In magnocellular oxytocin neurons of the SON, α-MSH acts at MC4 receptors to increase the intracellular calcium concentration; this increase directly evokes oxytocin release from the large dendrites of these neurons and also results in the production of endocannabinoids by the oxytocin neurons. Endocannabinoids produced in response to α-MSH act presynaptically to suppress glutamatergic afferent inputs to the oxytocin neurons. Thus, remarkably, the response of magnocellular oxytocin neurons to α-MSH is an increase in central release of oxytocin but a simultaneous suppression of electrical activity and hence a suppression of secretion into the systemic circulation (Sabatier and Leng, 2006).

Further evidence of an interaction between oxytocin and α-MSH is illustrated in the model of Sim1 heterozygous mice. In wild type mice, an agonist of α-MSH MC4 receptor (MC4R) reduced food intake, and induced Fos expression in PVN neurons, of which some co-express oxytocin and MC4R (Liu et al., 2003), and oxytocin and Sim1 (Kublaoui et al., 2008). However in Sim1 heterozygous mice, MC4R agonist had a much attenuated effect on both food intake and Fos expression in the PVN (Kublaoui et al., 2006a). This suggests that the α-MSH agonist actions on the PVN of Sim1$^{\pm}$ mice were impaired by the lack of oxytocin production in these mice (Michaud et al., 2001).

THE VENTROMEDIAL NUCLEUS OF THE HYPOTHALAMUS – A SITE OF ACTION OF OXYTOCIN

It seems possible that oxytocin released from the dendrites of magnocellular neurons is involved in the regulation of appetite, presumably reaching its targets by volume transmission. We have estimated that a release rate of just one vesicle per oxytocin cell every 10 s would be enough to achieve a mean basal concentration of ~260 pg/ml throughout the anterior hypothalamus within a minute (Leng and Ludwig, 2008). The half life of oxytocin in CSF is ~20 min – it is likely to be less than this in the extracellular fluid, but there are no clear data on this point. We have argued elsewhere that the effects of oxytocin depends less on its sites of release but rather on the location of its receptors (Sabatier et al., 2007). Thus it is likely that food intake is inhibited in various physiological conditions in which oxytocin is released from the dendrites of magnocellular neurons. Indeed, appetite is inhibited in rats subjected to dehydration or sodium loading (Flanagan et al., 1992a), two stimuli that result in a hyperosmolar environment, which is known to stimulate the dendritic release of oxytocin from supraoptic neurons (Neumann et al., 1993). The main physiological circumstances in which there is extensive central secretion of oxytocin is in lactation, when suckling-induced dendritic oxytocin release is an essential part of the milk-ejection reflex (Rossoni et al., 2008). Lactation is associated with a marked increase of food intake, rather than a reduction, but despite this, lactation is a time of negative energy balance, because the increased food intake does not adequately compensate for the energy demands of the suckling young. Accordingly, it seems that appetite during lactation is not increased to the degree needed to maintain energy homeostasis – and it may be that suppression of appetite during suckling is necessary to ensure that the mother nurses the young rather than searches for food.

One particularly intriguing potential target for dendritic oxytocin is the VMN. This large hypothalamic nucleus contains a very high density of oxytocin receptors, as shown by intense labeling both for oxytocin receptor binding sites (Tribollet et al., 1988) and oxytocin receptor mRNA expression (Yoshimura et al., 1993), particularly in the ventrolateral region. Oxytocin receptors in the VMN have an established role in sexual behavior in female rats (McCarthy et al., 1994), and we have previously suggested that they are involved in the reciprocal regulation of appetite and sexual behavior (Leng and Ludwig, 2008). Although the VMN has a high density of oxytocin receptors, it contains very few oxytocin fibers, and is therefore a likely target for oxytocin released from the dendrites of magnocellular oxytocin neurons (Leng and Ludwig, 2008).

The VMN is not a functionally homogeneous nucleus so it is not surprising that systemic injections of CCK have diverse effects on VMN neurons, but the most common effect of CCKon the electrical activity of VMN neurons is inhibitory (Sabatier and Leng, 2010); these responses varied particularly between different subpopulations of VMN that displayed contrasting electrophysiological features. To test whether the appetite-inhibiting effects of oxytocin and those of CCK converge at the level of the VMN, we have studied the effects of central icv injection of oxytocin on the electrical activity of VMN neurons *in vivo*, and compared these responses with those of the same neurons to CCK. As with CCK, the responses to oxytocin were diverse. About 30% of neurons responded to oxytocin, 78% with a significant increase in their mean firing rate (**Figure 1**), and again there were differences in the responses of electrophysiologically distinct subpopulations. However, when we compared the responses of the same neurons to CCK and oxytocin, we noted particularly that, while one subpopulation of neurons had clearly divergent responses to CCK and oxytocin, in all other subpopulations the responses were remarkably convergent – for most neuronal types in the VMN, the response to icv oxytocin was a very strong predictor of the response to systemic CCK (**Figure 2**), supporting the hypothesis that VMN neurons are part of a common pathway mediating satiety.

Finally, to test the feasibility of the hypothesis that oxytocin affects VMN neurons via dendritic release of oxytocin from magnocellular neurons, we studied the electrical activity of single VMN neurons while applying α-MSH directly to the ipsilateral SON by microdialysis to evoke dendritic oxytocin release. Like the effects of icv oxytocin, this too had long-lasting, mainly excitatory effects upon a subset of VMN neurons (**Figure 3**).

OXYTOCIN AND REWARD

In addition to the drive to eat for metabolizable energy and nutritional factors (homeostatic feeding), humans and many other animals attend selectively to palatable foods and are motivated to eat them for pleasure (hedonic feeding). In addition to its effects on homeostatic food intake, oxytocin may have a role in the modulation of hedonic food intake.

Activation of dopaminergic mesolimbic neurons of the ventral tegmental area (VTA) is currently thought to be closely associated with reward and motivation. During palatable food intake, dopamine is released in the VTA's target regions such as the nucleus accumbens (NAcc) and dopamine release in these structures can also be evoked by stimuli associated with or predictive of palatable food. It is likely that activation of this system equates with the motivation to attend to, pursue and consume rewarding stimuli like palatable food. Oxytocin-containing axons from the PVN contact mesolimbic neurons (Sofroniew, 1980; Succu

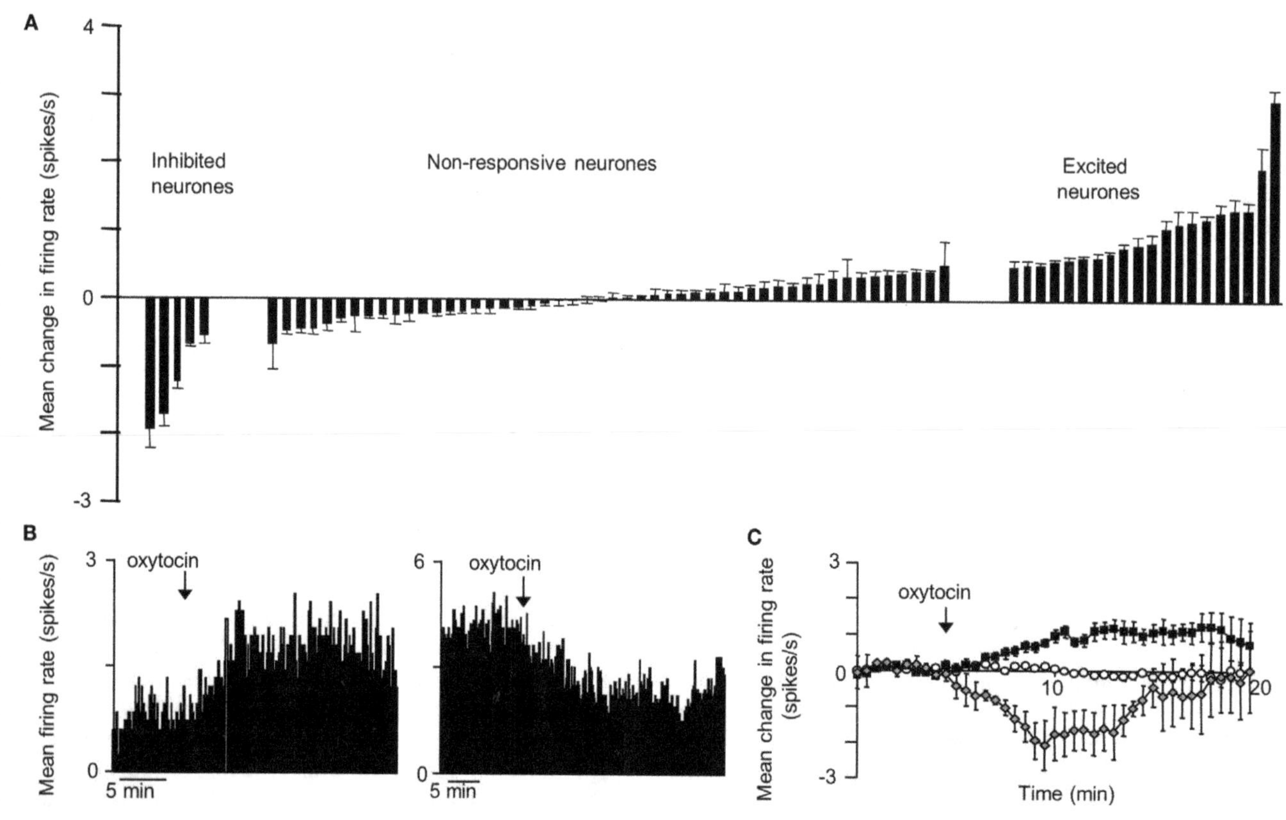

FIGURE 1 | Responses to icv oxytocin in VMN neurons *in vivo*. Single VMN neurons were recorded extracellularly from the VMN of urethane-anesthetized rats (Sabatier and Leng, 2008). **(A)** Each bar represent the mean change in firing rate (±SD) averaged over the first 10 min after icv injection of oxytocin (1–10 ng) in each VMN cell tested. The cells are ranked by response magnitude and are classed as inhibited, non-responsive, and excited according to whether the responses were significant or not. **(B)** Representative example of an inhibition (left panel) and activation (right panel) of the mean firing rate in response to icv oxytocin in a single VMN cell recorded extracellularly. **(C)** Mean change in firing rate (±SE) in the VMN cells that were significantly activated -■-; $n = 14$), significantly inhibited -◆-; $n = 4$), and not significantly affected -○-; $n = 43$) by icv oxytocin.

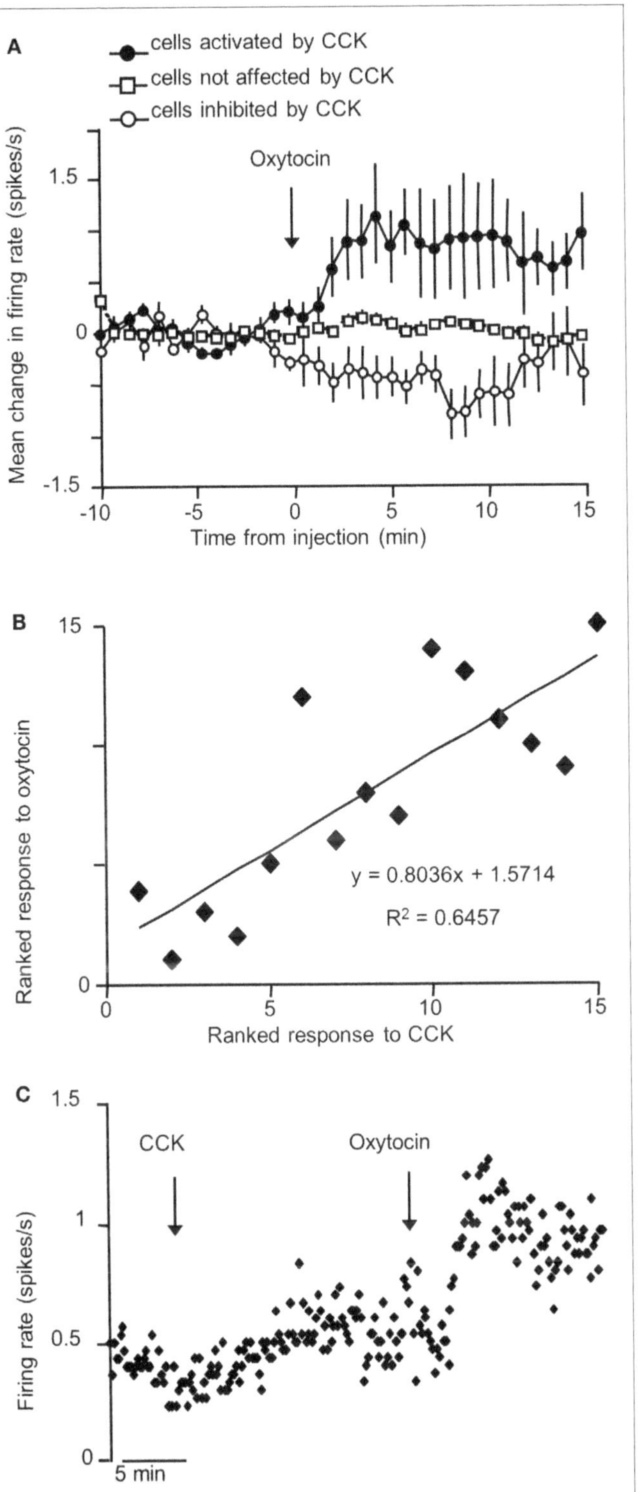

FIGURE 2 | Correlation of responses to icv oxytocin and iv CCK in VMN neurons *in vivo*. (A) Mean change in firing rate (±SE) in response to icv oxytocin (1–10 ng) in single VMN cells that were activated -●-; $n=5$), inhibited -□-; $n=4$), and not affected -○-; $n=6$) by iv CCK injection. **(B)** Rank correlation of responses to CCK and oxytocin (high ranks excited; low ranks inhibited). The solid line is the linear fit to the ranks ($r^2=0.65$). **(C)** Example of convergent responses to icv oxytocin (1–10 ng) and iv CCK (20 μg/kg) in a single VMN neuron.

et al., 2008) and likely have an inhibitory action as exogenous oxytocin activates NO synthase in mesolimbic dopaminergic neurons *in vivo* (Succu et al., 2008. Exogenous oxytocin also reduces amphetamine-evoked dopamine turnover in the NAcc (Qi et al., 2008) and inhibits the formation of a place-preference to methamphetamine when given into the NAcc core (Baracz et al., 2012). However, administration of oxytocin does not always lead to a reduction in dopamine release, administration into the ventral subiculum for example, a hippocampal region innervated by the PVN and potentially involved in restraining the stress response and reinstating non-food reward responding behavior, results in increased dopamine release in the NAcc (Melis et al., 2009). Inhibition of the PVN by optical stimulation of GABAergic fibers from arcuate NPY/AgRP/GABA neurons increases motivation to obtain sugar in a progressive ratio lever pressing task (Atasoy et al., 2012) suggesting that signals arising from the PVN may suppress the motivation for rewarding foods.

Consumption of readily catabolizable sugars seems to be innate in animals. Without training, rodents given a choice between water and sucrose will consume large volumes of a 10% sucrose solution [over 200 ml a day in adult male Sprague-Dawley rats (unpublished observations)] and voluntarily cease water drinking. Even transgenic mice lacking functional sweet taste receptors prefer sucrose over water (de Araujo et al., 2008) indicating that a post-ingestive reward is provided by sucrose. Transgenic mice lacking oxytocin show an enhanced preference for and consumption of sweet solutions over water in a two-bottle choice paradigm (Amico et al., 2005; Billings et al., 2006). The increase in intake is driven by a greater number of feeding bouts rather than by an increase in their duration (Sclafani et al., 2007). However, no such effect of oxytocin deficiency is seen on consumption of a palatable high-fat liquid formulation (Miedlar et al., 2007) or of a sucrose-containing solid food (Amico et al., 2005), though scheduled feeding of a high-sugar diet to rats increases oxytocin gene expression (Olszewski et al., 2009). Progressive ratio operant conditioning paradigms are often used as a measure of motivation to work for a reward. In contrast to an effect of oxytocin deficiency on freely available sweet solutions, there is less evidence that oxytocin-deficient mice have enhancements (or deficiencies) in motivation to work for food as they are not different to wild type mice in this task (Sclafani et al., 2007). In addition to Fos expression observed at the termination of bland food intake (Johnstone et al., 2006), Fos expression is also increased in PVN oxytocin neurons at the termination of a bout of feeding where only either sucrose or a high-fat food was available (Olszewski et al., 2010). In this study, hypothalamic oxytocin mRNA levels were higher in mice allowed access to a high-sugar diet compared to a high-fat diet despite both being palatable and readily consumed. Furthermore, oxytocin receptor antagonism led to an increase in sucrose consumption but has no effect on fat consumption when presented separately. Regular exposure in rats to a diet high in sugar reduces Fos expression in PVN and SON oxytocin neurons after a high- or low-sugar meal compared to animals regularly receiving a low-sugar diet (Mitra et al., 2010). This suggests that regular sugar consumption might blunt the activity of oxytocin neurons in response to any meal, whether high in sugar or not. Nonetheless, it may be that oxytocin has a satiating effect related to certain components of diet rather than a general effect.

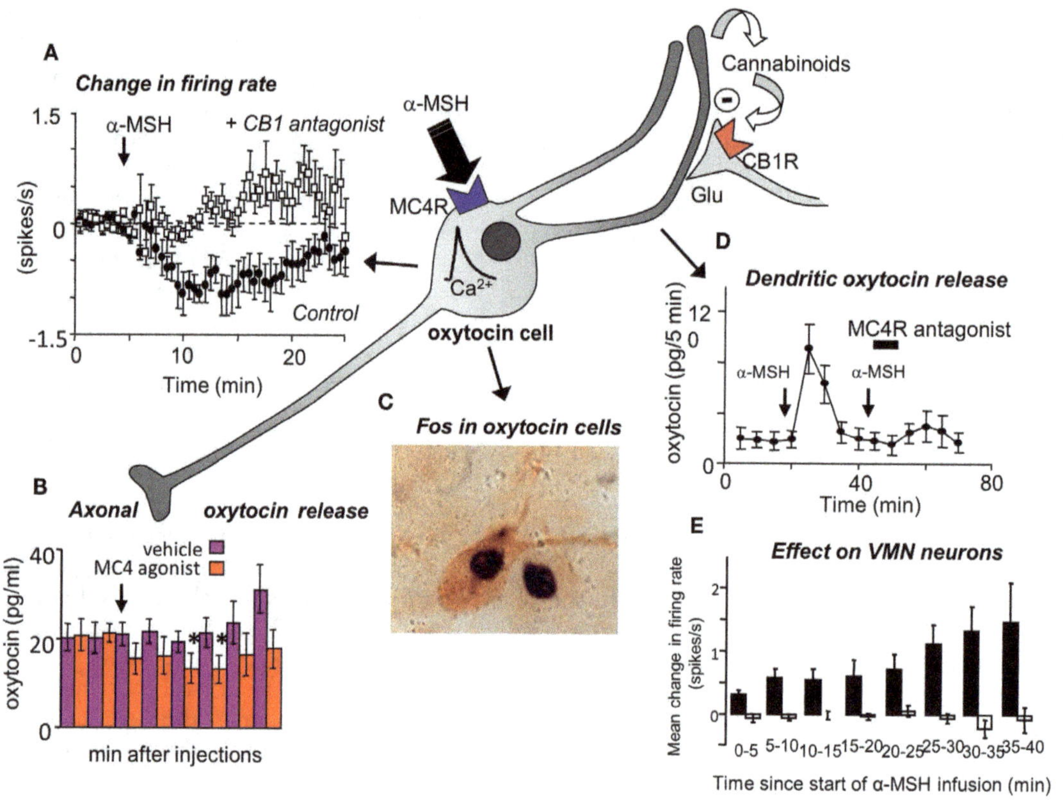

FIGURE 3 | (A) Magnocellular oxytocin neurons are inhibited by icv injections of α-MSH and this effect can be blocked by pre-administration of a CB1 cannabinoid antagonist (Sabatier et al., 2003). **(B)** Oxytocin secretion from the posterior pituitary gland is reduced by icv injection of MC4 agonists. **(C)** However, α-MSH and MC4 agonists induce Fos expression in magnocellular oxytocin neurons and **(D)** induce dendritic oxytocin release. **(E)** Application of α-MSH retrodialysis to the SON affects the electrical activity of VMN neurons *in vivo*. Mean change in firing rate (±SE) in VMN neurons that were not affected (open bars; $n = 13$), and activated (solid bars; $n = 8$; $P < 0.005$, 0–30 min vs. control) in the 30 min period from the start of α-MSH infusion (100 μM) on the SON.

Thus, the balance of evidence suggests that oxytocin might have a role in limiting the intake of palatable food by suppressing the activation of the reward pathway.

CONCLUSION

It now seems clear that oxytocin has a physiological role in energy balance through its actions in the caudal brainstem, but probably also through actions within the hypothalamus, including at the VMN, and possibly at other sites in the brain. While the actions in the brainstem appear to be part of a suite of autonomic regulatory functions exercised by parvocellular oxytocin neurons of the PVN, the hypothalamic actions appear to be more associated with motivational drive to eat, and are probably attributable to the magnocellular oxytocin system rather than the parvocellular system. It is possible that the inhibitory effects of oxytocin on appetite are closely linked to the stimulatory effects of oxytocin in sexual behavior and that this link reflects an evolutionarily conserved reciprocal regulation of these two key motivational drives (Caquineau et al., 2012). Whether it is possible to find a way of dissociating the appetite-inhibiting effects of oxytocin from the sexual arousal effects is unclear at present, but this may be the key to success in using the oxytocin system as a target for appetite-reducing drug therapies.

ACKNOWLEDGMENTS

Supported by the EU Seventh Framework program under grant agreements FP7-KBBE-2009-245009 (NeuroFAST) and FP7-KBBE-2010-266408 (Full4Health). This research was supported in part by a grant award to Dr. Nancy Sabatier from Medical Research Scotland (Grant award 316-FRG-L-0901).

REFERENCES

Adan, R. A., Tiesjema, B., Hillebrand, J. J., La Fleur, S. E., Kas, M. J., and de Krom, M. (2006). The MC4 receptor and control of appetite. *Br. J. Pharmacol.* 149, 815–827.

Alkemade, A. (2010). Central and peripheral effects of thyroid hormone signalling in the control of energy metabolism. *J. Neuroendocrinol.* 22, 56–63.

Amico, J. A., Vollmer, R. R., Cai, H. M., Miedlar, J. A., and Rinaman, L. (2005). Enhanced initial and sustained intake of sucrose solution in mice with an oxytocin gene deletion. *Am. J. Physiol. Regul. Integr. Comp. Physiol.* 289, R1798–R1806.

Archer, Z. A., and Mercer, J. G. (2007). Brain responses to obesogenic diets and diet-induced obesity. *Proc. Nutr. Soc.* 66, 124–130.

Arletti, R., Benelli, A., and Bertolini, A. (1990). Oxytocin inhibits food and fluid intake in rats. *Physiol. Behav.* 48, 825–830.

Atasoy, D., Betley, J. N., Su, H. H., and Sternson, S. M. (2012). Deconstruction of a neural circuit for hunger. *Nature* 488, 172–177.

Baracz, S. J., Rourke, P. I., Pardey, M. C., Hunt, G. E., McGregor, I. S., and Cornish, J. L. (2012). Oxytocin directly administered into the nucleus accumbens core or subthalamic nucleus attenuates methamphetamine-induced conditioned place preference. *Behav. Brain Res.* 228, 185–193.

Billings, L. B., Spero, J. A., Vollmer, R. R., and Amico, J. A. (2006). Oxytocin null mice ingest enhanced amounts of sweet solutions during light and dark cycles and during repeated shaker stress. *Behav. Brain Res.* 171, 134–141.

Blevins, J. E., Eakin, T. J., Murphy, J. A., Schwartz, M. W., and Baskin, D. G. (2003). Oxytocin innervation of caudal brainstem nuclei activated by cholecystokinin. *Brain Res.* 993, 30–41.

Bojanowska, E., and Stempniak, B. (2000). Effects of centrally or systemically injected glucagon-like peptide-1 (7-36) amide on release of neurohypophysial hormones and blood pressure in the rat. *Regul. Pept.* 91, 75–81.

Bosch, O. J., Meddle, S. L., Beiderbeck, D. I., Douglas, A. J., and Neumann, I. D. (2005). Brain oxytocin correlates with maternal aggression: link to anxiety. *J. Neurosci.* 25, 6807–6815.

Brogan, R. S., Grove, K. L., and Smith, M. S. (2000). Differential regulation of leptin receptor but not orexin in the hypothalamus of the lactating rat. *J. Neuroendocrinol.* 12, 1077–1086.

Caquineau, C., Douglas, A. J., and Leng, G. (2010). Effects of cholecystokinin in the supraoptic nucleus and paraventricular nucleus are negatively modulated by leptin in 24-h fasted lean male rats. *J. Neuroendocrinol.* 22, 446–452.

Caquineau, C., Leng, G., and Douglas, A. J. (2012). Sexual behaviour and neuronal activation in the vomeronasal pathway and hypothalamus of food-deprived male rats. *J. Neuroendocrinol.* 24, 712–723.

de Araujo, I. E., Oliveira-Maia, A. J., Sotnikova, T. D., Gainetdinov, R. R., Caron, M. G., Nicolelis, M. A., et al. (2008). Food reward in the absence of taste receptor signaling. *Neuron* 57, 930–941.

Deblon, N., Veyrat-Durebex, C., Bourgoin, L., Caillon, A., Bussier, A. L., Petrosino, S., et al. (2011). Mechanisms of the anti-obesity effects of oxytocin in diet-induced obese rats. *PLoS ONE* 6:e25565. doi:10.1371/journal.pone.0025565

Dombret, C., Nguyen, T., Schakman, O., Michaud, J. L., Hardin-Pouzet, H., Bertrand, M. J., et al. (2012). Loss of Maged1 results in obesity, deficits of social interactions, impaired sexual behavior and severe alteration of mature oxytocin production in the hypothalamus. *Hum. Mol. Genet.* 21, 4703–4717.

Dubois-Dauphin, M., Raggenbass, M., Widmer, H., Tribollet, E., and Dreifuss, J. J. (1992). Morphological and electrophysiological evidence for postsynaptic localization of functional oxytocin receptors in the rat dorsal motor nucleus of the vagus nerve. *Brain Res.* 575, 124–131.

Farooqi, I. S., and O'Rahilly, S. (2005). Monogenic obesity in humans. *Annu. Rev. Med.* 56, 443–458.

Ferguson, A. V., Latchford, K. J., and Samson, W. K. (2008). The paraventricular nucleus of the hypothalamus – a potential target for integrative treatment of autonomic dysfunction. *Expert Opin. Ther. Targets* 12, 717–727.

Fernando, R. N., Larm, J., Albiston, A. L., and Chai, S. Y. (2005). Distribution and cellular localization of insulin-regulated aminopeptidase in the rat central nervous system. *J. Comp. Neurol.* 487, 372–390.

Flanagan, L. M., Blackburn, R. E., Verbalis, J. G., and Stricker, E. M. (1992a). Hypertonic NaCl inhibits gastric motility and food intake in rats with lesions in the rostral AV3V region. *Am. J. Physiol.* 263, R9–R14.

Flanagan, L. M., Olson, B. R., Sved, A. F., Verbalis, J. G., and Stricker, E. M. (1992b). Gastric motility in conscious rats given oxytocin and an oxytocin antagonist centrally. *Brain Res.* 578, 256–260.

Foo, K. S., Brismar, H., and Broberger, C. (2008). Distribution and neuropeptide coexistence of nucleobindin-2 mRNA/nesfatin-like immunoreactivity in the rat CNS. *Neuroscience* 156, 563–579.

Gaetani, S., Fu, J., Cassano, T., Dipasquale, P., Romano, A., Righetti, L., et al. (2010). The fat-induced satiety factor oleoylethanolamide suppresses feeding through central release of oxytocin. *J. Neurosci.* 30, 8096–8101.

Garza, J. C., Kim, C. S., Liu, J., Zhang, W., and Lu, X. Y. (2008). Adeno-associated virus-mediated knockdown of melanocortin-4 receptor in the paraventricular nucleus of the hypothalamus promotes high-fat diet-induced hyperphagia and obesity. *J. Endocrinol.* 197, 471–482.

Hakansson, M. L., Brown, H., Ghilardi, N., Skoda, R. C., and Meister, B. (1998). Leptin receptor immunoreactivity in chemically defined target neurons of the hypothalamus. *J. Neurosci.* 18, 559–572.

Hakansson, M. L., and Meister, B. (1998). Transcription factor STAT3 in leptin target neurons of the rat hypothalamus. *Neuroendocrinology* 68, 420–427.

Herman, J. P., Figueiredo, H., Mueller, N. K., Ulrich-Lai, Y., Ostrander, M. M., Choi, D. C., et al. (2003). Central mechanisms of stress integration: hierarchical circuitry controlling hypothalamo-pituitary-adrenocortical responsiveness. *Front. Neuroendocrinol.* 24, 151–180.

Holder, J. L. Jr., Butte, N. F., and Zinn, A. R. (2000). Profound obesity associated with a balanced translocation that disrupts the SIM1 gene. *Hum. Mol. Genet.* 9, 101–108.

Huang, W., Lee, S. L., Arnason, S. S., and Sjoquist, M. (1996). Dehydration natriuresis in male rats is mediated by oxytocin. *Am. J. Physiol.* 270, R427–R433.

Jia, G., Yang, C. G., Yang, S., Jian, X., Yi, C., Zhou, Z., et al. (2008). Oxidative demethylation of 3-methylthymine and 3-methyluracil in single-stranded DNA and RNA by mouse and human FTO. *FEBS Lett.* 582, 3313–3319.

Johnstone, L. E., Fong, T. M., and Leng, G. (2006). Neuronal activation in the hypothalamus and brainstem during feeding in rats. *Cell Metab.* 4, 313–321.

Kalsbeek, A., La Fleur, S., Van Heijningen, C., and Buijs, R. M. (2004). Suprachiasmatic GABAergic inputs to the paraventricular nucleus control plasma glucose concentrations in the rat via sympathetic innervation of the liver. *J. Neurosci.* 24, 7604–7613.

Kc, P., and Dick, T. E. (2010). Modulation of cardiorespiratory function mediated by the paraventricular nucleus. *Respir. Physiol. Neurobiol.* 174, 55–64.

Kim, M. S., Rossi, M., Abusnana, S., Sunter, D., Morgan, D. G., Small, C. J., et al. (2000). Hypothalamic localization of the feeding effect of agouti-related peptide and alpha-melanocyte-stimulating hormone. *Diabetes* 49, 177–182.

Kirchgessner, A. L., Sclafani, A., and Nilaver, G. (1988). Histochemical identification of a PVN-hindbrain feeding pathway. *Physiol. Behav.* 42, 529–543.

Koves, K., Gorcs, T. J., Kausz, M., and Arimura, A. (1994). Present status of knowledge about the distribution and colocalization of PACAP in the forebrain. *Acta Biol. Hung.* 45, 297–321.

Kublaoui, B. M., Gemelli, T., Tolson, K. P., Wang, Y., and Zinn, A. R. (2008). Oxytocin deficiency mediates hyperphagic obesity of Sim1 haploinsufficient mice. *Mol. Endocrinol.* 22, 1723–1734.

Kublaoui, B. M., Holder, J. L. Jr., Gemelli, T., and Zinn, A. R. (2006a). Sim1 haploinsufficiency impairs melanocortin-mediated anorexia and activation of paraventricular nucleus neurons. *Mol. Endocrinol.* 20, 2483–2492.

Kublaoui, B. M., Holder, J. L. Jr., Tolson, K. P., Gemelli, T., and Zinn, A. R. (2006b). SIM1 overexpression partially rescues agouti yellow and diet-induced obesity by normalizing food intake. *Endocrinology* 147, 4542–4549.

Kutlu, S., Aydin, M., Alcin, E., Ozcan, M., Bakos, J., Jezova, D., et al. (2010). Leptin modulates noradrenaline release in the paraventricular nucleus and plasma oxytocin levels in female rats: a microdialysis study. *Brain Res.* 1317, 87–91.

Leibowitz, S. F., Hammer, N. J., and Chang, K. (1981). Hypothalamic paraventricular nucleus lesions produce overeating and obesity in the rat. *Physiol. Behav.* 27, 1031–1040.

Leng, G., and Ludwig, M. (2008). Neurotransmitters and peptides: whispered secrets and public announcements. *J. Physiol. (Lond.)* 586, 5625–5632.

Leng, G., Way, S., and Dyball, R. E. (1991). Identification of oxytoxin cells in the rat supraoptic nucleus by their response to cholecystokinin injection. *Neurosci. Lett.* 122, 159–162.

Liu, H., Kishi, T., Roseberry, A. G., Cai, X., Lee, C. E., Montez, J. M., et al. (2003). Transgenic mice expressing green fluorescent protein under the control of the melanocortin-4 receptor promoter. *J. Neurosci.* 23, 7143–7154.

Lo Verme, J., Gaetani, S., Fu, J., Oveisi, F., Burton, K., and Piomelli, D. (2005). Regulation of food intake by oleoylethanolamide. *Cell. Mol. Life Sci.* 62, 708–716.

Ludwig, M., and Leng, G. (2006). Dendritic peptide release and peptide-dependent behaviours. *Nat. Rev. Neurosci.* 7, 126–136.

Maejima, Y., Sedbazar, U., Suyama, S., Kohno, D., Onaka, T., Takano, E., et al. (2009). Nesfatin-1-regulated oxytocinergic signaling in the paraventricular nucleus causes anorexia through a leptin-independent melanocortin pathway. *Cell Metab.* 10, 355–365.

McCann, M. J., and Rogers, R. C. (1990). Oxytocin excites gastric-related neurones in rat dorsal vagal complex. *J. Physiol. (Lond.)* 428, 95–108.

McCann, S. M., Gutkowska, J., and Antunes-Rodrigues, J. (2003). Neuroendocrine control of body fluid homeostasis. *Braz. J. Med. Biol. Res.* 36, 165–181.

McCarthy, M. M., Kleopoulos, S. P., Mobbs, C. V., and Pfaff, D. W. (1994). Infusion of antisense oligodeoxynucleotides to the oxytocin receptor in the ventromedial hypothalamus reduces estrogen-induced sexual receptivity and oxytocin receptor binding in the female rat. *Neuroendocrinology* 59, 432–440.

Melis, M. R., Argiolas, A., and Gessa, G. L. (1986). Oxytocin-induced penile erection and yawning: site of action in the brain. *Brain Res.* 398, 259–265.

Melis, M. R., Succu, S., Sanna, F., Boi, A., and Argiolas, A. (2009). Oxytocin injected into the ventral subiculum or the posteromedial cortical nucleus of the amygdala induces penile erection and increases extracellular dopamine levels in the nucleus accumbens of male rats. *Eur. J. Neurosci.* 30, 1349–1357.

Michaud, J. L., Boucher, F., Melnyk, A., Gauthier, F., Goshu, E., Levy, E., et al. (2001). Sim1 haploinsufficiency causes hyperphagia, obesity and reduction of the paraventricular nucleus of the hypothalamus. *Hum. Mol. Genet.* 10, 1465–1473.

Michaud, J. L., Rosenquist, T., May, N. R., and Fan, C. M. (1998). Development of neuroendocrine lineages requires the bHLH-PAS transcription factor SIM1. *Genes Dev.* 12, 3264–3275.

Miedlar, J. A., Rinaman, L., Vollmer, R. R., and Amico, J. A. (2007). Oxytocin gene deletion mice overconsume palatable sucrose solution but not palatable lipid emulsions. *Am. J. Physiol. Regul. Integr. Comp. Physiol.* 293, R1063–R1068.

Mitra, A., Gosnell, B. A., Schioth, H. B., Grace, M. K., Klockars, A., Olszewski, P. K., et al. (2010). Chronic sugar intake dampens feeding-related activity of neurons synthesizing a satiety mediator, oxytocin. *Peptides* 31, 1346–1352.

Muscatelli, F., Abrous, D. N., Massacrier, A., Boccaccio, I., Le Moal, M., Cau, P., et al. (2000). Disruption of the mouse Necdin gene results in hypothalamic and behavioral alterations reminiscent of the human Prader-Willi syndrome. *Hum. Mol. Genet.* 9, 3101–3110.

Mutze, J., Roth, J., Gerstberger, R., and Hubschle, T. (2007). Nuclear translocation of the transcription factor STAT5 in the rat brain after systemic leptin administration. *Neurosci. Lett.* 417, 286–291.

Neumann, I. D. (2009). The advantage of social living: brain neuropeptides mediate the beneficial consequences of sex and motherhood. *Front. Neuroendocrinol.* 30, 483–496.

Neumann, I., Ludwig, M., Engelmann, M., Pittman, Q. J., and Landgraf, R. (1993). Simultaneous microdialysis in blood and brain: oxytocin and vasopressin release in response to central and peripheral osmotic stimulation and suckling in the rat. *Neuroendocrinology* 58, 637–645.

Nillni, E. A. (2010). Regulation of the hypothalamic thyrotropin releasing hormone (TRH) neuron by neuronal and peripheral inputs. *Front. Neuroendocrinol.* 31, 134–156.

Nishimori, K., Young, L. J., Guo, Q., Wang, Z., Insel, T. R., and Matzuk, M. M. (1996). Oxytocin is required for nursing but is not essential for parturition or reproductive behavior. *Proc. Natl. Acad. Sci. U.S.A.* 93, 11699–11704.

Olson, B. R., Drutarosky, M. D., Chow, M. S., Hruby, V. J., Stricker, E. M., and Verbalis, J. G. (1991a). Oxytocin and an oxytocin agonist administered centrally decrease food intake in rats. *Peptides* 12, 113–118.

Olson, B. R., Drutarosky, M. D., Stricker, E. M., and Verbalis, J. G. (1991b). Brain oxytocin receptor antagonism blunts the effects of anorexigenic treatments in rats: evidence for central oxytocin inhibition of food intake. *Endocrinology* 129, 785–791.

Olszewski, P. K., Fredriksson, R., Eriksson, J. D., Mitra, A., Radomska, K. J., Gosnell, B. A., et al. (2011). Fto colocalizes with a satiety mediator oxytocin in the brain and upregulates oxytocin gene expression. *Biochem. Biophys. Res. Commun.* 408, 422–426.

Olszewski, P. K., Klockars, A., Olszewska, A. M., Fredriksson, R., Schioth, H. B., and Levine, A. S. (2010). Molecular, immunohistochemical, and pharmacological evidence of oxytocin's role as inhibitor of carbohydrate but not fat intake. *Endocrinology* 151, 4736–4744.

Olszewski, P. K., Shaw, T. J., Grace, M. K., Hoglund, C. E., Fredriksson, R., Schioth, H. B., et al. (2009). Complexity of neural mechanisms underlying overconsumption of sugar in scheduled feeding: involvement of opioids, orexin, oxytocin and NPY. *Peptides* 30, 226–233.

Onaka, T., Takayanagi, Y., and Yoshida, M. (2012). Roles of oxytocin neurones in the control of stress, energy metabolism, and social behaviour. *J. Neuroendocrinol.* 24, 587–598.

Qi, J., Yang, J. Y., Song, M., Li, Y., Wang, F., and Wu, C. F. (2008). Inhibition by oxytocin of methamphetamine-induced hyperactivity related to dopamine turnover in the mesolimbic region in mice. *Naunyn Schmiedebergs Arch. Pharmacol.* 376, 441–448.

Qi, Y., Henry, B. A., Oldfield, B. J., and Clarke, I. J. (2010). The action of leptin on appetite-regulating cells in the ovine hypothalamus: demonstration of direct action in the absence of the arcuate nucleus. *Endocrinology* 151, 2106–2116.

Renaud, L. P., Tang, M., McCann, M. J., Stricker, E. M., and Verbalis, J. G. (1987). Cholecystokinin and gastric distension activate oxytocinergic cells in rat hypothalamus. *Am. J. Physiol.* 253, R661–R665.

Rinaman, L. (1998). Oxytocinergic inputs to the nucleus of the solitary tract and dorsal motor nucleus of the vagus in neonatal rats. *J. Comp. Neurol.* 399, 101–109.

Rogers, R. C., and Hermann, G. E. (1987). Oxytocin, oxytocin antagonist, TRH, and hypothalamic paraventricular nucleus stimulation effects on gastric motility. *Peptides* 8, 505–513.

Rossoni, E., Feng, J., Tirozzi, B., Brown, D., Leng, G., and Moos, F. (2008). Emergent synchronous bursting of oxytocin neuronal network. *PLoS Comput. Biol.* 4:e1000123. doi:10.1371/journal.pcbi.1000123.

Sabatier, N., Caquineau, C., Dayanithi, G., Bull, P., Douglas, A. J., Guan, X. M., et al. (2003). Alpha-melanocyte-stimulating hormone stimulates oxytocin release from the dendrites of hypothalamic neurons while inhibiting oxytocin release from their terminals in the neurohypophysis. *J. Neurosci.* 23, 10351–10358.

Sabatier, N., and Leng, G. (2006). Presynaptic actions of endocannabinoids mediate alpha-MSH-induced inhibition of oxytocin cells. *Am. J. Physiol. Regul. Integr. Comp. Physiol.* 290, R577–R584.

Sabatier, N., and Leng, G. (2008). Spontaneous discharge characteristic of neurons in the ventromedial nucleus of the rat hypothalamus in vivo. *Eur. J. Neurosci.* 28, 693–706.

Sabatier, N., and Leng, G. (2010). Responses to cholecystokinin in the ventromedial nucleus of the rat hypothalamus in vivo. *Eur. J. Neurosci.* 31, 1127–1135.

Sabatier, N., Rowe, I., and Leng, G. (2007). Central release of oxytocin and the ventromedial hypothalamus. *Biochem. Soc. Trans.* 35, 1247–1251.

Saper, C. B., Loewy, A. D., Swanson, L. W., and Cowan, W. M. (1976). Direct hypothalamo-autonomic connections. *Brain Res.* 117, 305–312.

Sawchenko, P. E., Swanson, L. W., and Vale, W. W. (1984). Corticotropin-releasing factor: co-expression within distinct subsets of oxytocin-, vasopressin-, and neurotensin-immunoreactive neurons in the hypothalamus of the male rat. *J. Neurosci.* 4, 1118–1129.

Sclafani, A., Rinaman, L., Vollmer, R. R., and Amico, J. A. (2007). Oxytocin knockout mice demonstrate enhanced intake of sweet and nonsweet carbohydrate solutions. *Am. J. Physiol. Regul. Integr. Comp. Physiol.* 292, R1828–R1833.

Shor-Posner, G., Azar, A. P., Insinga, S., and Leibowitz, S. F. (1985). Deficits in the control of food intake after hypothalamic paraventricular nucleus lesions. *Physiol. Behav.* 35, 883–890.

Simpson, K., Parker, J., Plumer, J., and Bloom, S. (2012). CCK, PYY and PP: the control of energy balance. *Handb. Exp. Pharmacol.* 209, 209–230.

Sims, J. S., and Lorden, J. F. (1986). Effect of paraventricular nucleus lesions on body weight, food intake and insulin levels. *Behav. Brain Res.* 22, 265–281.

Sofroniew, M. V. (1980). Projections from vasopressin, oxytocin, and neurophysin neurons to neural targets in the rat and human. *J. Histochem. Cytochem.* 28, 475–478.

Strader, A. D., and Woods, S. C. (2005). Gastrointestinal hormones and food intake. *Gastroenterology* 128, 175–191.

Succu, S., Sanna, F., Cocco, C., Melis, T., Boi, A., Ferri, G. L., et al. (2008). Oxytocin induces penile erection when injected into the ventral tegmental area of male rats: role of nitric oxide and cyclic GMP. *Eur. J. Neurosci.* 28, 813–821.

Swaab, D. F., Purba, J. S., and Hofman, M. A. (1995). Alterations in the hypothalamic paraventricular nucleus and its oxytocin neurons (putative satiety cells) in Prader-Willi syndrome: a study of five cases. *J. Clin. Endocrinol. Metab.* 80, 573–579.

Swanson, L. W., and Kuypers, H. G. (1980). The paraventricular nucleus of the hypothalamus: cytoarchitectonic subdivisions and organization of projections to the pituitary, dorsal vagal complex, and spinal cord as demonstrated by retrograde fluorescence double-labeling methods. *J. Comp. Neurol.* 194, 555–570.

Takayanagi, Y., Kasahara, Y., Onaka, T., Takahashi, N., Kawada, T., and Nishimori, K. (2008). Oxytocin receptor-deficient mice developed late-onset obesity. *Neuroreport* 19, 951–955.

Tolson, K. P., Gemelli, T., Gautron, L., Elmquist, J. K., Zinn, A. R., and Kublaoui, B. M. (2010). Postnatal Sim1 deficiency causes hyperphagic obesity and reduced Mc4r and oxytocin expression. *J. Neurosci.* 30, 3803–3812.

Tribollet, E., Barberis, C., Jard, S., Dubois-Dauphin, M., and Dreifuss, J. J. (1988). Localization and pharmacological characterization of high affinity binding sites for vasopressin and oxytocin in the rat brain by light microscopic autoradiography. *Brain Res.* 442, 105–118.

Valassi, E., Scacchi, M., and Cavagnini, F. (2008). Neuroendocrine control of food intake. *Nutr. Metab. Cardiovasc. Dis.* 18, 158–168.

Vanderhaeghen, J. J., Lotstra, F., Vandesande, F., and Dierickx, K. (1981). Coexistence of cholecystokinin and oxytocin-neurophysin in some magnocellular hypothalamo-hypophyseal neurons. *Cell Tissue Res.* 221, 227–231.

Verbalis, J. G., Mangione, M. P., and Stricker, E. M. (1991). Oxytocin produces natriuresis in rats at physiological plasma concentrations. *Endocrinology* 128, 1317–1322.

Verbalis, J. G., McCann, M. J., Mchale, C. M., and Stricker, E. M. (1986). Oxytocin secretion in response to cholecystokinin and food: differentiation of nausea from satiety. *Science* 232, 1417–1419.

Vrang, N., Larsen, P. J., Clausen, J. T., and Kristensen, P. (1999). Neurochemical characterization of hypothalamic cocaine- and amphetamine-regulated transcript neurons. *J. Neurosci.* 19, RC5.

Williams, T. D., Abel, D. C., King, C. M., Jelley, R. Y., and Lightman, S. L. (1986). Vasopressin and oxytocin responses to acute and chronic osmotic stimuli in man. *J. Endocrinol.* 108, 163–168.

Yarnell, D. O., Knight, D. S., Hamilton, K., Tulp, O., and Tso, P. (1998). Localization of leptin receptor immunoreactivity in the lean and obese Zucker rat brain. *Brain Res.* 785, 80–90.

Yokosuka, M., Kalra, P. S., and Kalra, S. P. (1999). Inhibition of neuropeptide Y (NPY)-induced feeding and c-Fos response in magnocellular paraventricular nucleus by a NPY receptor antagonist: a site of NPY action. *Endocrinology* 140, 4494–4500.

Yokosuka, M., Xu, B., Pu, S., Kalra, P. S., and Kalra, S. P. (1998). Neural substrates for leptin and neuropeptide Y (NPY) interaction: hypothalamic sites associated with inhibition of NPY-induced food intake. *Physiol. Behav.* 64, 331–338.

Yoshimura, R., Kiyama, H., Kimura, T., Araki, T., Maeno, H., Tanizawa, O., et al. (1993). Localization of oxytocin receptor messenger ribonucleic acid in the rat brain. *Endocrinology* 133, 1239–1246.

Yosten, G. L., and Samson, W. K. (2010). The anorexigenic and hypertensive effects of nesfatin-1 are reversed by pretreatment with an oxytocin receptor antagonist. *Am. J. Physiol. Regul. Integr. Comp. Physiol.* 298, R1642–R1647.

9

Arcuate AgRP neurons and the regulation of energy balance

Céline Cansell[1†], Raphaël G. P. Denis[1†], Aurélie Joly-Amado[1†], Julien Castel[1,2] and Serge Luquet[1,2]*

[1] Unité de Biologie Fonctionnelle et Adaptative, CNRS-EAC 4413, Sorbonne Paris Cité, Université Paris Diderot-Paris 7, Paris, France
[2] Centre National de la Recherche Scientifique EAC 4413, Paris, France

Edited by:
Hubert Vaudry, University of Rouen, France

Reviewed by:
Chris Scott, Charles Sturt University, Australia
Virginie Tolle, Institut National de la Santé et de la Recherche Médicale, France

***Correspondence:**
Serge Luquet, Unité de Biologie Fonctionnelle et Adaptative, CNRS-EAC 4413, Sorbonne Paris Cité, Université Paris Diderot-Paris 7, 4 rue Marie-Andrée Lagroua Weill-Hallé, Bâtiment Buffon, Case courrier 7126, 75205 Paris Cedex 13, France.
e-mail: serge.luquet@univ-paris-diderot.fr

† Céline Cansell, Raphaël G. P. Denis, and Aurélie Joly-Amado have contributed equally to this work.

The arcuate nucleus of the hypothalamus contains at least two populations of neurons that continuously monitor signals reflecting energy status and promote the appropriate behavioral and metabolic responses to changes in energy demand. Activation of neurons making pro-opiomelanocortin (POMC) decreases food intake and increases energy expenditure through activation of G protein-coupled melanocortin receptors via the release of α-melanocyte-stimulating hormone. Until recently, the prevailing idea was that the neighboring neurons [agouti-related protein (AgRP) neurons] co-expressing the orexigenic neuropeptides, AgRP, and neuropeptide Y increase feeding by opposing the anorexigenic actions of the POMC neurons. However, it has now been demonstrated that only AgRP neurons activation – not POMC neurons inhibition – is necessary and sufficient to promote feeding. Projections of AgRP-expressing axons innervate mesolimbic, midbrain, and pontine structures where they regulate feeding and feeding-independent functions such as reward or peripheral nutrient partitioning. AgRP neurons also make gamma aminobutyric acid , which is now thought to mediate many of critical functions of these neurons in a melanocortin-independent manner and on a timescale compatible with neuromodulation.

Keywords: neuropeptide Y, agouti-related protein, GABA, feeding behavior, metabolism, obesity, reward, dopamine

During the last several decade, the world has witnessed a pandemic expansion of pathologies related to high-fat and high-carbohydrate diets including obesity, diabetes, dyslipidemia, and cardiovascular diseases – collectively referred to as metabolic syndrome. Obesity is now considered by the World Health Organization (WHO) to be a worldwide epidemic, having more than doubled since 1980. In 2008, there were 1.5 billion overweight adults in both developed and developing countries (http://www.who.int/mediacentre/factsheets/fs311/en/). The WHO believes the fundamental cause of obesity and being overweight is an energy imbalance between calories consumed and calories expended. Appropriate energy balance is reached when energy intake and energy expenditure are adapted to meet energy demands and nutrient availability. It took billions of years for mammalian species to shape a highly responsive homeostatic system in which the multiple aspects of energy expenditure are exquisitely balanced with both hunger and the motivational component of feeding to ensure energy homeostasis. Disruption of this regulation gives rise to life-threatening conditions that include anorexia nervosa at one extreme and metabolic syndrome at the other.

During the last decade, a significant effort has been focused on the identification of neuronal pathways that control food intake and energy expenditure. This review focuses primarily on a tiny neuronal population of about ~1000 cells located in arcuate nucleus (ARC) of the hypothalamus, namely the neurons that produce agouti-related protein (AgRP), neuropeptide Y (NPY), and gamma aminobutyric acid (GABA; referred to here as AgRP neurons), and the recent conceptual advances that have been made studying their function in energy balance.

AgRP AND POMC NEURONS: TWO INTERMINGLED NEURONAL POPULATIONS DEFINING THE MELANOCORTIN SYSTEM

Agouti-related protein was discovered as an endogenously released neuropeptide that acts as an inverse agonist for the melanocortin receptors, MC3R/MC4R (Fan et al., 1997; Haskell-Luevano et al., 1999; Haskell-Luevano and Monck, 2001; Nijenhuis et al., 2001; Flier, 2006; Tolle and Low, 2008). Shortly after its discovery, Hahn et al. (1998) discovered that AgRP is co-expressed in hunger-activated neurons with NPY, another peptide that stimulates food intake and regulates weight gain (Tatemoto et al., 1982; Clark et al., 1984). The inhibitory nature of the NPY/AgRP neurons was further substantiated through the identification of GABA as their ionotropic neurotransmitter (Horvath et al., 1997). These neurons are now commonly referred to as AgRP neurons because, unlike NPY and GABA which are widely expressed in the nervous system, AgRP is uniquely produced by these neurons. It is a unique molecular signature that has been extensively exploited for the selective manipulation of these neurons. AgRP neurons are located in the ARC subdivision of the hypothalamus at the bottom of the third ventricle close to a circumventricular organ called median eminence (ME). The blood–brain barrier in this region is fenestrated and allows for facilitated blood–brain exchange. As a result, neurons that reside there are referred to as "first order neurons" because they would be the first to respond to the circulating signals of hunger and satiety.

Neurons in the ARC that make pro-opiomelanocortin (POMC) and cocaine- and amphetamine-related transcript (CART) secrete the melanocortin peptides adrenocorticotropic hormone (ACTH) and α, β, and γ-melanocyte-stimulating hormone (MSH), which are derived from post-translational processing of POMC. POMC and AgRP neurons are considered to be two functionally opposed components of the "central melanocortin system," a term that refers to as a set of hormonal, neuropeptidergic, and paracrine signaling pathways that are defined by components that include the five G protein-coupled melanocortin receptors (MCR1 to MCR5; Cone, 2005). These receptors are distributed throughout the body (Mountjoy and Wong, 1997; Liu et al., 2003). In the CNS, MC4R is broadly expressed while MC3R is mainly restricted to POMC and AgRP neurons (Jegou et al., 2000). The integral role of the melanocortin system in body weight homeostasis is supported by the fact that any mutation in the melanocortin signaling pathway including MC3R- or MC4R-null mutants (Huszar et al., 1997) and ectopic expression of MCR3/4 antagonist, agouti, in agouti lethal yellow (A^y) mutant mice (Miltenberger et al., 1997), results in hyperphagia, hypometabolism, hyperinsulinemia, and hyperglycemia in both rodents and humans (Hinney et al., 1999; Krude et al., 1999). The antagonistic relationship between POMC and AgRP neurons results from a tonic GABAergic inhibition from AgRP neurons onto POMC neurons (Horvath et al., 1992; Broberger and Hokfelt, 2001; Cowley et al., 2001; Williams et al., 2001; Pinto et al., 2004) and the interaction of NPY released by AgRP neurons with the NPY-Y1 receptor expressed on POMC neurons. The two populations project to several nuclei within the hypothalamus, including the paraventricular (PVN), ventromedial, dorsomedial, and lateral hypothalamus, and to the nucleus of tractus solitarii (NTS), the parabrachial nucleus (PBN) and the amygdala and the bed of the stria terminalis (BNST) which lie outside the hypothalamus (Broberger et al., 1998; **Figure 1**). In these regions AgRP- and NPY-containing fibers are found in close apposition to α-MSH-containing fibers and synapse onto second-order targets (Broberger et al., 1998). The release of α-MSH by POMC neurons and its binding to G-coupled MCR's initiates the central anorexic signaling pathway that results in decreased food intake and increased energy expenditure while AgRP exerts its orexigenic action partly by blocking the binding of α-MSH to its receptor there by preventing the α-MSH-induced anorexic pathway (Michaud et al., 1994; Ollmann et al., 1997; Shutter et al., 1997; Haskell-Luevano et al., 1999; Haskell-Luevano and Monck, 2001; Nijenhuis et al., 2001; Tolle and Low, 2008).

Thyroid-releasing hormone (TRH)-, oxytocin (OT)-, and corticotropin-releasing hormone (CRH)-expressing neurons located in the PVN all express MC4R (Lu et al., 2003). The binding of α-MSH to MC4R on these neurons has a positive action onto the hypothalamic–pituitary–thyroid (HPT) axis and the hypothalamic–corticotropic axis (HPA). During fasting, increased release of AgRP by AgRP neurons has been demonstrated to be a key mechanism for fasting-induced down regulation of the HPT axis and the consequent adaptation during negative energy balance (Fekete et al., 2000; Lechan and Fekete, 2006).

These observations promoted a dominant conceptual framework that, until recently envisioned the orexigenic and anabolic action of AgRP neurons as the result of POMC neuron antagonism (Palmiter, 2012).

However, there are several lines of evidence supporting a melanocortin-independent pathway for AgRP. For exemple, short- and long-term hyperphagic actions of AgRP are still observed in MC4R KO mice and some AgRP fibers—but not α-MSH fibers—have been found in close apposition to TRH-synthesizing neurons expressing MC4R (Fekete et al., 2000). Moreover, it has been shown that AgRP can act by a melanocortin-independent pathway that regulates glutamatergic neurons in the ventromedial hypothalamus (Fu and van den Pol, 2008). These data were first to suggest that AgRP, can exert an action as an agonist on unidentified receptors that are independent from the melanocortin signaling pathway.

Recent studies expand further the role of AgRP neurons to include melanocortin-independent mechanisms and non-feeding-related functions such as goal-directed behavior and peripheral nutrient partitioning.

AgRP NEURONS ARE NECESSARY AND SUFFICIENT TO INITIATE THE FULL FEEDING SEQUENCE

In 2005, several laboratories reported the selective ablation of AgRP neurons. Although the methods and the results differed somewhat, there was agreement that acute depletion of AgRP neurons in the adult mouse leads to life-threatening anorexia (Bewick et al., 2005; Gropp et al., 2005; Luquet et al., 2005; Xu et al., 2005). These experiments demonstrated that ablation of AgRP neurons in adult mice inhibits feeding and can lead to starvation. Ablation of AgRP neurons still caused severe anorexia when performed in the genetic context of A^y mice (Wu et al., 2008a), a model in which the melanocortin signaling pathway is already tonically inhibited by the ectopic expression of the melanocortin receptor antagonist, agouti (Miltenberger et al., 1997). These data indicated that the anorexia is not the direct consequence of unopposed melanocortin tone. Wu et al. (2008a) went on to show that acute loss of GABA signaling by AgRP neurons was responsible. Although ablation of AgRP neurons in adult mice leads to starvation, mice can adapt to the loss of AgRP neurons and continue to eat adequately. This was first shown by performing the ablation in neonatal mice, before AgRP neurons are mature (Luquet et al., 2005), but it was subsequently shown that this phenomenon can also occur in adult mice (Wu et al., 2009, 2012a,b).

Direct activation of AgRP neurons *in vivo* has been achieved through either forced expression of designer receptors exclusively activated by designer drugs (DREADD) or photoactivated channel rhodopsin allowing for chemical- or light-mediated activation of neurons (Hegemann and Moglich, 2011; Krashes et al., 2011). Using optogenetic techniques, Aponte et al. (2011) found that photoactivation of AgRP neurons promoted feeding in both wild-type and A^y mice. In a subsequent study, the Sternson group showed that photoactivation of feeding is mediated in part by activation of OT-expressing neurons in the PVN (Atasoy et al., 2012). They also confirmed that inhibition of POMC neurons is neither necessary nor sufficient to trigger feeding since co-stimulation of both POMC and AgRP neurons resulted in rapid feeding response.

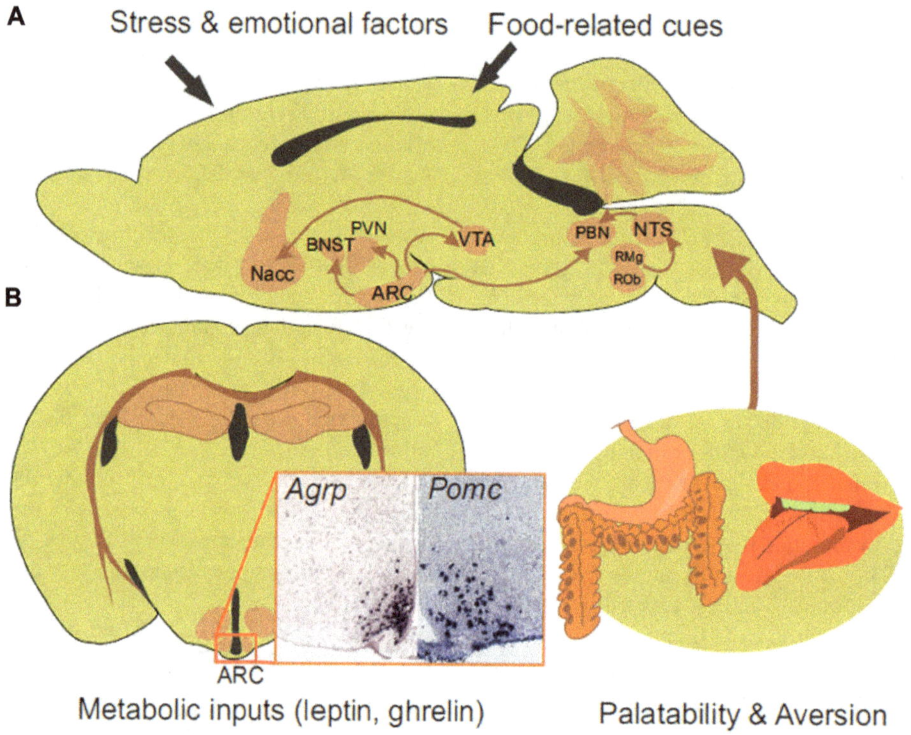

FIGURE 1 | Sagittal (A) and coronal section (B) of a mouse brain showing *in situ* hybridization for mRNA encoding *Agrp* or *Pomc* and the connections recently described for AgRP neurons. Arcuate neurons project to the PVN, BNST, PBN, and VTA of the midbrain. The dopaminergic neurons of the VTA project to the nucleus accumbens (Nacc) to process the reward and motivational aspect of feeding. Gut-initiated viscerosensitive information and taste-related cues are routed to the NTS. The NTS targets the PBN and also receives serotoninergic input from the raphe obscurus (ROb) and the raphe magnus (RMg) and exerts an anorectic action through the glutamatergic excitation of the PBN. AgRP neurons integrate metabolic input of hunger and have direct connections to brain regions processing reward and motivation together with food-related cues such as palatability and aversive aspect. *In situ* hybridization picture were downloaded from the Allen Mouse Brain Atlas [http://mouse.brain-map.org/Seattle (WA): Allen Institute for Brain Science (Lein et al., 2007). © 2009].

These results provide an entirely new perspective to the field by showing that extinction of α-MSH signaling cascade was not mandatory for AgRP neurons to initiate feeding.

PROCESSING OF TASTE AND VISCEROSENSORY INPUTS IN THE HYPOTHALAMUS–PONS–MEDULLA AXIS

By using Fos immunostaining to reveal neuron activation, Wu et al. (2008b) found that acute ablation of AgRP neurons in the PBN induces hyperactivity in all known targets of axonal projections from AgRP neurons. Moreover, they showed that GABA replacement in the PBN prevented anorexia and body weight loss after AgRP neuron ablation. This study demonstrated that GABA made by AgRP neurons was critically required to mediate their action in a melanocortin-independent manner (Wu et al., 2009; Wu and Palmiter, 2011) and put a new light on the PBN, a pontine structure that links gustatory sensory circuits to the brain center that processes the reward and motivational aspects of feeding (de Araujo, 2009; Suwabe and Bradley, 2009; Tokita et al., 2009; Oliveira-Maia et al., 2011). Gut-initiated viscerosensitive satiety or aversive signals together with food-related cues gathered by sensory neurons innervating the oral cavity are routed to the NTS primarily by the afferent portion of the vagus nerve (Schwartz et al., 1991, 1993; Moran et al., 2001; Schwartz and Moran, 2002). In the rodent, the PBN is a second-order target for NTS taste-related information. It serves as a relay structure for the encoding of the reward and motivational components of food-associated cues through the activation of the mesolimbic dopaminergic system (de Araujo, 2009; Suwabe and Bradley, 2009; Tokita et al., 2009; Oliveira-Maia et al., 2011). Looking for the source of excitatory inputs into the PBN that mediate its hyperactivity once the GABAergic tone from AgRP neurons is removed, Wu et al. (2012a) demonstrated that input to the PBN is glutamatergic and that it arises from a subpopulation of viscerosensitive NTS neurons. They also showed that the latter received tonic activation from serotoninergic neurons of the raphe obscurus and the raphe magnus (**Figures 1 and 2**).

The rostral NTS is also a target of descending projections from cognitive and emotional processing centers such as the insular and prefrontal cortex, the central nucleus of the amygdala, the lateral hypothalamus, and the BNST. The study from Wu et al. (2012a) provides an additional dimension to the hypothalamus–pons–medulla axis connection by suggesting a direct role for AgRP neurons in the ability of the medulla to relay rewarding and aversive information and integrate cognitive and emotional feedback from limbic structures (**Figure 1**). This Arc–pons–medulla axis could be instrumental in the gain of body weight that is often

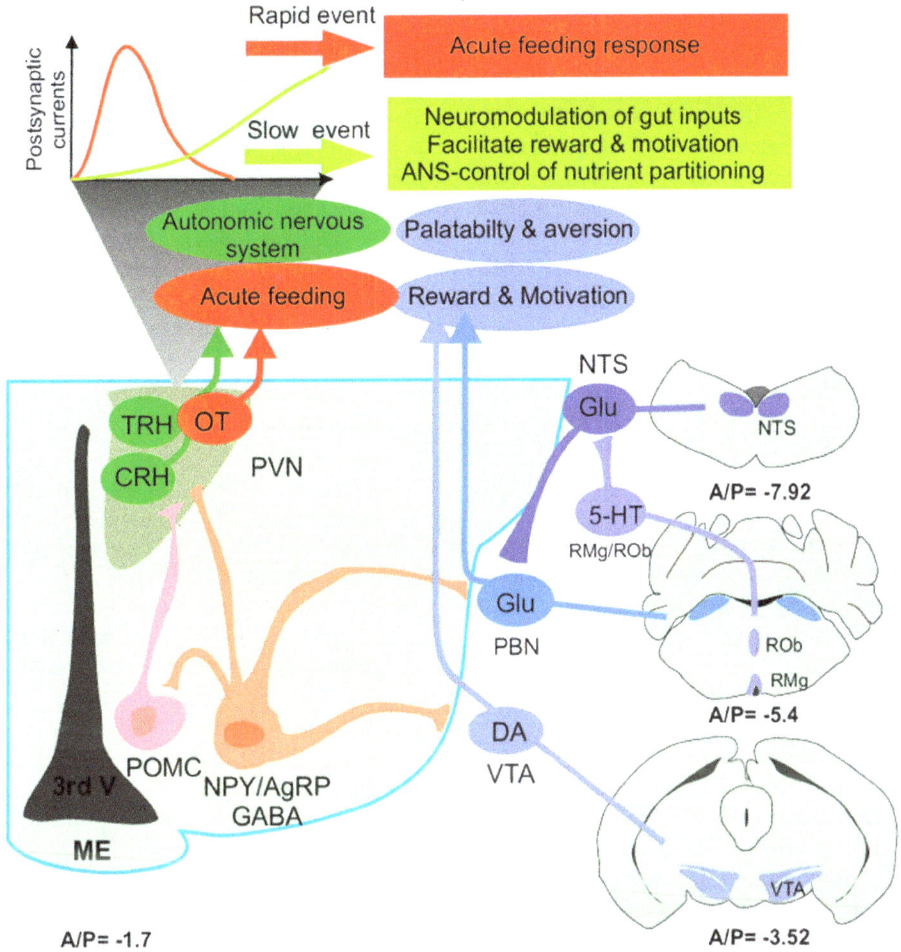

FIGURE 2 | Schematic representation of the feeding-neural circuitry. Arcuate AgRP neurons are located at the bottom of the third ventricle (3rd V) close to the circumventricular organs, the median eminence (ME). They exert a GABAergic tonic inhibition onto POMC-, OT-, CRH-, and TRH-expressing neurons from the PVN, the PBN and the dopaminergic neurons (DA) of the VTA. The PBN receives glutamatergic input from the NTS which is also a target for serotoninergic neurons of the raphe obscurus (ROb) and the raphe magnus (RMg). In the PVN, the synaptic properties of AgRP axons are such that GABA release could promote post-synaptic inhibition through the long after the propagation of action potential. The timescale of this electrical event is compatible with the neuromodulation of post-synaptic targets including the VTA, the PBN, and preganglionic structure of the PVN. Hence, hunger-activated neurons could have a role that extends beyond the acute regulation of feeding to autonomic control of nutrient partitioning, the modulation of gut-borne signals in the brainstem, and the fine tuning mesolimbic reward and motivational circuitry. (A/P) Antero-posterior stereotaxic coordinates are presented in mm from bregma below each section.

associated with the treatment of depression of bipolar disorders using selective serotonin re-uptake inhibitors.

Based on the circuitry described, one would expect that activation of AgRP neurons stimulate feeding by activating OT-expressing neurons in the PVN, while at the same time dampening activation of the PBN and thereby minimizing the influence of satiety and or visceral malaise. Photoactivation of AgRP axons in the PBN did not promote feeding, whereas activation of the PVN resulted in robust feeding (Atasoy et al., 2012). However, reducing satiety or visceral malaise would not necessarily promote robust feeding. Thus, the discrepancy may be resolved by considering the timescale at which the two events occur as well as their potential contribution to body weight maintenance. AgRP input to the PVN could convey an acute hunger-activated feeding response whereas AgRP input to the PBN could be more tonic in nature and involve longer-lasting actions that insure the proper excitatory balance of the PBN.

CONNECTING METABOLIC NEEDS AND GOAL-DIRECTED BEHAVIOR

A recent study provides evidence that AgRP neurons could directly participate in the dopaminergic encoding of goal-directed behavior independent from the actual retrieval of food. The reinforcing and motivational aspects of food are closely tied to the release of the neurotransmitter dopamine by midbrain dopamine neurons in the ventral tegmental area (VTA) that project to the nucleus accumbens, and other limbic brain regions. VTA-mediated dopamine release is stimulated by high-fat/high-sugar foods as well as by most other objects of desire (e.g., sex, drugs; Wise, 2006). The VTA–striatal network provides a crucial neural substrate upon which drugs of abuse (e.g., cocaine, nicotine, morphine) exert their effect; thus, this projection is often referred to as the brain "reward circuit" (Kelley et al., 2005).

Using a model in which AgRP neurons are either ablated from birth or rendered hypoactive through selective knockdown of the metabolic sensor of the sirtuin family Sirt1 (silent mating type information regulation 2 homolog), a direct role for AgRP neurons in modulation of dopamine signaling was revealed (Dietrich et al., 2012). They demonstrated a direct projection from AgRP neurons to the VTA and inactivation or ablation of AgRP neurons reduced GABAergic tone to VTA dopamine neurons. This translated to higher excitability of VTA neurons and facilitated the induction of long-term potentiation. Hence, a reduced activity of AgRP neurons resulted in enhanced dopamine-dependent encoding of reward and motivation. At the behavioral level, the two models showed an enhanced response to novelty and a stronger preference for an environment associated with cocaine injection (Dietrich et al., 2012; Palmiter, 2012).

One can therefore envision GABAergic tone from AgRP neurons to the PBN and the VTA as a necessary input to counteract gut-borne aversive input while reducing the threshold at which taste-related information is successfully transferred to cognitive, emotional, and rewarding processing centers in the brain (**Figure 1**). This mechanism could be central to the maintenance of the motivational and rewarding components of feeding when energy stores are low and when the food is deprived of reinforcing properties. The activity of AgRP neurons would be necessary to maintain metabolic need as a significant contributor of goal-directed behavior. Decreased AgRP neuronal input, tonic or phasic, could result in the progressive replacement of hunger by limbic-associated emotional inputs such as stress or anxiety. The overall consequence could be that a drive for reward seeking eventually prevails over metabolic demand in the control of feeding (Dallman et al., 2005; **Figure 2**).

ORCHESTRATING NUTRIENT PARTITIONING THROUGH TONIC CONTROL OF PREGANGLIONIC STRUCTURES

Agouti-related protein neurons project to several preganglionic structures (Broberger et al., 1998) including the regions involved in activating autonomic nervous system (ANS) output such as the PVN (Cowley et al., 1999). ANS innervation of peripheral tissues (pancreas, liver, visceral adipose tissue) has a distinct organization that can be tracked back to pre-autonomic hypothalamic neurons (Kreier et al., 2006). Nutrient partitioning (the integrated processes that control conversion, storage, and utilization of nutrients) relies on the ability of the brain to orchestrate peripheral organ activity through the modulation of the ANS. Using a model of neonatal depletion, we showed that the lack of AgRP neurons affects the relative balance between lipid and carbohydrate metabolism. As a consequence, mice lacking AgRP neurons became obese and hyperinsulinemic on regular chow but displayed reduced body weight gain and paradoxical improvement in glucose tolerance on high-fat diet (Joly-Amado et al., 2012). This action was independent from feeding, and involved GABAergic input to preganglionic structures and the consequent modulation of ANS output onto liver, muscle, and pancreas.

These findings indicate that AgRP neurons play a role that extends beyond the regulation of feeding, to the control of peripheral nutrient partitioning. In good agreement, a recent study showed that Sirt 1 inactivation selectively in AgRP neurons resulted in a shift in the overall metabolic profile, the impairment of metabolic adaptation induced by a fast, and a change in ghrelin-induced excitability of AgRP neurons (Dietrich et al., 2010). Importantly, we found that a $GABA_A$ receptor agonist normalized the metabolic profile in mice lacking AgRP neurons (Joly-Amado et al., 2012). These results suggest that, here too, GABA may be a crucial signaling molecule by which AgRP neurons control peripheral nutrient partitioning.

In conclusion, several recent studies have significantly broadened the spectrum of brain structure, mechanism, and timescale that underlie the action of AgRP neurons in the regulation of energy balance. The intrinsic nature of GABA release has received much attention and technological tools and approaches have allowed dissociation of the behavioral and metabolic actions of AgRP from the melanocortin signaling pathway. Long-lasting inhibitory currents that persist long after the action potential indicate a putative function for AgRP neurons in the neuromodulation of post-synaptic targets. A second era is just beginning for this neurocircuitry that will likely provide fundamental insights into the mechanisms that underlie not only food-related but also non-food-related behavior including cognitive, emotional, and reward processes.

ACKNOWLEDGMENTS

This work was supported by young investigator ATIP grant from the CNRS, a research fellowship from and a grant by the "Agence Nationale de la Recherche" ANR-09-BLAN-0267-02. Céline Cansell received a PhD fellowship from the Centre National de la Recherche Scientifique (CNRS) and a research grant from the Société Francophone du Diabète-Roche (SFD). Aurélie Joly-Amado received a National Merit Scholarship from the French Department of National Education and Research and a research grant from the SFNEP-ANTADIR. Raphaël G. P. Denis received a research fellowship from the Region Île-de-France. We would like to express our gratitude to Richard D. Palmiter and Diane Durnam for fruitful comments on the manuscript and for editing.

REFERENCES

Aponte, Y., Atasoy, D., and Sternson, S. M. (2011). AGRP neurons are sufficient to orchestrate feeding behavior rapidly and without training. *Nat. Neurosci.* 14, 351–355.

Atasoy, D., Betley, J. N., Su, H. H., and Sternson, S. M. (2012). Deconstruction of a neural circuit for hunger. *Nature* 488, 172–177.

Bewick, G. A., Gardiner, J. V., Dhillo, W. S., Kent, A. S., White, N. E., Webster, Z., et al. (2005). Post-embryonic ablation of AgRP neurons in mice leads to a lean, hypophagic phenotype. *FASEB J.* 19, 1680–1682.

Broberger, C., and Hokfelt, T. (2001). Hypothalamic and vagal neuropeptide circuitries regulating food intake. *Physiol. Behav.* 74, 669–682.

Broberger, C., Johansen, J., Johansson, C., Schalling, M., and Hokfelt, T. (1998). The neuropeptide Y/agouti gene-related protein (AGRP) brain circuitry in normal, anorectic, and monosodium glutamate-treated mice. *Proc. Natl. Acad. Sci. U.S.A.* 95, 15043–15048.

Clark, J. T., Kalra, P. S., Crowley, W. R., and Kalra, S. P. (1984). Neuropeptide Y and human pancreatic polypeptide stimulate feeding behavior in rats. *Endocrinology* 115, 427–429.

Cone, R. D. (2005). Anatomy and regulation of the central melanocortin system. *Nat. Neurosci.* 8, 571–578.

Cowley, M. A., Pronchuk, N., Fan, W., Dinulescu, D. M., Colmers, W. F., and Cone, R. D. (1999). Integration of NPY, AGRP, and melanocortin signals in the hypothalamic paraventricular nucleus: evidence of a cellular basis for the adipostat. *Neuron* 24, 155–163.

Cowley, M. A., Smart, J. L., Rubinstein, M., Cerdan, M. G., Diano, S., Horvath, T. L. et al. (2001). Leptin activates anorexigenic POMC neurons through a neural network in the arcuate nucleus. *Nature* 411, 480–484.

Dallman, M. F., Pecoraro, N. C., and La Fleur, S. E. (2005). Chronic stress and comfort foods: self-medication and abdominal obesity. *Brain Behav. Immun.* 19, 275–280.

de Araujo, I. E. (2009). Gustatory and homeostatic functions of the rodent parabrachial nucleus. *Ann. N. Y. Acad. Sci.* 1170, 383–391.

Dietrich, M. O., Antunes, C., Geliang, G., Liu, Z. W., Borok, E., Nie, Y., et al. (2010). Agrp neurons mediate Sirt1's action on the melanocortin system and energy balance: roles for Sirt1 in neuronal firing and synaptic plasticity. *J. Neurosci.* 30, 11815–11825.

Dietrich, M. O., Bober, J., Ferreira, J. G., Tellez, L. A., Mineur, Y. S., Souza, D. O., et al. (2012). AgRP neurons regulate development of dopamine neuronal plasticity and nonfood-associated behaviors. *Nat. Neurosci.* 15, 1108–1110.

Fan, W., Boston, B. A., Kesterson, R. A., Hruby, V. J., and Cone, R. D. (1997). Role of melanocortinergic neurons in feeding and the agouti obesity syndrome. *Nature* 385, 165–168.

Fekete, C., Legradi, G., Mihaly, E., Huang, Q. H., Tatro, J. B., Rand, W. M., et al. (2000). alpha-Melanocyte-stimulating hormone is contained in nerve terminals innervating thyrotropin-releasing hormone-synthesizing neurons in the hypothalamic paraventricular nucleus and prevents fasting-induced suppression of prothyrotropin-releasing hormone gene expression. *J. Neurosci.* 20, 1550–1558.

Flier, J. S. (2006). AgRP in energy balance: will the real AgRP please stand up? *Cell Metab.* 3, 83–85.

Fu, L. Y., and van den Pol, A. N. (2008). Agouti-related peptide and MC3/4 receptor agonists both inhibit excitatory hypothalamic ventromedial nucleus neurons. *J. Neurosci.* 28, 5433–5449.

Gropp, E., Shanabrough, M., Borok, E., Xu, A. W., Janoschek, R., Buch, T., et al. (2005). Agouti-related peptide-expressing neurons are mandatory for feeding. *Nat. Neurosci.* 8, 1289–1291.

Hahn, T. M., Breininger, J. F., Baskin, D. G., and Schwartz, M. W. (1998). Coexpression of Agrp and NPY in fasting-activated hypothalamic neurons. *Nat. Neurosci.* 1, 271–272.

Haskell-Luevano, C., Chen, P., Li, C., Chang, K., Smith, M. S., Cameron, J. L., et al. (1999). Characterization of the neuroanatomical distribution of agouti-related protein immunoreactivity in the rhesus monkey and the rat. *Endocrinology* 140, 1408–1415.

Haskell-Luevano, C., and Monck, E. K. (2001). Agouti-related protein functions as an inverse agonist at a constitutively active brain melanocortin-4 receptor. *Regul Pept.* 99, 1–7.

Hegemann, P., and Moglich, A. (2011). Channelrhodopsin engineering and exploration of new optogenetic tools. *Nat. Methods* 8, 39–42.

Hinney, A., Schmidt, A., Nottebom, K., Heibult, O., Becker, I., Ziegler, A., et al. (1999). Several mutations in the melanocortin-4 receptor gene including a nonsense and a frameshift mutation associated with dominantly inherited obesity in humans. *J. Clin. Endocrinol. Metab.* 84, 1483–1486.

Horvath, T. L., Bechmann, I., Naftolin, F., Kalra, S. P., and Leranth, C. (1997). Heterogeneity in the neuropeptide Y-containing neurons of the rat arcuate nucleus: GABAergic and non-GABAergic subpopulations. *Brain Res.* 756, 283–286.

Horvath, T. L., Naftolin, F., Kalra, S. P., and Leranth, C. (1992). Neuropeptide-Y innervation of beta-endorphin-containing cells in the rat mediobasal hypothalamus: a light and electron microscopic double immunostaining analysis. *Endocrinology* 131, 2461–2467.

Huszar, D., Lynch, C. A., Fairchild-Huntress, V., Dunmore, J. H., Fang, Q., Berkemeier, L. R., et al. (1997). Targeted disruption of the melanocortin-4 receptor results in obesity in mice. *Cell* 88, 131–141.

Jegou, S., Boutelet, I., and Vaudry, H. (2000). Melanocortin-3 receptor mRNA expression in pro-opiomelanocortin neurones of the rat arcuate nucleus. *J. Neuroendocrinol.* 12, 501–505.

Joly-Amado, A., Denis, R. G., Castel, J., Lacombe, A., Cansell, C., Rouch, C., et al. (2012). Hypothalamic AgRP-neurons control peripheral substrate utilization and nutrient partitioning. *EMBO J.* 31, 4276–4288.

Kelley, A. E., Baldo, B. A., and Pratt, W. E. (2005). A proposed hypothalamic-thalamic-striatal axis for the integration of energy balance, arousal, and food reward. *J. Comp. Neurol.* 493, 72–85.

Krashes, M. J., Koda, S., Ye, C., Rogan, S. C., Adams, A. C., Cusher, D. S., et al. (2011). Rapid, reversible activation of AgRP neurons drives feeding behavior in mice. *J. Clin. Invest.* 121,1424–1428.

Kreier, F., Kap, Y. S., Mettenleiter, T. C., Van Heijningen, C., Van Der Vliet, J., Kalsbeek, A., et al. (2006). Tracing from fat tissue, liver, and pancreas: a neuroanatomical framework for the role of the brain in type 2 diabetes. *Endocrinology* 147, 1140–1147.

Krude, H., Schnabel, D., Luck, W., and Gruters, A. (1999). Implications of the phenotype of POMC deficiency for the role of POMC-derived peptides in skin physiology. *Ann. N. Y. Acad. Sci.* 885, 419–421.

Lechan, R. M., and Fekete, C. (2006). The TRH neuron: a hypothalamic integrator of energy metabolism. *Prog. Brain Res.* 153, 209–235.

Lein, E. S., Hawrylycz, M. J., Ao, N., Ayres, M., Bensinger, A., Bernard, A., et al. (2007). Genome-wide atlas of gene expression in the adult mouse brain. *Nature* 445, 168–176.

Liu, H., Kishi, T., Roseberry, A. G., Cai, X., Lee, C. E., Montez, J. M., et al. (2003). Transgenic mice expressing green fluorescent protein under the control of the melanocortin-4 receptor promoter. *J. Neurosci.* 23, 7143–7154.

Lu, X. Y., Barsh, G. S., Akil, H., and Watson, S. J. (2003). Interaction between alpha-melanocyte-stimulating hormone and corticotropin-releasing hormone in the regulation of feeding and hypothalamo-pituitary-adrenal responses. *J. Neurosci.* 23, 7863–7872.

Luquet, S., Perez, F. A., Hnasko, T. S., and Palmiter, R. D. (2005). NPY/AgRP neurons are essential for feeding in adult mice but can be ablated in neonates. *Science* 310, 683–685.

Michaud, E. J., Bultman, S. J., Klebig, M. L., Van Vugt, M. J., Stubbs, L. J., Russell, L. B., et al. (1994). A molecular model for the genetic and phenotypic characteristics of the mouse lethal yellow (Ay) mutation. *Proc. Natl. Acad. Sci. U.S.A.* 91, 2562–2566.

Miltenberger, R. J., Mynatt, R. L., Wilkinson, J. E., and Woychik, R. P. (1997). The role of the agouti gene in the yellow obese syndrome. *J. Nutr.* 127, 1902S–1907S.

Moran, T. H., Ladenheim, E. E., and Schwartz, G. J. (2001). Within-meal gut feedback signaling. *Int. J. Obes. Relat. Metab. Disord.* 25(Suppl. 5), S39–S41.

Mountjoy, K. G., and Wong, J. (1997). Obesity, diabetes and functions for proopiomelanocortin-derived peptides. *Mol. Cell. Endocrinol.* 128, 171–177.

Nijenhuis, W. A., Oosterom, J., and Adan, R. A. (2001). AgRP(83-132) acts as an inverse agonist on the human-melanocortin-4 receptor. *Mol. Endocrinol.* 15, 164–171.

Oliveira-Maia, A. J., Roberts, C. D., Simon, S. A., and Nicolelis, M. A. (2011). Gustatory and reward brain circuits in the control of food intake. *Adv. Tech. Stand. Neurosurg.* 36, 31–59.

Ollmann, M. M., Wilson, B. D., Yang, Y. K., Kerns, J. A., Chen, Y., Gantz, I., et al. (1997). Antagonism of central melanocortin receptors in vitro and in vivo by agouti-related protein. *Science* 278, 135–138.

Palmiter, R. D. (2012). New game for hunger neurons. *Nat. Neurosci.* 15, 1060–1061.

Pinto, S., Roseberry, A. G., Liu, H., Diano, S., Shanabrough, M., Cai, X., et al. (2004). Rapid rewiring of arcuate nucleus feeding circuits by leptin. *Science* 304, 110–115.

Schwartz, G. J., Mchugh, P. R., and Moran, T. H. (1991). Integration of vagal afferent responses to gastric loads and cholecystokinin in rats. *Am. J. Physiol.* 261, R64–R69.

Schwartz, G. J., Mchugh, P. R., and Moran, T. H. (1993). Gastric loads and cholecystokinin synergistically stimulate rat gastric vagal afferents. *Am. J. Physiol.* 265, R872–R876.

Schwartz, G. J., and Moran, T. H. (2002). Leptin and neuropeptide y have opposing modulatory effects on nucleus of the solitary tract neurophysiological responses to gastric loads: implications for the control of food intake. *Endocrinology* 143, 3779–3784.

Shutter, J. R., Graham, M., Kinsey, A. C., Scully, S., Luthy, R., and Stark, K. L. (1997). Hypothalamic expression of ART, a novel gene related to agouti, is up-regulated in obese and diabetic mutant mice. *Genes Dev.* 11, 593–602.

Suwabe, T., and Bradley, R. M. (2009). Characteristics of rostral solitary tract nucleus neurons with identified afferent connections that project to the parabrachial nucleus in rats. *J. Neurophysiol.* 102, 546–555.

Tatemoto, K., Carlquist, M., and Mutt, V. (1982). Neuropeptide Y – a novel brain peptide with structural similarities to peptide YY and pancreatic polypeptide. *Nature* 296, 659–660.

Tokita, K., Inoue, T., and Boughter, J. D. Jr. (2009). Afferent connections of the parabrachial nucleus in C57BL/6J mice. *Neuroscience* 161, 475–488.

Tolle, V., and Low, M. J. (2008). In vivo evidence for inverse agonism of Agouti-related peptide in the central nervous system of proopiomelanocortin-deficient mice. *Diabetes* 57, 86–94.

Williams, G., Bing, C., Cai, X. J., Harrold, J. A., King, P. J., and Liu, X. H. (2001). The hypothalamus and the control of energy homeostasis: different circuits, different purposes. *Physiol. Behav.* 74, 683–701.

Wise, R. A. (2006). Role of brain dopamine in food reward and reinforcement. *Philos. Trans. R. Soc. Lond. B Biol. Sci.* 361, 1149–1158.

Wu, Q., Boyle, M. P., and Palmiter, R. D. (2009). Loss of GABAergic signaling by AgRP neurons to the parabrachial nucleus leads to starvation. *Cell* 137, 1225–1234.

Wu, Q., Clark, M. S., and Palmiter, R. D. (2012a). Deciphering a neuronal circuit that mediates appetite. *Nature* 483, 594–597.

Wu, Q., Whiddon, B. B., and Palmiter, R. D. (2012b). Ablation of neurons expressing agouti-related protein, but not melanin concentrating hormone, in leptin-deficient mice restores metabolic functions and fertility. *Proc. Natl. Acad. Sci. U.S.A.* 109, 3155–3160.

Wu, Q., Howell, M. P., Cowley, M. A., and Palmiter, R. D. (2008a). Starvation after AgRP neuron ablation is independent of melanocortin signaling. *Proc. Natl. Acad. Sci. U.S.A.* 105, 2687–2692.

Wu, Q., Howell, M. P., and Palmiter, R. D. (2008b). Ablation of neurons expressing agouti-related protein activates fos and gliosis in postsynaptic target regions. *J. Neurosci.* 28, 9218–9226.

Wu, Q., and Palmiter, R. D. (2011). GABAergic signaling by AgRP neurons prevents anorexia via a melanocortin-independent mechanism. *Eur. J. Pharmacol.* 660, 21–27.

Xu, A. W., Kaelin, C. B., Morton, G. J., Ogimoto, K., Stanhope, K., Graham, J., et al. (2005). Effects of hypothalamic neurodegeneration on energy balance. *PLoS Biol.* 3:e415. doi: 10.1371/journal.pbio.0030415

10

Activation of somatostatin 2 receptors in the brain and the periphery induces opposite changes in circulating ghrelin levels: functional implications

Andreas Stengel[1]* and Yvette Taché[2]*

[1] Division Psychosomatic Medicine and Psychotherapy, Department of Medicine, Obesity Center Berlin, Charité, Universitätsmedizin Berlin, Berlin, Germany
[2] Digestive Diseases Division, CURE: Digestive Diseases Research Center, Center for Neurobiology of Stress and Women's Health, Department of Medicine, VA Greater Los Angeles Health Care System, University of California at Los Angeles, Los Angeles, CA, USA

Edited by:
Hubert Vaudry, University of Rouen, France

Reviewed by:
Rafael Vazquez-Martinez, University of Cordoba, Spain
Francisco Gracia-Navarro, University of Cordoba, Spain

***Correspondence:**
Andreas Stengel, Division Psychosomatic Medicine and Psychotherapy, Department of Medicine, Obesity Center Berlin, Charité, Universitätsmedizin Berlin, Luisenstr. 13a, 10117 Berlin, Germany.
e-mail: andreas.stengel@charite.de;
Yvette Taché, Digestive Diseases Division, CURE: Digestive Diseases Research Center, Center for Neurobiology of Stress and Women's Health, Department of Medicine, VA Greater Los Angeles Health Care System, University of California at Los Angeles, CURE Building 115, Room 117, 11301 Wilshire Boulevard, Los Angeles, CA 90073, USA.
e-mail: ytache@mednet.ucla.edu

Somatostatin is an important modulator of neurotransmission in the central nervous system and acts as a potent inhibitor of hormone and exocrine secretion and regulator of cell proliferation in the periphery. These pleiotropic actions occur through interaction with five G protein-coupled somatostatin receptor subtypes (sst_{1-5}) that are widely expressed in the brain and peripheral organs. The characterization of somatostatin's effects can be investigated by pharmacological or genetic approaches using newly developed selective sst agonists and antagonists and mice lacking specific sst subtypes. Recent evidence points toward a divergent action of somatostatin in the brain and in the periphery to regulate circulating levels of ghrelin, an orexigenic hormone produced by the endocrine X/A-like cells in the rat gastric mucosa. Somatostatin interacts with the sst_2 in the brain to induce an increase in basal ghrelin plasma levels and counteracts the visceral stress-related decrease in circulating ghrelin. By contrast, stimulation of peripheral somatostatin-sst_2 signaling results in the inhibition of basal ghrelin release and mediates the postoperative decrease in circulating ghrelin. The peripheral sst_2-mediated reduction of plasma ghrelin is likely to involve a paracrine action of D cell-derived somatostatin acting on sst_2 bearing X/A-like ghrelin cells in the gastric mucosa. The other member of the somatostatin family, named cortistatin, in addition to binding to sst_{1-5} also directly interacts with the ghrelin receptor and therefore may simultaneously modulate ghrelin release and actions at target sites bearing ghrelin receptors representing a link between the ghrelin and somatostatin systems.

Keywords: X/A-like cell, somatostatin receptor subtypes, ghrelin cell, somatostatin receptor agonists and antagonist, cortistatin

INTRODUCTION

In 1972, Guillemin's group – while searching for additional releasing factors in hypothalamic extracts after their identification of thyrotropin-releasing hormone (TRH) – identified a novel negative regulator of pituitary somatotropic cells releasing growth hormone (GH; Brazeau et al., 1973). The cyclo peptide was named somatostatin (somatotropin release-inhibiting factor, SRIF), in keeping with its hypophysiotropic action (Guillemin, 2011). Somatostatin was found to be expressed in two biologically active isoforms: the tetradecapeptide somatostatin-14 (Brazeau et al., 1973) and the amino terminally extended octacosapeptide somatostatin-28 generated by differential post-translational processing from a common precursor molecule (Pradayrol et al., 1980). Thereafter, a flow of articles in rodents and humans established the ubiquitous distribution of somatostatin in various brain areas (Finley et al., 1981; Johansson et al., 1984; Uhl et al., 1985) and peripheral organs including the gastrointestinal tract (Costa et al., 1977; Walsh, 1994). This was followed by the identification and characterization of five distinct, high-affinity, specific somatostatin receptors (sst) encoded by five distinct genes (Gahete et al., 2010a). Structurally, these receptors belong to the so-called "superfamily" of membrane G protein-coupled (GPC) receptors. The sst_{1-5} have distinct as well as overlapping patterns of distribution in the brain (Fehlmann et al., 2000; Spary et al., 2008) and gut (Schafer and Meyerhof, 1999; Ludvigsen et al., 2004; Corleto et al., 2006) with a prominent expression of sst_2 in the gastrointestinal tract (Sternini et al., 1997). Studies using new pharmacological tools, namely selective sst subtype agonists and antagonists (Grace et al., 2006; Cescato et al., 2008; Erchegyi et al., 2008, 2009; **Table 1**) point toward the role of different sst_{1-5} in mediating the large spectrum of somatostatin biological actions, mostly inhibitory in nature. Multiple effects of somatostatin can also result from the ability of sst to form both homodimers or heterodimers (sst_5 with sst_1 or dopamine D_2 receptor, sst_{2a} with sst_3, D_2 or μ opioid receptor subtype 1) resulting in the activation of different intracellular signaling cascades (Rocheville et al., 2000; Baragli et al., 2007; Siehler et al., 2008).

Of interest to neuroendocrinologists, somatostatin's inhibitory action on pituitary GH release was soon extended to a wide range of hypophyseal hormones including prolactin, thyrotropin (thyroid-stimulating hormone, TSH), and adrenocorticotropic hormone (ACTH; Brown et al., 1984; Bertherat et al., 1995;

Table 1 | Structure and receptor binding affinity of somatostatin and somatostatin receptor agonists.

Peptide	Structure	Receptor binding affinity (IC_{50}, nM)[a]				
		sst_1	sst_2	sst_3	sst_4	sst_5
Somatostatin-14 (Viollet et al., 1995)	Ala-Gly-c[Cys-Lys-Asn-Phe-Phe-Trp-Lys-Thr-Phe-Thr-Ser-Cys]-OH	0.1–1.5	1.7	1.7	1.0–1.6	0.2–2.2
Somatostatin-28 (Viollet et al., 1995)	Ser-Ala-Asn-Ser-Asn-Pro-Ala-Met-Ala-Pro-Arg-Glu-Arg-Lys-Ala-Gly-c[Cys-Lys-Asn-Phe-Phe-Trp-Lys-Thr-Phe-Thr-Ser-Cys]-OH	0.1–4.7	0.4–5.2	0.2	0.3–1.1	0.05–0.19
Octreotide (Grace et al., 2008)	H-(D)-Phe^2-c[Cys^3-Phe^7-$DTrp^8$-Lys^9-Thr^{10}-Cys^{14}]-Thr^{15}(ol)	>1K	1.9 ± 0.3	39 ± 14	>1K	5.1 ± 1.1
ODT8-SST (Erchegyi et al., 2008)	des-$AA^{1,2,4,5,12,13}$-($DTrp^8$)-SST	27.0 ± 3.4	41.0 ± 8.7	13.0 ± 3.2	1.8 ± 0.7	46.0 ± 27.0
Cortistatin-17 (Fukusumi et al., 1997)	Asp-Arg-Met-Pro-cyclo-[Cys-Arg-Asn-Phe-Phe-Trp-Lys-Thr-Phe-Ser-Ser-Cys]Lys	0.3–7.0	0.6–0.9	0.4–0.6	0.5–0.6	0.3–0.4
sst_1 agonist (Erchegyi et al., 2009)	des-$AA^{1,4-6,10,12,13}$-[$DTyr^2$,D-Agl(NMe,2naphtoyl)^8, $IAmp^9$]-SST-Thr-NH_2	0.19 ± 0.04	>1K	158.0 ± 14.0	27.0 ± 7.5	>1K
sst_2 agonist (Grace et al., 2006)	des-$AA^{1,4-6,11-13}$-[$DPhe^2$,Aph^7(Cbm),$DTrp^8$]-Cbm-SST-Thr-NH_2	>1K	7.5–20	942–1094	872–957	109–260
sst_2 antagonist (Cescato et al., 2008)	des-$AA^{1,4-6,11-13}$-[pNO_2-Phe^2,$DCys^3$,Tyr^7,DAph(Cbm)^8]-SST-2Nal-NH_2	>1K	2.6 ± 0.7	384.0 ± 97.0	>1K	>1K

Receptor affinities were derived from competitive radioligand displacement assays in cells stably expressing the cloned human receptor using ^{125}I-[Leu^8 $DTrp^{22}$ Tyr^{25}] SST-28 (Grace et al., 2006, 2008; Cescato et al., 2008; Erchegyi et al., 2008, 2009) except for somatostatin-14 (Viollet et al., 1995), somatostatin-28 (Viollet et al., 1995), and cortistatin (Fukusumi et al., 1997).

Shimon et al., 1997) as well as a large number of hormones secreted from endocrine cells of the gastrointestinal tract including gastrin (Lloyd et al., 1997), cholecystokinin (CCK; Shiratori et al., 1991), secretin (Shiratori et al., 1991), gastric inhibitory peptide (GIP; Pederson et al., 1975), and neurotensin (Rokaeus, 1984), and from the pancreas glucagon (Marco et al., 1983; Strowski et al., 2000), insulin (Pederson et al., 1975; Marco et al., 1983; Strowski et al., 2000), and pancreatic polypeptide (PP; Marco et al., 1983). Studies to characterize the somatostatin receptor subtypes established that sst_2 is primarily involved and, to a smaller extent, sst_5 in the broad inhibitory effects of somatostatin on endocrine secretion (Lloyd et al., 1997; Strowski et al., 2000; de Heer et al., 2008). Of clinical relevance was also the compelling evidence that the majority of neuroendocrine tumors (NETs) expressed increased levels of sst_2 leading to the development of radiolabeled peptides and peptide receptor radionuclides as diagnostic and therapeutic tools respectively for NETs (van der Hoek et al., 2010; Culler et al., 2011; Giovacchini et al., 2012; Jawiarczyk et al., 2012).

In the past decade, a significant breakthrough came from the identification of a 28-amino-acid octanoylated peptide, ghrelin in the endocrine cells of the gastric mucosa as the cognate ligand for the GH-secretagogue receptor 1a (GHS-R_{1a}, later renamed ghrelin receptor, GRLN-R; Kojima et al., 2001; Davenport et al., 2005). Ghrelin's interaction with the GRLN-R represents a third independent regulatory pathway controlling the pulsatile release of pituitary GH besides the GH-releasing hormone (GHRH) and somatostatin (Kojima et al., 2001; Malagon et al., 2003; Kineman and Luque, 2007).

Consistent with ghrelin, being predominantly produced by the endocrine cells of the stomach (Ariyasu et al., 2001), recent studies also documented that gastrointestinal NETs released ghrelin (Corbetta et al., 2003; Tsolakis et al., 2004). Therefore the regulation of ghrelin release by somatostatin will be of clinical relevance. The present review focuses on recent evidence that somatostatin signaling in the brain and the periphery exerts opposite influence on circulating ghrelin levels. The sst receptor subtype(s) involved and functional relevance of somatostatin-induced altered ghrelin plasma levels in the context of orexigenic and gastric prokinetic actions of the peptide (Kojima and Kangawa, 2005) will also be addressed.

SOMATOSTATIN AND ITS RECEPTORS: EXPRESSION AND MODULATION OF FEEDING BEHAVIOR AND GASTROINTESTINAL MOTILITY

EXPRESSION OF SOMATOSTATIN AND sst

Somatostatin is expressed throughout the brain except in the cerebellum (Finley et al., 1981; Johansson et al., 1984). Peptide distribution has been investigated by immunohistochemistry indicating the expression in the cortex, limbic system, central nucleus of the amygdala, sensory structures, hypothalamus (including the arcuate, ventromedial, and paraventricular nucleus), and the periaqueductal central gray (Finley et al., 1981; Johansson et al., 1984; Moga and Gray, 1985). Similarly, sst receptor mRNA expression is widely detected in the rat brain including the deep layers of the cerebral cortex, bed nucleus of the stria terminalis, basolateral amygdaloid nucleus, medial amygdaloid nucleus, paraventricular thalamic nucleus, medial preoptic nucleus, dorsomedial and ventromedial hypothalamic nucleus, arcuate and paraventricular nucleus of the hypothalamus, substantia nigra, dorsal raphe nucleus, granular layer of the cerebellum, locus coeruleus, nucleus of the solitary tract, and the dorsal motor nucleus of the vagus nerve (Fehlmann et al., 2000; Spary et al., 2008). The wide distribution of the ligand along with the receptors is consistent with the pleiotropic action of the sst signaling systems.

Somatostatin is widely expressed in the gastrointestinal tract and the pancreas, namely in endocrine mucosal D cells scattered within the stomach, small and large intestine, and in δ-cells of the pancreatic islets of Langerhans (Walsh, 1994). In addition, somatostatin is also detected in neurons of the gut enteric nervous system within both the submucosal and myenteric plexus (Costa et al., 1977). Similar to the ligand, sst receptor subtypes are widely expressed in the gastrointestinal tract. In rats, mRNA expression of sst_1, sst_2, sst_3, and sst_4 is detected in the small and large intestine without any clear predominance to one segment (Schafer and Meyerhof, 1999). The sst_1 is the predominant form in gastrointestinal tract of mice, whereas the sst_5 was almost undetectable (Schafer and Meyerhof, 1999). In human colon, a differential expression has been reported with sst_2 mRNA expression on circular smooth muscle cells and sst_{1-3} mRNA on longitudinal muscle layer cells (Corleto et al., 2006). Interestingly, in the pancreas protein expression of all sst_{1-5} receptor subtypes has been identified on every major endocrine cell type, namely α, β, δ, and PP cells with a differential expression pattern between species (Ludvigsen et al., 2004).

BRAIN ACTIONS OF SOMATOSTATIN

The first function assigned to somatostatin was the inhibition of GH release (Brazeau et al., 1973). Now somatostatin is recognized to exert several central extrapituitary actions such as the regulation of other pituitary endocrine hormones especially those responsive to stress, parasympathetic and sympathetic outflow, thermogenesis, visceral functions, and behaviors. Namely, intracerebroventricular (icv) injection of somatostatin-28 inhibited the tail suspension stress-induced rise of circulating ACTH (Brown et al., 1984). This effect was mimicked by the stable pan-somatostatin agonist, ODT8-SST but not by somatostatin-14 (Brown et al., 1984). The sst_2 seems to play a pivotal role in these regulatory processes as sst_2 receptor knockout mice display an increased ACTH release compared to their wild type littermates (Viollet et al., 2000).

With regard to the central actions of somatostatin to affect visceral functions, recent studies have focused on the gastrointestinal tract. ODT8-SST injected intracisternally (ic) in rats accelerated gastric emptying of a liquid non-nutrient solution. This effect is mimicked by somatostatin-28 and the sst_5 preferring agonist, BIM-23052 but not somatostatin-14 or the agonists preferring sst_1, CH-275, sst_2, DC-32-87, sst_3, BIM-23056, and sst_4, L-803,087 (Martinez et al., 2000) indicating a prominent role of brain sst_5 activation to induce a gastroprokinetic effect. This contention is further corroborated by the prominent mRNA expression of sst_5 in the dorsal motor nucleus of the vagus nerve (Thoss et al., 1995). Since sst receptors are also expressed in hypothalamic brain nuclei regulating colonic functions (Mönnikes et al., 1993; Mönnikes et al., 1994; Tebbe et al., 2005) including the arcuate (sst_{1-5}; Fehlmann et al., 2000; Schulz et al., 2000) and paraventricular nucleus of the hypothalamus (sst_{2-4}; Fehlmann et al., 2000; Schulz et al., 2000) and the locus coeruleus (sst_{2-4}; Fehlmann et al., 2000; Schulz et al., 2000), several studies investigated whether activation of central somatostatin signaling influences colonic motor functions. Stressing mice by short exposure to anesthesia vapor and icv injection of vehicle robustly stimulated propulsive colonic motor function shown by a 99% increase in fecal pellet output (Stengel et al., 2011a). This effect was completely abolished by icv pretreatment with ODT8-SST, somatostatin-28 and the selective sst_1 agonist, whereas sst_2 or sst_4 agonists or octreotide (**Table 1**) had no effect. These data suggest that activation of brain sst_1 can prevent the stress-related stimulation of colonic propulsive motor function in mice (Stengel et al., 2011a).

Central somatostatin alters food intake with a divergent action depending on the doses used: an increase is induced by icv injection of lower (picomolar) doses and a decrease following high (nanomolar) in rats (Feifel and Vaccarino, 1990). The stable pan-somatostatin agonist, ODT8-SST (Erchegyi et al., 2008) icv stimulated food intake in rats under basal as well as already stimulated conditions during the dark phase with a rapid onset (during the first hour) and a long duration of action (lasting for 4 h; Stengel et al., 2010a). ODT8-SST's orexigenic action is sst_2 mediated as it is reproduced by icv injection of the selective peptide sst_2 agonist (Stengel et al., 2010d) and blocked by the selective peptide sst_2 antagonist (Stengel et al., 2010a). This represents a central action since injected intraperitoneally at a 30-fold higher dose, the peptide did not influence food intake (Stengel et al., 2010d). The orexigenic effect of central sst_2 stimulation observed in rats has been recently expanded to mice (Stengel et al., 2010c). A detailed analysis of the food intake microstructure using an automated food intake monitoring device showed that icv injection of the sst_2 agonist increased the number of meals, shortened inter-meal intervals, and induced a higher rate of ingestion, whereas meal sizes were not altered (Stengel et al., 2010c). Collectively, these data indicate that brain activation of sst_2 signaling pathways in rodents induces a rapid orexigenic response by decreasing satiety (number of meals), without influencing satiation indicated by normal meal sizes (Stengel et al., 2010c). The physiological role of brain sst_2 signaling in modulating food intake is also supported by the decrease of nocturnal food intake induced by the peptide sst_2 antagonist injected icv at the beginning of the dark phase (Stengel et al., 2010d). In addition, hypothalamic somatostatin shows a circadian rhythm with a peak in the early dark phase and a nadir in the early light phase (Gardi et al., 1999). Moreover, food restriction increases pituitary somatostatin release (Ishikawa et al., 1997) which could increase the drive to eat under these conditions.

PERIPHERAL ACTIONS OF SOMATOSTATIN

Contrasting to the central effects, somatostatin's actions in the periphery are largely inhibitory. In the stomach, somatostatin delays emptying of the food (Smedh et al., 1999) and inhibits gastric acid secretion which is mediated directly by an interaction with acid producing parietal cells but also via the reduced release of histamine from ECL cells and gastrin from G cells (Walsh, 1994). The acid-antisecretory action of somatostatin is no longer observed in sst_2 knockout mice, indicative of a primary role of the sst_2 (Piqueras et al., 2003). Similarly, in the small intestine somatostatin reduces intestinal peristalsis in cats, rabbits and rats, while stimulating the duodenal, jejunal, and ileal contractile response in dogs (Tansy et al., 1979). In line with the findings in rodents, somatostatin increases gastrointestinal transit time in humans (Gregersen et al., 2011). The effects on colonic motility are likely mediated by the sst_1 and sst_2 based on *in vitro* studies using circular and longitudinal human colonic smooth muscle cells (Corleto et al., 2006). In addition, somatostatin reduces visceral sensitivity with the sst_2 playing a key role as indicated by visceral hypersensitivity to both mechanical and chemical stimulation in the jejunum of sst_2 knockout mice (Rong et al., 2007). This finding is likely to be relevant in humans as well. Patients with irritable bowel syndrome injected subcutaneously with octreotide display an anti-hyperalgesic response as shown by the increased threshold of discomfort and pain using rectal barostat manometry compared to injection of placebo (Bradette et al., 1994; Schwetz et al., 2004).

GHRELIN AND ITS RECEPTOR: EXPRESSION AND PHYSIOLOGICAL OREXIGENIC AND PROKINETIC ACTIONS

EXPRESSION AND REGULATION OF GHRELIN AND GHRELIN RECEPTOR

Ghrelin bears a unique fatty acid (*n*-octanoyl) residue on the third amino acid which is essential for affinity and binding to the GRLN-R (Kojima et al., 1999; Kojima and Kangawa, 2005). Other dietary fatty acids of medium length can also serve as a direct source for the acylation of ghrelin (Nishi et al., 2005). The enzyme catalyzing the acylation of ghrelin was unknown for several years and just recently identified in mouse and human as a member of the membrane-bound *O*-acyltransferases (MBOATs), namely MBOAT4 which was subsequently renamed ghrelin-*O*-acyltransferase (GOAT; Gutierrez et al., 2008; Yang et al., 2008). GOAT mRNA and protein are prominently expressed in rodent and human gastric mucosa in ghrelin expressing cells (Sakata et al., 2009; Stengel et al., 2010f). In addition, GOAT protein has been detected in rodent and human intestine, pancreatic duct, gallbladder, hypothalamus and pituitary gland (Gahete et al., 2010b; Lim et al., 2011; Kang et al., 2012), rodent plasma (Stengel et al., 2010f) and human visceral and subcutaneous adipocytes (Rodriguez et al., 2012) leading to the speculation of additional acylation sites of ghrelin.

Unlike ghrelin, desacyl ghrelin, which does not bear the hydrophobic residue on the third amino acid, is the main circulating form. The acyl:desacyl ghrelin ratio is 1:3 as recently reported using an optimized blood processing protocol to improve the yield of acylated ghrelin in rats (Stengel et al., 2009). Although desacyl ghrelin does not bind to and activate the GRLN-R (Kojima et al., 1999), recent studies indicate that the peptide exerts several biological actions to influence food intake (Stengel et al., 2010e), reduce inflammatory somatic pain (Sibilia et al., 2012), muscle cachexia produced by injury in rats (Sheriff et al., 2012) and basal autophagy in human visceral adipocytes (Rodriguez et al., 2012). However, the understanding of the physiological function of this peptide is hampered by the fact that the desacyl ghrelin receptor mediating its effects is still to be identified.

Blood levels of ghrelin vary in relation with the meal pattern with an increase before meals and a decrease thereafter (Cummings et al., 2001; Tschöp et al., 2001a). In addition, fasting also increases ghrelin mRNA expression (Toshinai et al., 2001; Kim et al., 2003; Xu et al., 2009) and reduces ghrelin peptide content in the stomach (Toshinai et al., 2001; Kim et al., 2003) indicative of a stimulated production and release under conditions of food deprivation. Ghrelin levels are not only regulated by short-term variations in energy status associated with meal patterns but also by long-term changes in body weight. Ghrelin plasma levels are elevated under conditions of reduced body weight such as anorexia nervosa or tumor cachexia and reduced in obesity (Tschöp et al., 2000, 2001b; Cummings et al., 2002). Similar to the ligand, the ghrelin acylating enzyme, GOAT is regulated by the metabolic status with an increased GOAT mRNA and protein expression in rodent gastric mucosa, hypothalamus, and pituitary following a 12- or 24-h fast (Gonzalez et al., 2008; Gahete et al., 2010b; Stengel et al., 2010f). Under conditions of obesity induced by high fat diet or leptin deficiency in *ob/ob* mice, a down-regulation of GOAT mRNA occurred in the mouse pituitary, unlike the stomach or hypothalamus (Gahete et al., 2010b), while patients with obesity-associated type 2 diabetes showed higher levels of GOAT in visceral adipose tissue (Rodriguez et al., 2012). This indicates a tissue specific regulation of GOAT under conditions of obesity.

OREXIGENIC AND PROKINETIC EFFECTS OF GHRELIN

Ghrelin is well established to stimulate food intake in line with its regulation by changes in energy status in many species including humans (Wren et al., 2000; Tang-Christensen et al., 2004; Druce et al., 2005). It is so far the only known peripherally produced and centrally acting orexigenic peptide, contrasting with the numerous anorexigenic peptides in the gut (Suzuki et al., 2011). Ghrelin's action is blocked by pharmacological or genetic approaches using GRLN-R antagonists (Salome et al., 2009) and GRLN-R knockout mice (Sun et al., 2004; Zigman et al., 2005) indicating a key role of ghrelin-GRLN-R interaction in mediating the orexigenic response. The food intake stimulatory action can result from ghrelin crossing the blood–brain barrier and binding to GRLN-R expressed on food intake regulatory brain nuclei (Banks et al., 2002; Pan et al., 2006) or acting directly on vagal afferents which also bear the ghrelin receptor (Date et al., 2002; Sakata et al., 2003). The respective role of these pathways under nutritional changes is still to be delineated. In addition to the stimulation of food intake, ghrelin is also involved in the regulation of body weight inducing an increase of body weight following chronic infusion of the peptide. This occurs through combined actions of stimulating appetite along with increasing fat storage and reducing lipid mobilization (Tschöp et al., 2000; Strassburg et al., 2008; Davies et al., 2009). Further corroborating these findings, ghrelin and GRLN-R double knockout mice display an increased energy expenditure leading to a reduction of body weight (Pfluger et al., 2008) which, however, could not be reproduced with a single genetic deletion of either ghrelin (Sun et al., 2003; Pfluger et al., 2008) or the GRLN-R (Pfluger et al., 2008). These differential phenotypes may reflect the functional relevance of the high constitutive activity of the GRLN-R (Damian et al., 2012) and also give rise to the speculation that additional ligands for the receptor may exist (Deghenghi et al., 2001a).

DIFFERENTIAL MODULATION OF GH RELEASE BY GHRELIN AND SOMATOSTATIN

Ghrelin exerts endocrine actions opposite to somatostatin by stimulating anterior pituitary release of GH (Kojima et al., 1999; Yamazaki et al., 2002; Kojima and Kangawa, 2011), prolactin, and ACTH (Lanfranco et al., 2010). Somatostatin's GH inhibitory effect is mediated by the sst_2 (Briard et al., 1997), sst_5 (Saveanu et al., 2001) and also sst_1 (Kreienkamp et al., 1999). The GH releasing effect of ghrelin is blunted by intravenous (iv) infusion of somatostatin in healthy volunteers (Di Vito et al., 2002) and was completely blocked in pig pituitary cells *in vitro* (Malagon et al., 2003). The GH releasing action of ghrelin is likely to not only result from inhibiting somatostatin release (Feng et al., 2011) but also from direct activation of GH release (Veldhuis et al., 2006). In addition, ghrelin and somatostatin antagonistically interact on hypothalamic arcuate cells to regulate the release of GHRH with an activation of these neurons following ghrelin and a reduction after application of somatostatin *in vitro* (Mori et al., 2010).

ACTIVATION OF BRAIN sst_2 SIGNALING INCREASES BASAL AND PREVENTS VISCERAL STRESS-INDUCED SUPPRESSION OF CIRCULATING GHRELIN

Based on the established centrally sst_2-mediated orexigenic action of somatostatin (Stengel et al., 2010a,d), we further investigated whether changes in circulating ghrelin may play a role. We found that the pan-somatostatin peptide, ODT8-SST (**Table 1**) injected icv increased basal plasma acyl ghrelin levels in *ad libitum* fed rats (Stengel et al., 2010a). However, the rise was observed at 3 h postinjection and therefore unlikely to underlie the initial increase in food intake response to central ODT8-SST which occurred within the first hour. However, it may contribute to the sustained significant increase in cumulative food intake still maintained at 4 h after icv injection of ODT8-SST (Stengel et al., 2010a). Other studies showed that activation of brain sst_2 receptor prevents the decline in circulating ghrelin induced by visceral stress. Abdominal surgery reproducibly decreased the fasting plasma levels of acyl and desacyl ghrelin with a rapid onset and long lasting effect in rats (Stengel et al., 2010b, 2011b,c). Such a response was completely prevented by the ic injection of ODT8-SST as monitored 50 min postsurgery at a time where the peptide induces a 31 and 46% rise in fasting circulating acyl and desacyl ghrelin, respectively in sham animals (Stengel et al., 2011b). In addition, the sst_2 selective peptide agonist injected ic also prevented the postoperative decline in plasma levels of acyl ghrelin, whereas sst_1 and sst_4 agonists (**Table 1**) did not when tested under the same conditions (Stengel et al., 2011b).

Of interest was the demonstration that ic ODT8-SST or sst_2 agonist in addition to preventing the decline in acyl ghrelin induced by abdominal surgery also blunted the postoperative suppression of food intake (Stengel et al., 2011b). However, the observed prevention of declining circulating ghrelin levels is not the main factor for the restoration of the orexigenic response postsurgically. The peripheral blockade of the GRLN-R using the GRLN-R antagonist ([D-Lys^3]-GHRP-6) injected intraperitoneally did not modify the food intake stimulating effect of ic ODT8-SST (Stengel et al., 2011b). ODT8-SST injected icv also restored gastric emptying inhibited by abdominal surgery to levels observed under basal conditions, an effect mimicked by the sst_5 but not the sst_1, sst_2, and sst_4 agonists in rats (Stengel et al., 2011b). Similar to the effect on food intake, this action was not mediated by acyl ghrelin as the intraperitoneal injection of the GRLN-R antagonist did not influence the gastroprokinetic action of ODT8-SST postsurgery (Stengel et al., 2011b).

Taken together, these data indicate that the central activation of sst_2 increases basal or prevents the surgical inhibition of circulating levels of ghrelin and food intake while activation of sst_5 restores postoperative gastric ileus in rats. It also points to a differential role of brain sst subtypes 2 and 5 in preventing the stress-related suppression of ghrelin release/food intake and gastric emptying, respectively. In addition, the restoration of suppressed circulating acyl ghrelin levels after surgery does not play a major role as underlying mechanisms through which ODT8-SST injected into the brain exerts its prokinetic and orexigenic effects. Other studies showed that activation of sst_2 and sst_5 receptors in the brain inhibits stimulated CRF release in the hypothalamus and acute stress-related CRF mediated ACTH release (Brown et al., 1984; Tizabi and Calogero, 1992; Saegusa et al., 2011; Tringali et al., 2012). Brain CRF acting on CRF receptors is involved in the stress-related decrease in feeding behavior, ghrelin secretion, and gastric emptying (Hotta et al., 1999; Sekino et al., 2004; Taché and Bonaz, 2007; Yakabi et al., 2011). Therefore, it may be speculated that central activation of sst_2 and/or sst_5 dampens hypothalamic CRF activated by abdominal surgery (Wang et al., 2011) which may have a bearing with preventing the reduction in feeding, gastric emptying, and circulating ghrelin induced by abdominal surgery (Stengel et al., 2011b).

ACTIVATION OF PERIPHERAL sst_2 SIGNALING INHIBITS CIRCULATING GHRELIN

In contrast to the rise in circulating ghrelin induced by central administration of somatostatin agonists, convergent *in vivo* and *in vitro* rodent studies established that somatostatin or the stable agonists octreotide and SOM230 act peripherally through the sst_2 to reduce ghrelin release (Seoane et al., 2007; Iwakura et al., 2010; Lu et al., 2012) resulting in lower circulating levels (Shimada et al., 2003; Silva et al., 2005; de la Cour et al., 2007). Such a response is in line with the inhibitory effects of somatostatin-sst_2 on the endocrine secretion of other intestinal hormones (Pederson et al., 1975; Marco et al., 1983; Rokaeus, 1984; Shiratori et al., 1991; Strowski et al., 2000). Likewise, in humans, peripherally injected somatostatin (Broglio et al., 2002; Norrelund et al., 2002) and somatostatin agonists such as octreotide (Barkan et al., 2003) reduce circulating ghrelin in healthy subjects. Of relevance, chronic subcutaneous infusion of the $sst_2/sst_3/sst_5$ agonist octreotide-induced suppression of ghrelin plasma levels is not subject to rapid desensitization in rats and is likely to be sst_2 mediated based on the prominent sst_2 mRNA expression in the rat stomach (Silva et al., 2005). Further support for a role of sst_2 came from immunofluorescent double labeling studies detecting the protein expression of sst_2 on ghrelin-producing X/A-like cells of the rat stomach (Stengel et al., 2011c) and similarly on human ghrelin-producing gastric mucosal P/D_1 cells (Fischer et al., 2008). Moreover, the selective peptide sst_2 agonist (**Table 1**) injected intravenously decreased circulating levels of acyl and desacyl ghrelin with a rapid onset (0.5 h) and a long duration of action (still visible at 2 h; Stengel et al., 2011c). Lastly, the selective peptide sst_2 antagonist (**Table 1**) injected intravenously prevents the decline in circulating ghrelin induced by the stimulation of endogenous peripheral somatostatin in rats (Stengel et al., 2011c).

The physiological role of peripheral somatostatin-sst_2 signaling in the regulation of ghrelin was investigated under conditions of stimulation of endogenous gastric somatostatin. Urethane is well established to stimulate gastric somatostatin mRNA expression and peptide release in rats (Yang et al., 1990). Under these conditions, plasma ghrelin levels are decreased and the selective peptide sst_2 antagonist (**Table 1**) injected intravenously prevents the decline in circulating ghrelin induced by urethane (Stengel et al., 2011c). Convergent reports showed that abdominal surgery induces a rapid and sustained inhibition of circulating levels of ghrelin in rats (Stengel et al., 2010b, 2011b,c). Likewise, iv injection of the selective peptide sst_2 antagonist (**Table 1**) blocked the abdominal surgery-induced decrease of plasma ghrelin at 0.5 h postsurgery (Stengel et al., 2011c). The peptide is likely to act through paracrine transmission since somatostatin positive D cells directly contact ghrelin immunoreactive X/A-like cells in the rat stomach (Shimada et al., 2003). Interestingly, following abdominal surgery, acyl ghrelin was reduced more rapidly compared to desacyl ghrelin which was associated with a reduction of gastric as well as plasma concentrations of GOAT (Stengel et al., 2011c). Since blockade of peripheral sst_2 signaling restores circulating levels of ghrelin (Stengel et al., 2011c), these data collectively suggest that peripheral somatostatin may blunt gastric GOAT mRNA expression and thereby negatively affect the acylation of ghrelin. In primary pituitary cell cultures somatostatin was reported to reduce GOAT mRNA expression and somatostatin knockout mice showed higher GOAT mRNA expression in the pituitary gland than the wild type (Gahete et al., 2010b). Based on these findings, somatostatin may influence ghrelin signaling not only *via* a direct inhibition of secretion but also by modulating the ghrelin activating enzyme GOAT. Further support for a physiological inhibitory action of peripheral somatostatin on ghrelin signaling came from somatostatin knockout mice that displayed an increased gastric ghrelin expression and higher circulating ghrelin levels compared to their wild type littermates (Luque et al., 2006a). These data indicate that endogenous somatostatin exerts a physiological inhibitory tone on gastric ghrelin synthesis and release.

During the past years, several clinical studies described ghrelin-producing NETs (Papotti et al., 2001; Volante et al., 2002; Taal and Visser, 2004) including six insulinomas, gastrinomas, vasoactive intestinal polypeptide (VIP)omas, non-functioning tumors (Volante et al., 2002) and as part of the multiple endocrine neoplasia type 1 (MEN-1; Iwakura et al., 2002; Raffel et al., 2005; Ekeblad et al., 2007). Moreover, ghrelinomas have been identified to originate from the stomach or pancreas and were associated with very high ghrelin levels (Corbetta et al., 2003; Tsolakis et al., 2004). Growing evidence from clinical reports indicates that in addition to the surgical, chemotherapeutic, alpha-interferon, and local radiation treatments, the use of somatostatin or somatostatin analog is an established treatment option for gastroenteropancreatic NETs (Pavel and Wiedenmann, 2011). Based on the evidence described above, the determination of the sst subtype expressed on those ghrelinoma tumor cells followed by the use of peripherally acting selective sst compounds may result in an even more targeted approach.

INTERACTION OF CORTISTATIN WITH GHRELIN SIGNALING

In 1996, the discovery of a new peptide sharing 11 of its 14 amino acids with somatostatin-14 was named cortistatin based on its predominant cortical expression and ability to depress cortical activity (de Lecea et al., 1996). Despite the chemical structure homology with somatostatin, both peptides are derived from distinct genes (de Lecea et al., 1997b). Similar to pro-somatostatin, processing of cortistatin precursor generated two mature products, cortistatin-14 and -29 in rodents and cortistatin-17 and -29 in humans (Fukusumi et al., 1997; Spier and de Lecea, 2000). Cortistatin is widely expressed in the brain, namely in the cortex and hippocampus, and although regional overlap exists, the distribution pattern differs from that of somatostatin (de Lecea et al., 1997a). Likewise, the peripheral expression pattern of cortistatin (e.g., in adrenal, thyroid, and parathyroid gland, testis, pancreas, kidney, lung, liver, stomach, ileum, jejunum, colon, endothelial, and immune cells) does not fully match that of somatostatin (Papotti et al., 2003; Dalm et al., 2004; Xidakis et al., 2007). Consistent with being a close somatostatin endogenous analog, cortistatin contains the FWKT tetramer crucial for sst binding, and therefore displays high-affinity (1–2 nM) to all five sst subtypes where the peptide acts as an agonist (Fukusumi et al., 1997; Siehler et al., 2008). However, emerging evidence indicates that cortistatin induces distinct central and peripheral effects that differ from those exerted by the somatostatin-sst interaction such as central acetylcholine release, reduction of locomotor activity, depression of cortical activity, induction of slow wave sleep, anti-inflammatory and immunomodulatory effects, and reduction of vascular calcium deposition (for review, see Spier and de Lecea, 2000; Broglio et al., 2007; Gonzalez-Rey and Delgado, 2008).

The existence of a specific cortistatin receptor has not been identified yet but differential actions between somatostatin and cortistatin may possibly reside in the ability of cortistatin to bind and to activate the GRLN-R, whereas somatostatin does not (Deghenghi et al., 2001b; Muccioli et al., 2001). Divergent from native somatostatin, however, synthetic somatostatin agonists, lanreotide, octreotide, and vapreotide bind to the GRLN-R in human pituitary tissue (Deghenghi et al., 2001c) in addition to their selective affinity for $sst_2 > sst_5 > sst_3$ (Bauer et al., 1982; Reichlin, 1983; Redding and Schally, 1984). In addition to binding studies, few functional findings also support the possibility that cortistatin may be another endogenous high-affinity ligand of the

GRLN-R. Cortistatin has been reported to inhibit vascular calcification induced experimentally in rats through activation of the GRLN-R receptor rather than sst or Mrg X2 (Liu et al., 2010). Of interest was the demonstration that cortistatin selectively upregulates the GRLN-R mRNA expression in cultured rat vascular smooth muscle cells, further indicative of an interaction between cortistatin and ghrelin signaling (Liu et al., 2010). Other studies in primates and mice demonstrated that endogenous cortistatin, unlike somatostatin, is involved in the stimulation of pituitary prolactin release, an effect that is blocked *in vitro* by the GRLN-R antagonist (Cordoba-Chacon et al., 2011). However, most of the endocrine studies performed *in vivo* or *in vitro* showed parallel inhibitory responses between cortistatin and somatostatin consistent with the activation of classical sst subtypes (Broglio et al., 2008) with some exceptions (Prodam et al., 2008). This is further corroborated by the finding that cortistatin knockout mice display elevated circulating acyl ghrelin levels associated with an upregulated gastric ghrelin and GOAT expression (Cordoba-Chacon et al., 2011) indicating an inhibitory tone of endogenous cortistatin on ghrelin signaling.

To further delineate the actions of cortistatin mediated *via* the GRLN-R another peptide, cortistatin-8, has been shown to bind to the GRLN-R while being devoid of affinity to the sst subtypes (Luque et al., 2006b). However, in one clinical study cortistatin-8 did not influence spontaneous pituitary hormone secretion (GH, prolactin, and ACTH) and did not interfere with ghrelin's endocrine responses when given in equimolar dose ratios in healthy human subjects (Prodam et al., 2008). Therefore, additional specific tools may be needed to characterize a possible direct link between the ghrelin and somatostatin signaling system *via* interaction on the GRLN-R.

SUMMARY

In summary, somatostatin robustly affects circulating levels of ghrelin through interaction with the sst_2. However, alterations vary with the site of action. Central somatostatin elevates plasma levels of acyl and desacyl ghrelin *via* interaction with brain sst_2 and counteracts the visceral stress-related decrease in circulating ghrelin through pathways still to be elucidated in rodents. By contrast, the activation of peripheral somatostatin-sst_2 inhibits circulating ghrelin levels in experimental and clinical studies and mediates the decline in circulating ghrelin induced by abdominal surgery in rodents likely *via* a paracrine action of somatostatin on sst_2-bearing ghrelin cells in the stomach. Of interest, cortistatin, the other member of the somatostatin family, in addition to binding to sst_{1-5}, also binds to and activates the GRLN-R. There is evidence that the peptide can exert a dual influence on ghrelin, by inhibiting its release through interaction with sst_2 located on gastric ghrelin cells while activating GRLN-R at ghrelin's tissue targets.

ACKNOWLEDGMENTS

This work was supported by NIH R01 DK-33061, NIH Center Grant DK-41301 (Animal Core), VA Research Career Scientist and VA Merit grant (to Yvette Taché), German Research Foundation STE 1765/3-1 (to Andreas Stengel), and Charité University Funding UFF 89-441-176 (to Andreas Stengel).

REFERENCES

Ariyasu, H., Takaya, K., Tagami, T., Ogawa, Y., Hosoda, K., Akamizu, T., et al. (2001). Stomach is a major source of circulating ghrelin, and feeding state determines plasma ghrelin-like immunoreactivity levels in humans. *J. Clin. Endocrinol. Metab.* 86, 4753–4758.

Banks, W. A., Tschöp, M., Robinson, S. M., and Heiman, M. L. (2002). Extent and direction of ghrelin transport across the blood–brain barrier is determined by its unique primary structure. *J. Pharmacol. Exp. Ther.* 302, 822–827.

Baragli, A., Alturaihi, H., Watt, H. L., Abdallah, A., and Kumar, U. (2007). Heterooligomerization of human dopamine receptor 2 and somatostatin receptor 2 co-immunoprecipitation and fluorescence resonance energy transfer analysis. *Cell. Signal.* 19, 2304–2316.

Barkan, A. L., Dimaraki, E. V., Jessup, S. K., Symons, K. V., Ermolenko, M., and Jaffe, C. A. (2003). Ghrelin secretion in humans is sexually dimorphic, suppressed by somatostatin, and not affected by the ambient growth hormone levels. *J. Clin. Endocrinol. Metab.* 88, 2180–2184.

Bauer, W., Briner, U., Doepfner, W., Haller, R., Huguenin, R., Marbach, P., et al. (1982). SMS 201–995: a very potent and selective octapeptide analogue of somatostatin with prolonged action. *Life Sci.* 31, 1133–1140.

Bertherat, J., Bluet-Pajot, M. T., and Epelbaum, J. (1995). Neuroendocrine regulation of growth hormone. *Eur. J. Endocrinol.* 132, 12–24.

Bradette, M., Delvaux, M., Staumont, G., Fioramonti, J., Bueno, L., and Frexinos, J. (1994). Octreotide increases thresholds of colonic visceral perception in IBS patients without modifying muscle tone. *Dig. Dis. Sci.* 39, 1171–1178.

Brazeau, P., Vale, W., Burgus, R., Ling, N., Butcher, M., Rivier, J., et al. (1973). Hypothalamic polypeptide that inhibits the secretion of immunoreactive pituitary growth hormone. *Science* 179, 77–79.

Briard, N., Dutour, A., Epelbaum, J., Sauze, N., Slama, A., and Oliver, C. (1997). Species differences between male rat and ram pituitary somatostatin receptors involved in the inhibition of growth hormone secretion. *Eur. J. Endocrinol.* 137, 545–555.

Broglio, F., Grottoli, S., Arvat, E., and Ghigo, E. (2008). Endocrine actions of cortistatin: in vivo studies. *Mol. Cell. Endocrinol.* 286, 123–127.

Broglio, F., Papotti, M., Muccioli, G., and Ghigo, E. (2007). Brain–gut communication: cortistatin, somatostatin and ghrelin. *Trends Endocrinol. Metab.* 18, 246–251.

Broglio, F., Van Koetsveld, P., Benso, A., Gottero, C., Prodam, F., Papotti, M., et al. (2002). Ghrelin secretion is inhibited by either somatostatin or cortistatin in humans. *J. Clin. Endocrinol. Metab.* 87, 4829–4832.

Brown, M. R., Rivier, C., and Vale, W. (1984). Central nervous system regulation of adrenocorticotropin secretion: role of somatostatins. *Endocrinology* 114, 1546–1549.

Cescato, R., Erchegyi, J., Waser, B., Piccand, V., Maecke, H. R., Rivier, J. E., et al. (2008). Design and in vitro characterization of highly sst2-selective somatostatin antagonists suitable for radiotargeting. *J. Med. Chem.* 51, 4030–4037.

Corbetta, S., Peracchi, M., Cappiello, V., Lania, A., Lauri, E., Vago, L., et al. (2003). Circulating ghrelin levels in patients with pancreatic and gastrointestinal neuroendocrine tumors: identification of one pancreatic ghrelinoma. *J. Clin. Endocrinol. Metab.* 88, 3117–3120.

Cordoba-Chacon, J., Gahete, M. D., Culler, M. D., Castano, J. P., Kineman, R. D., and Luque, R. M. (2012). Somatostatin dramatically stimulates growth hormone release from primate somatotrophs acting at low doses via somatostatin receptor 5 and cyclic AMP. *J. Neuroendocrinol.* 24, 453–463.

Cordoba-Chacon, J., Gahete, M. D., Pozo-Salas, A. I., Martinez-Fuentes, A. J., de Lecea, L., Gracia-Navarro, F., et al. (2011). Cortistatin is not a somatostatin analogue but stimulates prolactin release, and inhibits GH and ACTH in a gender-dependent fashion: potential role of ghrelin. *Endocrinology* 152, 4800–4812.

Corleto, V. D., Severi, C., Romano, G., Tattoli, I., Weber, H. C., Stridsberg, M., et al. (2006). Somatostatin receptor subtypes mediate contractility on human colonic smooth muscle cells. *Neurogastroenterol. Motil.* 18, 217–225.

Costa, M., Patel, Y., Furness, J. B., and Arimura, A. (1977). Evidence that some intrinsic neurons of the intestine contain somatostatin. *Neurosci. Lett.* 6, 215–222.

Culler, M. D., Oberg, K., Arnold, R., Krenning, E. P., Sevilla, I., and Diaz, J. A. (2011). Somatostatin analogs for the treatment of neuroendocrine tumors. *Cancer Metastasis Rev.* 30(Suppl. 1), 9–17.

Cummings, D. E., Purnell, J. Q., Frayo, R. S., Schmidova, K., Wisse, B. E., and Weigle, D. S. (2001). A preprandial rise in plasma ghrelin levels suggests a role in meal initiation in humans. *Diabetes.* 50, 1714–1719.

Cummings, D. E., Weigle, D. S., Frayo, R. S., Breen, P. A., Ma, M. K., Dellinger, E. P., et al. (2002). Plasma ghrelin levels after diet-induced weight loss or gastric bypass surgery. *N. Engl. J. Med.* 346, 1623–1630.

Dalm, V. A., Van Hagen, P. M., de Krijger, R. R., Kros, J. M., Van Koetsveld, P. M., Van Der Lely, A. J., et al. (2004). Distribution pattern of somatostatin and cortistatin mRNA in human central and peripheral tissues. *Clin. Endocrinol. (Oxf.)* 60, 625–629.

Damian, M., Marie, J., Leyris, J. P., Fehrentz, J. A., Verdie, P., Martinez, J., et al. (2012). High constitutive activity is an intrinsic feature of ghrelin receptor protein: a study with a functional monomeric GHS-R1a receptor reconstituted in lipid discs. *J. Biol. Chem.* 287, 3630–3641.

Date, Y., Murakami, N., Toshinai, K., Matsukura, S., Niijima, A., Matsuo, H., et al. (2002). The role of the gastric afferent vagal nerve in ghrelin-induced feeding and growth hormone secretion in rats. *Gastroenterology* 123, 1120–1128.

Davenport, A. P., Bonner, T. I., Foord, S. M., Harmar, A. J., Neubig, R. R., Pin, J. P., et al. (2005). International Union of Pharmacology. LVI. Ghrelin receptor nomenclature, distribution, and function. *Pharmacol. Rev.* 57, 541–546.

Davies, J. S., Kotokorpi, P., Eccles, S. R., Barnes, S. K., Tokarczuk, P. F., Allen, S. K., et al. (2009). Ghrelin induces abdominal obesity via GHS-R-dependent lipid retention. *Mol. Endocrinol.* 23, 914–924.

Deghenghi, R., Avallone, R., Torsello, A., Muccioli, G., Ghigo, E., and Locatelli, V. (2001a). Growth hormone-inhibiting activity of cortistatin in the rat. *J. Endocrinol. Invest.* 24, RC31–RC33.

Deghenghi, R., Papotti, M., Ghigo, E., and Muccioli, G. (2001b). Cortistatin, but not somatostatin, binds to growth hormone secretagogue (GHS) receptors of human pituitary gland. *J. Endocrinol. Invest.* 24, RC1–RC33.

Deghenghi, R., Papotti, M., Ghigo, E., Muccioli, G., and Locatelli, V. (2001c). Somatostatin octapeptides (lanreotide, octreotide, vapreotide, and their analogs) share the growth hormone-releasing peptide receptor in the human pituitary gland. *Endocrine* 14, 29–33.

de Heer, J., Rasmussen, C., Coy, D. H., and Holst, J. J. (2008). Glucagon-like peptide-1, but not glucose-dependent insulinotropic peptide, inhibits glucagon secretion via somatostatin (receptor subtype 2) in the perfused rat pancreas. *Diabetologia* 51, 2263–2270.

de la Cour, C. D., Norlen, P., and Hakanson, R. (2007). Secretion of ghrelin from rat stomach ghrelin cells in response to local microinfusion of candidate messenger compounds: a microdialysis study. *Regul. Pept.* 143, 118–126.

de Lecea, L., Criado, J. R., Prospero-Garcia, O., Gautvik, K. M., Schweitzer, P., Danielson, P. E., et al. (1996). A cortical neuropeptide with neuronal depressant and sleep-modulating properties. *Nature* 381, 242–245.

de Lecea, L., del Rio, J. A., Criado, J. R., Alcantara, S., Morales, M., Danielson, P. E., et al. (1997a). Cortistatin is expressed in a distinct subset of cortical interneurons. *J Neurosci.* 17, 5868–5880.

de Lecea, L., Ruiz-Lozano, P., Danielson, P. E., Peelle-Kirley, J., Foye, P. E., Frankel, W. N., et al. (1997b). Cloning, mRNA expression, and chromosomal mapping of mouse and human preprocortistatin. *Genomics* 42, 499–506.

Di Vito, L., Broglio, F., Benso, A., Gottero, C., Prodam, F., Papotti, M., et al. (2002). The GH-releasing effect of ghrelin, a natural GH secretagogue, is only blunted by the infusion of exogenous somatostatin in humans. *Clin. Endocrinol. (Oxf.)* 56, 643–648.

Druce, M. R., Wren, A. M., Park, A. J., Milton, J. E., Patterson, M., Frost, G., et al. (2005). Ghrelin increases food intake in obese as well as lean subjects. *Int. J. Obes. (Lond.)* 29, 1130–1136.

Ekeblad, S., Lejonklou, M. H., Grimfjard, P., Johansson, T., Eriksson, B., Grimelius, L., et al. (2007). Co-expression of ghrelin and its receptor in pancreatic endocrine tumours. *Clin. Endocrinol. (Oxf.)* 66, 115–122.

Erchegyi, J., Cescato, R., Grace, C. R., Waser, B., Piccand, V., Hoyer, D., et al. (2009). Novel, potent, and radio-iodinatable somatostatin receptor 1 (sst_1) selective analogues. *J. Med. Chem.* 52, 2733–2746.

Erchegyi, J., Grace, C. R., Samant, M., Cescato, R., Piccand, V., Riek, R., et al. (2008). Ring size of somatostatin analogues (ODT-8) modulates receptor selectivity and binding affinity. *J. Med. Chem.* 51, 2668–2675.

Fehlmann, D., Langenegger, D., Schuepbach, E., Siehler, S., Feuerbach, D., and Hoyer, D. (2000). Distribution and characterisation of somatostatin receptor mRNA and binding sites in the brain and periphery. *J. Physiol. Paris* 94, 265–281.

Feifel, D., and Vaccarino, F. J. (1990). Central somatostatin: a re-examination of its effects on feeding. *Brain Res.* 535, 189–194.

Feng, D. D., Yang, S. K., Loudes, C., Simon, A., Al-Sarraf, T., Culler, M., et al. (2011). Ghrelin and obestatin modulate growth hormone-releasing hormone release and synaptic inputs onto growth hormone-releasing hormone neurons. *Eur. J. Neurosci.* 34, 732–744.

Finley, J. C., Maderdrut, J. L., Roger, L. J., and Petrusz, P. (1981). The immunocytochemical localization of somatostatin-containing neurons in the rat central nervous system. *Neuroscience* 6, 2173–2192.

Fischer, T., Doll, C., Jacobs, S., Kolodziej, A., Stumm, R., and Schulz, S. (2008). Reassessment of sst2 somatostatin receptor expression in human normal and neoplastic tissues using the novel rabbit monoclonal antibody UMB-1. *J. Clin. Endocrinol. Metab.* 93, 4519–4524.

Fukusumi, S., Kitada, C., Takekawa, S., Kizawa, H., Sakamoto, J., Miyamoto, M., et al. (1997). Identification and characterization of a novel human cortistatin-like peptide. *Biochem. Biophys. Res. Commun.* 232, 157–163.

Gahete, M. D., Cordoba-Chacon, J., Duran-Prado, M., Malagon, M. M., Martinez-Fuentes, A. J., Gracia-Navarro, F., et al. (2010a). Somatostatin and its receptors from fish to mammals. *Ann. N. Y. Acad. Sci.* 1200, 43–52.

Gahete, M. D., Cordoba-Chacon, J., Salvatori, R., Castano, J. P., Kineman, R. D., and Luque, R. M. (2010b). Metabolic regulation of ghrelin O-acyl transferase (GOAT) expression in the mouse hypothalamus, pituitary, and stomach. *Mol. Cell. Endocrinol.* 317, 154–160.

Gardi, J., Obal, F. Jr., Fang, J., Zhang, J., and Krueger, J. M. (1999). Diurnal variations and sleep deprivation-induced changes in rat hypothalamic GHRH and somatostatin contents. *Am. J. Physiol.* 277, R1339–R1344.

Giovacchini, G., Nicolas, G., and Forrer, F. (2012). Peptide receptor radionuclide therapy with somatostatin analogues in neuroendocrine tumors. *Anticancer Agents Med. Chem.* 12, 526–542.

Gonzalez, C. R., Vazquez, M. J., Lopez, M., and Dieguez, C. (2008). Influence of chronic undernutrition and leptin on GOAT mRNA levels in rat stomach mucosa. *J. Mol. Endocrinol.* 41, 415–421.

Gonzalez-Rey, E., and Delgado, M. (2008). Emergence of cortistatin as a new immunomodulatory factor with therapeutic potential in immune disorders. *Mol. Cell. Endocrinol.* 286, 135–140.

Grace, C. R., Erchegyi, J., Koerber, S. C., Reubi, J. C., Rivier, J., and Riek, R. (2006). Novel sst2-selective somatostatin agonists. Three-dimensional consensus structure by NMR. *J. Med. Chem.* 49, 4487–4496.

Grace, C. R., Erchegyi, J., Samant, M., Cescato, R., Piccand, V., Riek, R., et al. (2008). Ring size in octreotide amide modulates differently agonist versus antagonist binding affinity and selectivity. *J. Med. Chem.* 51, 2676–2681.

Gregersen, T., Gronbaek, H., Worsoe, J., Schlageter, V., Laurberg, S., and Krogh, K. (2011). Effects of Sandostatin LAR on gastrointestinal motility in patients with neuroendocrine tumors. *Scand. J. Gastroenterol.* 46, 895–902.

Guillemin, R. (2011). Neuroendocrinology: a short historical review. *Ann. N. Y. Acad. Sci.* 1220, 1–5.

Gutierrez, J. A., Solenberg, P. J., Perkins, D. R., Willency, J. A., Knierman, M. D., Jin, Z., et al. (2008). Ghrelin octanoylation mediated by an orphan lipid transferase. *Proc. Natl. Acad. Sci. U.S.A.* 105, 6320–6325.

Hotta, M., Shibasaki, T., Arai, K., and Demura, H. (1999). Corticotropin-releasing factor receptor type 1 mediates emotional stress-induced inhibition of food intake and behavioral changes in rats. *Brain Res.* 823, 221–225.

Ishikawa, M., Mizobuchi, M., Takahashi, H., Bando, H., and Saito, S. (1997). Somatostatin release as measured by in vivo microdialysis: circadian variation and effect of prolonged food deprivation. *Brain Res.* 749, 226–231.

Iwakura, H., Hosoda, K., Doi, R., Komoto, I., Nishimura, H., Son, C., et al. (2002). Ghrelin expression in islet cell tumors: augmented expression of ghrelin in a case of glucagonoma with multiple endocrine neoplasm type I. *J. Clin. Endocrinol. Metab.* 87, 4885–4888.

Iwakura, H., Li, Y., Ariyasu, H., Hosoda, H., Kanamoto, N., Bando, M., et al. (2010). Establishment of a novel ghrelin-producing cell line. *Endocrinology* 151, 2940–2945.

Jawiarczyk, A., Bolanowski, M., Syrycka, J., Bednarek-Tupikowska, G., Kaluzny, M., Kolodziejczyk, A., et al. (2012). Effective therapy of insulinoma by using long-acting somatostatin analogue. A case report and literature review. *Exp. Clin. Endocrinol. Diabetes* 120, 68–72.

Johansson, O., Hokfelt, T., and Elde, R. P. (1984). Immunohistochemical distribution of somatostatin-like immunoreactivity in the central nervous system of the adult rat. *Neuroscience* 13, 265–339.

Kang, K., Schmahl, J., Lee, J. M., Garcia, K., Patil, K, Chen, A., et al. (2012). Mouse ghrelin-O-acyltransferase (GOAT) plays a critical role in bile acid reabsorption. *FASEB J.* 26, 259–271.

Kim, M. S., Yoon, C. Y., Park, K. H., Shin, C. S., Park, K. S., Kim, S. Y., et al. (2003). Changes in ghrelin and ghrelin receptor expression according to feeding status. *Neuroreport* 14, 1317–1320.

Kineman, R. D., and Luque, R. M. (2007). Evidence that ghrelin is as potent as growth hormone (GH)-releasing hormone (GHRH) in releasing GH from primary pituitary cell cultures of a nonhuman primate (*Papio anubis*), acting through intracellular signaling pathways distinct from GHRH. *Endocrinology* 148, 4440–4449.

Kojima, M., Hosoda, H., Date, Y., Nakazato, M., Matsuo, H., and Kangawa, K. (1999). Ghrelin is a growth-hormone-releasing acylated peptide from stomach. *Nature* 402, 656–660.

Kojima, M., Hosoda, H., Matsuo, H., and Kangawa, K. (2001). Ghrelin: discovery of the natural endogenous ligand for the growth hormone secretagogue receptor. *Trends Endocrinol. Metab.* 12, 118–122.

Kojima, M., and Kangawa, K. (2005). Ghrelin: structure and function. *Physiol Rev.* 85, 495–522.

Kojima, M., and Kangawa, K. (2011). The discovery of ghrelin: with a little luck and great passion. *Peptides* 32, 2153–2154.

Kreienkamp, H. J., Akgun, E., Baumeister, H., Meyerhof, W., and Richter, D. (1999). Somatostatin receptor subtype 1 modulates basal inhibition of growth hormone release in somatotrophs. *FEBS Lett.* 462, 464–466.

Lanfranco, F., Motta, G., Baldi, M., Gasco, V., Grottoli, S., Benso, A., et al. (2010). Ghrelin and anterior pituitary function. *Front. Horm. Res.* 38, 206–211.

Lim, C. T., Kola, B., Grossman, A., and Korbonits, M. (2011). The expression of ghrelin O-acyltransferase (GOAT) in human tissues. *Endocr. J.* 8, 707–710.

Liu, Y., Zhou, Y. B., Zhang, G. G., Cai, Y., Duan, X. H., Teng, X., et al. (2010). Cortistatin attenuates vascular calcification in rats. *Regul. Pept.* 159, 35–43.

Lloyd, K. C., Amirmoazzami, S., Friedik, F., Chew, P., and Walsh, J. H. (1997). Somatostatin inhibits gastrin release and acid secretion by activating sst2 in dogs. *Am. J. Physiol.* 272, G1481–G1488.

Lu, X., Zhao, X., Feng, J., Liou, A. P., Anthony, S., Pechhold, S., et al. (2012). Postprandial inhibition of gastric ghrelin secretion by long-chain fatty acid (LCFA) through GPR 120 in isolated gastric ghrelin cells and mice. *Am. J. Physiol. Gastrointest. Liver Physiol.* 303, G367–G376.

Ludvigsen, E., Olsson, R., Stridsberg, M., Janson, E. T., and Sandler, S. (2004). Expression and distribution of somatostatin receptor subtypes in the pancreatic islets of mice and rats. *J. Histochem. Cytochem.* 52, 391–400.

Luque, R. M., Gahete, M. D., Hochgeschwender, U., and Kineman, R. D. (2006a). Evidence that endogenous SST inhibits ACTH and ghrelin expression by independent pathways. *Am. J. Physiol. Endocrinol. Metab.* 291, E395–E403.

Luque, R. M., Peinado, J. R., Gracia-Navarro, F., Broglio, F., Ghigo, E., Kineman, R. D., et al. (2006b). Cortistatin mimics somatostatin by inducing a dual, dose-dependent stimulatory and inhibitory effect on growth hormone secretion in somatotropes. *J. Mol. Endocrinol.* 36, 547–556.

Malagon, M. M., Luque, R. M., Ruiz-Guerrero, E., Rodriguez-Pacheco, F., Garcia-Navarro, S., Casanueva, F. F., et al. (2003). Intracellular signaling mechanisms mediating ghrelin-stimulated growth hormone release in somatotropes. *Endocrinology* 144, 5372–5380.

Marco, J., Correas, I., Zulueta, M. A., Vincent, E., Coy, D. H., Comaru-Schally, A. M., et al. (1983). Inhibitory effect of somatostatin-28 on pancreatic polypeptide, glucagon and insulin secretion in normal man. *Horm. Metab. Res.* 15, 363–366.

Martinez, V., Rivier, J., Coy, D., and Taché, Y. (2000). Intracisternal injection of somatostatin receptor 5-preferring agonists induces a vagal cholinergic stimulation of gastric emptying in rats. *J. Pharmacol. Exp. Ther.* 293, 1099–1105.

Moga, M. M., and Gray, T. S. (1985). Evidence for corticotropin-releasing factor, neurotensin, and somatostatin in the neural pathway from the central nucleus of the amygdala to the parabrachial nucleus. *J. Comp. Neurol.* 241, 275–284.

Mönnikes, H., Raybould, H. E., Schmidt, B., and Taché, Y. (1993). CRF in the paraventricular nucleus of the hypothalamus stimulates colonic motor activity in fasted rats. *Peptides* 14, 743–747.

Mönnikes, H., Schmidt, B. G., Tebbe, J., Bauer, C., and Taché, Y. (1994). Microinfusion of corticotropin releasing factor into the locus coeruleus/subcoeruleus nuclei stimulates colonic motor function in rats. *Brain Res.* 644, 101–108.

Mori, K., Kim, J., and Sasaki, K. (2010). Electrophysiological effect of ghrelin and somatostatin on rat hypothalamic arcuate neurons in vitro. *Peptides* 31, 1139–1145.

Muccioli, G., Papotti, M., Locatelli, V., Ghigo, E., and Deghenghi, R. (2001). Binding of ^{125}I-labeled ghrelin to membranes from human hypothalamus and pituitary gland. *J. Endocrinol. Invest.* 24, RC7–RC9.

Nishi, Y., Hiejima, H., Hosoda, H., Kaiya, H., Mori, K., Fukue, Y., et al. (2005). Ingested medium-chain fatty acids are directly utilized for the acyl modification of ghrelin. *Endocrinology* 146, 2255–2264.

Norrelund, H., Hansen, T. K., Orskov, H., Hosoda, H., Kojima, M., Kangawa, K., et al. (2002). Ghrelin immunoreactivity in human plasma is suppressed by somatostatin. *Clin. Endocrinol. (Oxf)* 57, 539–546.

Pan, W., Tu, H., and Kastin, A. J. (2006). Differential BBB interactions of three ingestive peptides: obestatin, ghrelin, and adiponectin. *Peptides* 27, 911–916.

Papotti, M., Cassoni, P., Volante, M., Deghenghi, R., Muccioli, G., and Ghigo, E. (2001). Ghrelin-producing endocrine tumors of the stomach, and intestine. *J. Clin. Endocrinol. Metab.* 86, 5052–5059.

Papotti, M., Tarabra, E., Allia, E., Bozzalla-Cassione, F., Broglio, F., Deghenghi, R., et al. (2003). Presence of cortistatin in the human pancreas. *J. Endocrinol. Invest.* 26, RC15–RC18.

Pavel, M. E., and Wiedenmann, B. (2011). Novel therapeutic agents for the treatment of gastroenteropancreatic neuroendocrine tumors. *Horm. Metab. Res.* 43, 844–853.

Pederson, R. A., Dryburgh, J. R., and Brown, J. C. (1975). The effect of somatostatin on release and insulinotropic action of gastric inhibitory polypeptide. *Can. J. Physiol. Pharmacol.* 53, 1200–1205.

Pfluger, P. T., Kirchner, H., Gunnel, S., Schrott, B., Perez-Tilve, D., Fu, S., et al. (2008). Simultaneous deletion of ghrelin and its receptor increases motor activity and energy expenditure. *Am. J. Physiol. Gastrointest. Liver Physiol.* 294, G610–G618.

Piqueras, L., Taché, Y., and Martinez, V. (2003). Somatostatin receptor type 2 mediates bombesin-induced inhibition of gastric acid secretion in mice. *J. Physiol.* 549, 889–901.

Pradayrol, L., Jornvall, H., Mutt, V., and Ribet, A. (1980). N-terminally extended somatostatin: the primary structure of somatostatin-28. *FEBS Lett.* 109, 55–58.

Prodam, F., Benso, A., Gramaglia, E., Lucatello, B., Riganti, F., van der Lely, A. J., et al. (2008). Cortistatin-8, a synthetic cortistatin-derived ghrelin receptor ligand, does not modify the endocrine responses to acylated ghrelin or hexarelin in humans. *Neuropeptides* 42, 89–93.

Raffel, A., Krausch, M., Cupisti, K., Gerharz, C. D., Eisenberger, C. F., and Knoefel, W. T. (2005). Ghrelin expression in neuroendocrine tumours of the gastrointestinal tract with multiple endocrine neoplasia type 1. *Horm. Metab. Res.* 37, 653–655.

Redding, T. W., and Schally, A. V. (1984). Inhibition of growth of pancreatic carcinomas in animal models by analogs of hypothalamic hormones. *Proc. Natl. Acad. Sci. U.S.A.* 81, 248–252.

Reichlin, S. (1983). Somatostatin. *N. Engl. J. Med.* 309, 1495–1501.

Rocheville, M., Lange, D. C., Kumar, U., Sasi, R., Patel, R. C., and Patel, Y. C. (2000). Subtypes of the somatostatin receptor assemble as functional homo- and heterodimers. *J. Biol. Chem.* 275, 7862–7869.

Rodriguez, A., Gomez-Ambrosi, J., Catalan, V., Rotellar, F., Valenti, V., Silva, C., et al. (2012). The ghrelin O-acyltransferase-ghrelin system reduces TNF-alpha-induced apoptosis and autophagy in human visceral adipocytes. *Diabetologia* 55, 3038–3050.

Rokaeus, A. (1984). Increase in neurotensin-like immunoreactivity in rat plasma after administration of calcium, bombesin and fat and its inhibition by somatostatin. *Acta Physiol. Scand.* 122, 261–267.

Rong, W., Winchester, W. J., and Grundy, D. (2007). Spontaneous hypersensitivity in mesenteric afferent nerves of mice deficient in the sst2 subtype of somatostatin receptor. *J. Physiol.* 581, 779–786.

Saegusa, Y., Takeda, H., Muto, S., Nakagawa, K., Ohnishi, S., Sadakane, C., et al. (2011). Decreased plasma ghrelin contributes to anorexia following novelty stress. *Am. J. Physiol. Endocrinol. Metab.* 301, E685–E696.

Sakata, I., Yamazaki, M., Inoue, K., Hayashi, Y., Kangawa, K., and Sakai, T. (2003). Growth hormone secretagogue receptor expression in the cells of the stomach-projected afferent nerve in the rat nodose ganglion. *Neurosci. Lett.* 342, 183–186.

Sakata, I., Yang, J., Lee, C. E., Osborne-Lawrence, S., Rovinsky, S. A., Elmquist, J. K., et al. (2009). Colocalization of ghrelin *O*-acyltransferase and ghrelin in gastric mucosal cells. *Am. J. Physiol. Endocrinol. Metab.* 297, E134–E141.

Salome, N., Haage, D., Perrissoud, D., Moulin, A., Demange, L., Egecioglu, E., et al. (2009). Anorexigenic and electrophysiological actions of novel ghrelin receptor (GHS-R1A) antagonists in rats. *Eur. J. Pharmacol.* 612, 167–173.

Saveanu, A., Gunz, G., Dufour, H., Caron, P., Fina, F., Ouafik, L., et al. (2001). Bim-23244, a somatostatin receptor subtype 2- and 5-selective analog with enhanced efficacy in suppressing growth hormone (GH) from octreotide-resistant human GH-secreting adenomas. *J. Clin. Endocrinol. Metab.* 86, 140–145.

Schafer, J., and Meyerhof, W. (1999). sst1 mRNA is the prominent somatostatin receptor mRNA in the rat gastrointestinal tract: reverse transcription polymerase chain reaction and in situ-hybridization study. *Neuropeptides* 33, 457–463.

Schulz, S., Handel, M., Schreff, M., Schmidt, H., and Hollt, V. (2000). Localization of five somatostatin receptors in the rat central nervous system using subtype-specific antibodies. *J. Physiol. Paris* 94, 259–264.

Schwetz, I., Naliboff, B., Munakata, J., Lembo, T., Chang, L., Matin, K., et al. (2004). Anti-hyperalgesic effect of octreotide in patients with irritable bowel syndrome. *Aliment. Pharmacol. Ther.* 19, 123–131.

Sekino, A., Ohata, H., Mano-Otagiri, A., Arai, K., and Shibasaki, T. (2004). Both corticotropin-releasing factor receptor type 1 and type 2 are involved in stress-induced inhibition of food intake in rats. *Psychopharmacology (Berl.)* 76, 30–38.

Seoane, L. M., Al-Massadi, O., Barreiro, F., Dieguez, C., and Casanueva, F. F. (2007). Growth hormone and somatostatin directly inhibit gastric ghrelin secretion. An in vitro organ culture system. *J. Endocrinol. Invest.* 30, RC22–RC25.

Sheriff, S., Kadeer, N., Joshi, R., Friend, L. A., James, J. H., and Balasubramaniam, A. (2012). Des-acyl ghrelin exhibits pro-anabolic and anti-catabolic effects on C2C12 myotubes exposed to cytokines and reduces burn-induced muscle proteolysis in rats. *Mol. Cell. Endocrinol.* 351, 286–295.

Shimada, M., Date, Y., Mondal, M. S., Toshinai, K., Shimbara, T., Fukunaga, K., et al. (2003). Somatostatin suppresses ghrelin secretion from the rat stomach. *Biochem. Biophys. Res. Commun.* 302, 520–525.

Shimon, I., Taylor, J. E., Dong, J. Z., Bitonte, R. A., Kim, S., Morgan, B., et al. (1997). Somatostatin receptor subtype specificity in human fetal pituitary cultures. Differential role of SSTR2 and SSTR5 for growth hormone, thyroid-stimulating hormone, and prolactin regulation. *J. Clin. Invest.* 99, 789–798.

Shiratori, K., Watanabe, S., and Takeuchi, T. (1991). Somatostatin analog, SMS 201–995, inhibits pancreatic exocrine secretion and release of secretin and cholecystokinin in rats. *Pancreas* 6, 23–30.

Sibilia, V., Pagani, F., Mrak, E., Dieci, E., Tulipano, G., and Ferrucci, F. (2012). Pharmacological characterization of the ghrelin receptor mediating its inhibitory action on inflammatory pain in rats. *Amino Acids* 43, 1751–1759.

Siehler, S., Nunn, C., Hannon, J., Feuerbach, D., and Hoyer, D. (2008). Pharmacological profile of somatostatin and cortistatin receptors. *Mol. Cell. Endocrinol.* 286, 26–34.

Silva, A. P., Bethmann, K., Raulf, F., and Schmid, H. A. (2005). Regulation of ghrelin secretion by somatostatin analogs in rats. *Eur. J. Endocrinol.* 152, 887–894.

Smedh, U., Kaplan, J. M., Bjorkstrand, E., and Uvnas-Moberg, K. (1999). Dual effects of somatostatin analog octreotide on gastric emptying during and after intragastric fill. *Am. J. Physiol.* 277, R1291–R1296.

Spary, E. J., Maqbool, A., and Batten, T. F. (2008). Expression and localisation of somatostatin receptor subtypes sst1-sst5 in areas of the rat medulla oblongata involved in autonomic regulation. *J. Chem. Neuroanat.* 35, 49–66.

Spier, A. D., and de Lecea, L. (2000). Cortistatin: a member of the somatostatin neuropeptide family with distinct physiological functions. *Brain Res. Brain Res. Rev.* 33, 228–241.

Stengel, A., Coskun, T., Goebel, M., Wang, L., Craft, L., Alsina-Fernandez, J., et al. (2010a). Central injection of the stable somatostatin analog ODT8-SST induces a somatostatin2 receptor-mediated orexigenic effect: role of neuropeptide Y and opioid signaling pathways in rats. *Endocrinology* 151, 4224–4235.

Stengel, A., Goebel, M., Luckey, A., Yuan, P. Q., Wang, L., and Taché, Y. (2010b). Cold ambient temperature reverses abdominal surgery-induced delayed gastric emptying, and decreased plasma ghrelin levels in rats. *Peptides* 31, 2229–2235.

Stengel, A., Goebel, M., Wang, L., Rivier, J., Kobelt, P., Mönnikes, H., et al. (2010c). Activation of brain somatostatin(2) receptors stimulates feeding in mice: analysis of food intake microstructure. *Physiol. Behav.* 101, 614–622.

Stengel, A., Goebel, M., Wang, L., Rivier, J., Kobelt, P., Mönnikes, H., et al. (2010d). Selective central activation of somatostatin2 receptor increases food intake, grooming behavior and rectal temperature in rats. *J. Physiol. Pharmacol.* 61, 399–407.

Stengel, A., Goebel, M., Wang, L., and Taché, Y. (2010e). Ghrelin, des-acyl ghrelin, and nesfatin-1 in gastric X/A-like cells: role as regulators of food intake and body weight. *Peptides* 31, 357–369.

Stengel, A., Goebel, M., Wang, L., Taché, Y., Sachs, G., and Lambrecht, N. W. (2010f). Differential distribution of ghrelin-*O*-acyltransferase (GOAT) immunoreactive cells in the mouse and rat gastric oxyntic mucosa. *Biochem. Biophys. Res. Commun.* 392, 67–71.

Stengel, A., Goebel-Stengel, M., Wang, L., Larauche, M., Rivier, J., and Taché, Y. (2011a). Central somatostatin receptor 1 activation reverses acute stress-related alterations of gastric, and colonic motor function in mice. *Neurogastroenterol. Motil.* 23, e223–e236.

Stengel, A., Goebel-Stengel, M., Wang, L., Luckey, A., Hu, E., Rivier, J., et al. (2011b). Central administration of pan-somatostatin agonist ODT8-SST prevents abdominal surgery-induced inhibition of circulating ghrelin, food intake and gastric emptying in rats. *Neurogastroenterol. Motil.* 23, e294–e308.

Stengel, A., Goebel-Stengel, M., Wang, L., Shaikh, A., Lambrecht, N. W., Rivier, J. E., et al. (2011c). Abdominal surgery inhibits circulating acyl ghrelin, and ghrelin-*O*-acyltransferase levels in rats: role of the somatostatin receptor subtype 2. *Am. J. Physiol. Gastrointest. Liver Physiol.* 301, G239–G248.

Stengel, A., Keire, D., Goebel, M., Evilevitch, L., Wiggins, B., Taché, Y., et al. (2009). The RAPID method for blood processing yields new insight in plasma concentrations and molecular forms of circulating gut peptides. *Endocrinology* 150, 5113–5118.

Sternini, C., Wong, H., Wu, S. V., de Giorgio, R., Yang, M., Reeve, J. Jr., et al. (1997). Somatostatin 2A receptor is expressed by enteric neurons, and by interstitial cells of Cajal and enterochromaffin-like cells of the gastrointestinal tract. *J. Comp. Neurol.* 386, 396–408.

Strassburg, S., Anker, S., Castaneda, T., Burget, L., Perez-Tilve, D., Pfluger, P. T., et al. (2008). Long-term effects of ghrelin and ghrelin receptor agonists on energy balance in rats. *Am. J. Physiol. Endocrinol. Metab.* 295, E78–E84.

Strowski, M. Z., Parmar, R. M., Blake, A. D., and Schaeffer, J. M. (2000). Somatostatin inhibits insulin and glucagon secretion via two receptors subtypes: an in vitro study of pancreatic islets from somatostatin receptor 2 knockout mice. *Endocrinology* 141, 111–117.

Sun, Y., Ahmed, S., and Smith, R. G. (2003). Deletion of ghrelin impairs neither growth nor appetite. *Mol. Cell. Biol.* 23, 7973–7981.

Sun, Y., Wang, P., Zheng, H., and Smith, R. G. (2004). Ghrelin stimulation of growth hormone release and appetite is mediated through the growth hormone secretagogue receptor. *Proc. Natl. Acad. Sci. U.S.A.* 101, 4679–4684.

Suzuki, K., Jayasena, C. N., and Bloom, S. R. (2011). The gut hormones in appetite regulation. *J. Obes.* 2011, 528401.

Taal, B. G., and Visser, O. (2004). Epidemiology of neuroendocrine tumours. *Neuroendocrinology* 80 (Suppl. 1), 3–7.

Taché, Y., and Bonaz, B. (2007). Corticotropin-releasing factor receptors and stress-related alterations of gut motor function. *J. Clin. Invest.* 117, 33–40.

Tang-Christensen, M., Vrang, N., Ortmann, S., Bidlingmaier, M., Horvath,

T. L., and Tschöp, M. (2004). Central administration of ghrelin and agouti-related protein (83–132) increases food intake and decreases spontaneous locomotor activity in rats. *Endocrinology* 45, 4645–4652.

Tansy, M. F., Martin, J. S., Landin, W. E., and Kendall, F. M. (1979). Species difference in GI motor response to somatostatin. *J. Pharm. Sci.* 68, 1107–1113.

Tebbe, J. J., Pasat, I. R., Mönnikes, H., Ritter, M., Kobelt, P., and Schafer, M. K. (2005). Excitatory stimulation of neurons in the arcuate nucleus initiates central CRF-dependent stimulation of colonic propulsion in rats. *Brain Res.* 1036, 130–138.

Thoss, V. S., Perez, J., Duc, D., and Hoyer, D. (1995). Embryonic and postnatal mRNA distribution of five somatostatin receptor subtypes in the rat brain. *Neuropharmacology* 34, 1673–1688.

Tizabi, Y., and Calogero, A. E. (1992). Effect of various neurotransmitters and neuropeptides on the release of corticotropin-releasing hormone from the rat cortex in vitro. *Synapse* 10, 341–348.

Toshinai, K., Mondal, M. S., Nakazato, M., Date, Y., Murakami, N., Kojima, M., et al. (2001). Upregulation of ghrelin expression in the stomach upon fasting, insulin-induced hypoglycemia, and leptin administration. *Biochem. Biophys. Res. Commun.* 281, 1220–1225.

Tringali, G., Greco, M. C., Lisi, L., Pozzoli, G., and Navarra, P. (2012). Cortistatin modulates the expression and release of corticotrophin releasing hormone in rat brain. Comparison with somatostatin and octreotide. *Peptides* 34, 353–359.

Tschöp, M., Smiley, D. L., and Heiman, M. L. (2000). Ghrelin induces adiposity in rodents. *Nature* 407, 908–913.

Tschöp, M., Wawarta, R., Riepl, R. L., Friedrich, S., Bidlingmaier, M., Landgraf, R., et al. (2001a). Post-prandial decrease of circulating human ghrelin levels. *J. Endocrinol. Invest.* 24, RC19–RC21.

Tschöp, M., Weyer, C., Tataranni, P. A., Devanarayan, V., Ravussin, E., and Heiman, M. L. (2001b). Circulating ghrelin levels are decreased in human obesity. *Diabetes* 50, 707–709.

Tsolakis, A. V., Portela-Gomes, G. M., Stridsberg, M., Grimelius, L., Sundin, A., Eriksson, B. K., et al. (2004). Malignant gastric ghrelinoma with hyperghrelinemia. *J. Clin. Endocrinol. Metab.* 89, 3739–3744.

Uhl, G. R., Tran, V., Snyder, S. H., and Martin, J. B. (1985). Somatostatin receptors: distribution in rat central nervous system and human frontal cortex. *J. Comp. Neurol.* 240, 288–304.

van der Hoek, J., Lamberts, S. W., and Hofland, L. J. (2010). The somatostatin receptor subtype 5 in neuroendocrine tumours. *Expert Opin. Investig. Drugs* 19, 385–399.

Veldhuis, J. D., Iranmanesh, A., Mielke, K., Miles, J. M., Carpenter, P. C., and Bowers, C. Y. (2006). Ghrelin potentiates growth hormone secretion driven by putative somatostatin withdrawal and resists inhibition by human corticotropin-releasing hormone. *J. Clin. Endocrinol. Metab.* 91, 2441–2446.

Viollet, C., Prevost, G., Maubert, E., Faivre-Bauman, A., Gardette, R., Kordon, C., et al. (1995). Molecular pharmacology of somatostatin receptors. *Fundam. Clin. Pharmacol.* 9, 107–113.

Viollet, C., Vaillend, C., Videau, C., Bluet-Pajot, M. T., Ungerer, A., L'Heritier, A., et al. (2000). Involvement of sst2 somatostatin receptor in locomotor, exploratory activity and emotional reactivity in mice. *Eur. J. Neurosci.* 12, 3761–3770.

Volante, M., Allia, E., Gugliotta, P., Funaro, A., Broglio, F., Deghenghi, R., et al. (2002). Expression of ghrelin and of the GH secretagogue receptor by pancreatic islet cells and related endocrine tumors. *J. Clin. Endocrinol. Metab.* 87, 1300–1308.

Walsh, J. (1994). "Somatostatin," in *Physiology of the Gastrointestinal Tract*, ed. L. R. Johnson (New York: Raven Press), 31–48.

Wang, L., Goebel-Stengel, M., Stengel, A., Wu, S. V., Ohning, G., and Taché, Y. (2011). Comparison of CRF-immunoreactive neurons distribution in mouse and rat brains and selective induction of Fos in rat hypothalamic CRF neurons by abdominal surgery. *Brain Res.* 1415, 34–46.

Wren, A. M., Small, C. J., Ward, H. L., Murphy, K. G., Dakin, C. L., Taheri, S., et al. (2000). The novel hypothalamic peptide ghrelin stimulates food intake and growth hormone secretion. *Endocrinology* 141, 4325–4328.

Xidakis, C., Mastrodimou, N., Notas, G., Renieri, E., Kolios, G., Kouroumalis, E., et al. (2007). RT-PCR and immunocytochemistry studies support the presence of somatostatin, cortistatin and somatostatin receptor subtypes in rat Kupffer cells. *Regul. Pept.* 143, 76–82.

Xu, G., Li, Y., An, W., Li, S., Guan, Y., Wang, N., et al. (2009). Gastric mammalian target of rapamycin signaling regulates ghrelin production and food intake. *Endocrinology* 150, 3637–3644.

Yakabi, K., Noguchi, M., Ohno, S., Ro, S., Onouchi, T., Ochiai, M., et al. (2011). Urocortin 1 reduces food intake and ghrelin secretion via CRF(2) receptors. *Am. J. Physiol. Endocrinol. Metab.* 301, E72–E82.

Yamazaki, M., Nakamura, K., Kobayashi, H., Matsubara, M., Hayashi, Y., Kangawa, K., et al. (2002). Regulational effect of ghrelin on growth hormone secretion from perfused rat anterior pituitary cells. *J. Neuroendocrinol.* 14, 156–162.

Yang, H., Wong, H., Wu, V., Walsh, J. H., and Taché, Y. (1990). Somatostatin monoclonal antibody immunoneutralization increases gastrin and gastric acid secretion in urethane-anesthetized rats. *Gastroenterology* 99, 659–665.

Yang, J., Brown, M. S., Liang, G., Grishin, N. V., and Goldstein, J. L. (2008). Identification of the acyltransferase that octanoylates ghrelin, an appetite-stimulating peptide hormone. *Cell* 132, 387–396.

Zigman, J. M., Nakano, Y., Coppari, R., Balthasar, N., Marcus, J. N., Lee, C. E., et al. (2005). Mice lacking ghrelin receptors resist the development of diet-induced obesity. *J. Clin. Invest.* 115, 3564–3572.

11

Development of the hypothalamic melanocortin system

Berengere Coupe*[1,2] *and Sebastien G. Bouret*[1,2]*

[1] *Neuroscience Program, The Saban Research Institute, Children's Hospital Los Angeles, University of Southern California, Los Angeles, CA, USA*
[2] *U837, Neurobese Lab, INSERM, Jean-Pierre Aubert Research Center, University Lille 2, Lille, France*

Edited by:
Hubert Vaudry, University of Rouen, France

Reviewed by:
Robert Dores, University of Minnesota, USA
James A. Carr, Texas Tech University, USA

****Correspondence:***
Sebastien G. Bouret, Neuroscience Program, The Saban Research Institute, Children's Hospital Los Angeles, University of Southern California, 4650 Sunset Boulevard, MS#135, Los Angeles, CA 90027, USA.
e-mail: sbouret@chla.usc.edu

The melanocortin system is a critical component of the forebrain and hindbrain regulatory systems involved in energy balance. This system is composed of pro-opiomelanocortin (POMC) neurons that act, in part, through the melanocortin-4 receptor (MC4R). Although the importance of the melanocortin system in controlling feeding has been established for two decades, the understanding of the developmental substrates underlying POMC and MC4R neuron development and function has just begun to emerge. The formation of the melanocortin system involves several discrete developmental steps that include the birth and fate specification of POMC- and MC4R-containing neurons and the extension and guidance of POMC axons to their MC4R-expressing target nuclei. Each of these developmental processes appears to require specific sets of genes and developmental cues that include perinatal hormones. Recent evidence has also highlighted the importance of perinatal nutrition in controlling the ultimate architecture of the melanocortin system.

Keywords: pro-opiomelanocortin, αMSH, MC4R, hypothalamus, development, hormones, axon guidance, neurogenesis

INTRODUCTION

Pro-opiomelanocortin (POMC) neurons control a variety of physiological functions, the most characterized of which is the regulation of energy balance. They reduce food intake and increase energy expenditure by releasing α-melanocyte-stimulating hormone (αMSH), a product of POMC processing (Cone, 2006; Ellacott and Cone, 2006). More recent targeted deletion studies have specifically shown the importance of POMC neurons in mediating the physiological actions of metabolic hormones, such as leptin and insulin (Belgardt and Brüning, 2010; Williams and Elmquist, 2012). POMC neurons have a limited distribution across the central nervous system (CNS). POMC cell bodies are found only in two CNS nuclei: the arcuate nucleus of the hypothalamus (ARH) in the forebrain and the nucleus of the tractus solitarius (NTS) in the brain stem (Joseph et al., 1983; Cone, 2005). Recent data indicated that while hypothalamic POMC neurons appear to be more involved in integrating long-term adiposity signals, the contribution of hindbrain POMC neurons seem to be more specific to the integration of short-term satiety signals (Zhan et al., 2013). POMC neurons provide extensive projections to various parts of the brain, especially to the paraventricular (PVH) and dorsomedial (DMH) nuclei of the hypothalamus, the lateral hypothalamic area (LHA), and the ventral tegmental area (VTA). Each of these nuclei and areas also plays a major role in the central regulation of feeding behavior and energy balance (King and Hentges, 2011) (**Figure 1**).

Of the five known melanocortin receptors (MCRs), αMSH binds with various affinities to MC1R, MC3R, MC4R, and MC5R. However, it is the MC4R subtype that has been primarily implicated in the regulation of energy balance. The observation that deletion of the MC4R results in a phenotype that is a virtual carbon copy of POMC-deficient mice (including late onset of obesity and diabetes) strongly supports this idea (Huszar et al., 1997; Yaswen et al., 1999; Butler et al., 2001; Challis et al., 2004). Notably, mutations in the MC4R gene are the most common monogenic disorders that cause obesity in humans (Coll et al., 2007). MC4R is a G-protein-coupled receptor that has a widespread distribution throughout the CNS. MC4R mRNA is found in virtually every part of the brain, including the hypothalamus, thalamus, cortex, brainstem, and spinal cord (Mountjoy et al., 1994; Kishi et al., 2003). Soon after the cloning of the MC4R, agouti-related protein (AgRP), which is synthesized in the ARH, has been identified as an endogenous antagonist of the MC4R (Huszar et al., 1997; Ollmann et al., 1997).

This review attempts to summarize our current understanding of the development of the melanocortin system within the context of metabolic programing. Because of the lack of data on the development of POMC neurons in the NTS, this review will largely focus on the development of arcuate POMC neurons and their related hypothalamic MC4R pathways.

DEVELOPMENT OF THE MELANOCORTIN SYSTEM

The developmental processes that produce the melanocortin system can fall into two broad categories: the birth and determination of the neuronal phenotype of POMC- and MC4R-containing neurons and the formation of functional circuits, which includes POMC axon growth and synaptogenesis onto MC4R-responsive targets.

NEUROGENESIS

Classic experiments that used birth dating tools, such as the thymidine analog bromodeoxyuridine, revealed that the majority of POMC neurons in the mouse ARH are born primarily on embryonic day (E)11–E12 (Khachaturian et al., 1985; Padilla et al., 2010). However, some POMC neurons, which are located more laterally in the ARH, are generated as late as E13. Gene expression

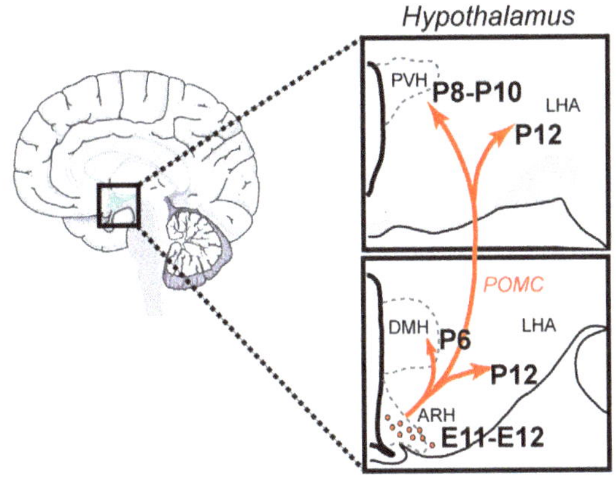

FIGURE 1 | Architecture and development of the POMC neural system in the mouse. POMC neurons located in the arcuate nucleus of the hypothalamus (ARH) send direct projections to discrete populations of neurons located in the dorsomedial (DMH) and paraventricular nuclei (PVH) of the hypothalamus and to the lateral hypothalamic area (LHA). Each of these regions plays a major role in the control of energy balance and feeding behavior. ARH POMC neurons are born at E11–E12 and innervate their target nuclei primarily during the first 2 weeks of postnatal life.

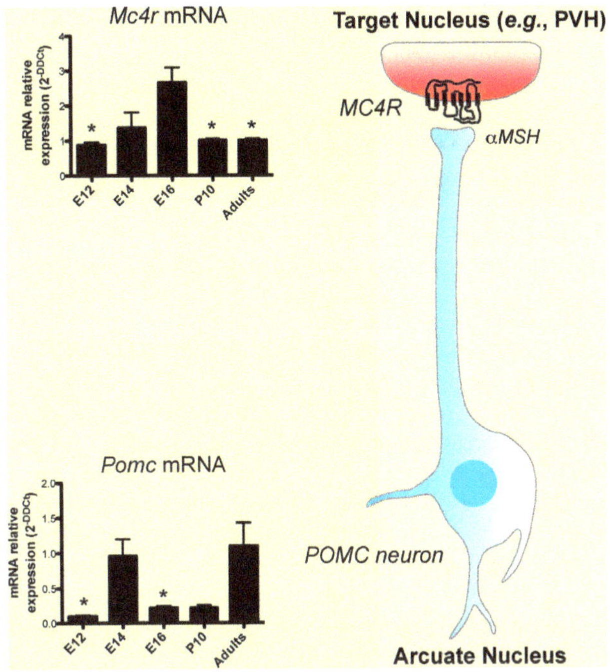

FIGURE 2 | Developmental regulation of the melanocortin system. Low levels of *Pomc* mRNA are found in the hypothalamus as early as embryonic day (E)12, i.e., soon after the birth of POMC neurons. *Pomc* mRNA exhibits a peak of expression on E14. POMC neurons act in part through the melanocortin-4 receptor (MC4R) to exert their effects. *Mc4r* mRNA is also found in the hypothalamus as early as on E12 and display a peak of expression on E16.

studies have also shown that neurons in the presumptive ARH first express POMC mRNA on E10–E12 (Padilla et al., 2010) (**Figure 2**), which is consistent with early determination of cell fate. Recent genetic cell lineage tracing studies confirmed this hypothesis and revealed that POMC neurons acquire their terminal phenotype at approximately E15 (Padilla et al., 2010). However, only a portion of embryonic *Pomc*-expressing precursors adopts a POMC fate in adult mice. Half of *Pomc*-expressing precursors acquire a non-POMC fate in adult mice and nearly one quarter of the mature NPY neurons in the ARH share a common progenitor with POMC cells (Padilla et al., 2010). These data show the unique property of *Pomc*-expressing progenitors with respect to giving rise to antagonistic neuronal populations.

DEVELOPMENT OF POMC-CONTAINING AXONAL PROJECTION

The ontogeny of the POMC neuronal projections remains to be determined specifically. However, axonal tract tracing experiments in mice have revealed that ARH projections are largely immature at birth and develop postnatally during the first 2 weeks of postnatal life. By P6, ARH projections extend through the periventricular zone of the hypothalamus to provide inputs to the DMH first, followed by inputs to the PVH between P8 and P10. Projections from the ARH to the LHA develop significantly later, with the mature pattern of innervation first apparent on P12. Not until P18 does the pattern of ARH axonal projections achieve a distribution that resembles that seen in the adult (Bouret et al., 2004a). These findings suggest that the development of ARH POMC axonal projections toward each of their target nuclei does not occur until the second week of postnatal life, i.e., at a time that is far removed from the birth of these neurons (E11–E12). At the synaptic levels, Colmers and collaborators showed that there is an age-dependent increase in the electrophysiological response of specific sets of PVH neurons to melanocortin, with a maximal response observed at P28–P35 (Melnick et al., 2007). These results suggest that synapses between POMC axons and PVH MC4R-containing neurons are not structurally and functionally mature until puberty.

DEVELOPMENTAL REGULATION OF MC4R

In spite of the importance of MC4R in energy balance regulation, we still know relatively little about the exact time point at which the assembly of this system is fully established. For example, we still do not know when MC4R neurons are born or when MC4R becomes functional and able to signal. Nevertheless, the fact that peripheral injection of the MCR agonist MTII reduces milk intake and body weight as early as during the first 2 weeks of postnatal life suggests that MC4R receptors might be present and functional in the hypothalamus at this age (Glavas et al., 2007). Consistent with this idea, *in situ* hybridization analysis shows that MC4R mRNA is abundant in the hypothalamus and especially in the PVH at P10 (**Figure 2**). That peripheral injection of MTII induces strong activation of cFos immunoreactivity (a marker of neuronal activation) in the PVH at P5–P15 further supports the functionality of MC4R in the PVH during early postnatal life (Glavas et al., 2007). At the molecular level, it was shown that MC4R mRNA is first expressed at E12 in the proliferative zone surrounding the lower portion of the third ventricle (also known as the neurepithelium) and that this mRNA expression peaks at E16 (**Figure 2**) (Mountjoy and Wild, 1998). These findings are particularly interesting because it is known that neurons that compose various hypothalamic nuclei in adults are primarily derived from precursors that originate from this proliferative zone, raising the possibility that MC4R could be involved in hypothalamic neurogenesis. Supporting this hypothesis, melanocortins stimulate astrocyte proliferation *in vitro* (Zohar and Salomon, 1992). Other brains sites express MC4R during embryonic development. In addition to being expressed in the diencephalic neurepithelium, MC4R mRNA is also found in the telencephalon and the lamina terminalis at E14 (Mountjoy and Wild, 1998). By E19, MC4R mRNA is widely expressed throughout the brain (Mountjoy and Wild, 1998).

HORMONAL REGULATION OF POMC NEURONS DURING EARLY LIFE

Accumulating evidence suggests that there are physiological differences in the regulation of energy balance between adults and neonates. For example, in sharp contrast to the effects of leptin on adults, several groups have reported that exogenous leptin does not significantly inhibit growth, food intake, or energy expenditure until after weaning (Mistry et al., 1999; Ahima and Hileman, 2000; Schmidt et al., 2001; Proulx et al., 2002). Similarly, in contrast to the well-known orexigenic effects of ghrelin in mature animals, exogenous ghrelin does not significantly promote milk intake in the first 2–3 postnatal weeks (Piao et al., 2008; Steculorum and Bouret, 2011a). The general thinking has been that the neonatal brain is relatively insensitive to metabolic hormones. However, both leptin and ghrelin receptors are expressed in the ARH during early postnatal life (Caron et al., 2010; Steculorum and Bouret, 2011a) and these receptors can initiate cellular responses, particularly in POMC neurons. First, acute peripheral leptin treatment in mice on P10 induces phosphorylation of STAT3 and ERK (two major leptin receptor signaling pathways) in 20–35% of ARH POMC neurons (Caron et al., 2010; Bouret et al., 2012). The same leptin treatment increases *Pomc* mRNA levels in the rat ARH (Proulx et al., 2002). Second, acute peripheral ghrelin treatment in P10 mice causes a reduction in *Pomc* gene expression in the ARH (Steculorum and Bouret, 2011a). Collectively, these findings provide convincing evidence that POMC neurons contain functional receptors for metabolic hormones such as leptin and ghrelin during the postnatal period, and suggest that the "hormone insensitivity" observed during this period could instead be from a failure of these cells to relay hormonal signals to other parts of the hypothalamus.

MECHANISMS UNDERLYING POMC NEURON DEVELOPMENT

The process of developing highly specialized cellular structures, such as POMC neurons require tight temporal and regional regulation of expression for specific sets of genes and developmental cues. A variety of genetic tools are now available to specifically identify the cellular and molecular pathways that are involved in POMC neuronal development.

MECHANISMS UNDERLYING CELL FATE SPECIFICATION: THE ROLE OF TRANSCRIPTION FACTORS

While the specific programs involved in the determination of POMC terminal fates are unknown, recent data investigating the role of the Mash1-neurogenin 3 (Ngn3) pathway provides some clues as to the role of these transcription factors in the differentiation of the POMC lineage. Using a mouse model of Mash1 deficiency (Mash1−/− mice), McNay et al. (2006) found that this basic helix-loop-helix transcription factor has a pro-neural function and act upstream of Ngn3 to regulate neurogenesis in the ventral hypothalamus. Loss of Mash1 blunts Ngn3 expression in ARH progenitors and is associated with a dramatic reduction in the number of POMC-expressing cells at E12. More recent genetic fate mapping and loss of function studies in mice further demonstrated that the expression of Ngn3 in progenitor cells promotes the development of arcuate POMC neurons (Pelling et al., 2011). Based on the recent observations that a subset of *Pomc*-expressing progenitors in the ARH differentiates into functional mature NPY neurons (Padilla et al., 2010), it would also be interesting to determine the molecular mechanisms that underlie this developmental switch.

CUES INVOLVED IN AXON GROWTH AND AXON GUIDANCE

The precise molecular mechanisms that are responsible for the formation of POMC circuits are only beginning to be understood. In general, axon development comprises two aspects: the physical act of extension and the molecular mechanisms underlying this process. Axons grow by sending out a highly plastic and sensitive structure called a "growth cone," which travels toward the target and trails behind it the elongating neurite. As noted above, neonatal POMC neurons express LepRb, and the administration of leptin to mouse neonates results in the activation of major LepRb signaling pathways, including pSTAT3 and pERK in POMC neurons, specifically (Caron et al., 2010; Bouret et al., 2012). Recent anatomical data showed that one of the key factors in controlling the development of POMC neural circuits appears to be the expression of LepRb by POMC neurons (**Table 1**). Direct exposure of ARH explants *in vitro* to leptin promotes axon growth (Bouret et al., 2004b). In addition, mice or rats that lack functional LepRb signaling ($Lepr^{db}/Lepr^{db}$ mice and fa/fa rats, respectively) display a reduced density of ARH POMC projections to the PVH (Bouret and Simerly, 2007; Bouret et al., 2012). Similarly, the density of αMSH-immunoreactive fibers is also markedly reduced in the PVH of s/s mice that lack functional LepRb → STAT3 signaling (Bouret et al., 2012). This observation raises the importance of this signaling pathway, specifically, in the development of POMC neural projections. However, not all LepRb signaling pathways play a role in the formation of POMC projections. For example,

Table 1 | List of genetic and pathological conditions that alter development of POMC-derived neural projections.

Animal model	Reference
Leptin-deficient (Lep^{ob}/Lep^{ob}) mouse	Bouret et al. (2004b)
Leptin receptor ($Lepr^{db}/Lepr^{db}$) null mouse	Bouret et al. (2012)
LepRb → pSTAT3 (s/s) null mouse	Bouret et al. (2012)
Obese (fa/fa) Zucker rat	Bouret and Simerly (2007)
Obesity-prone DIO rat	Bouret et al. (2008)
Maternal obesity	Kirk et al. (2009)
Maternal diabetes	Steculorum and Bouret (2011b)
Maternal caloric restriction	Delahaye et al. (2008)
Maternal low-protein diet	Coupe et al. (2010)
Postnatal overfeeding	Bouret et al. (2007)

mice that lack LepRb → ERK signaling (l/l mice) display comparable densities of αMSH-immunoreactive fibers in the PVH compared to wild-type mice (Bouret et al., 2012). Of particular importance is the fact that leptin appears to exert its developmental action on POMC neural projections during a discrete developmental critical period. POMC neuronal projections are disrupted in leptin-deficient (Lep^{ob}/Lep^{ob}) mice, and exogenous leptin treatment during the first 2 weeks of postnatal life rescues these projections (Bouret et al., 2004b). In contrast, the treatment of adult Lep^{ob}/Lep^{ob} mice with leptin is relatively ineffective and does not increase the density of αMSH fibers in the PVH to levels that are characteristic of wild-type mice (Bouret et al., 2004b).

Growing POMC axons must then choose a path to follow and must decide the direction to go on this path to innervate the proper nucleus (e.g., the PVH). The pathways are defined by cell–cell interactions and diffusible chemorepulsive and chemoattractive cues (Tessier-Lavigne and Goodman, 1996). Notably, the diffusible axon guidance cues Netrin, Slit, and Semaphorins are highly expressed in the PVH during development (Xu and Fan, 2008), and POMC terminals express the semaphorin receptor neuropilin 1 (LeGuern and Bouret, unpublished data). Supporting a role for neuropilins/semaphorins in POMC axon guidance, a loss of neuropilin 1 receptors in POMC neurons disrupts the development of POMC axonal projections to the PVH, specifically (LeGuern and Bouret, unpublished data). The formation of POMC neural connections also likely involves cell adhesion molecules. Supporting this idea, mice that are deficient in contactin, a cell adhesion molecule that is involved in the formation of axonal projections, display reduced density of αMSH-immunoreactive fibers in the PVH during postnatal development (Fetissov et al., 2005).

CELLULAR MECHANISMS INVOLVED IN POMC NEURON DEVELOPMENT: ROLE OF AUTOPHAGY

The development of POMC neurons also requires massive cytoplasmic remodeling. Autophagy is one of the major cellular degradation processes in which parts of the cytoplasm and intracellular organelles are engulfed within double-membraned vesicles, known as autophagosomes (Klionsky, 2007). An important function of autophagy is to promote cell growth, development, and homeostasis, by maintaining a balance between the synthesis, degradation, and subsequent recycling of cellular components (Levine and Klionsky, 2004; Maiuri et al., 2007; Cecconi and Levine, 2008). Recent morphological data revealed that autophagy is constitutively present in the hypothalamus during important periods of development, including in POMC neuron perikarya and processes such as dendrites (Coupe et al., 2012). Consistent with a functional role for autophagy in POMC neurons, conditional deletion of essential autophagy genes, such as the autophagy-related gene (Atg) 7, results in obesity and impaired glucose homeostasis (Coupe et al., 2012; Kaushik et al., 2012; Quan et al., 2012). These metabolic disturbances are associated with neurodevelopmental abnormalities. Neonates lacking ATG7 in POMC neurons display a reduced density of POMC-containing projections to each of their target nuclei, including the PVH, DMH, and LHA (Coupe et al., 2012). These structural abnormalities persist throughout adult life and appear to be the result of a diminished capacity of POMC neurons for extending axons (Coupe et al., 2012). However, not all of the developmental processes are affected by autophagy deficiency. No changes in POMC cell numbers were reported in mice that lacked autophagy in POMC neurons (Coupe et al., 2012; Kaushik et al., 2012; Quan et al., 2012), which suggests that autophagy does not influence neurogenesis or programed cell death and that instead it has a specific role in axon growth.

PATHOLOGICAL CONDITIONS THAT ALTER MELANOCORTIN SYSTEM DEVELOPMENT

MATERNAL OBESITY AND/OR DIABETES

In the United States, epidemiological studies have estimated that 20% of women are obese when they conceive (Johnson et al., 2006). This disturbing observation highlights the importance of evaluating the outcomes of maternal obesity in the offspring. Maternal high-fat diet (HFD) feeding during pregnancy is most likely the most widely used approach for studying the consequences of maternal obesity. Notably, offspring born to obese females fed an HFD (45–60% of calories from fat) during gestation only or during both gestation and lactation become progressively overweight, hyperphagic, and glucose intolerant, and they display an increase in adiposity (Chen et al., 2009; Kirk et al., 2009). The model of diet-induced obesity (DIO) developed by Levin et al. (1997) also provides a valuable tool for the study of obesity, in part because Levin's DIO rats share several features with human obesity, including polygenic inheritance. This animal model is therefore particularly well suited for the study of the relative contribution of genetic versus environmental factors in metabolic programing. Impaired organization of POMC neural circuits is a common feature of maternal obesity (**Table 1**). Animals born to either high-fat fed or obese-prone DIO dams display a reduced density of αMSH fibers innervating the PVH (Bouret et al., 2008; Kirk et al., 2009). In DIO rats, the abnormal development of POMC projections appears to be the result of a diminished response to the neurotrophic action of leptin during the early postnatal period (Bouret et al., 2008). In addition, a significant remodeling of synapses onto POMC neurons has been observed in DIO rats, particularly in response to nutritional challenges (Horvath et al., 2010). DIO rats fed a chow diet display increased inhibitory inputs to POMC neurons compared to obesity-resistant DR rats. In addition, DIO rats fed a HFD display a loss of synapses onto POMC neurons, whereas high-fat feeding in control (DR) rats causes an increase in POMC synaptic coverage (Horvath et al., 2010).

However, one caveat to keep in mind is that almost all of the animal models of maternal obesity are also hyperglycemic and insulin-resistant. This complication makes it difficult to differentiate the detrimental effects of maternal obesity *per se* as opposed to maternal diabetes. Nevertheless, the manipulation of glucose and insulin levels without an alteration of the diet can be performed experimentally by injecting streptozotocin, a pancreatic beta-cell toxin. Using this approach, we recently found that maternal diabetes alone (i.e., without maternal obesity) can cause a reduction in the density of αMSH-immunoreactive projections to the PVH (Steculorum and Bouret, 2011b) (**Table 1**).

Importantly, an increase in the POMC cell number is observed in the ARH of pups that were born to diabetic dams (Steculorum and Bouret, 2011b), which supports the hypothesis that the low density of POMC-derived fibers is more likely the result of alterations in POMC axon growth as opposed to a reduction in cell numbers.

MATERNAL MALNUTRITION

Interest in maternal malnutrition is also particularly high given its high prevalence in underdeveloped countries and the evidence regarding its disease-promoting potential in offspring. Animal models commonly used to study the consequences of maternal malnutrition include caloric restriction and a low-protein diet during pregnancy and lactation. Maternal malnutrition (caused either by caloric restriction or a low-protein diet) affects the overall organization of POMC neural circuits by altering the density of αMSH-containing axons (Delahaye et al., 2008; Coupe et al., 2010) (**Table 1**). However, if pups born to malnourished dams do not exhibit a rapid catch-up growth, this reduction of POMC innervation is associated with an increased sensitivity to the anorexigenic effect of the melanocortin agonist MTII (Stocker et al., 2012). Therefore, the timing of catch-up growth appears to be an important determinant for the lifelong regulation of the melanocortin system. Supporting this hypothesis, although early catch-up growth ameliorates the abnormal organization of POMC pathways observed in pups born to protein-restricted dams and is highly beneficial for markers of brain development, including markers of cell adhesion and axon elongation, late catch-up growth causes permanent structural defects of POMC neural projections (Coupe et al., 2010).

POSTNATAL OVERFEEDING/OBESITY

Because of the importance of hypothalamic development during postnatal life, including the melanocortin system, in rodents, animal models of postnatal metabolic programing are particularly relevant. An animal model that has proven to be extremely fruitful for the study of postnatal overfeeding is the divergent litter size model. In this model, pups are raised in small litters (SL) from birth to weaning to induce accelerated growth during the pre-weaning period. Postnatally overfed animals show increased adult body weight and an accelerated and exacerbated weight gain when fed an HFD (Glavas et al., 2010). Chronic postnatal overfeeding is associated with a reduced activity of the melanocortin system. For example, rats raised in SL display an overall decrease in the expression of *Pomc* gene expression (Srinivasan et al., 2008; Chen et al., 2009). The observed changes appear to reflect an acquired mechanism that originates from a malprograming of the hypothalamic melanocortin system during early life rather than being a consequence of metabolic dysfunctions, such as overweight and hyperphagia. Consistent with this idea, changes in POMC innervation to the PVH are observed as early as during the first postnatal weeks in neonatally overfed mice, i.e., prior to the development of overweight and hyperphagia (Bouret et al., 2007). In addition to its adverse effects on the *Pomc* gene expression, postnatal overfeeding affects the neuronal response to melanocortins. For example, PVH neurons of chronically overfed pups display reduced electrophysiological responses to αMSH (Davidowa et al., 2003).

EPIGENETIC CHANGES

Epigenetic mechanisms of gene regulation, such as DNA methylation and histone modifications (e.g., methylation, acetylation, ubiquitination) can regulate gene expression in response to environmental stimuli. Given that *Pomc* expression can be affected by the prenatal or early postnatal diet (see above) many groups have investigated whether epigenetic modifications of the POMC promoter occur during the neonatal period in response to nutritional insults. Using a bisulfite sequencing approach, Plagemann and colleagues studied the methylation status of CpG dinucleotides of the *Pomc* promoter in rats that were raised in SL and found that postnatal overfeeding causes hypermethylation of the *Pomc* promoter. Interestingly, this hypermethylation occurs within the two Sp1-related binding sequences of the *Pomc* promoter (Sp1, NF-KB), which are essential for mediating the effect of leptin and insulin on *Pomc* gene expression (Plagemann et al., 2009). Similarly, recent human studies showed that childhood obesity is associated with POMC hypermethylation (Kuehnen et al., 2012). In contrast, methylation of the fetal hypothalamic *Pomc* promoter is reduced in underfed sheep, which is associated with reduced DNA methyltransferase activity and altered histone methylation and acetylation (Begum et al., 2012). In addition, rat neonates from protein-restricted dams display a reduction of hypothalamic Dnmt1 and Dmnt3a mRNA expression (Coupe et al., 2010).

CONCLUSION

At a time when obesity, including in children, is reaching epidemic proportions, it appears crucial to better understand the biological processes that mediate the development of metabolic systems. The melanocortin system plays an important role in this process, and recent studies are providing knowledge on how POMC- and MC4R-containing neurons develop. These studies have also revealed that changes in the hormonal and nutritional milieu during critical periods of life can permanently influence the development and functional activity of the melanocortin system. This finding could represent a key mechanism for effecting long-term changes in weight regulation in response to perinatal insults. It also opens new avenues for understanding congenital eating disorders, such as Prader–Willi syndrome. However, if we want to design therapeutic interventions to reverse the metabolic programing of the fetus and/or neonate, it remains to show the periods of vulnerability for the melanocortin system in humans, which most likely proceeds on a timeline of months, compared to days in rodents.

ACKNOWLEDGMENTS

Work in the authors' laboratory is supported by grants from the National Institute of Health (Grant DK84142), the Foundation for Prader–Willi Research, the "Fondation pour la Recherche Médicale," the EU FP7 integrated project (grant agreement no. 266408, "Full4Health"), and the "Agence Nationale de la Recherche" (Grants ANR-08-JCJC-0055-01 and ANR-11-BSV1-021-02).

REFERENCES

Ahima, R. S., and Hileman, S. M. (2000). Postnatal regulation of hypothalamic neuropeptide expression by leptin: implications for energy balance and body weight regulation. *Regul. Pept.* 92, 1–7.

Begum, G., Stevens, A., Smith, E. B., Connor, K., Challis, J. R. G., Bloomfield, F., et al. (2012). Epigenetic changes in fetal hypothalamic energy regulating pathways are associated with maternal undernutrition and twinning. *FASEB J.* 26, 1694–1703.

Belgardt, B. F., and Brüning, J. C. (2010). CNS leptin and insulin action in the control of energy homeostasis. *Ann. N. Y. Acad. Sci.* 1212, 97–113.

Bouret, S., and Simerly, R. B. (2007). Development of leptin-sensitive circuits. *J. Neuroendocrinol.* 19, 575–582.

Bouret, S. G., Bates, S. H., Chen, S., Myers, M. G., and Simerly, R. B. (2012). Distinct roles for specific leptin receptor signals in the development of hypothalamic feeding circuits. *J. Neurosci.* 32, 1244–1252.

Bouret, S. G., Burt-Solorzano, C., Wang, C.-H., and Simerly, R. B. (2007). "Impact of neonatal nutrition on development of brain metabolic circuits in mice," in *Proceedings of the 37th Annual Meeting the Society for Neuroscience*, San Diego.

Bouret, S. G., Draper, S. J., and Simerly, R. B. (2004a). Formation of projection pathways from the arcuate nucleus of the hypothalamus to hypothalamic regions implicated in the neural control of feeding behavior in mice. *J. Neurosci.* 24, 2797–2805.

Bouret, S. G., Draper, S. J., and Simerly, R. B. (2004b). Trophic action of leptin on hypothalamic neurons that regulate feeding. *Science* 304, 108–110.

Bouret, S. G., Gorski, J. N., Patterson, C. M., Chen, S., Levin, B. E., and Simerly, R. B. (2008). Hypothalamic neural projections are permanently disrupted in diet-induced obese rats. *Cell Metab.* 7, 179–185.

Butler, A. A., Marks, D. L., Fan, W., Kuhn, C. M., Bartolome, M., and Cone, R. D. (2001). Melanocortin-4 receptor is required for acute homeostatic responses to increased dietary fat. *Nat. Neurosci.* 4, 605–611.

Caron, E., Sachot, C., Prevot, V., and Bouret, S. G. (2010). Distribution of leptin-sensitive cells in the postnatal and adult mouse brain. *J. Comp. Neurol.* 518, 459–476.

Cecconi, F., and Levine, B. (2008). The role of autophagy in mammalian development: cell makeover rather than cell death. *Dev. Cell* 15, 344–357.

Challis, B. G., Coll, A. P., Yeo, G. S. H., Pinnock, S. B., Dickson, S. L., Thresher, R. R., et al. (2004). Mice lacking pro-opiomelanocortin are sensitive to high-fat feeding but respond normally to the acute anorectic effects of peptide-YY3-36. *Proc. Natl. Acad. Sci. U.S.A.* 101, 4695–4700.

Chen, H., Simar, D., and Morris, M. J. (2009). Hypothalamic neuroendocrine circuitry is programmed by maternal obesity: interaction with postnatal nutritional environment. *PLoS ONE* 4:e6259. doi:10.1371/journal.pone.0006259

Coll, A. P., Farooqi, I. S., and O'Rahilly, S. (2007). The hormonal control of food intake. *Cell* 129, 251–262.

Cone, R. D. (2005). Anatomy and regulation of the central melanocortin system. *Nat. Neurosci.* 8, 571–578.

Cone, R. D. (2006). Studies on the physiological functions of the melanocortin system. *Endocr. Rev.* 27, 736–749.

Coupe, B., Amarger, V., Grit, I., Benani, A., and Parnet, P. (2010). Nutritional programming affects hypothalamic organization and early response to leptin. *Endocrinology* 151, 702–713.

Coupe, B., Ishii, Y., Dietrich, M. O., Komatsu, M., Horvath, T. L., and Bouret, S. G. (2012). Loss of autophagy in pro-opiomelanocortin neurons perturbs axon growth and causes metabolic dysregulation. *Cell Metab.* 15, 247–255.

Davidowa, H., Li, Y., and Plagemann, A. (2003). Altered responses to orexigenic (AGRP, MCH) and anorexigenic (a-MSH, CART) neuropeptides of paraventricular hypothalamic neurons in early postnatally overfed rats. *Eur. J. Neurosci.* 18, 613–621.

Delahaye, F., Breton, C., Risold, P.-Y., Enache, M., Dutriez-Casteloot, I., Laborie, C., et al. (2008). Maternal perinatal undernutrition drastically reduces postnatal leptin surge and affects the development of arcuate nucleus proopiomelanocortin neurons in neonatal male rat pups. *Endocrinology* 149, 470–475.

Ellacott, K., and Cone, R. (2006). The role of the central melanocortin system in the regulation of food intake and energy homeostasis: lessons from mouse models. *Philos. Trans. R. Soc. Lond. B Boil. Sci.* 361, 1265–1274.

Fetissov, S. O., Bergstrom, U., Johansen, J. E., Hokfelt, T., Schalling, M., and Ranscht, B. (2005). Alterations of arcuate nucleus neuropeptidergic development in contactin-deficient mice: comparison with anorexia and food-deprived mice. *Eur. J. Neurosci.* 22, 3217–3228.

Glavas, M. M., Joachim, S. E., Draper, S. J., Smith, M. S., and Grove, K. L. (2007). Melanocortinergic activation by melanotan II inhibits feeding and increases uncoupling protein 1 messenger ribonucleic acid in the developing rat. *Endocrinology* 148, 3279–3287.

Glavas, M. M., Kirigiti, M. A., Xiao, X. Q., Enriori, P. J., Fisher, S. K., Evans, A. E., et al. (2010). Early overnutrition results in early-onset arcuate leptin resistance and increased sensitivity to high-fat diet. *Endocrinology* 151, 1598–1610.

Horvath, T. L., Sarman, B., García-Cáceres, C., Enriori, P. J., Sotonyi, P., Shanabrough, M., et al. (2010). Synaptic input organization of the melanocortin system predicts diet-induced hypothalamic reactive gliosis and obesity. *Proc. Natl. Acad. Sci. U.S.A.* 107, 14875–14880.

Huszar, D., Lynch, C. A., Fairchild-Huntress, V., Dunmore, J. H., Fang, Q., Berkemeier, L. R., et al. (1997). Targeted disruption of the melanocortin-4 receptor results in obesity in mice. *Cell* 88, 131–141.

Johnson, K., Posner, S. F., Biermann, J., Cordero, J. F., Atrash, H. K., Parker, C. S., et al. (2006). Recommendations to improve preconception health and health care – United States. A report of the CDC/ATSDR preconception care work group and the select panel on preconception care. *MMWR Recomm. Rep.* 55, 1–23.

Joseph, S. A., Pilcher, W. H., and Bennett-Clarke, C. (1983). Immunocytochemical localization of ACTH perikarya in nucleus tractus solitarius: evidence for a second opiocortin neuronal system. *Neurosci. Lett.* 38, 221–225.

Kaushik, S., Arias, E., Kwon, H., Lopez, N. M., Athonvarangkul, D., Sahu, S., et al. (2012). Loss of autophagy in hypothalamic POMC neurons impairs lipolysis. *EMBO Rep.* 13, 258–265.

Khachaturian, H., Alessi, N. E., Lewis, M. E., Munfakh, N., Fitzsimmons, M. D., and Watson, S. J. (1985). Development of hypothalamic opioid neurons: a combined immunocytochemical and [3H]thymidine autoradiographic study. *Neuropeptides* 5, 477–480.

King, C. M., and Hentges, S. T. (2011). Relative number and distribution of murine hypothalamic proopiomelanocortin neurons innervating distinct target sites. *PLoS ONE* 6:e25864. doi:10.1371/journal.pone.0025864

Kirk, S. L., Samuelsson, A.-M., Argenton, M., Dhonye, H., Kalamatianos, T., Poston, L., et al. (2009). Maternal obesity induced by diet in rats permanently influences central processes regulating food intake in offspring. *PLoS ONE* 4:e5870. doi:10.1371/journal.pone.0005870

Kishi, T., Aschkenasi, C. J., Lee, C. E., Mountjoy, K. G., Saper, C. B., and Elmquist, J. K. (2003). Expression of melanocortin 4 receptor mRNA in the central nervous system of the rat. *J. Comp. Neurol.* 457, 213–235.

Klionsky, D. J. (2007). Autophagy: from phenomenology to molecular understanding in less than a decade. *Nat. Rev. Mol. Cell Biol.* 8, 931–937.

Kuehnen, P., Mischke, M., Wiegand, S., Sers, C., Horsthemke, B., Lau, S., et al. (2012). An Alu element-associated hypermethylation variant of the POMC gene is associated with childhood obesity. *PLoS Genet.* 8:e1002543. doi:10.1371/journal.pgen.1002543

Levin, B. E., Dunn-Meynell, A. A., Balkan, B., and Keesey, R. E. (1997). Selective breeding for diet-induced obesity and resistance in Sprague-Dawley rats. *Am. J. Physiol. Regul. Integr. Comp. Physiol.* 273, R725–R730.

Levine, B., and Klionsky, D. J. (2004). Development by self-digestion: molecular mechanisms and biological functions of autophagy. *Dev. Cell* 6, 463–477.

Maiuri, M. C., Zalckvar, E., Kimchi, A., and Kroemer, G. (2007). Self-eating and self-killing: crosstalk between autophagy and apoptosis. *Nat. Rev. Mol. Cell Biol.* 8, 741–752.

McNay, D. E. G., Pelling, M., Claxton, S., Guillemot, F. O., and Ang, S.-L. (2006). Mash1 is required for generic and subtype differentiation of hypothalamic neuroendocrine cells. *Mol. Endocrinol.* 20, 1623–1632.

Melnick, I., Pronchuck, N., Cowley, M. A., Grove, K. L., and Colmers, W. F. (2007). Developmental switch in neuropeptide Y and melanocortin effects in the paraventricular nucleus of the hypothalamus. *Neuron* 56, 1103–1115.

Mistry, A., Swick, A., and Romsos, D. (1999). Leptin alters metabolic rates before acquisition of its anorectic effect in developing neonatal mice. *Am. J. Physiol.* 277, R742–R747.

Mountjoy, K. G., Mortrud, M. T., Low, M. J., Simerly, R. B., and Cone,

R. D. (1994). Localization of the melanocortin-4 receptor (MC4-R) in neuroendocrine and autonomic control circuits in the brain. *Mol. Endocrinol.* 8, 1298–1308.

Mountjoy, K. G., and Wild, J. M. (1998). Melanocortin-4 receptor mRNA expression in the developing autonomic and central nervous systems. *Brain Res. Dev. Brain Res.* 107, 309–314.

Ollmann, M. M., Wilson, B. D., Yang, Y.-K., Kerns, J. A., Chen, Y., Gantz, I., et al. (1997). Antagonism of central melanocortin receptors in vitro and in vivo by agouti-related protein. *Science* 278, 135–138.

Padilla, S. L., Carmody, J. S., and Zeltser, L. M. (2010). Pomc-expressing progenitors give rise to antagonistic neuronal populations in hypothalamic feeding circuits. *Nat. Med.* 16, 403–405.

Pelling, M., Anthwal, N., McNay, D., Gradwohl, G., Leiter, A. B., Guillemot, F., et al. (2011). Differential requirements for neurogenin 3 in the development of POMC and NPY neurons in the hypothalamus. *Dev. Biol.* 349, 406–416.

Piao, H., Hosoda, H., Kangawa, K., Murata, T., Narita, K., and Higuchi, T. (2008). Ghrelin stimulates milk intake by affecting adult type feeding behaviour in postnatal rats. *J. Neuroendocrinol.* 20, 330–334.

Plagemann, A., Harder, T., Brunn, M., Harder, A., Roepke, K., Wittrock-Staar, M., et al. (2009). Hypothalamic proopiomelanocortin promoter methylation becomes altered by early overfeeding: an epigenetic model of obesity and the metabolic syndrome. *J. Physiol. (Lond.)* 587, 4963–4976.

Proulx, K., Richard, D., and Walker, C.-D. (2002). Leptin regulates appetite-related neuropeptides in the hypothalamus of developing rats without affecting food intake. *Endocrinology* 143, 4683–4692.

Quan, W., Kim, H.-K., Moon, E.-Y., Kim, S. S., Choi, C. S., Komatsu, M., et al. (2012). Role of hypothalamic proopiomelanocortin neuron autophagy in the control of appetite and leptin response. *Endocrinology* 153, 1817–1826.

Schmidt, I., Fritz, A., Scholch, C., Schneider, D., Simon, E., and Plagemann, A. (2001). The effect of leptin treatment on the development of obesity in overfed suckling Wistar rats. *Int. J. Obes. Relat. Metab. Disord.* 25, 1168–1174.

Srinivasan, M., Mitrani, P., Sadhanandan, G., Dodds, C., Shbeir-Eldika, S., Thamotharan, S., et al. (2008). A high-carbohydrate diet in the immediate postnatal life of rats induces adaptations predisposing to adult-onset obesity. *J. Endocrinol.* 197, 565–574.

Steculorum, S. M., and Bouret, S. G. (2011a). Developmental effects of ghrelin. *Peptides* 32, 2362–2366.

Steculorum, S. M., and Bouret, S. G. (2011b). Maternal diabetes compromises the organization of hypothalamic feeding circuits and impairs leptin sensitivity in offspring. *Endocrinology* 152, 4171–4179.

Stocker, C. J., Wargent, E. T., Martin-Gronert, M. S., Cripps, R. L., O'Dowd, J. F., Zaibi, M. S., et al. (2012). Leanness in postnatally nutritionally programmed rats is associated with increased sensitivity to leptin and a melanocortin receptor agonist and decreased sensitivity to neuropeptide Y. *Int. J. Obes.* 36, 1040–1046.

Tessier-Lavigne, M., and Goodman, C. S. (1996). The molecular biology of axon guidance. *Science* 274, 1123–1133.

Williams, K. W., and Elmquist, J. K. (2012). From neuroanatomy to behavior: central integration of peripheral signals regulating feeding behavior. *Nat. Neurosci.* 15, 1350–1355.

Xu, C., and Fan, C.-M. (2008). Expression of Robo/Slit and Semaphorin/Plexin/Neuropilin family members in the developing hypothalamic paraventricular and supraoptic nuclei. *Gene Expr. Patterns* 8, 502–507.

Yaswen, L., Diehl, N., Brennan, M. B., and Hochgeschwender, U. (1999). Obesity in the mouse model of pro-opiomelanocortin deficiency. *Nat. Med.* 5, 1066–1070.

Zhan, C., Zhou, J., Feng, Q., Zhang, J., Lin, S., Bao, J., et al. (2013). Acute and long-term suppression of feeding behavior by POMC neurons in the brainstem and hypothalamus, respectively. *J. Neurosci.* 33, 3624–3632.

Zohar, M., and Salomon, Y. (1992). Melanocortins stimulate proliferation and induce morphological changes in cultured rat astrocytes by distinct transducing mechanisms. *Brain Res.* 576, 49–58.

12

GHS-R1a constitutive activity and its physiological relevance

Yves Mear[1], Alain Enjalbert[1,2] and Sylvie Thirion[1]*

[1] CNRS, CRN2M UMR7286, Aix Marseille University, Marseille, France
[2] Molecular Biology Laboratory, Conception Hospital, AP-HM, Marseille, France

Edited by:
María M. Malagón, University of Cordoba, Spain

Reviewed by:
Rhonda D. Kineman, University of Illinois at Chicago, USA
Jesus P. Camiña, Hospital Clínico Universitario de Santiago, Spain

***Correspondence:**
Sylvie Thirion, Faculté de Médecine Nord, CRN2M - Neurobiology and Neurophysiological Research Center of Marseille, UMR CNRS 7286, Aix-Marseille University, Bd Pierre Dramard-CS 80011, 13344 Marseille Cedex 15, France
e-mail: sylvie.thirion@univ-amu.fr

Abundant evidences have shown that ghrelin, by its binding to GHS-R1a, plays an important role for fundamental physiological functions. Increasing attention is given to the GHS-R1a unusually high constitutive activity and its contribution to downstream signaling and physiological processes. Here, we review recent lines of evidences showing that the interaction between ligand-binding pocket TM domains and the ECL2 could be partially responsible for this high constitutive activity. Interestingly, GHSR-1a constitutive activity activates in turn the downstream PLC, PKC, and CRE signaling pathways and this activation is reversed by the inverse agonist [D-Arg^{1}, D-Phe^{5}, D-Trp^{7,9}, Leu^{11}]-substance P (MSP). Noteworthy, GHSR-1a exhibits a C-terminal-dependent constitutive internalization. Non-sense GHS-R1a mutation (Ala204Glu), first discovered in Moroccan patients, supports the role of GHSR-1a constitutive activity in physiological impairments. Ala204Glu-point mutation, altering exclusively the GHSR-1a constitutive activity, was associated with familial short stature syndrome. Altogether, these findings suggest that GHS-R1a constitutive activity could contribute to GH secretion or body weight regulation. Consequently, future research on basic and clinical applications of GHS-R1a inverse agonists will be challenging and potentially rewarding.

Keywords: ghrelin receptor, GPCR, constitutive activity, signaling pathway, PLC, β-arrestin

INTRODUCTION

The secretion of growth hormone (GH) by the anterior pituitary is under complex control. Small synthetic molecules termed GH secretagogues (GHS) are synthetic, peptidyl, and non-peptidyl molecules which possess strong and dose-dependent GH-releasing activity *in vivo* in several species and in humans (Cheng et al., 1989; Bowers et al., 1991; Cheng et al., 1991). The cloning of the GH secretagogue receptor (GHS-R1a, now called ghrelin receptor) in 1996 (Howard et al., 1996; Pong et al., 1996), led to the isolation of the endogenous ligand, ghrelin in 1999 (Kojima et al., 1999).

Ghrelin is a 28 amino acid peptide that differs from all other peptide hormones known by an octanoylation. This fatty acid modification is essential both for the binding to and activation of the receptor and for its pharmacokinetic properties (Kojima et al., 2001). Ghrelin strongly stimulates GH release in humans (Bowers et al., 1991), and it is much more potent than Growth Hormone-Releasing Hormone (GHRH) under similar conditions. Ghrelin potently increase food intake and weight gain, and also regulates energy homeostasis and metabolism following central and systemic administration (Castañeda et al., 2010; Stengel and Taché, 2012).

The GHS-R1a is a G protein-coupled receptor (GPCR) of 366 amino acids with the characteristic seven transmembrane-spanning domains (7TM receptor; for review Schwartz et al., 2006; Cruz and Smith, 2008). Signal transduction from the extracellular environment via 7TM receptors in general requires a conformational change from an inactive (R) to a active state (R*). Certain 7TM receptors are stabilized in an active conformation without any ligand present. The ability to propagate the intracellular signal in the absence of agonist is commonly known as constitutive activity.

Constitutive activity is described for mostly all GPCR, however for a large part of them the level of constitutive activity is very low (Arvanitakis et al., 1998; Smit et al., 2007).

The GHS-R1a exhibits unusual high constitutive activity (Holst et al., 2003) as it signal with ~50% of its maximal capacity in the absence of the agonist, ghrelin. This article aims to review the current knowledge on GHS-R1a ligand-independent constitutive activity and its functions.

GHS-R1a AND ITS CONSTITUTIVE ACTIVITY

MOLECULAR BASIS

For several years, it has been noted that mostly all GPCRs exhibit intrinsic constitutive activity (Arvanitakis et al., 1998; Smit et al., 2007). In 1999, studies performed on the β_2-adrenergic receptor suggested that this ligand-independent activity could involve an inward movement of the extracellular segments of the transmembrane domains (TMs) VI and VII toward TM III in the ligand-binding pocket (Elling et al., 1999).

Holst and colleagues performed a structural analysis of GHS-R1a and revealed the crucial role of an aromatic cluster formed by three residues (*Phe VI:16, Phe VII:06, and Phe VII:09*) on the inner face of the extracellular ends of GHS-R1a TMs VI and VII. Their close spatial proximity and the formation of this cluster allow GHS-R1a to stabilize in its active conformation in absence of agonist (Holst et al., 2004; Mokrosinski and Holst, 2010).

The residue in position *VI:16* is central for the constitutive activity level that can gradually be increased or decreased depending on the size and hydrophobic properties of the side chain of the amino acid. It has also been suggested that the aromatic residue *VI:16* may work as a tethered agonist located strategically at the interface between TM III TM VI and TM VII, blocking these extracellular TM segments in a conformation promoting GHS-R1a high constitutive activity (Schwartz et al., 2006).

A conserved aromatic lock crucial for GHS-R1a high basal signaling level is formed by the Trp *VI:13* and Phe *V:13* residues (Holst et al., 2004). The Trp *VI:13* (=Trp276) is located in the conserved motif CWxP in the middle of TM VI and is supposed to act as a global toggle switch model allowing the inward movement of this domain, and the GHS-R1a high basal activation level (Schwartz et al., 2006; Floquet et al., 2010).

Specific residues in the vinicity of this cluster have been proposed to orchestrate finely tuned microswitches critical for the activation level in absence of ligand (Holst et al., 2004; Valentin-Hansen et al., 2012).

In order to study the importance of this core peptide in the GHS-R1a constitutive activity, Gozé et al. introduced the mutation Trp276Ala and mutated the two surrounding amino acid residues Val131 and Ile134. Their results revealed that the mutation Trp276A1a dramatically impairs the ligand-independent activity whereas Val131Leu and Ile134Met highly increase GHS-R1a basal activity. According to these results, the three residues Trp276, Val131, and Ile134 could also significantly impact on GHS-R1a constitutive signaling (Gozé et al., 2010).

In 2006, Pantel et al. reported a mutation (Ala204Glu) in the extracellular loop II (ECL2) of the human GHS-R1a affecting selectively the ligand-independent activity (Pantel et al., 2006). The ECL2 structure function analysis revealed that by restricting this segment, and so possibly TM V/TM III, movements either by mutation or by ligand binding, reduces the constitutive signaling level (Mokrosinski et al., 2012), showing that the high GHS-R1a basal signaling level depends on the flexibility in these segments. Other studies showed that a single mutation or space generating a substitution in the GHS-R1a sequence or in the ligand peptide sequence can change the ligand properties from agonist to inverse agonist or from inverse agonist to agonist depending on the residue mutated (Holst et al., 2007; Els et al., 2012).

TM VI and TM VII movements into their inward-bend promoting the ligand-independent active conformation can be stoically blocked, using a modified substance P (MSP) inverse agonist, [D-Arg^{1}, D-Phe^{5}, D-Trp^{7,9}, Leu^{11}]-substance P (often referred in the literature as SPA, for substance P analog). The systematic analysis of this peptide structure-function relationship identified the C-terminal heptapeptide (fQwFwLL) as its active core, the D-Phe^{5} residue being apparently crucial for the inverse agonist property and the binding affinity (Holst et al., 2006). Unlike ghrelin that only interacts with the middle part of the ligand-binding pocket, the inverse agonist binds to an extended-binding pocket comprising all the seven TM domains of the receptor except for the first one. In addition, the space-generating mutants located relatively deep in the binding pocket at key positions within the TM III, TM IV, and TM V, upregulate the effects of MSP, suggesting that this molecule could prevent the spontaneous receptor activation across the binding pocket extend (Holst et al., 2006; Mokrosinski and Holst, 2010).

INTRACELLULAR PATHWAYS AND CONSTITUTIVE INTERNALIZATION

Inositol phosphate (IP) signaling pathway, through Phospholipase C (PLC) activation, was the first specifically associated with the GHS-R1a ligand-dependent activity (Adams et al., 1995; Lei et al., 1995; Chen et al., 1996; Petersenn, 2002) inducing intracellular calcium mobilization (Herrington and Hille, 1994). Consequently, this pathway has been investigated for determining the receptor constitutive signaling. PLC activation was demonstrated comparing heterologous HEK-293 and COS-7 cells overexpressing the GHS-R1a to cells transfected with the motilin receptor (that is the closest GPCR homolog of GHS-R1a without constitutive activity; Holst et al., 2003). The unusualy high GHS-R1a ligand-independent signaling level was similar to that of the most famous highly constitutively active GPCR, the virally encoded ORF74 receptor. To note, this paper allowed characterizing MSP as a full GHS-R1a inverse agonist. Indeed, this compound inhibits the GHS-R1a constitutive ligand-independent IP accumulation and decreases the IP level to that of cells transfected with the empty vector (Holst et al., 2003). Lau et al. reported that GHS-R1a constitutive activity could reduce apoptosis in HEK-293 overexpressing the (seabream) sbGHS-R1a, through PKC-dependent caspase-3 inhibition (Lau et al., 2009).

Gq/11-coupled GHS-R1a constitutive activity also resulted in a dose-dependent but ligand-independent increase in the CRE luciferase reporter while the full inverse agonist MSP partially reversed this effect. To note, heterotrimeric Gq/11 protein-coupled receptors have previously been reported to phosphorylate the cAMP responsive element-binding protein (CREB) by activating the CRE pathway as a result of calcium/calmoduline kinase IV (CaMK IV) and/or protein kinase C (PKC) activation (Matthews et al., 1994; Poulin et al., 2009) (**Figure 1**). Finally, performing serum responsive element (SRE) reporter assay on HEK-293 cells transfected with GHS-R1a revealed a 10-fold increase in the ligand-independent signaling compared to the cells transfected with the empty plasmid.

While many other signaling pathways have been shown to play a role in the GHS-R1a ligand-dependent activation, the GHS-R1a ligand-independent activation has not been investigated. Indeed, Gi/o heterotrimeric pathway was clearly associated with beta-arrestin-mediated ERK1/2 activation following GHS-R1a activation by ghrelin (Camiña et al., 2007). Similarly, c-Src that is involved in the GHS-R1a ghrelin-dependent Akt activation (via Gi/o-protein; Lodeiro et al., 2009) has not been studied for the high basal level associated signaling pathways.

Since GHS-R1a exhibits an unusually high constitutive activity, it could be hypothesized that the downstream signaling level could reflect the membrane expression level. In this context, a better understanding of the mechanisms underlying and modulating its plasma membrane expression was necessary. To this end, GHS-R1a was tagged using M2 anti-FLAG antibody labeling, thus allowing following the intracellular movement of

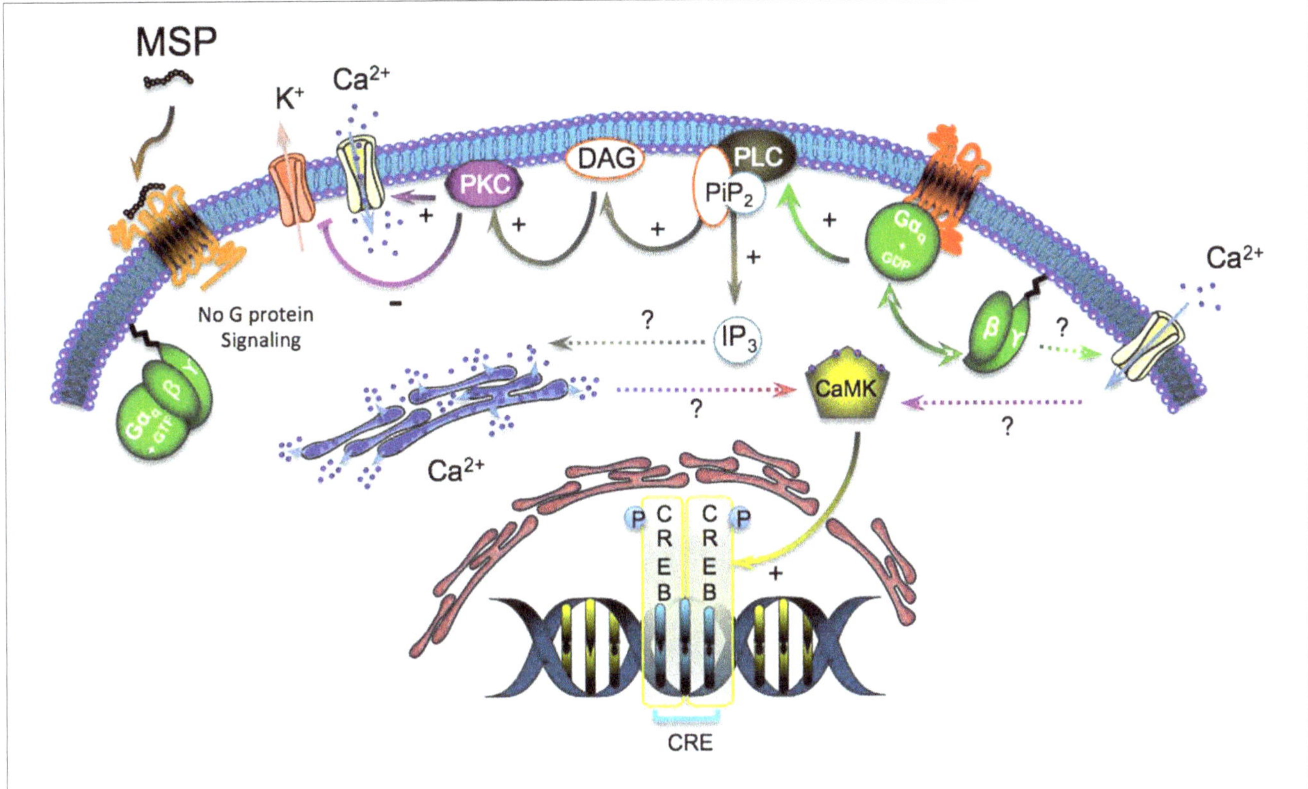

FIGURE 1 | GHS-R1a constitutive activity leads to the dissociation of α and βγ subunits of heterotrimeric G-proteins. The free Gq subunit activates the PLC that cleaves PiP_2 into IP3 and DAG. DAG activates the PKC, which in turn actives the Ca^{2+} channels and inhibits the K^+ channels (continuous line). The effects of IP3 on the intracellular Ca^{2+} mobilization and the origin of the Ca^{2+} that activates the Ca^{2+} calmodulin kinase (CaMK) remain unclear and will need further investigations (dotted line). The binding of the inverse agonist MSP to the GHS-R1a inhibits the G-protein signaling and decreases the IP3 (via PLC) and CRE pathway (via phosphorylated CREB) constitutive activation.

GHS-R1a. These experiments revealed a GHS-R1a constitutive ligand-independent internalization and the receptor could be trapped at the cell surface by the inverse agonist MSP. The punctiform receptor intracellular labeling co-localizes with clathrin-coated vesicles and recycling endosome markers (Holst et al., 2003).

Unlike the GHS-R1a, GPR-39 receptor, a member of the ghrelin receptor family, is not constitutively internalized but it displays a high ligand-independent signaling level (Holst et al., 2003). Based on these observations, Holliday et al. developed an elegant approach by switching the GHS-R1a C tail with that of the GPR-39. The chimera, named GhR-39, was constitutively active through the PLC pathway but its internalization was impaired. Components supporting the constitutive activity could be necessary but not sufficient for GHS-R1a endocytosis and additional regulatory elements in the C-terminal domain may be involved (Holliday et al., 2007).

GHS-R1a constitutive internalization requires the sequential activation of the monomeric G proteins Rab5 and Rab11. Rab proteins control various important cellular processes, such as endocytosis, trafficking, endosome fusion. and exocytosis (Seachrist and Ferguson, 2003). These proteins regulate vesicle transport and fusion with specific target compartments, the early endosomes for Rab5, and the endosomal recycling compartments such as the perinuclear recycling compartment (PNRC) for Rab11. MSP-induced GHS-R1a membrane plasma anchorage is blocked by the constitutive expression of GTP-binding mutants of Rab_s (Rab5 Gln79Leu or Rab11 Gln70Leu) confirming that MSP naturally inhibits GHS-R1a internalization rather than activates GHS-R1a neosynthesis and trafficking (Holliday et al., 2007).

β-arrestin recruitment has been obviously investigated as it appears as the most widely standard adaptor for GPCR endocytosis (Lefkowitz, 1998) (**Figure 2**). Only ghrelin stimulation induces GHSR-1a phosphorylation and β-arrestin 2 recruitment. Besides, dominant-negative β-arrestin 2 construct, which competes for clathrin interaction, does not inhibit the constitutive endocytosis, supporting the hypothesis of a GHS-R1a β-arrestin-independent constitutive internalization. These results suggest that the aromatic residue *VI:16*, already mentioned above, could act as "tethered biased agonist" rather than "tethered agonist" because it blocks the receptor in a conformation that only induces the Gq/11 protein activation without β-arrestin 2 recruitment (Shukla et al., 2011; Reiter et al., 2012). To note, β-arrestin 2 recruitment has been reported to active the MAPK pathway. In this context, the absence of β-arrestin 2 recruitment in basal condition has been proposed to explain the absence of MAPK pathway activation (Holliday et al., 2007).

Purified GHS-R1a monomers in a lipid disc showed that the ghrelin receptor *per se* activates Gq/11 in the absence of agonist,

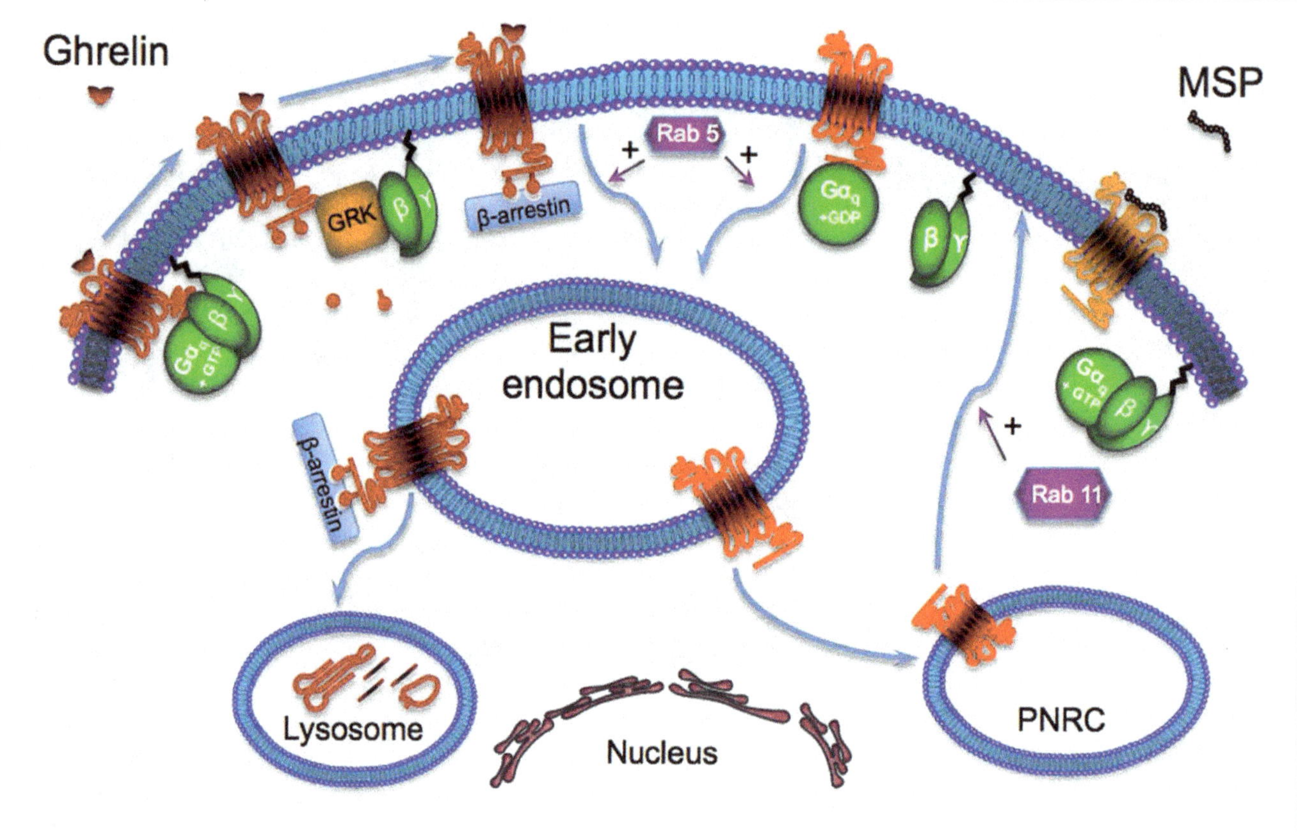

FIGURE 2 | GHS-R1a activation by its endogenous ligand ghrelin leads to the dissociation of α and βγ subunits of heterotrimeric G-proteins. The βγ dimer recruits G-protein-receptor kinases (such as GRK_2 or GRK_3) to the receptor, where they phosphorylate the agonist-bound receptor. These phosphorylations lead to the recruitment of β-arrestins and activation of the monomeric G-protein RAb_5 that targets the receptor to early endosomes. Then the receptor is addressed to the lysosome for degradation. GHS-R1a constitutive activation recruits Rab_5 without activation of the GRK, inducing subsequent phosphorylation and β-arrestin recruitment. This constitutive activation of Rab_5 explains the receptor ligand-independent internalization that is first addressed to the early endosome then to the PNRC (perinuclear recycling compartment) where it activates the monomeric G-protein Rab_{11}.

and that GHS-R1a constitutive activity is an intrinsic property of the protein and is not influenced by its cellular environment (Damian et al., 2012). In this context, the receptor isolated in lipid discs recruits arrestin-2 in an agonist-dependent manner (Mary et al., 2012), whereas it interacts with μ-AP2 (plasma membrane-localized clathrin adaptor subunit) in the absence of ligand or in the presence of ghrelin (Damian et al., 2012). Thus, μ-AP2 could be involved in the basal regulation of GHS-R1a trafficking.

PHYSIOLOGICAL RELEVANCE

Many types of GPCR display a high ligand-independent signaling *in vitro* (Seifert and Wenzel-Seifert, 2002). Among them, GHS-R1a has been shown to display both the highest basal activation of Gq/11 (about 50% of its maximal activity) *in vitro* (Holst et al., 2004), and substantial basal signaling for food intake and weight control *in vivo* (Petersen et al., 2009; Els et al., 2012). Pantel et al., who reported naturally occurring mutations in the GHS-R1a sequence, have first shown a putative link with physiological impairments in 2006. They reported a substitution mutation located within the first GHS-R1a exon, predicting the substitution of Alanine by Glutamate (Ala204Glu) in two independent Moroccan families. This missense mutation is located in the GHS-R1a ECL2 and affects a fully conserved amino acid. HEK-293 cells stably transfected with WT and Ala204Glu-mutant GHS-R1a showed, using POU1F1-luciferase reporter assay that this mutation selectively abolishes the GHS-R1a ligand-independent signaling without altering the Ghrelin-dependent activity. Noteworthy, mutations altering exclusively the constitutive activity are associated with familial short stature syndrome and the latter can be partially reversed with GH treatment (Pantel et al., 2006, 2009; Inoue et al., 2011). Wang reported another uncharacterized GHS-R1a mutation affecting the Phe 279 residue (Phe *VI:16*) recently identified as being of particular interest for GHS-R1a constitutive activity. Noteworthy, the phenotype of patients expressing this mutation is characterized by an increased obesity and short stature (Wang, 2004). Regarding these different but functionally similar mutations, Holst and Schwartz proposed that the absence of GHS-R1a constitutively active signaling results in a syndrome, characterized, not only by a short stature, but also by obesity (Holst and Schwartz, 2006). This suggestion has been confirmed recently using icv MSP administration that significantly decreased the food intake, body weight, and neuropeptide Y (NPY) and uncoupling protein 2 (UCP2) gene expression in the hypothalamus (Petersen et al., 2009).

Ligand-dependent GHS-R1a heterodimerizations have been reported for the subtype 1 dopamine receptor that increases dopamine signaling (Jiang et al., 2006), the somatostatin receptor-5 that regulates insulin release (Park et al., 2012) and the melanocortin-3 receptor that is involved in body weight regulation and energy balance (Rediger et al., 2011, 2012). Also, the dimerization of the GHS-R1a with the dopamine D2 receptor has recently been shown to regulate appetite (Kern et al., 2012).

Its dimerization with the melanocortin-3 receptor, the D1 receptor, and the newly discovered 5-HT_{2C} receptor may be central in modulating and controlling GHS-R1a-mediated downstream signaling and subsequent satiety and appetite signaling, as well as the rewarding and motivational aspects of food intake (Schellekens et al., 2013). The understanding of the underlying mechanisms leading to these activations may ultimately lead to the development of new therapeutic strategies.

On the other hand, ghrelin and GHS-R1a knockout mice explorations may allow the emergence of new regulatory properties of the ghrelin receptor constitutive activity. For example, GHS-R1a constitutive activity increases limbic seizures in rodents, the endogenous ligand being naturally anticonvulsive (Portelli et al., 2012). In the mouse brain, deficits in spontaneous receptor activity cause marked functional impairment in learning and memory (Albarran-Zeckler et al., 2012). GHS-R1a signaling is necessary for hippocampal-dependent learning and habituated feeding responses (Davis et al., 2011). Ghrelin plays also a role in sleep whereas the GHS-R1a will be more implicated in arousal (Esposito et al., 2012).

To move beyond putative redundant compensation mechanisms, further *in vivo* investigations targetting the receptor constitutive activity with appropriate pharmacological tools (Mokrosinski and Holst, 2010; Sivertsen et al., 2011) would be needed to determine the underlying physiological functions linked to this constitutive activity.

CONCLUSION

Abundant evidence currently indicates that ghrelin, by its binding to GHS-R1a, plays a role in various physiological functions that led to the development of clinical trials to translate basic research findings to human disease treatment and diagnosis (for review Akamizu and Kangawa, 2012). Concerning the GHS-R1a constitutive activity, most of the studies performed so far focused on the molecular aspects. Even if some physiological relevance are emerging for food intake regulation (see paragraph above), further studies remain necessary to confirm the role played by the GHS-R1a constitutive activity in the regulation of the GH axis. Pituitary somatotroph adenomas express higher GHS-R1a transcript and protein levels than normal pituitary (Korbonits et al., 1998; Barlier et al., 1999). Moreover, Pantel et al. (2006) have shown that a reduced GHS-R1a constitutive activity impairs the GH secretion. Thus, it should be interesting to test if the GHS-R1a constitutive activity disrupts the GH hypersecretion observed in acromegalic patients with somatotroph tumors (Acunzo et al., 2008; Roche et al., 2012).

The signaling pathways associated with this high constitutive activity should also be addressed. Knowing that the heterogeneity of the coupling on the signaling varies depending on the tissue or cell type, it is crucial to address now these questions in physiological or pathophysiological models. Depending on the model, does the GHS-R1a ligand-independent CRE activation pass through the calcium/calmodulin kinase? And/or via the cAMP/PKA pathways?

These issues are part of the many questions pending in this field. Some of them may support the development of clinical applications of GHS-R1a inverse agonists in physiological disorders in the future, allowing developing novel and unique therapies for various disorders, including intractable and serious diseases. Indeed, research on basic and clinical applications of GHS-R1a inverse agonists will be challenging and potentially rewarding.

ACKNOWLEDGMENTS

We thank very gratefully Prof. Isabelle Limon for helpful criticisms and careful corrections of the manuscript. We acknowledge Dr. Marie-Pierre Blanchard for her manuscript reading. This work was supported by Aix-Marseille University and CNRS.

REFERENCES

Acunzo, J., Thirion, S., Roche, C., Saveanu, A., Gunz, G., Germanetti, A. L., et al. (2008). Somatostatin receptor sst2 decreases cell viability and hormonal hypersecretion and reverses octreotide resistance of human pituitary adenomas. *Cancer Res.* 68, 10163–10170.

Adams, E. F., Petersen, B., Lei, T., Buchfelder, M., and Fahlbusch, R. (1995). The growth hormone secretagogue, L-692, 429, induces phosphatidylinositol hydrolysis and hormone secretion by human pituitary tumors. *Biochem. Biophys. Res. Commun.* 208, 555–561.

Akamizu, T., and Kangawa, K. (2012). The physiological significance and potential clinical applications of ghrelin. *Eur. J. Intern. Med.* 23, 197–202.

Albarran-Zeckler, R. G., Brantley, A. F., and Smith, R. G. (2012). Growth hormone secretagogue receptor (GHS-R1a) knockout mice exhibit improved spatial memory and deficits in contextual memory. *Behav. Brain Res.* 232, 13–19.

Arvanitakis, L., Geras-Raaka, E., and Gershengorn, M. C. (1998). Constitutively signaling G-protein-coupled receptors and human disease. *Trends Endocrinol. Metab.* 9, 27–31.

Barlier, A., Zamora, A. J., Grino, M., Gunz, G., Pellegrini-Bouiller, I., Morange-Ramos, I., et al. (1999). Expression of functional growth hormone secretagogue receptors in human pituitary adenomas: polymerase chain reaction, triple *in-situ* hybridization and cell culture studies. *J. Neuroendocrinol.* 11, 491–502.

Bowers, C. Y., Sartor, A. O., Reynolds, G. A., and Badger, T. M. (1991). On the actions of the growth hormone-releasing hexapeptide, GHRP. *Endocrinology* 128, 2027–2035.

Camiña, J. P., Lodeiro, M., Ischenko, O., Martini, A. C., and Casanueva, F. F. (2007). Stimulation by ghrelin of p42/p44 mitogen-activated protein kinase through the GHS-R1a receptor: role of G-proteins and beta-arrestins. *J. Cell. Physiol.* 213, 187–200.

Castañeda, T. R., Tong, J., Datta, R., Culler, M., and Tschöp, M. H. (2010). Ghrelin in the regulation of body weight and metabolism. *Front. Neuroendocrinol.* 31, 44–60. doi: 10.1016/j.yfrne.2009.10.008

Chen, C., Wu, D., and Clarke, I. J. (1996). Signal transduction systems employed by synthetic GH-releasing peptides in somatotrophs. *J. Endocrinol.* 148, 381–386.

Cheng, K., Chan, W. W., Barreto, A., Convey, E. M., and Smith, R. G. (1989). The synergistic effects of His-D-Trp-Ala-Trp-D-Phe-Lys-NH2 on growth hormone (GH)-releasing factor-stimulated GH release and intracellular adenosine 3′, 5′-monophosphate accumulation in rat primary pituitary cell culture. *Endocrinology* 124, 2791–2798.

Cheng, K., Chan, W. W., Butler, B., Barreto, A., and Smith, R. G. (1991). Evidence for a role of protein kinase-C in His-D-Trp-Ala-Trp-D-Phe-Lys-NH2-induced growth hormone release from rat primary pituitary cells. *Endocrinology* 129, 3337–3342.

Cruz, C. R. Y., and Smith, R. G. (2008). The growth hormone secretagogue receptor. *Vitam. Horm.* 77, 47–88.

Damian, M., Marie, J., Leyris, J. P., Fehrentz, J. A., Verdié, P., Martinez, J., et al. (2012). High constitutive activity is an intrinsic feature of ghrelin receptor protein: a study with a functional monomeric GHS-R1a receptor reconstituted in lipid discs. *J. Biol. Chem.* 287, 3630–3641.

Davis, J. F., Choi, D. L., Clegg, D. J., and Benoit, S. C. (2011). Signaling through the ghrelin receptor modulates hippocampal function and meal anticipation in mice. *Physiol. Behav.* 103, 39–43.

Elling, C. E., Thirstrup, K., Holst, B., and Schwartz, T. W. (1999). Conversion of agonist site to metal-ion chelator site in the beta(2)-adrenergic receptor. *Proc. Natl. Acad. Sci. U.S.A.* 96, 12322–12327.

Els, S., Schild, E., Petersen, P. S., Kilian, T. M., Mokrosinski, J., Frimurer, T. M., et al. (2012). An aromatic region to induce a switch between agonism and inverse agonism at the ghrelin receptor. *J. Med. Chem.* 55, 7437–7449.

Esposito, M., Pellinen, J., Kapás, L., and Szentirmai, É. (2012). Impaired wake-promoting mechanisms in ghrelin receptor-deficient mice. *Eur. J. Neurosci.* 35, 233–243.

Floquet, N., M'Kadmi, C., Perahia, D., Gagne, D., Bergé, G., Marie, J., et al. (2010). Activation of the ghrelin receptor is described by a privileged collective motion: a model for constitutive and agonist-induced activation of a sub-class A G-protein coupled receptor (GPCR). *J. Mol. Biol.* 395, 769–784.

Gozé, C., Bergé, G., M'Kadmi, C., Floquet, N., Gagne, D., Galleyrand, J. C., et al. (2010). Involvement of tryptophan W276 and of two surrounding amino acid residues in the high constitutive activity of the ghrelin receptor GHS-R1a. *Eur. J. Pharmacol.* 643, 153–161.

Herrington, J., and Hille, B. (1994). Growth hormone-releasing hexapeptide elevates intracellular calcium in rat somatotropes by two mechanisms. *Endocrinology* 135, 1100–1108.

Holliday, N. D., Holst, B., Rodionova, E. A., Schwartz, T. W., and Cox, H. M. (2007). Importance of constitutive activity and arrestin-independent mechanisms for intracellular trafficking of the ghrelin receptor. *Mol. Endocrinol.* 21, 3100–3112.

Holst, B., Cygankiewicz, A., Jensen, T. H., Ankersen, M., and Schwartz, T. W. (2003). High constitutive signaling of the ghrelin receptor–identification of a potent inverse agonist. *Mol. Endocrinol.* 17, 2201–2210.

Holst, B., Holliday, N. D., Bach, A., Elling, C. E., Cox, H. M., and Schwartz, T. W. (2004). Common structural basis for constitutive activity of the ghrelin receptor family. *J. Biol. Chem.* 279, 53806–53817.

Holst, B., Lang, M., Brandt, E., Bach, A., Howard, A., Frimurer, T. M., et al. (2006). Ghrelin receptor inverse agonists: identification of an active peptide core and its interaction epitopes on the receptor. *Mol. Pharmacol.* 70, 936–946.

Holst, B., Mokrosinski, J., Lang, M., Brandt, E., Nygaard, R., Frimurer, T. M., et al. (2007). Identification of an efficacy switch region in the ghrelin receptor responsible for interchange between agonism and inverse agonism. *J. Biol. Chem.* 282, 15799–15811.

Holst, B., and Schwartz, T. W. (2006). Ghrelin receptor mutations—too little height and too much hunger. *J. Clin. Invest.* 116, 637–641.

Howard, A. D., Feighner, S. D., Cully, D. F., Arena, J. P., Liberator, P. A., Rosenblum, C. I., et al. (1996). A receptor in pituitary and hypothalamus that functions in growth hormone release. *Science* 273, 974–977.

Inoue, H., Kangawa, N., Kinouchi, A., Sakamoto, Y., Kimura, C., Horikawa, R., et al. (2011). Identification and functional analysis of novel human growth hormone secretagogue receptor (GHSR) gene mutations in Japanese subjects with short stature. *J. Clin. Endocrinol. Metab.* 96, E373–E378.

Jiang, H., Betancourt, L., and Smith, R. G. (2006). Ghrelin amplifies dopamine signaling by cross talk involving formation of growth hormone secretagogue receptor/dopamine receptor subtype 1 heterodimers. *Mol. Endocrinol.* 20, 1772–1785.

Kern, A., Albarran-Zeckler, R., Walsh, H. E., and Smith, R. G. (2012). Apo-ghrelin receptor forms heteromers with DRD2 in hypothalamic neurons and is essential for anorexigenic effects of DRD2 agonism. *Neuron* 73, 317–332.

Kojima, M., Hosoda, H., Date, Y., Nakazato, M., Matsuo, H., and Kangawa, K. (1999). Ghrelin is a growth-hormone-releasing acylated peptide from stomach. *Nature* 402, 656–660.

Kojima, M., Hosoda, H., Matsuo, H., and Kangawa, K. (2001). Ghrelin: discovery of the natural endogenous ligand for the growth hormone secretagogue receptor. *Trends Endocrinol. Metab.* 12, 118–122.

Korbonits, M., Jacobs, R. A., Aylwin, S. J., Burrin, J. M., Dahia, P. L., Monson, J. P., et al. (1998). Expression of the growth hormone secretagogue receptor in pituitary adenomas and other neuroendocrine tumors. *J. Clin. Endocrinol. Metab.* 83, 3624–3630.

Lau, P. N., Chow, K. B. S., Chan, C. B., Cheng, C. H. K., and Wise, H. (2009). The constitutive activity of the ghrelin receptor attenuates apoptosis via a protein kinase C-dependent pathway. *Mol. Cell. Endocrinol.* 299, 232–239.

Lefkowitz, R. J. (1998). G Protein-coupled Receptors. *J. Biol. Chem.* 273, 18677–18680.

Lei, T., Buchfelder, M., Fahlbusch, R., and Adams, E. F. (1995). Growth hormone releasing peptide (GHRP-6) stimulates phosphatidylinositol (PI) turnover in human pituitary somatotroph cells. *J. Mol. Endocrinol.* 14, 135–138.

Lodeiro, M., Theodoropoulou, M., Pardo, M., Casanueva, F. F., and Camiña, J. P. (2009). c-Src regulates Akt signaling in response to ghrelin via beta-arrestin signaling-independent and -dependent mechanisms. *PLoS ONE* 4:e4686. doi: 10.1371/journal.pone.0004686

Mary, S., Damian, M., Louet, M., Floquet, N., Fehrentz, J., Marie, J., et al. (2012). Ligands and signaling proteins govern the conformational landscape explored by a G protein-coupled receptor. *Proc. Natl. Acad. Sci. U.S.A.* 109, 8304–8309.

Matthews, R. P., Guthrie, C. R., Wailes, L. M., Zhao, X., Means, A. R., and McKnight, G. S. (1994). Calcium/calmodulin-dependent protein kinase types II and IV differentially regulate CREB-dependent gene expression. *Mol. Cell. Biol.* 14, 6107–6116.

Mokrosinski, J., Frimurer, T. M., Sivertsen, B., Schwartz, T. W., and Holst, B. (2012). Modulation of constitutive activity and signaling bias of the ghrelin receptor by conformational constraint in the second extracellular loop. *J. Biol. Chem.* 287, 33488–33502.

Mokrosinski, J., and Holst, B. (2010). Modulation of the constitutive activity of the ghrelin receptor by use of pharmacological tools and mutagenesis. *Methods Enzymol.* 484, 53–73.

Pantel, J., Legendre, M., Cabrol, S., Hilal, L., Hajaji, Y., Nivot, S., et al. (2006). Loss of constitutive activity of the growth hormone secretagogue receptor in familial short stature. *J. Clin. Invest.* 116, 760–768.

Pantel, J., Legendre, M., Nivot, S., Morisset, S., Vie-Luton, M. P., Le Bouc, Y., et al. (2009). Recessive isolated growth hormone deficiency and mutations in the ghrelin receptor. *J. Clin. Endocrinol. Metab.* 94, 4334–4341.

Park, S., Jiang, H., Zhang, H., and Smith, R. G. (2012). Modification of ghrelin receptor signaling by somatostatin receptor-5 regulates insulin release. *Proc. Natl. Acad. Sci. U.S.A.* 109, 19003–19008.

Petersen, P. S., Woldbye, D. P. D., Madsen, A. N., Egerod, K. L., Jin, C., Lang, M., et al. (2009). *In vivo* characterization of high Basal signaling from the ghrelin receptor. *Endocrinology* 150, 4920–4930.

Petersenn, S. (2002). Structure and regulation of the growth hormone secretagogue receptor. *Minerva Endocrinol.* 27, 243–256.

Pong, S. S., Chaung, L. Y., Dean, D. C., Nargund, R. P., Patchett, A. A., and Smith, R. G. (1996). Identification of a new G-protein-linked receptor for growth hormone secretagogues. *Mol. Endocrinol.* 10, 57–61.

Portelli, J., Thielemans, L., Ver Donck, L., Loyens, E., Coppens, J., Aourz, N., et al. (2012). Inactivation of the constitutively active ghrelin receptor attenuates limbic seizure activity in rodents. *Neurotherapeutics* 9, 658–672.

Poulin, B., Maccario, H., Thirion, S., Junoy, B., Boyer, B., Enjalbert, A., et al. (2009). Ubiquitination as a priming process of PKC alpha and PKC epsilon degradation in the alphaT3-1 gonadotrope cell line. *Neuroendocrinology* 89, 252–266.

Rediger, A., Piechowski, C. L., Habegger, K., Grüters, A., Krude, H., Tschöp, M. H., et al. (2012). MC4R dimerization in the paraventricular nucleus and GHSR/MC3R heterodimerization in the arcuate nucleus: is there relevance for body weight regulation? *Neuroendocrinology* 95, 277–288.

Rediger, A., Piechowski, C. L., Yi, C. X., Tarnow, P., Strotmann, R., Grüters, A., et al. (2011). Mutually opposite signal modulation by hypothalamic heterodimerization of ghrelin and melanocortin-3 receptors. *J. Biol. Chem.* 286, 39623–39631.

Reiter, E., Ahn, S., Shukla, A. K., and Lefkowitz, R. J. (2012). Molecular mechanism of β-arrestin-biased agonism at seven-transmembrane receptors. *Annu. Rev. Pharmacol. Toxicol.* 52, 179–197.

Roche, C., Rasolonjanahary, R., Thirion, S., Goddard, I., Fusco, A., Figarella-Branger, D., et al. (2012). Inactivation of transcription factor pit-1 to target tumoral somatolactotroph cells. *Hum. Gene Ther.* 23, 104–114.

Schellekens, H., Van Oeffelen, W. E., Dinan, T. G., and Cryan, J. F. (2013). Promiscuous dimerization of the growth hormone secretagogue receptor (GHS-R1a) attenuates ghrelin-mediated signaling. *J. Biol. Chem.* 288, 181–191.

Schwartz, T. W., Frimurer, T. M., Holst, B., Rosenkilde, M. M., and Elling, C. E. (2006). Molecular mechanism of 7TM receptor activation–a global toggle switch model. *Annu. Rev. Pharmacol. Toxicol.* 46, 481–519.

Seachrist, J. L., and Ferguson, S. S. (2003). Regulation of G protein-coupled receptor endocytosis and trafficking by Rab GTPases. *Life Sci.* 74, 225–235.

Seifert, R., and Wenzel-Seifert, K. (2002). Constitutive activity of G-protein-coupled receptors: cause of disease and common property of wild-type receptors. *Arch. Pharmacol.* 366, 381–416.

Shukla, A. K., Xiao, K., and Lefkowitz, R. J. (2011). Emerging paradigms of β-arrestin-dependent seven transmembrane receptor signaling. *Trends Biochem. Sci.* 36, 457–469.

Sivertsen, B., Lang, M., Frimurer, T. M., Holliday, N. D., Bach, A., Els, S., et al. (2011). Unique interaction pattern for a functionally biased ghrelin receptor agonist. *J. Biol. Chem.* 286, 20845–20860.

Smit, M. J., Vischer, H. F., Bakker, R. A., Jongejan, A., Timmerman, H., Pardo, L., et al. (2007). Pharmacogenomic and structural analysis of constitutive g protein-coupled receptor activity. *Annu. Rev. Pharmacol. Toxicol.* 47, 53–87.

Stengel, A., and Taché, Y. (2012). Ghrelin—a pleiotropic hormone secreted from endocrine x/a-like cells of the stomach. *Front. Neurosci.* 6:24. doi: 10.3389/fnins.2012.00024

Valentin-Hansen, L., Holst, B., Frimurer, T. M., and Schwartz, T. W. (2012). PheVI:09 (Phe6.44) as a sliding microswitch in seven-transmembrane (7TM) G protein-coupled receptor activation. *J. Biol. Chem.* 287, 43516–43526.

Wang, H. J. (2004). Ghrelin receptor gene: identification of several sequence variants in extremely obese children and adolescents, healthy normal-weight and underweight students, and children with short normal stature. *J. Clin. Endocrinol. Metab.* 89, 157–162.

13

Neurotensin and its receptors in the control of glucose homeostasis

Jean Mazella**, Sophie Béraud-Dufour, Christelle Devader, Fabienne Massa and Thierry Coppola*

Institut de Pharmacologie Moléculaire et Cellulaire, UMR 7275, Centre National de la Recherche Scientifique, Université de Nice-Sophia Antipolis, Valbonne, France

Edited by:
Hubert Vaudry, University of Rouen, France

Reviewed by:
Isabelle Dubuc, Université de Rouen, France
Gina Leinninger, Michigan State University, USA

***Correspondence:**
Jean Mazella and Thierry Coppola, Institut de Pharmacologie Moléculaire et Cellulaire, UMR 7275, Centre National de la Recherche Scientifique, Université de Nice-Sophia Antipolis, 660 route des Lucioles, Sophia Antipolis, 06560 Valbonne, France.
e-mail: mazella@ipmc.cnrs.fr; coppola@ipmc.cnrs.fr

The pharmacological roles of the neuropeptide neurotensin through its three known receptors are various and complex. Neurotensin is involved in several important biological functions including analgesia and hypothermia in the central nervous system and also food intake and glucose homeostasis in the periphery. This review focuses on recent works dealing with molecular mechanisms regulating blood glucose level and insulin secretion upon neurotensin action. Investigations on crucial cellular components involved in the protective effect of the peptide on beta cells are also detailed. The role of xenin, a neurotensin-related peptide, on the regulation of insulin release by glucose-dependent insulinotropic polypeptide is summarized. The last section comments on the future research areas which should be developed to address the function of new effectors of the neurotensinergic system in the endocrine pancreas.

Keywords: neurotensin, G protein-coupled receptor, pancreas, beta cell, sortilin

INTRODUCTION

The endogenous peptide neurotensin (NT) was discovered in 1973 in bovine hypothalami by Carraway and Leeman (1973) for its ability to induce vasodilatation. This property added to its cerebral expression indicated that the peptide could fulfill a dual function, as a neurotransmitter/neuromodulator in the central nervous system, and as a hormone in the periphery. NT is expressed in the central nervous system where it is located in neuronal synaptic vesicles (Uhl and Snyder, 1976; Bayer et al., 1991) and in the gastrointestinal tract (Goedert and Emson, 1983) in neuroendocrine cells (Atoji et al., 1995). NT is synthesized from a precursor following excision by prohormone convertases (Kitabgi, 2006).

The pharmacological and physiological effects of NT are triggered following its interaction, depending on the tissue or the cell type, by three known receptors (NTSRs). Two of them, NTSR1 and NTSR2, are classical neuropeptide receptors coupled to G-proteins (GPCR) bearing seven transmembrane domains (Vincent et al., 1999; Myers et al., 2009). The third one, NTSR3 also called sortilin (Petersen et al., 1997; Mazella et al., 1998), is a type I receptor with a single transmembrane domain, non-coupled to G-proteins, which belongs to the Vps10p containing domain receptor family (Mazella, 2001; Hermey, 2009). The heterogeneity in the structure of NTSRs, added to their ability to form homo and/or heterodimers (Martin et al., 2002; Beraud-Dufour et al., 2009; Hwang et al., 2010), underlines the complexity to study the neurotensinergic system both in the brain and in peripheral tissues.

In the central nervous system, the effects of NT include the interaction of the peptide with the dopaminergic system (Studler et al., 1988) and its ability to induce opioid-independent analgesia (Dubuc et al., 1999) and hypothermia (Popp et al., 2007). The latter property could allow the use of bioavailable NT analogs to reduce the risk of brain damage following hypoxia (Choi et al., 2012). The anti-psychotic and hypothermia effects of NT are mediated through NTSR1 (Dobner, 2005; Hadden et al., 2005; Choi et al., 2012), whereas NT-induced analgesia involves both NTSR1 and NTSR2 (Dubuc et al., 1999; Smith et al., 2012). NTSR3/sortilin is responsible for the migration and the release of cytokines and chemokines from microglial cells induced by NT (Martin et al., 2003; Dicou et al., 2004).

At the neuroendocrine point of view, the actions of NT as a regulator of anterior pituitary secretions and food intake has been recently well reviewed (Rostene and Alexander, 1997; Stolakis et al., 2010; Kalafatakis and Triantafyllou, 2011). For this reason, these sections will be only summarized at the beginning of this review focusing essentially on the role of NT in the control of glucose homeostasis. The roles of NT in insulin regulation and pancreatic cell growth have been initiated by several works (Kaneto et al., 1978; Dolais-Kitabgi et al., 1979; Wood et al., 1988). However, molecular characterization of the signaling pathways and the receptors involved in both pancreatic cell proliferation and beta cell secretion have been only recently investigated (Guha et al., 2003; Friess et al., 2003; Kisfalvi et al., 2005; Elghazi et al., 2006; Beraud-Dufour et al., 2010).

In addition, we will present the role of a NT-related peptide, named xenin, in the regulation of glucose homeostasis. Xenin is a peptide of 25 amino acids discovered in 1992 (Feurle et al., 1992), and which is synthesized from a precursor of 35 amino acids (Hamscher et al., 1996). Intriguingly, the sequence of this precursor is 100% identical to the N-terminal sequence of the mammalian coat protein α (α-COP; Chow and Quek, 1996), a cytoplasmic protein which cannot be released.

NT AND METABOLISM

The energetic balance is regulated by the control of satiety, a domain which has evoluted following the discovery of leptin. This peptide is secreted by adipocytes and acts as a hormone directly on specific hypothalamic areas involved in the control of food intake (Jequier, 2002). Interestingly, several works reported that the effects of leptin are controlled by NT expressing neurons (Cui et al., 2006). Indeed, the anorectic effect of leptin is impaired in NTSR1-deficient mice (Kim et al., 2008), suggesting that the complex NT-NTSR1 is crucial for the action of leptin. Moreover, Leinninger et al. (2011) published an elegant demonstration showing that the action of leptin via NT neurons controls orexin release, the mesolimbic dopamine system and energy balance. In conclusion, the control of food intake is mediated by leptin on NT expressing neurons through NTSR1.

The other important aspect of the neurotensinergic system in the periphery concerns the control of nutrient absorption. Rapidly following its discovery, it was observed that the level of circulating NT increased several minutes after a meal, and this increase was more important when the food was enriched with fatty acid (Leeman and Carraway, 1982). Recently, Gui and Carraway (2001) completed this observation by demonstrating that NT acts as a hormone released from intestine following ingestion of fat, and facilitates lipid digestion by stimulating pancreatic secretion. It was also demonstrated that NT enhanced taurocholate absorption from proximal rat small intestine indicating a role in the regulation of enterohepatic circulation. This effect is largely mediated by the release of mast cell mediators, and is regulated by NO (Gui and Carraway, 2004). In conclusion, NT acting as a neurotransmitter or as a hormone, regulates food intake (satiety) and lipids absorption indicating a general role for NT in the regulation of energy balance and in the control of homeostasis.

NT AND PANCREAS

Immunoreactive-NT (IR-NT) has been detected in plasma extracts and plasma IR-NT elevation occurs in response to nutrient stimuli (Rosell and Rokaeus, 1979). This suggested that NT may influence pancreatic regulation by a hormonal mechanism. IR-NT is present in the pancreas (Fernstrom et al., 1981) and a direct (paracrine) influence on islet hormone secretion was suggested. The presence of NT in the circulation and in the pancreas can be correlated to its effects on insulin and glucagon release (Dolais-Kitabgi et al., 1979) and on the growth of ductal adenocarcinoma of the pancreas (Reubi et al., 1998). Actually, we know that the action of NT on islet secretion is the consequence of the expression of the three NTSRs in normal endocrine pancreas (Beraud-Dufour et al., 2010). By contrast, NTSRs are not expressed in normal exocrine pancreas, their expression being linked with the development of tumors (Kitabgi, 2002; Myers et al., 2009).

Administration of NT increased pancreatic weight, DNA, RNA, and protein contents as well as lipase concentration (Feurle et al., 1987). The proliferative effect of NT on the pancreas has been also demonstrated by Wood et al. (1988). The role of NT and other gastrointestinal hormones like cholecystokinin or gastrin releasing peptide in the growth of normal and neoplastic tissues, including pancreas, has been well documented in a review article (Thomas et al., 2003).

NT AND PANCREATIC CANCER GROWTH

It is now well established that NT receptors are expressed in exocrine pancreatic tumors and chronic pancreatitis whereas these receptors were not found in normal exocrine pancreatic tissues (Reubi et al., 1998; Wang et al., 2000). Numerous studies have demonstrated that NT stimulates mitogenic signaling pathways and DNA synthesis in human pancreatic cancer cell lines including PANC-1 and MIA PaCa-2 cells (Herzig et al., 1999; Ehlers et al., 2000; Ryder et al., 2001; Guha et al., 2002; Falciani et al., 2010). These growth effects are mediated through NTSR1 stimulation (Iwase et al., 1997). However, a recent study concluded that NT-induced migration of pancreatic ductal adenocarcinoma cells *in vitro* occurs via NTSR3/sortilin pathways (Mijatovic et al., 2007).

NT AND ENDOCRINE PANCREAS

The first *in vivo* observation that NT displayed a role in glucose homeostasis was performed in the rat where the peptide produced hypoinsulinemia and consequently hyperglycemia (Brown and Vale, 1976). Then after, a more detailed work performed on rat islets of Langerhans demonstrated that NT regulates endocrine pancreatic hormones release (Dolais-Kitabgi et al., 1979). In this study, NT was shown to stimulate insulin and glucagon release at low glucose concentration whereas at high glucose or arginine levels, NT inhibits the release of both peptides. However, in another study performed on isolated neonatal rat islets, NT was unable to alter insulin secretion under high glucose concentration (Fujimoto, 1981). This result may be due to the absence of some NTSRs at this stage of development (Zsurger et al., 1992). The involvement of NT in the regulation of glucose homeostasis has been confirmed in a clinical study dealing with healthy elderly and young subjects. It was demonstrated that in addition to hyperinsulinemia and hypergastrinemia, the postprandial responses for NT were significantly higher in the aged subjects (Arnalich et al., 1990). However, no abnormality in the content of NT was detected in human diabetes, as demonstrated in insulin-dependent diabetic patients and in lean or obese non-insulin-dependent diabetic patients (Service et al., 1986).

MOLECULAR MECHANISMS OF NT ACTION ON BETA CELLS

PROTECTION OF BETA CELLS

Although there is a lack of evidence for a role of NT in diabetes, there are convincing data for its implication in glucose homeostasis. Surprisingly, no more important studies have been carried out to identify the NT receptor(s) involved in the effects observed. Only very recently our studies investigated the molecular mechanisms involved in the activation of the signaling pathways responsible for NT functions in cultured beta cells. We first demonstrated that all the identified NTSRs are expressed in murine Langerhans islets and in beta cell lines (Coppola et al., 2008; Beraud-Dufour et al., 2009). We demonstrated that NT efficiently protects beta cells from external cytotoxic agents (staurosporine, IL-1beta) through the PI3 kinase pathway (Coppola et al., 2008; **Figure 1**). The NTSR2 partial agonist levocabastine exerts a protective effect similar to that of NT whereas the NTSR1 antagonist SR48692 is unable to block the effect of NT suggesting the predominant involvement of the NTSR2 in the protective action of NT on beta cells. Moreover, we showed that this effect is mediated by NTSR2 via the protein complex formed between the GPCR NTSR2 and the type I receptor NTSR3/sortilin (Beraud-Dufour et al., 2009; **Figure 1**). In this case, the role of NTSR3/sortilin has been postulated to direct NTSR2 to its functional plasma membrane compartment as shown for NTSR1 in HT29 cells (Martin et al., 2002) and for the potassium channel TREK-1 in neurons (Mazella et al., 2010).

The protective action of NT on beta cells is of importance since in diabetes beta cell death is generally the consequence of prolonged hyperglycemia and/or hyperlipidemia. Therefore taking into account that NT is released in the circulation after a meal, in particular after lipid absorption, the neurotensinergic system may save endocrine pancreas as previously demonstrated for glucagon-like peptide 1 (for review Desgraz et al., 2011).

REGULATION OF INSULIN SECRETION

From experiments carried out on rat beta cell lines, we confirmed the dual action of NT, which is able to increase insulin secretion at low glucose concentration and also to decrease the glucose-induced insulin release (Dolais-Kitabgi et al., 1979; Beraud-Dufour et al., 2010). At the cellular level NT, as well as the NTSR2 selective ligand levocabastine, rapidly and transiently increases the intracellular concentration of calcium in Ins1-E cell line. NT-evoked calcium regulation involves PKC and the translocation of PKCα and PKCε to the plasma membrane. A similar response is obtained with levocabastine, indicating that NTSR2 triggers the effect of NT both on insulin secretion and calcium concentration (**Figure 1**). This result is in total agreement with a study from 1978 in which the hyperglycemia action of NT was shown to be mediated through histamine since blockers of both H1 and H2 histamine receptors were able to inhibit the effect of NT (Nagai and Frohman, 1978). Indeed, it is important to remember that levocabastine, originally developed against H1 histamine receptors (Kitabgi et al., 1987), is a selective ligand of NTSR2 (Chalon et al., 1996; Mazella et al., 1996). Moreover, we demonstrated that the propeptide issued from the maturation of the precursor form of NTSR3/sortilin (Munck Petersen et al., 1999) triggers an increase of intracellular calcium and insulin secretion as observed for NT and levocabastine (Beraud-Dufour et al., 2010). The propeptide acts as an antagonist of NTSR3/sortilin (Martin et al., 2003), however it does not block the NT effect. This

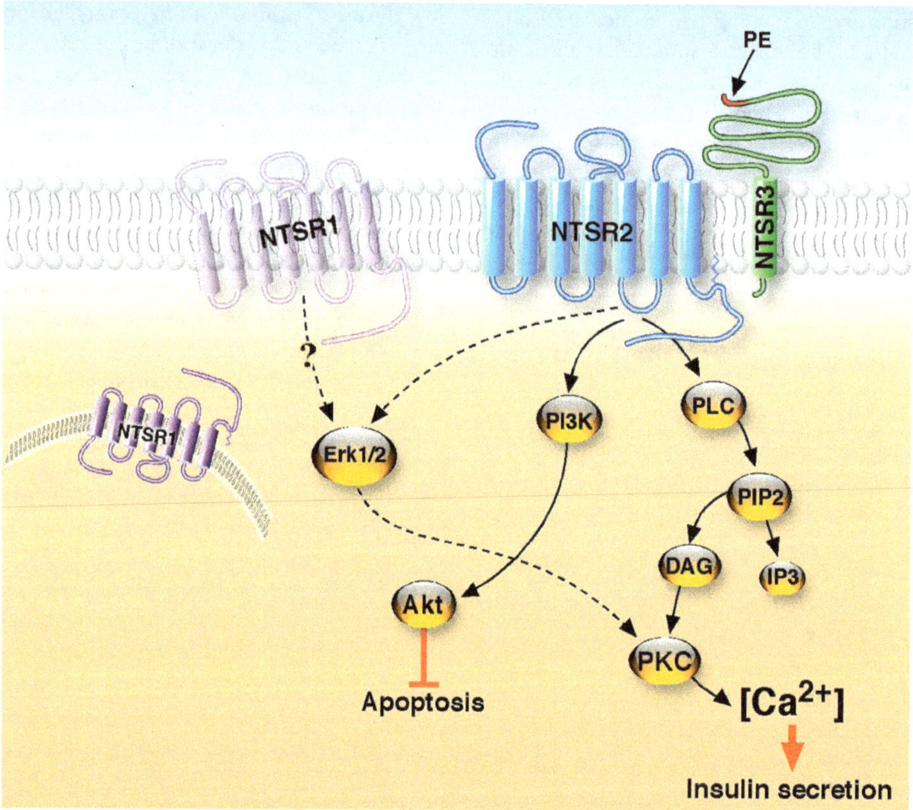

FIGURE 1 | Neurotensin receptors signaling in beta cells.
Two G protein-coupled receptors, NTSR1 and NTSR2, and one type I receptor, NTSR3, are expressed in beta cells. In one hand, the binding of NT to the complex NTSR2/NTSR3 leads to the stimulation of phospholipase C to enhance the intracellular concentration of calcium responsible for the secretion of insulin. In a second hand, the interaction of NT with the same receptor complex activates the PI3 kinase, resulting in the phosphorylation of Akt to protect beta cells from the apoptosis induced by cytotoxic external agents. Although NTSR1 is expressed in beta cells, an unusual positioning or the absence of the receptor at the plasma membrane may explain the absence of interaction with NT. The propeptide (PE) which is released from the precursor form of NTSR3 displays agonist activity to increase intracellular calcium concentration.

suggests that NTSR3/sortilin may be also involved, in combination with NTSR2, in the action of NT. We know that NTSR2 and NTSR3/sortilin form heterodimers in these beta cells (Beraud-Dufour et al., 2009). However, we do not know the exact role of NTSR3 in this complex. NTSR3 may regulate the membrane expression of NTSR2, as reported for NTSR1 (Martin et al., 2002) and the two pore potassium channel TREK-1 (Mazella et al., 2010), and so only NTSR2 selective ligand may activate the receptor complex to trigger the effect. NTSR3/sortilin selective ligands (i.e., the propeptide) may also contribute to the final activation. Further studies carried out on NTSR KO animal models would be crucial for a better understanding of the role of each receptor on insulin secretion.

Interestingly, xenin, a peptide related to NT (Feurle et al., 1992) and co-secreted with glucose-dependent insulinotropic polypeptide (GIP) from intestinal K-cells (Anlauf et al., 2000), regulates glucose homeostasis and potentiates the action of GIP on glucose-mediated insulin release (Taylor et al., 2010; Wice et al., 2010). Xenin enhances GIP-mediated insulin release by a mechanism which does not involve direct action on beta cells. Rather, the effect of xenin appears to be mediated by activating non-ganglionic cholinergic neurons that innervate islets (Wice et al., 2010). The effect of xenin in combination with molecules regulating insulin secretion rates is observed only in humans with normal or impaired glucose tolerance but not with type 2 diabetes (Wice et al., 2012). However, although xenin has been suggested to interact with NTSR1 in guinea pig enteral smooth muscles (Feurle et al., 2002) and in the effect of the peptide in food intake (Kim and Mizuno, 2010), evidence for non-neurotensin receptor-mediated effects of xenin has also been documented in rat intestine (Heuser et al., 2002). In the absence of demonstration that xenin interacts directly with one of the three known NTSRs, the effects of this peptide could be mediated by a system which is, at least partly, independent from the neurotensinergic system for the regulation of insulin secretion.

CONCLUSION AND FUTURE

From the overall data obtained on pancreatic beta cells and islets, it is clear that although the three NT receptors are expressed, the effects of NT involve both NTSR2 and NTSR3/sortilin but not NTSR1 (**Figure 1**). This is intriguing since the majority of the actions of NT both in the brain and in the periphery involves, at least partly, NTSR1, a receptor which was always shown to be expressed and functional at the plasma membrane of NT target cells. One possible explanation of its lack of implication in beta cells could be that although NTSR1 is detected by PCR and Western blot, the protein is absent or not correctly sorted at the plasma membrane. One of the arguments in favor of this hypothesis is that the binding of iodinated NT measured on membrane homogenate from beta cells is totally displaced by levocabastine (personal observation). Unfortunately, in the absence of efficient antibodies directed against NTSR1 for immunocytochemistry, sub-cellular localization of protein expression appears difficult to be correctly investigated.

On another hand, the presence of NTSR3/sortilin, as well as the effect of the propeptide on the intracellular concentration of calcium in beta cells, may be also of importance. Indeed, the role of NTSR3/sortilin as a sorting protein and its ability to be translocated to the plasma membrane upon activation by NT (Chabry et al., 1993; Navarro et al., 2001) where the propeptide can be released could serve as a new system of regulation of endocrine hormone release. Moreover, NTSR3/sortilin is also expressed on adipocytes and skeletal muscles, targets of insulin, in which its translocation to the cell surface has been also demonstrated (Lin et al., 1997; Shi and Kandror, 2007). Here again, the propeptide can be released in the circulation and then can

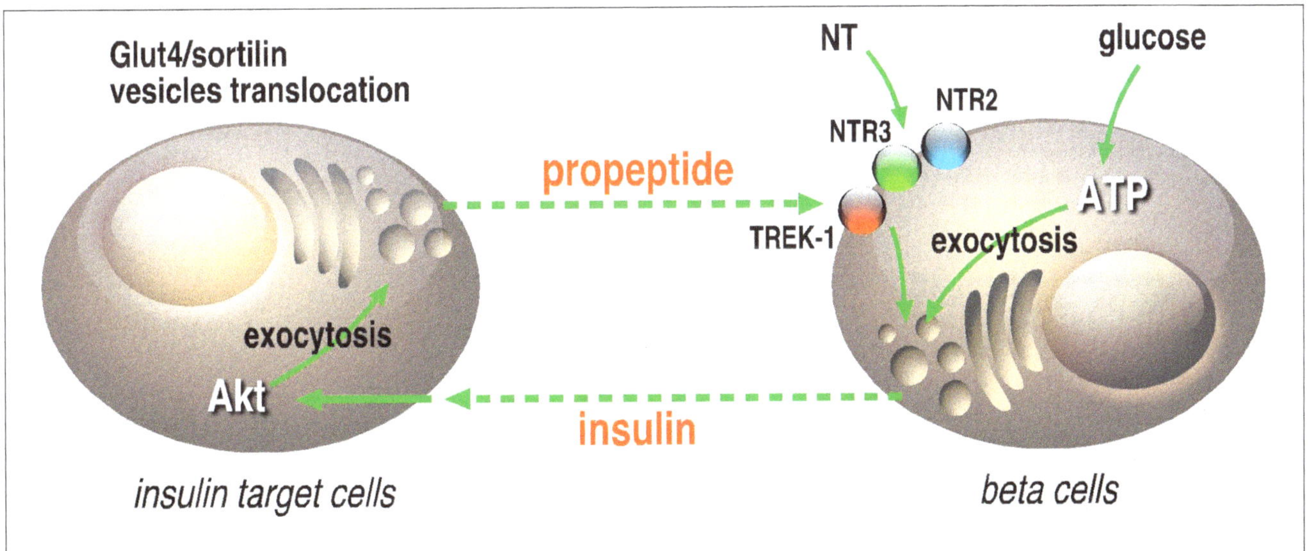

FIGURE 2 | Regulation loop between insulin secreting and target cells. In beta cells, insulin can be secreted in the circulation by glucose, NT and also by the propeptide (PE) likely through its interaction with NTSR2 or the potassium channel TREK-1 through NTSR3. In insulin target cells, the activation of insulin receptor by insulin leads to the Akt-dependent translocation of Glut4/NTSR3/sortilin containing vesicles to the plasma membrane where the propeptide can be released in the circulation. This loop of regulation between insulin secreting and insulin target cells is likely involved in fine tuning of glucose homeostasis.

regulate by feedback the secretion of insulin by interacting with NTSR3/sortilin and TREK-1 (**Figure 2**). Taken together, these observations refine the regulation scheme of glucose homeostasis through NT and its receptors and will lead to novel research areas with new components and new functions like the propeptide release and action.

ACKNOWLEDGMENTS

This work was supported by the Centre National de la Recherche Scientifique and by grants from the Plan National de la Recherche sur le Diabète, INSERM (grant no. PNRD0701) and Association pour la Recherche sur le Diabète (ARD). We thank Franck Aguila for artwork.

REFERENCES

Anlauf, M., Weihe, E., Hartschuh, W., Hamscher, G., and Feurle, G. E. (2000). Localization of xenin-immunoreactive cells in the duodenal mucosa of humans and various mammals. *J. Histochem. Cytochem.* 48, 1617–1626.

Arnalich, F., Hernanz, A., Arribas, J. R., Codoceo, R., Grande, C., and Vazquez, J. J. (1990). Gut regulatory peptides and pancreatic beta-cell response to nutritional stimuli in the elderly. *J. Med.* 21, 323–330.

Atoji, Y., Hirasawa, Y., Yamamoto, Y., and Suzuki, Y. (1995). Distribution of neurotensin-immunoreactive neurons in the digestive tract of the chicken. *J. Auton. Nerv. Syst.* 53, 185–194.

Bayer, V. E., Towle, A. C., and Pickel, V. M. (1991). Vesicular and cytoplasmic localization of neurotensin-like immunoreactivity (NTLI) in neurons postsynaptic to terminals containing NTLI and/or tyrosine hydroxylase in the rat central nucleus of the amygdala. *J. Neurosci. Res.* 30, 398–413.

Beraud-Dufour, S., Abderrahmani, A., Noel, J., Brau, F., Waeber, G., Mazella, J., et al. (2010). Neurotensin is a regulator of insulin secretion in pancreatic beta-cells. *Int. J. Biochem. Cell Biol.* 42, 1681–1688.

Beraud-Dufour, S., Coppola, T., Massa, F., and Mazella, J. (2009). Neurotensin receptor-2 and -3 are crucial for the anti-apoptotic effect of neurotensin on pancreatic beta-TC3 cells. *Int. J. Biochem. Cell Biol.* 41, 2398–2402.

Brown, M., and Vale, W. (1976). Effects of neurotensin and substance P on plasma insulin, glucagon and glucose levels. *Endocrinology* 98, 819–822.

Carraway, R., and Leeman, S. E. (1973). The isolation of a new hypotensive peptide, neurotensin, from bovine hypothalami. *J. Biol. Chem.* 248, 6854–6861.

Chabry, J., Gaudriault, G., Vincent, J. P., and Mazella, J. (1993). Implication of various forms of neurotensin receptors in the mechanism of internalization of neurotensin in cerebral neurons. *J. Biol. Chem.* 268, 17138–17144.

Chalon, P., Vita, N., Kaghad, M., Guillemot, M., Bonnin, J., Delpech, B., et al. (1996). Molecular cloning of a levocabastine-sensitive neurotensin binding site. *FEBS Lett.* 386, 91–94.

Choi, K. E., Hall, C. L., Sun, J. M., Wei, L., Mohamad, O., Dix, T. A., et al. (2012). A novel stroke therapy of pharmacologically induced hypothermia after focal cerebral ischemia in mice. *FASEB J.* 26, 2799–2810.

Chow, V. T., and Quek, H. H. (1996). HEP-COP, a novel human gene whose product is highly homologous to the alpha-subunit of the yeast coatomer protein complex. *Gene* 169, 223–227.

Coppola, T., Beraud-Dufour, S., Antoine, A., Vincent, J. P., and Mazella, J. (2008). Neurotensin protects pancreatic beta cells from apoptosis. *Int. J. Biochem. Cell Biol.* 40, 2296–2302.

Cui, H., Cai, F., and Belsham, D. D. (2006). Leptin signaling in neurotensin neurons involves STAT, MAP kinases ERK1/2, and p38 through c-Fos and ATF1. *FASEB J.* 20, 2654–2656.

Desgraz, R., Bonal, C., and Herrera, P. L. (2011). Beta-cell regeneration: the pancreatic intrinsic faculty. *Trends Endocrinol. Metab.* 22, 34–43.

Dicou, E., Vincent, J. P., and Mazella, J. (2004). Neurotensin receptor-3/sortilin mediates neurotensin-induced cytokine/chemokine expression in a murine microglial cell line. *J. Neurosci. Res.* 78, 92–99.

Dobner, P. R. (2005). Multitasking with neurotensin in the central nervous system. *Cell. Mol. Life Sci.* 62, 1946–1963.

Dolais-Kitabgi, J., Kitabgi, P., Brazeau, P., and Freychet, P. (1979). Effect of neurotensin on insulin, glucagon, and somatostatin release from isolated pancreatic islets. *Endocrinology* 105, 256–260.

Dubuc, I., Sarret, P., Labbe-Jullie, C., Botto, J. M., Honore, E., Bourdel, E., et al. (1999). Identification of the receptor subtype involved in the analgesic effect of neurotensin. *J. Neurosci.* 19, 503–510.

Ehlers, R. A., Zhang, Y., Hellmich, M. R., and Evers, B. M. (2000). Neurotensin-mediated activation of MAPK pathways and AP-1 binding in the human pancreatic cancer cell line, MIA PaCa-2. *Biochem. Biophys. Res. Commun.* 269, 704–708.

Elghazi, L., Balcazar, N., and Bernal-Mizrachi, E. (2006). Emerging role of protein kinase B/Akt signaling in pancreatic beta-cell mass and function. *Int. J. Biochem. Cell Biol.* 38, 157–163.

Falciani, C., Lelli, B., Brunetti, J., Pileri, S., Cappelli, A., Pini, A., et al. (2010). Modular branched neurotensin peptides for tumor target tracing and receptor-mediated therapy: a proof-of-concept. *Curr. Cancer Drug Targets* 10, 695–704.

Fernstrom, M. H., Mirski, M. A., Carraway, R. E., and Leeman, S. E. (1981). Immunoreactive neurotensin levels in pancreas: elevation in diabetic rats and mice. *Metabolism* 30, 853–855.

Feurle, G. E., Hamscher, G., Kusiek, R., Meyer, H. E., and Metzger, J. W. (1992). Identification of xenin, a xenopsin-related peptide, in the human gastric mucosa and its effect on exocrine pancreatic secretion. *J. Biol. Chem.* 267, 22305–22309.

Feurle, G. E., Metzger, J. W., Grudinki, A., and Hamscher, G. (2002). Interaction of xenin with the neurotensin receptor of guinea pig enteral smooth muscles. *Peptides* 23, 1519–1525.

Feurle, G. E., Muller, B., and Rix, E. (1987). Neurotensin induces hyperplasia of the pancreas and growth of the gastric antrum in rats. *Gut* 28(Suppl.), 19–23.

Friess, H., Zhu, Z., Liard, V., Shi, X., Shrikhande, S. V., Wang, L., et al. (2003). Neurokinin-1 receptor expression and its potential effects on tumor growth in human pancreatic cancer. *Lab. Invest.* 83, 731–742.

Fujimoto, W. Y. (1981). Effect of gut peptides on glucose-stimulated insulin release by monolayer cultures of neonatal rat islet cells. *Horm. Metab. Res.* 13, 135–138.

Goedert, M., and Emson, P. C. (1983). The regional distribution of neurotensin-like immunoreactivity in central and peripheral tissues of the cat. *Brain Res.* 272, 291–297.

Guha, S., Lunn, J. A., Santiskulvong, C., and Rozengurt, E. (2003). Neurotensin stimulates protein kinase C-dependent mitogenic signaling in human pancreatic carcinoma cell line PANC-1. *Cancer Res.* 63, 2379–2387.

Guha, S., Rey, O., and Rozengurt, E. (2002). Neurotensin induces protein kinase C-dependent protein kinase D activation and DNA synthesis in human pancreatic carcinoma cell line PANC-1. *Cancer Res.* 62, 1632–1640.

Gui, X., and Carraway, R. E. (2001). Enhancement of jejunal absorption of conjugated bile acid by neurotensin in rats. *Gastroenterology* 120, 151–160.

Gui, X., and Carraway, R. E. (2004). Involvement of mast cells in basal and neurotensin-induced intestinal absorption of taurocholate in rats. *Am. J. Physiol. Gastrointest. Liver Physiol.* 287, G408–416.

Hadden, M. K., Orwig, K. S., Kokko, K. P., Mazella, J., and Dix, T. A. (2005). Design, synthesis, and evaluation of the antipsychotic potential of orally bioavailable neurotensin (8-13) analogues containing non-natural arginine and lysine residues. *Neuropharmacology* 49, 1149–1159.

Hamscher, G., Meyer, H. E., and Feurle, G. E. (1996). Identification of proxenin as a precursor of the peptide xenin with sequence homology to yeast and mammalian coat protein alpha. *Peptides* 17, 889–893.

Hermey, G. (2009). The Vps10p-domain receptor family. *Cell. Mol. Life Sci.* 66, 2677–2689.

Herzig, M. C., Chapman, W. G., Sheridan, A., Rake, J. B., and Woynarowski, J. M. (1999). Neurotensin receptor-mediated inhibition of pancreatic cancer cell growth by the neurotensin antagonist SR 48692. *Anticancer Res.* 19, 213–219.

Heuser, M., Kleiman, I., Popken, O., Nustede, R., and Post, S. (2002). Evidence for non-neurotensin receptor-mediated effects of xenin (1-25) – focus on intestinal microcirculation. *Regul. Pept.* 107, 23–27.

Hwang, J. R., Baek, M. W., Sim, J., Choi, H. S., Han, J. M., Kim, Y. L., et al. (2010). Intermolecular cross-talk between NTR1 and NTR2 neurotensin receptor promotes intracellular sequestration and functional inhibition of NTR1 receptors. *Biochem. Biophys. Res. Commun.* 391, 1007–1013.

Iwase, K., Evers, B. M., Hellmich, M. R., Kim, H. J., Higashide, S.,

Gully, D., et al. (1997). Inhibition of neurotensin-induced pancreatic carcinoma growth by a nonpeptide neurotensin receptor antagonist, SR48692. *Cancer* 79, 1787–1793.

Jequier, E. (2002). Leptin signaling, adiposity, and energy balance. *Ann. N. Y. Acad. Sci.* 967, 379–388.

Kalafatakis, K., and Triantafyllou, K. (2011). Contribution of neurotensin in the immune and neuroendocrine modulation of normal and abnormal enteric function. *Regul. Pept.* 170, 7–17.

Kaneto, A., Kaneko, T., Kajinuma, H., and Kosaka, K. (1978). Effects of substance P and neurotensin infused intrapancreatically on glucagon and insulin secretion. *Endocrinology* 102, 393–401.

Kim, E. R., Leckstrom, A., and Mizuno, T. M. (2008). Impaired anorectic effect of leptin in neurotensin receptor 1-deficient mice. *Behav. Brain Res.* 194, 66–71.

Kim, E. R., and Mizuno, T. M. (2010). Role of neurotensin receptor 1 in the regulation of food intake by neuromedins and neuromedin-related peptides. *Neurosci. Lett.* 468, 64–67.

Kisfalvi, K., Guha, S., and Rozengurt, E. (2005). Neurotensin and EGF induce synergistic stimulation of DNA synthesis by increasing the duration of ERK signaling in ductal pancreatic cancer cells. *J. Cell. Physiol.* 202, 880–890.

Kitabgi, P. (2002). Targeting neurotensin receptors with agonists and antagonists for therapeutic purposes. *Curr. Opin. Drug Discov. Dev.* 5, 764–776.

Kitabgi, P. (2006). Differential processing of pro-neurotensin/neuromedin N and relationship to pro-hormone convertases. *Peptides* 27, 2508–2514.

Kitabgi, P., Rostene, W., Dussaillant, M., Schotte, A., Laduron, P. M., and Vincent, J. P. (1987). Two populations of neurotensin binding sites in murine brain: discrimination by the antihistamine levocabastine reveals markedly different radioautographic distribution. *Eur. J. Pharmacol.* 140, 285–293.

Leeman, S. E., and Carraway, R. E. (1982). Neurotensin: discovery, isolation, characterization, synthesis and possible physiological roles. *Ann. N. Y. Acad. Sci.* 400, 1–16.

Leinninger, G. M., Opland, D. M., Jo, Y. H., Faouzi, M., Christensen, L., Cappellucci, L. A., et al. (2011). Leptin action via neurotensin neurons controls orexin, the mesolimbic dopamine system and energy balance. *Cell Metab.* 14, 313–323.

Lin, B. Z., Pilch, P. F., and Kandror, K. V. (1997). Sortilin is a major protein component of Glut4-containing vesicles. *J. Biol. Chem.* 272, 24145–24147.

Martin, S., Navarro, V., Vincent, J. P., and Mazella, J. (2002). Neurotensin receptor-1 and -3 complex modulates the cellular signaling of neurotensin in the HT29 cell line. *Gastroenterology* 123, 1135–1143.

Martin, S., Vincent, J. P., and Mazella, J. (2003). Involvement of the neurotensin receptor-3 in the neurotensin-induced migration of human microglia. *J. Neurosci.* 23, 1198–1205.

Mazella, J. (2001). Sortilin/neurotensin receptor-3: a new tool to investigate neurotensin signaling and cellular trafficking? *Cell Signal.* 13, 1–6.

Mazella, J., Botto, J. M., Guillemare, E., Coppola, T., Sarret, P., and Vincent, J. P. (1996). Structure, functional expression, and cerebral localization of the levocabastine-sensitive neurotensin/neuromedin N receptor from mouse brain. *J. Neurosci.* 16, 5613–5620.

Mazella, J., Petrault, O., Lucas, G., Deval, E., Beraud-Dufour, S., Gandin, C., et al. (2010). Spadin, a sortilin-derived peptide, targeting rodent TREK-1 channels: a new concept in the antidepressant drug design. *PLoS Biol.* 8, e1000355. doi: 10.1371/journal.pbio.1000355

Mazella, J., Zsurger, N., Navarro, V., Chabry, J., Kaghad, M., Caput, D., et al. (1998). The 100-kDa neurotensin receptor is gp95/sortilin, a non-G-protein-coupled receptor. *J. Biol. Chem.* 273, 26273–26276.

Mijatovic, T., Gailly, P., Mathieu, V., De Neve, N., Yeaton, P., Kiss, R., et al. (2007). Neurotensin is a versatile modulator of *in vitro* human pancreatic ductal adenocarcinoma cell (PDAC) migration. *Cell. Oncol.* 29, 315–326.

Munck Petersen, C., Nielsen, M. S., Jacobsen, C., Tauris, J., Jacobsen, L., Gliemann, J., et al. (1999). Propeptide cleavage conditions sortilin/neurotensin receptor-3 for ligand binding. *EMBO J.* 18, 595–604.

Myers, R. M., Shearman, J. W., Kitching, M. O., Ramos-Montoya, A., Neal, D. E., and Ley, S. V. (2009). Cancer, chemistry, and the cell: molecules that interact with the neurotensin receptors. *ACS Chem. Biol.* 4, 503–525.

Nagai, K., and Frohman, L. A. (1978). Neurotensin hyperglycemia: evidence for histamine mediation and the assessment of a possible physiologic role. *Diabetes* 27, 577–582.

Navarro, V., Martin, S., Sarret, P., Nielsen, M. S., Petersen, C. M., Vincent, J., et al. (2001). Pharmacological properties of the mouse neurotensin receptor 3. Maintenance of cell surface receptor during internalization of neurotensin. *FEBS Lett.* 495, 100–105.

Petersen, C. M., Nielsen, M. S., Nykjaer, A., Jacobsen, L., Tommerup, N., Rasmussen, H. H., et al. (1997). Molecular identification of a novel candidate sorting receptor purified from human brain by receptor-associated protein affinity chromatography. *J. Biol. Chem.* 272, 3599–3605.

Popp, E., Schneider, A., Vogel, P., Teschendorf, P., and Bottiger, B. W. (2007). Time course of the hypothermic response to continuously administered neurotensin. *Neuropeptides* 41, 349–354.

Reubi, J. C., Waser, B., Friess, H., Buchler, M., and Laissue, J. (1998). Neurotensin receptors: a new marker for human ductal pancreatic adenocarcinoma. *Gut* 42, 546–550.

Rosell, S., and Rokaeus, A. (1979). The effect of ingestion of amino acids, glucose and fat on circulating neurotensin-like immunoreactivity (NTLI) in man. *Acta Physiol. Scand.* 107, 263–267.

Rostene, W. H., and Alexander, M. J. (1997). Neurotensin and neuroendocrine regulation. *Front. Neuroendocrinol.* 18, 115–173.

Ryder, N. M., Guha, S., Hines, O. J., Reber, H. A., and Rozengurt, E. (2001). G protein-coupled receptor signaling in human ductal pancreatic cancer cells: neurotensin responsiveness and mitogenic stimulation. *J. Cell. Physiol.* 186, 53–64.

Service, F. J., Jay, J. M., Rizza, R. A., O'Brien, P. C., and Go, V. L. (1986). Neurotensin in diabetes and obesity. *Regul. Pept.* 14, 85–92.

Shi, J., and Kandror, K. V. (2007). The luminal Vps10p domain of sortilin plays the predominant role in targeting to insulin-responsive Glut4-containing vesicles. *J. Biol Chem.* 282, 9008–9016.

Smith, K. E., Boules, M., Williams, K., and Richelson, E. (2012). NTS1 and NTS2 mediate analgesia following neurotensin analog treatment in a mouse model for visceral pain. *Behav. Brain Res.* 232, 93–97.

Stolakis, V., Kalafatakis, K., Botis, J., Zarros, A., and Liapi, C. (2010). The regulatory role of neurotensin on the hypothalamic-anterior pituitary axons: emphasis on the control of thyroid-related functions. *Neuropeptides* 44, 1–7.

Studler, J. M., Kitabgi, P., Tramu, G., Herve, D., Glowinski, J., and Tassin, J. P. (1988). Extensive co-localization of neurotensin with dopamine in rat meso-cortico-frontal dopaminergic neurons. *Neuropeptides* 11, 95–100.

Taylor, A. I., Irwin, N., McKillop, A. M., Patterson, S., Flatt, P. R., and Gault, V. A. (2010). Evaluation of the degradation and metabolic effects of the gut peptide xenin on insulin secretion, glycaemic control and satiety. *J. Endocrinol.* 207, 87–93.

Thomas, R. P., Hellmich, M. R., Townsend, C. M. Jr., and Evers, B. M. (2003). Role of gastrointestinal hormones in the proliferation of normal and neoplastic tissues. *Endocr. Rev.* 24, 571–599.

Uhl, G. R., and Snyder, S. H. (1976). Regional and subcellular distributions of brain neurotensin. *Life Sci.* 19, 1827–1832.

Vincent, J. P., Mazella, J., and Kitabgi, P. (1999). Neurotensin and neurotensin receptors. *Trends Pharmacol. Sci.* 20, 302–309.

Wang, L., Friess, H., Zhu, Z., Graber, H., Zimmermann, A., Korc, M., et al. (2000). Neurotensin receptor-1 mRNA analysis in normal pancreas and pancreatic disease. *Clin. Cancer Res.* 6, 566–571.

Wice, B. M., Reeds, D. N., Tran, H. D., Crimmins, D. L., Patterson, B. W., Dunai, J., et al. (2012). Xenin-25 amplifies GIP-mediated insulin secretion in humans with normal and impaired glucose tolerance but not type 2 diabetes. *Diabetes* 61, 1793–1800.

Wice, B. M., Wang, S., Crimmins, D. L., Diggs-Andrews, K. A., Althage, M. C., Ford, E. L., et al. (2010). Xenin-25 potentiates glucose-dependent insulinotropic polypeptide action via a novel cholinergic relay mechanism. *J. Biol. Chem.* 285, 19842–19853.

Wood, J. G., Hoang, H. D., Bussjaeger, L. J., and Solomon, T. E. (1988). Effect of neurotensin on pancreatic and gastric secretion and growth in rats. *Pancreas* 3, 332–339.

Zsurger, N., Chabry, J., Coquerel, A., and Vincent, J. P. (1992). Ontogenesis and binding properties of high-affinity neurotensin receptors in human brain. *Brain Res.* 586, 303–310.

14

The role of melanin-concentrating hormone and its receptors in energy homeostasis

Douglas J. MacNeil *

Department of In Vitro Pharmacology, Merck Research Laboratories, Kenilworth, NJ, USA

Edited by:
Hubert Vaudry, University of Rouen, France

Reviewed by:
Jean Albert Boutin, Institut de Recherches Servier, France
Olivier Civelli, University of California Irvine, USA

***Correspondence:**
Douglas J. MacNeil, Department of In Vitro Pharmacology, Merck Research Laboratories, K15-3-309D, 2015 Galloping Hill Road, Kenilworth, NJ 07033, USA.
e-mail: doug.macneil@merck.com

Extensive studies in rodents with melanin-concentrating hormone (MCH) have demonstrated that the neuropeptide hormone is a potent orexigen. Acutely, MCH causes an increase in food intake, while chronically it leads to increased weight gain, primarily as an increase in fat mass. Multiple knockout mice models have confirmed the importance of MCH in modulating energy homeostasis. Animals lacking MCH, MCH-containing neurons, or the MCH receptor all are resistant to diet-induced obesity. These genetic and pharmacologic studies have prompted a large effort to identify potent and selective MCH receptor antagonists, initially as tool compounds to probe pharmacology in models of obesity, with an ultimate goal to identify novel anti-obesity drugs. In animal models, MCH antagonists have consistently shown efficacy in reducing food intake acutely and inhibiting body-weight gain when given chronically. Five compounds have proceeded into clinical testing. Although they were reported as well-tolerated, none has advanced to long-term efficacy and safety studies.

Keywords: MCH, neuropeptide, MCHR1, orexigenic, obesity, KO mice, antagonist, clinical study

INTRODUCTION

The mammalian form of melanin-concentrating hormone (MCH), is a 19-amino acid cyclic peptide encoded within a 165-amino acid preprohormone (**Figure 1**) (Vaughan et al., 1989). MCH has been associated with a wide variety of behaviors (see recent reviews by Saito and Nagasaki, 2008; Antal-Zimanyi and Khawaja, 2009; Chung et al., 2011), but the focus of this review is the role of MCH in energy homeostasis. The amino acid sequence of MCH is identical in all mammals evaluated and alternative processing of the preproMCH peptide can generate two additional putative peptides, designated neuropeptide E-I (NEI) and neuropeptide G-E (NGE) (Nahon et al., 1989). Several *in vivo* studies have shown that MCH plays a role in a variety of physiologic processes mediated within the central nervous system (CNS), including energy homeostasis sleep and arousal, and emotionality (Yumiko and Nagasaki, 2008; Torterolo et al., 2009). Although less studied, MCH may also have a role in peripheral tissues such as in gut and pancreatic islet function (Pissios et al., 2007; Kokkotou et al., 2008).

Two MCH G-protein coupled receptors (GPCRs) have been characterized (Pissios et al., 2006; Chung et al., 2011). MCHR1 is found in all vertebrates, while MCHR2 is found in non-rodent higher species, including primates (Hill et al., 2001; Sailer et al., 2001).

Neurobiology, rodent genetics, and rodent pharmacologic studies all demonstrate that MCH and the MCH receptors are involved in regulating body weight (Gomori et al., 2003, 2007; Hervieu, 2006; Bednarek, 2007; Antal-Zimanyi and Khawaja, 2009; Johansson, 2011; Cheon, 2012). On the basis of this information, many pharmaceutical companies have pursued the development of MCHR1 antagonists for the treatment of obesity (for a recent review, see Johansson, 2011). Unfortunately, although a few MCHR1 antagonists have entered development, no compound has successfully demonstrated anti-obesity efficacy in a clinical trial. It remains unclear if this lack of clinical efficacy is due to a lack of efficacy via the MCH1R pathway or to the inability of teams to identify safe and well-tolerated compounds with sufficient potency and pharmacodynamics properties to test the hypothesis. This review summarizes the evidence for a role of MCH and its receptors in energy homeostasis and the progress made to date toward identifying small-molecule antagonists to treat obesity.

MCH ACTS THROUGH TWO G-PROTEIN COUPLED RECEPTORS

Originally described as the orphan receptor SLC-1/GPR24 (Kolakowski et al., 1996), MCHR1 was later shown by five groups to be activated by MCH (Pissios et al., 2006). The 402-amino acid rodent and human MCHR1 receptors are highly homologous, sharing ~95% identity (Pissios and Maratos-Flier, 2003), and the highest expression of the receptors is within the brain (Saito et al., 1999; Hill et al., 2001). Like many family A GPCRs, the MCHR1 receptors have consensus *N*-glycosylation sites at the amino terminus and several potential phosphorylation sites in the intracellular loops (Lakaye et al., 1998).

In recombinant cell lines, the natural ligand, MCH, binds to MCHR1 with ~1 nM affinity, and it couples to Gi, Go, and Gq proteins (Hawes et al., 2000; Pissios et al., 2003). Thus, activation of MCHR1 leads to an increase in intracellular Ca^{++} accumulation acting through the Gq-coupled pathway and/or to lowered cyclic adenosine monophosphate (cAMP) levels via the Gi/o-coupled pathway. Further analyses of the signaling of MCHR1 in recombinant cell lines and in brain slices demonstrates that activation of MCHR1 also leads to ERK phosphorylation (Pissios et al., 2003). In 3T3-L1 adipocytes, MCH rapidly induced a threefold to fivefold

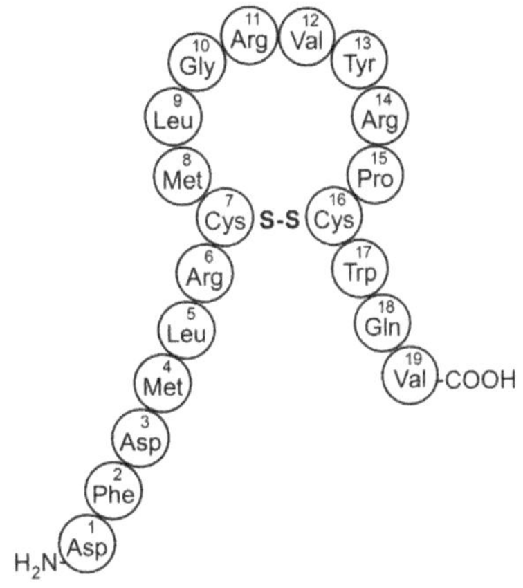

FIGURE 1 | The amino acid structure of mammalian MCH.

increase in MAPK pathway activities (Bradley et al., 2002). It is unclear if all, or some, of these signaling pathways contribute to MCH-mediated events *in vivo*.

A second MCHR was later identified and termed MCHR2 by six groups (Antal-Zimanyi and Khawaja, 2009). The functional role of MCHR2 is not well defined, in part because it is not expressed in rodents and related species (hamsters, guinea pigs, or rabbits), but it is expressed in humans, dogs, ferrets, and monkeys (Tan et al., 2002). The amino acid sequence identity between MCHR1 and MCHR2 is low, ~38%, with the highest homology in the seven-transmembrane domains that form the ligand binding pocket (Sailer et al., 2001). Although MCH binds to MCHR1 and MCHR2 with a similar nanomolar affinity, the signal transduction mechanism of MCHR2 is limited to the Gq-mediated increase in intracellular Ca^{++} levels (Sailer et al., 2001). MCHR2 is largely co-expressed with MCHR1 in the CNS (Sailer et al., 2001), although peripheral expression was also found in adipocytes, pancreas, prostate, and intestine (An et al., 2001). The phylogenetic tree of MCH-related receptors contains opioid, somatostatin, galanin, urotensin 2, and orphan receptors (Sailer et al., 2001). MCH receptors have the highest homology (about 40%) with the somatostatin receptors (Sailer et al., 2001).

NEUROANATOMY OF MCH AND MCH RECEPTORS

Melanin-concentrating hormone has been implicated in many behaviors. The hypothalamus is one of the primary sites in which MCH-containing nerve fibers and MCH receptors are extensively expressed (Gao, 2009). Although most of the MCH neurons are located within the incerto-hypothalamic and lateral hypothalamic area (LHA), a recent review by Bittencourt details the locations throughout the brain of MCH nerve terminals (Bittencourt, 2011). Neural signaling by MCH via its receptors has been implicated in the control of energy balance, but due to the wide distribution of MCH-containing fibers throughout the brain, the critical sites of action for particular behaviors have not been identified (Zheng et al., 2005). In male rats, neurons expressing MCH are found in the LHA and medial zona incerta, as well as, sparsely, in the olfactory tubercle and pontine reticular formation. The wide distribution of MCH fibers suggests the involvement of this neuropeptide in a variety of functions, including arousal, neuroendocrine control, and energy homeostasis (Rondini et al., 2007).

Melanin-concentrating hormone-expressing neurons in the LHA play an integrative role between signals from the periphery, acting via first-order neurons in the arcuate nucleus, and then from extra-hypothalamic systems, which modulate regulation of feeding, drinking, and seeking behaviors (Guyon et al., 2009). Factors from the periphery affect brain activity, resulting in changes in food intake and energy expenditure. Neurons from the arcuate nucleus detect changes in homeostatic parameters and transmit information to other brain areas, including the LHA. These secondary area neurons have widespread projections throughout the brain, and their activation leads to coordinated and altered behaviors (Guyon et al., 2009). About 25% of the LHA neurons projecting to the pedunculopontine tegmental (PPT) nucleus are immunoreactive for MCH, and 75% of the LHA neurons projecting to the cerebral motor cortex also contain MCH (Elias et al., 2008). Also, 15% of the incerto-hypothalamic neurons projecting to the PPT express MCH immunoreactivity. The MCH neurons express glutamic acid decarboxylase mRNA, a gamma-aminobutyric acid (GABA) synthesizing enzyme, indicating that the MCH/GABA neurons are involved in inhibitory modulation and their activation may lead to decreased motor activity in states of negative energy balance (Elias et al., 2008). Like MCH, vasopressin and oxytocin can influence energy homeostasis and other behaviors. Whole-cell recording in hypothalamic brain slices from the MCH-green fluorescent protein transgenic mouse revealed that both vasopressin and oxytocin evoked a substantial excitatory effect on MCH-expressing cells (Yao et al., 2012). Both neuropeptides reversibly increased spike frequency and depolarized the membrane potential in a concentration-dependent manner, suggesting that vasopressin or oxytocin exerts a robust excitatory effect on presumptive GABA cells that contain MCH (Yao et al., 2012).

Interestingly, projections to ventral medullary sites apparently play a role in the inhibitory effect of MCH on energy expenditure, but not food intake (Zheng et al., 2005). In the rat, a significant proportion (5–15%) of primarily perifornical and far-lateral hypothalamic MCH neurons project to the dorsal vagal complex. Retrograde tracing in the caudal brainstem demonstrated that MCH-immunoreactive axons are distributed densely in the nucleus of the solitary tract, in the dorsal motor nucleus of the vagus, and in sympathetic premotor areas in the ventral medulla (Zheng et al., 2005). In medulla slice preparations, MCH inhibited the amplitude of excitatory postsynaptic currents. Administration of MCH in the fourth ventricle in freely moving rats decreased core body temperature, but it did not change locomotor activity or food and water intake (Zheng et al., 2005).

The MCH pathways from the lateral hypothalamus to the mammillary nucleus may also enable the animal to look for food during the initial moments of appetite stimulation (Casatti et al., 2002). Injection of the retrograde tracer True Blue in the medial mammillary nucleus led to MCH/True Blue double-labeled neurons in the LHA, the rostromedial zona incerta, and the dorsal tuberomammillary nucleus. The afferents were confirmed using implants of the anterograde tracer *Phaseolus vulgaris* leucoagglutinin. The

MCH projections may participate in spatial memory processing mediated by the medial mammillary nucleus (Casatti et al., 2002).

In addition to the LHA, the nucleus accumbens shell (AcSh) is a brain region important for food intake. The AcSh contains high levels of receptor for MCH. MCH receptor activation in the AcSh increases food intake, while AcSh MCH receptor blockade reduces feeding. Moreover, *in vivo* recordings confirm that MCH reduces neuronal activity in the AcSh in freely moving animals, consistent with a model from other pharmacological and electrophysiological studies whereby reduced AcSh neuronal firing leads to food intake (Sears et al., 2010). Since the AcSh mediates reinforcing properties of food, MCH may modulate motivational aspects of feeding. Indeed, chronic loss of rat MCH decreased food intake predominantly via a reduction in meal size during development and reduced high-fat food reinforced operant response in adult rats (Mul et al., 2011). Also, chronic loss of ProMCH in the rat affects the limbic dopamine system, since adult $Pmch^{-/-}$ rats showed increased *ex vivo* electrically evoked dopamine release (Mul et al., 2011). Thus, MCH actions in the AcSh mediate motivational aspects of feeding behavior.

MCHR1 is widely distributed in the brain (Hervieu et al., 2000; Able et al., 2009). Hervieu et al. (2000) used *in situ* hybridization histochemistry and immunohistochemistry to determine that *Mchr1* mRNA and protein were widely expressed throughout the rat brain. Similar to the distribution of MCH, *Mchr1* signals were observed in the cerebral cortex, caudate-putamen, hippocampal formation, amygdala, hypothalamus, and thalamus, as well as in various nuclei of the mesencephalon and rhombencephalon (Hervieu et al., 2000). Able et al. (2009) used an MCHR1-specific radioligand to demonstrate highly MCHR1-specific binding in the rat nucleus accumbens, caudate-putamen, and preform cortex, as well as lower levels of binding in the hippocampus and amygdala. Surprisingly, and in contrast to Hervieu et al. (2000) and Able et al. (2009) did not detect MCHR1 binding in the hypothalamus.

The distribution of MCHR2 in the primate brain nearly overlaps that of MCHR1, but the latter shows much higher relative levels and a wider distribution pattern (Mori et al., 2001). *MCHR2* is expressed in several human brain areas, including the hippocampus and amygdala, although its distribution in the hypothalamus remains controversial. Specifically, *MCHR2* mRNA was reported to be mainly expressed in the arcuate nucleus and ventromedial hypothalamic nucleus in African green monkeys by *in situ* hybridization (Sailer et al., 2001), while three other reports did not detect its expression in the human hypothalamus by RT-PCR (Hill et al., 2001; Mori et al., 2001) or Northern blot analysis (Rodriguez et al., 2001).

HUMAN GENETICS OF MCH AND ENERGY HOMEOSTASIS

Genetic analysis of obese subjects has identified several variants of MCH and the MCH receptors, but no alterations have been conclusively linked to obesity or leanness. In an association study, among 106 subjects with severe early onset obesity and a history of hyperphagia, two missense variants were found in *MCHR1*: Y181H and R248Q (Gibson et al., 2004). Neither of these was found in 192 normal-weight controls. R248Q co-segregated with obesity across two generations, but family data were unavailable for Y181H. When tested for functional response, the R248Q variant showed no evidence of constitutive activation, alteration in cAMP signaling, or ligand hypersensitivity (Gibson et al., 2004). Two common single-nucleotide polymorphisms (SNPs) were found to be in linkage disequilibrium, but no association between either of these and obesity-related phenotypes was found among a population cohort of 541 whites. Only two rare, non-coding variants were found in *MCHR2*. However, the relationship of these *MCHR2* variants to metabolic phenotypes has not been clarified (Gibson et al., 2004). Genomic screening of 13.4 kb encompassing the *MCHR1* in extremely obese German children and adolescents identified 11 infrequent variations and two SNPs in the *MCHR1* coding sequence and 18 SNPs (eight were novel) in the flanking sequence. Although an association of an *MCHR1* haplotype (SNPs rs133072 and rs133073) with obesity was observed in two cohorts of German children and adolescents, it was not confirmed in five independent cohorts (Wermter et al., 2005). To investigate the possible polygenic role of *MCHR1*, six common SNPs (minor allele frequency >5%) found in the sequenced regions were screened in 557 morbidly obese adults, 552 obese children, and 1195 non-obese non-diabetic control subjects (Bell et al., 2005). The plausible promoter SNP, rs133068, was found to be associated with protection against obesity in obese children only (Bell et al., 2005).

A functional analysis of 11 MCHR1 variants that had been reported previously in the literature identified two mutant receptors, R210H and P377S, that failed to respond to MCH (Goldstein et al., 2010). Five other variants showed significant alterations in MCH efficacy, ranging from 44 to 142% of the wild-type value. Both inactive receptors had cell surface expression that was comparable to wild-type (Goldstein et al., 2010). It is of note that the two loss-of-function mutants were identified in markedly underweight individuals, raising the possibility that a lean phenotype may be linked to deficient MCHR1 signaling (Goldstein et al., 2010). Additional association studies with larger cohorts are needed to explore the extent to which signaling-deficient MCHR1 variants influence the maintenance of body weight.

The association between *MCHR2* variation and human obesity was investigated in 141 obese children and 24 non-obese adult subjects by DNA sequencing, and by case-control analyses using 628 severely obese children and 1401 controls (Ghoussaini et al., 2007). None of the *MCHR2* variants showed an association with adult severe obesity, but the A76A SNP was associated with severe obesity ($P = 0.01$) and overeating in obese children ($P = 0.02$) (Ghoussaini et al., 2007). Validation of an association of *MCHR2* with obesity requires replication in other cohorts.

The common allele of the *ProMCH* gene, rs7973796, may be associated with a higher body mass index (BMI) in olanzapine-treated patients with schizophrenia. In a subgroup of subjects under 50 years of age among 300 schizophrenia patients, the rs7973796 genotype was associated with an effect on BMI among patients taking olanzapine (interaction $P = 0.025$) (Chagnon et al., 2007). Olanzapine-treated patients with schizophrenia carrying the homozygote genotype showed a higher BMI for rs7973796 ($P = 0.016$ with the least-squares means t-test) than the variant homozygotes. The G allele was associated with an increase in the odds of obesity in schizophrenic patients taking olanzapine (Chagnon et al., 2007).

RODENT GENETICS INDICATE A ROLE FOR MCH IN ENERGY HOMEOSTASIS

Multiple mouse knockout (KO) models have been constructed to explore the role of MCH in energy homeostasis and other MCH-mediated behaviors. The KO models include multiple constructs that prevent synthesis of MCH and the MCHR1 receptor. Studies of these mice show that loss of MCH function leads to leanness and resistance to obesity.

MCH KO MICE

Strong evidence that MCH mediates energy homeostasis came from studies of mice in which the *Promch* gene was inactivated. Mice constructed with targeted inactivation of the *Promch* gene in a mixed C57BL/6 × 129SvJ genetic background had reduced body weight and leanness due to hypophagia (reduced feeding) and an increased metabolic rate, despite reduced amounts of both leptin and arcuate nucleus proopiomelanocortin mRNA (Shimada et al., 1998). Evaluation of *Promch* inactivation in pure genetic backgrounds confirmed that *Promch* deficiency increased energy expenditure and promoted increased running-wheel activity (Kokkotou et al., 2005; Zhou et al., 2005). As observed previously on a mixed background, the C57BL/6 *Promch* KO mice were hypophagic; however, the 129SvEv *Promch* KOs were hyperphagic, relative to wild-type. In both C57BL/6 and 129SvEv backgrounds, deletion of *Promch* led to reduced adiposity, attenuated weight gain, and increased locomotor activity, compared with wild-type counterparts. The relative increase in activity was greater on a high-fat diet (HFD) than on regular chow (Kokkotou et al., 2005). The lean phenotype of the *Promch* KO mice persisted as the mice aged. At 19 months, C57BL/6 *Promch*$^{-/-}$ male and female mice weighed about 25% less than their wild-type counterparts as a result of reduced fat mass in *Promch*$^{-/-}$ mice. The aged *Promch*$^{-/-}$ mice exhibited improved glucose tolerance in intraperitoneal glucose tolerance tests, were more insulin sensitive, and were more active compared with wild-type controls (Jeon et al., 2006).

Further confirmation of the role of MCH in energy homeostasis came from studies of *Promch* neuron-ablated mice, generated using toxin (ataxin-3)-mediated ablation strategy in an FVB/n background (Alon and Friedman, 2006). In these mice, the *Promch* gene is present throughout development, but 60–70% of MCH-expressing neurons degenerate in the first few weeks of life (Alon and Friedman, 2006). After 7 weeks of age, the mice developed reduced body weight, body length, fat mass, lean mass, and leptin levels. As observed in the C57BL/6 *Promch*$^{-/-}$ mice, leanness was characterized by hypophagia and increased energy expenditure. In leptin-deficient *ob/ob* mice, loss of either *Promch* or MCH-containing neurons improved obesity, diabetes, and hepatic steatosis, suggesting that MCH is an important mediator of the response to leptin deficiency (Segal-Lieberman et al., 2003; Alon and Friedman, 2006).

Promch tg MICE

The phenotype of *Promch* tg mice overexpressing MCH also supports a role for MCH in energy homeostasis. Ludwig et al. (2001) constructed transgenic mice that overexpressed *Promch* in the lateral hypothalamus at ~twofold higher levels than normal mice. On an FVB background, the homozygous transgenic mice fed a HFD ate 10% more and were 12% heavier than wild-type animals. Blood glucose levels were higher both preprandially and after an intraperitoneal glucose injection, and the transgenic mice were insulin-resistant (Ludwig et al., 2001). *Promch* tg heterozygous mice on a C57Bl/6 background were hyperphagic on regular chow, heavier, and insulin-resistant, but did not have elevated blood glucose (Ludwig et al., 2001).

Mchr1$^{-/-}$ MICE

As the gene for preproMCH encodes two additional peptides, NEI and NGE of unknown function (Nahon et al., 1989), studies with *Mchr1* KO mice provided clarification and confirmation of the role of MCH in energy homeostasis. Three groups independently produced *Mchr1*$^{-/-}$ mice. Chen et al. (2002) reported that *Mchr1* KO mice on a C57BL/6 × 129SvJ mixed background were resistant to diet-induced obesity and had fat mass that was significantly lower in both male (4.7 ± 0.6 vs. 9.6 ± 1.2 g) and female (3.9 ± 0.2 vs. 5.8 ± 0.5 g) mice than that of the wild-type control. The mice were hyperphagic on a HFD, but had a 28% higher metabolic rate than wild-type. Both leptin and insulin levels were significantly lower in male *Mchr1*$^{-/-}$ mice than in the wild-type controls, but there were no detectable differences in glucose levels. No differences were observed between heterozygotes and wild-type mice (Chen et al., 2002). Marsh et al. (2002) observed that *Mchr1*$^{-/-}$ mice also constructed on a C57BL/6 × 129SvJ mixed background had normal body weights, yet they had reduced fat mass and were hyperphagic when maintained on regular chow. In agreement with Chen et al. (2002) they observed that *Mchr1*$^{-/-}$ mice were less susceptible to diet-induced obesity, and the KO leanness was a consequence of hyperactivity and altered metabolism (Marsh et al., 2002). A later study by Zhou et al. (2005) showed that the *Mchr1* KO mice had a dramatic 250% increase in running-wheel activity along with hyperphagia (Antal-Zimanyi and Khawaja, 2009). Astrand et al. (2004) also independently generated *Mchr1*$^{-/-}$ mice on a mixed C57BL/6 × 129SvJ background and observed that the mice had an elevated metabolic rate and were hyperactive, hyperphagic, and lean. A >12% increase in heart rate without any change in blood pressure was noted (Astrand et al., 2004). Two groups studied *Mchr1* KO mice after backcrossing onto a C57BL/6 background (Bjursell et al., 2006; Ahnaou et al., 2011). In leptin-deficient *ob/ob* mice, loss of *Mchr1* reduced adiposity (although body weights were not statistically different), improved the response in an oral glucose tolerance test (OGTT), increased spontaneous movement, and improved thermoregulation upon exposure to cold, suggesting that MCH is an important mediator of the response to leptin deficiency (Bjursell et al., 2006).

The role of MCHR2 has not been investigated in animal models. MCHR2 is absent in rodents but is present in higher species, including primates (Hill et al., 2001; Sailer et al., 2001). The role of MCHR2 might be studied in MCHR2-humanized mice, but no such model has been described. Alternatively, *in vivo* studies with MCHR1- and MCHR2-selective agonists could be used to study the role of MCHR2 in non-rodent species with a functional MCHR2. Indeed, it is surprising that *in vivo* pharmacological studies with selective ligands have not been performed, in light of the availability of MCH peptides that are potent dual MCHR1/R2 agonists, selective MCHR1 agonists, MCHR2-preferring agonists, and

Table 1 | Mouse genetic models supporting a role for MCH in energy homeostasis.

Genotype	Phenotype	Reference
Promch$^{-/-}$C57BL/6 × 129SvJ	Hypophagic, reduced adiposity, increased metabolic rate, and reduced weight	Shimada et al. (1998)
Promch$^{-/-}$ C57BL/6	Normophagic, reduced adiposity, increased activity and metabolic rate, and reduced weight	Zhou et al. (2005), Kokkotou et al. (2005)
Promch$^{-/-}$C57BL/6 × 129SvEv	Hyperphagic, reduced adiposity, increased activity and metabolic rate, and reduced weight	Kokkotou et al. (2005)
Promch;ataxin-3 FVB/n	Hypophagic, reduced adiposity, increased metabolic rate, normo-activity, and reduced weight	Alon and Friedman (2006)
Promch;ataxin-3;ob/ob (FVB/nXC57BL/6)	Hyperphagic, reduced adiposity, reduced glucose, reduced steatosis, and reduced weight	Alon and Friedman (2006)
Promch$^{-/-}$*;ob/ob* C57BL/6	Reduced adiposity, reduced glucose, increased metabolic rate, increased activity, and reduced weight	Segal-Lieberman et al. (2003)
Promch tg/tg FVB	Increased weight, hyperphagic on HFD, increased glucose, and insulin-resistant	Ludwig et al. (2001)
Promch tg/+ C57BL/6	Increased weight, hyperphagic on chow, normo-glucose, and insulin-resistant	Ludwig et al. (2001)
Mchr1$^{-/-}$ C57BL/6 × 129SvJ	Reduced adiposity, hyperphagic, hyperactive, reduced weight, higher metabolic rate, and reduced insulin	Marsh et al. (2002), Chen et al. (2002), Astrand et al. (2004), Zhou et al. (2005)
Mchr1$^{-/+}$ C57BL/6 × 129SvJ	No differences vs. wild-type	Chen et al. (2002)
Mchr1$^{-/-}$ C57BL/6	Reduced insulin, improved OGTT, and elevated body temperature	Bjursell et al. (2006), Ahnaou et al. (2011)
Mchr1$^{-/-}$*;ob/ob* C57BL/6	Decreased adiposity, reduced insulin, improved OGTT, increased activity	Bjursell et al. (2006)

potent MCHR1/R2 antagonists (MacNeil and Bednarek, 2009). At this point, it is unclear if MCHR1 and MCHR2 play redundant or unique roles in MCH signaling in primates, or whether MCHR2 plays any significant role in energy homeostasis in humans.

Multiple mouse models show that disruption of the MCH system, via either the peptide ligand or the receptor, results in altered energy homeostasis (**Table 1**). In general, loss of MCH signaling leads to a lean, diet-induced obese (DIO)-resistant phenotype due primarily to increased energy expenditure, and in some models, lower food intake.

PHARMACOLOGIC STUDIES CONFIRM A ROLE FOR MCH IN ENERGY HOMEOSTASIS

In vivo studies have shown that MCH or MCH analogs increase food intake and body weight, while, conversely, studies with MCHR1 antagonists reduce body weight and associated comorbidities.

IN VIVO EFFECTS OF MCH PEPTIDE AGONISTS

Melanin-concentrating hormone, and occasionally MCH derivatives, have been used to evaluate the role of MCH in energy homeostasis. Most studies have utilized acute injections of MCH into either specific brain nuclei or, more commonly, the third or fourth ventricle. These injections almost certainly lead to supraphysiologic levels of MCH in at least some of the MCH receptor-containing nuclei. Qu et al. (1996) were the first to show that intracerebroventricular (ICV) MCH increased food intake. In multiple experiments ICV injections of 5 or 30 μg into Long Evans rats increased 2-, 4-, and 6-h food intake between 150 and 200% (Qu et al., 1996). ICV injection of MCH into the third ventricle of either Wistar or Sprague-Dawley rats also increased food intake (Qu et al., 1996; Della-Zuana et al., 2002; Shearman et al., 2003). The orexigenic effects of ICV MCH were maximal at 2 h post injection (Della-Zuana et al., 2002). In Wistar rats, low doses (0.1 and 0.5 μg/rat) were ineffective, while higher doses (1, 5, and 10 μg/rat) were equally effective, leading to an approximate doubling of food intake over 2–4 h (Della-Zuana et al., 2002). In Sprague-Dawley rats, only the two highest doses led to significant increases in food intake (Della-Zuana et al., 2002). When presented with sucrose solutions after ICV injection of MCH (2 nmol), Sprague-Dawley rats increased their intake of sucrose solution by increasing the rate of licking (Baird et al., 2006). The role of MCH in energy homeostasis was also confirmed in sheep, which have both MCHR1 and MCHR2; acute ICV doses of MCH increased food intake (Whitlock et al., 2005). Potent MCH analogs ($IC_{50} < 25$ nM), but not the weak analogs ($IC_{50} > 1000$ nM), reduced 2-h food intake after ICV administration of 4.4 nmol to Wistar rats (Suply et al., 2001). In a separate study in Sprague-Dawley rats using a smaller, potent MCH analog, Shearman et al. (2003) observed dose-dependent increases in 6-h food intake after an ICV injection of an MCH agonist (1 μg/rat, +68%; 5 μg/rat, +76%; 15 μg/rat, +122%). Guesdon et al. (2008) confirmed that the smaller MCH analog, when given ICV at 5 μg/rat, increased food intake in Wistar rats threefold over a 2-h period.

Intracerebroventricular injection of MCH into the third ventricle of rats significantly increased the ingestion of sucrose and glucose solution, but not of saccharin, indicating that the MCH-induced dipsogenic response is more related to caloric content than to sweet taste *per se* (Sakamaki et al., 2005). Injections of MCH into several brain nuclei led to increases in food intake. MCH (0.6 nmol) elicited a rapid and significant increase in feeding in satiated rats following injection into the arcuate nucleus, the paraventricular nucleus, or the dorsomedial nucleus (Abbott et al., 2003). However, no significant alteration in feeding was observed following injection into other brain regions associated with energy homeostasis, including the supraoptic nucleus, LHA, medial preoptic area, anterior hypothalamic area, or ventromedial nucleus of the hypothalamus (Abbott et al., 2003).

In a side-by-side comparison, MCH was found to be a weaker orexigen than two other hypothalamic neuropeptides. In lean rats, 1 and 3 nmol of the ICV-injected orexigenic peptides, neuropeptide Y (NPY) and agouti-related protein (AGRP), showed robust increases in intake of a sucrose solution, but 3 nmol of MCH mediated only a non-significant trend toward increased feeding (Semjonous et al., 2009). The importance of forebrain hypothalamic regions for MCH action was apparent when injection of 6 nmol of MCH into the fourth ventricle of lean rats or sheep failed to induce increased food intake, while control injections of NPY did increase food intake (Whitlock et al., 2005; Baird et al., 2007). Administration of LiCl, a potent inducer of conditioned taste aversion (CTA), to rats leads to an upregulation of *Mch* and *Mchr1* mRNA (Mitra et al., 2012). However, when MCH was injected prior to the induction of CTA with LiCl, as well as later during the CTA retrieval, MCH treatment did not reduce the magnitude of CTA upon subsequent presentations of the aversive tastant (Mitra et al., 2012). Thus, MCH is not critical to the development of CTA.

Although most ICV studies leading to an increase in food intake utilized injection into the third ventricle, Georgescu et al. (2005) demonstrated that direct injection of 1 μg of MCH into the AcSh, a region rich in MCHR1, resulted in a robust increase in food intake by Sprague-Dawley rats lasting at least 4 h. Guesdon et al. (2008) used a potent, truncated MCH analog and also observed that injection of 5 μg into the AcSh of Wistar rats increased food intake of regular chow threefold during the 2 h following injection.

Agonist studies in preproMCH-deficient rats confirmed that the orexigenic actions of MCH are independent of two other preproMCH encoded peptides, NGE and NEI. Acute AcSh administration of NGE and NEI, or chronic ICV infusion of NEI, did not affect feeding behavior in adult *Promch*$^{+/+}$ or *Promch*$^{-/-}$ rats (Mul et al., 2011). However, acute administration of MCH to the AcSh of adult *Promch*$^{-/-}$ rats elevated feeding behavior toward wild-type levels (Mul et al., 2011).

In addition to the effects of MCH on food intake, the role of MCH in mediating energy expenditure was also compared with that of two other orexigenic peptides, AGRP and orexin. Both AGRP and orexin, administered ICV (1 nmol/mouse), significantly decreased oxygen consumption compared with artificial cerebrospinal fluid (aCSF) treated controls; in contrast, MCH (1 nmol/mouse) had no significant effect compared with aCSF-treated controls (Asakawa et al., 2002). However, an effect of MCH on oxygen consumption might not have been detected, since only a relatively low dose of peptide was tested.

Chronic ICV infusions of MCH into rodents were shown to not only increase food intake, but to also cause obesity (Della-Zuana et al., 2002; Gomori et al., 2003; Ito et al., 2003); while MCH-induced insulin resistance in rats was observed acutely in the absence of weight changes (Pereira-da-Silva et al., 2005). Chronic infusions of MCH (8 μg/rat/day) over 12 days led to an increase in body weight of about 20 g more than did control aCSF infusions in both Wistar or Sprague-Dawley rats (Della-Zuana et al., 2002). After a 14-day infusion of MCH into the third ventricle of C57BL/6J mice (10 μg/day), no significant increase in food intake was observed in mice fed a regular chow, but on a moderately high-fat diet (MHF), the mice ate about 15% more food (Gomori et al., 2003). Mice on both diets were significantly heavier than control mice, with the largest increase in body weight observed in the MCH infused mice on a MHF diet; these mice gained 17% more weight than the control infused mice on an MHF diet (Gomori et al., 2003). Glick et al. (2009) also observed that chronic infusion of 10 μg/day of MCH for 14 days into C57BL/6 mice fed regular chow led to a 34% increase in food intake and a 15% increase in body weight after a 14-day infusion. In a separate study, C57BL/6J mice on an MHF diet infused with a lower amount of MCH (3 μg/day for 7 days) also were hyperphagic and gained 350% more weight than did the vehicle control mice, with no detectable changes in activity (Ito et al., 2003). In addition, a small, potent, MCH analog given chronically ICV (30 μg/day) to Sprague-Dawley rats increased food intake by 23% and body weight by 38% more than in the vehicle controls (Shearman et al., 2003).

Intracerebroventricular-injected MCH has metabolic effects beyond increases in food intake and body weight. The acute effects of single MCH injections probably identify direct effects from increased MCH signaling in the brain, while the chronic effects may be subsequent to increased adiposity associated with body-weight gain. A single ICV injection of MCH into Wistar rats (3 nmol) inhibited the thyroid axis (Kennedy et al., 2001) by suppressing release of thyroid hormone from the hypothalamus, leading to a suppression of plasma thyroid-stimulating hormone (Kennedy et al., 2001). ICV injections of 4 nmol of MCH into Wistar rats for 4 days resulted in an ~10% increase in fasting plasma glucose (Pereira-da-Silva et al., 2005). Guesdon et al. (2008) used a potent, truncated MCH analog and found that injection of 5 μg into the AcSh or the third ventricle of Wistar rats did not significantly increase energy expenditure, but it did increase glucose oxidation and reduce lipid oxidation in the period 3 h after injection.

Chronic ICV infusions of MCH into C57BL/6J mice resulted in increased fat pad weights (~100%), leptin (~300%), liver triglycerides (~120%), fasting plasma glucose (~10%), and insulin (~100%) (Gomori et al., 2003). Glick et al. (2009) also observed that chronic infusion of 10 μg/day of MCH for 14 days into C57BL/6 mice led to a 4.5-fold increase in adiposity, about a 0.4°C drop in body temperature during the active dark phase, a 15% decrease in oxygen utilization, and a 26% increase in plasma insulin-like growth factor 1 levels. Chronic

MCH agonist infusions into Sprague-Dawley rats also led to increases in insulin (~200%) and leptin (~400%) (Shearman et al., 2003).

IN VIVO EFFECTS OF MCH RECEPTOR ANTAGONISTS

As discussed above, rodent genetic models clearly show a role for MCH in energy homeostasis. However, the applicability of these studies to understanding the physiological role and disease states associated with MCH signaling may be limited due to developmental effects of MCH inactivation or neuronal loss affecting other neuromodulators. Moreover, the relevance of *in vivo* pharmacology studies is complicated, because they utilize MCH and MCH agonists administered ICV at what are probably supraphysiologic levels. To better understand the role of MCH in energy homeostasis, a series of *in vivo* studies utilized MCHR1-specific antagonists. Because many pathways can affect food intake and body weight, *in vivo* effects of MCHR1 antagonists might be due to non-specific effects; however, in a few cases, researchers have demonstrated MCHR1 specificity by showing that an antagonist is inactive in *Mchr1*$^{-/-}$ mice.

Studies with MCHR1 peptidic antagonists

Studies on truncated and substituted MCH analogs identified key amino acids for activation of the MCH receptors and led to synthesis of potent antagonist derivatives (Bednarek et al., 2002; Audinot et al., 2009). Several *in vivo* studies employed Ac-(Ava$^{9-10}$, Ava$^{14-15}$)-MCH(6–16)-NH_2, a truncated, cyclic MCH analog containing γ-aminovaleric acid which is a potent (Kb 4 nM) antagonist (MacNeil and Bednarek, 2009). Shearman et al. (2003) reported that the peptide antagonist given ICV (10 μg) did not significantly reduce spontaneous feeding, affect feeding duration or locomotor activity, or alter overnight body-weight gain in lean male Sprague-Dawley rats. However, the peptide antagonist blocked the initial 2- or 3-h hyperphagic activity of an MCH agonist (Shearman et al., 2003; Mashiko et al., 2005). Chronic ICV infusion of the antagonist at 48 μg/day for 14 days reduced cumulative food intake by 13% and body-weight gain by 33%, relative to vehicle controls (Shearman et al., 2003). In male C57BL/6J mice fed an MHF diet, 28-day ICV infusion of the peptide antagonist at 7.5 μg/day decreased cumulative food intake 15% and the antagonist-treated mice weighed 13% less than the vehicle-infused controls (Mashiko et al., 2005). The antagonist treatment led to improvements in other metabolic parameters, including reductions in plasma glucose, leptin, insulin, and total cholesterol, as well as reductions in fat pad and liver weights (Mashiko et al., 2005). The specificity of the MCHR1 peptide antagonist was confirmed using *Mchr1*$^{-/-}$ mice, as infusion of the antagonist for 2 weeks had no effect on body weight, fat mass, or cumulative food intake in the KO mice (Mashiko et al., 2005). In contrast to *Mchr1* KO mouse models (**Table 1**), no changes were noted in activity after a 4-week infusion of the MCHR1 antagonist (Mashiko et al., 2005). Obese, aged, male C57BL/6J mice fed a HFD for 1 y (body weight ~60 g) were subjected to a 4-week ICV infusion with the peptide antagonist at 7.5 μg/day (Ito et al., 2008). The antagonist-infused mice lost 21% of their weight, while vehicle-infused mice gained 6% more weight. Not surprisingly, given the large differences in body weight, the MCHR1 antagonist-treated mice showed significant reductions in serum leptin and insulin (Ito et al., 2008). Also, the liver weights of the antagonist-treated DIO mice decreased by about 50%, while the serum liver markers showed improvements (Ito et al., 2008). In a follow-up study to explore the role of MCH in modulating accumulation of triglycerides in liver, male C57BL/6J mice were fed a diet deficient in methionine and choline to induce steatohepatitis; ICV treatment with the MCHR1 antagonist (7.5 μg/day for 10 days) did not result in any body-weight difference vs. vehicle control, but accumulation of triglycerides in liver was reduced 33% (Ito et al., 2008). The ability of MCHR1 antagonist treatment to improve hepatic steatosis was confirmed in a female model of obesity in which ovariectomized mice were fed a regular chow diet. Thirty weeks after the ovariectomy, the female C57BL/6J mice weighed about 25% more than did the sham treated mice (Gomori et al., 2007). When these obese mice were treated ICV with the MCHR1 peptide antagonist for 4 weeks at 7.5 μg/day, they lost 13% of their body weight and 32% of their liver triglycerides (Gomori et al., 2007).

Studies with S38151 in multiple rodent models of obesity resulted in significant effects on food intake and body weight. S38151 [*p*-guanidinobenzoyl-[des-Gly^{10}]-MCH(7–17)] is a modified and truncated 11-amino acid MCH analog which is a potent (Kb = 4 nM) MCHR1 antagonist (Audinot et al., 2009). Injection of this peptidic MCHR1 antagonist into the AcSh reduced food intake (Georgescu et al., 2005). Over a 6-h period, in male Wistar rats, S38151 administered ICV dose dependently inhibited the orexigenic effects of previously injected MCH (Audinot et al., 2009). The highest doses of S38151, 30 and 50 nmol per rat, completely blocked MCH-induced food intake for 6 h (Audinot et al., 2009). The orexigenic effect of proMCH (131–165), which is more potent than MCH in stimulating feeding, was blocked for 2 h by 50 nmol/kg of S38151 administered ICV (Maulon-Feraille et al., 2002; Della-Zuana et al., 2012). Once daily ICV injections of 20 nmol/kg of S38151 into male Zucker *fa/fa* rats, reduced food intake, water intake, motility, and body weight (Della-Zuana et al., 2012). A single injection of 20 μmol/kg of S38151 intraperitoneally (i.p.), reduced cumulative food intake in Zucker *fa/fa* rats for 24 h (Della-Zuana et al., 2012). S38151 was administered i.p. at 30 mg/kg for 5 days into two mouse models of obesity, female *ob/ob* and female C57BL/6J DIO mice, resulting in reductions in body weight and cumulative food intake. The S38151 effects on energy homeostasis were MCH1R based, since no changes in food intake or body weight were observed after 5 days of i.p. injection into female *Mchr1* KO mice (Della-Zuana et al., 2012).

Studies with non-peptide MCHR1 antagonists

The overwhelming set of genetic and physiologic data demonstrating that MCHR1 modulates energy homeostasis attracted the interest of a many medicinal chemistry groups who have synthesized numerous structurally distinct MCHR1 antagonists (see a recent review by Cheon, 2012). In all, 23 different companies have published more than 100 medicinal chemistry papers and patents describing attempts to optimize MCHR1 antagonist hit compounds toward drug candidates (see the recent review of the patent literature by Johansson, 2011). Many of the

Table 2 | Acute effects of non-peptide MCH1R antagonists on food intake.

Feeding model*	Time of measurement			Reference
	2 h	4, 5, or 6 h	24 h	
MCH-INDUCED HYPERPHAGIA IN RAT				
Male Sprague-Dawley		−90%		Takekawa et al. (2002)
Male Sprague-Dawley	−72%			Moriya et al. (2009)
Male Sprague-Dawley	−75%	−75%		Nagasaki et al. (2009)
Male Wistar	−70%			Borowsky et al. (2002)
FASTING-INDUCED FEEDING				
Male Wistar rats	−35%	−30%	−25%	Huang et al. (2005)
Mice (strain and gender unknown)	−80%	−40%		Balavoine et al. (2007)
DIO male C57BL/6NCrl:BR mice	−35%	−32%	−22%	McBriar et al. (2006)
DIO mice (strain and gender unknown)		−17%	−14%	Palani et al. (2005)
DIO mice (strain and gender unknown)	−12%	−20%	−9%	Sasikumar et al. (2006)
SPONTANEOUS FEEDING				
Male Sprague-Dawley rats			−30%	Kamata et al. (2011)
Female KK*Ay* mice	−63%			Kamata et al. (2011)
DIO C57BL/6J mice (gender unknown)			−19%	Haga et al. (2011)
DIO mice (strain and gender unknown)			−21%	Xu et al. (2006)
DIO male F344/Jcl rats			−30%	Kasai et al. (2012)
DIO male F344/Jcl rats		−28%		Kasai et al. (2011)
DIO male Sprague-Dawley rats			−31%	Kowalski and Sasikumar (2007)
Male Sprague-Dawley rats, ingestion of condensed milk[#]	−45%			Borowsky et al. (2002)

**Data shown for the most potent analog in the cited reference at the highest dose tested.*
[#]Measured at 20 min.

resulting optimized lead compounds, representing a diverse set of non-peptide MCHR1 antagonists, have been evaluated *in vivo*. Non-peptide MCHR1 antagonists are effective in different models of acute food intake in a variety of different rodent strains (**Table 2**) (Borowsky et al., 2002; Takekawa et al., 2002; Huang et al., 2005; Palani et al., 2005; McBriar et al., 2006; Sasikumar et al., 2006; Xu et al., 2006; Balavoine et al., 2007; Kowalski and Sasikumar, 2007; Moriya et al., 2009; Nagasaki et al., 2009; Haga et al., 2011; Kamata et al., 2011; Kasai et al., 2011, 2012). In general, MCHR1 antagonists potently block up to 75% of MCH-induced food intake (Borowsky et al., 2002; Takekawa et al., 2002; Moriya et al., 2009; Nagasaki et al., 2009), but they have more modest effects on reducing fasting-induced feeding and spontaneous feeding.

Multiple MCHR1 antagonists have also shown dose-dependent and sustained efficacy in chronic models of obesity (Kym et al., 2005; Souers et al., 2005a,b, 2007; Vasudevan et al., 2005a,b; Carpenter et al., 2006; Hertzog et al., 2006; Tavares et al., 2006a,b; Mendez-Andino and Wos, 2007; Mendez-Andino et al., 2007; Gehlert et al., 2009; Ito et al., 2009; Semple et al., 2009; Suzuki et al., 2009; Hadden et al., 2010; Mihalic et al., 2012; Sasmal et al., 2012a,b). At the highest dose tested in DIO mice, ranging from 10 to 100 mpk, weight loss ranged from 5% at 5 days to 33% at 238 days (Ito et al., 2009; Mihalic et al., 2012). In several cases, weight loss was shown to be primarily due to the loss of fat mass (Souers et al., 2005a,b, 2007; Vasudevan et al., 2005a; Mendez-Andino et al., 2007). The mechanism of weight loss appears to involve a combination of reduced food intake, which was observed in six studies (**Table 3**), and increased energy expenditure with no increase in activity (Kowalski et al., 2006; Gehlert et al., 2009).

As shown above with peptides, and in **Tables 2** and **3** with non-peptide compounds, many different MCHR1 antagonists have demonstrated modest to robust efficacy in a variety of rodent obesity models, suggesting that MCHR1 antagonists may have potential for treating human obesity. One caveat for the data is that in most cases, the antagonists have not demonstrated the ability to induce weight loss through an MCHR1-specific mode of action, since efficacy in *Mchr1* KO mice has not been evaluated. In fact, in one report of robust weight loss, the authors caution that some weight loss at the highest dose tested maybe due to non-specific mechanisms, since the compound resulted in high brain levels, 6.46 μg/g (Kym et al., 2005). However, in four reports, the MCHR1-specific efficacy of antagonists was confirmed, since the antagonists lacked efficacy in DIO *Mchr1* KO mice, but they showed body-weight loss in DIO wild-type mice (Gehlert et al., 2009; Della-Zuana et al., 2012; Mashiko et al., 2005; Mihalic et al., 2012). Further support for an MCHR1 mechanism based-weight loss has been reported for three compounds, for which efficacy was correlated with brain MCHR1 receptor occupancy (Hervieu et al., 2003; Kowalski et al., 2006; Ito et al., 2009).

Studies with MCHR2 antagonists

The absence of the *Mchr2* in rodents has limited the interest in developing MCHR2-selective compounds. Only one paper has disclosed a potent MCHR2-selective non-peptide small-molecule

Table 3 | Chronic effects of non-peptide MCH1R antagonists in rodents.

Rodent model of energy homeostasis*			
	Reduced food intake vs. vehicle (%)	**Time (days)**	**Reference**
REDUCED CUMULATIVE FOOD INTAKE IN MICE			
Male DIO C57BL/6J	16	5	Ito et al. (2009)
DIO (strain and gender unknown)	11	10	Mendez-Andino et al. (2007)
DIO (strain and gender unknown)	37	13	Kym et al. (2005)
DIO (strain and gender unknown)	13	14	Souers et al. (2005b)
Male DIO C57BL/6NCrl:BR	18	28	Kowalski et al. (2006)
REDUCED CUMULATIVE FOOD INTAKE IN RATS			
DIO Long Evans (gender unknown)	16	14	Gehlert et al. (2009)
	Weight loss vs. vehicle (%)	**Time (days)**	**Reference**
REDUCED BODY WEIGHT IN MICE			
DIO C57BL/6J male	5	5	Ito et al. (2009)
DIO C57BL/6J male	6	5	Surman et al. (2010)
DIO C57BL/6J male	6	6	Hadden et al. (2010)
DIO (strain and gender unknown)	8	7	Mendez-Andino and Wos (2007)
DIO (strain and gender unknown)	5	10	Mendez-Andino et al. (2007)
DIO AKR/J (gender unknown)	13	12	Hertzog et al. (2006)
DIO (strain and gender unknown)	18	13	Kym et al. (2005)
DIO C57BL/6J male	8	13	Suzuki et al. (2009)
DIO C57BL/6J (gender unknown)	6	14	Vasudevan et al. (2005b)
DIO C57BL/6J (gender unknown)	12	14	Sasmal et al. (2012a)
DIO C57BL/6J (gender unknown)	13	14	Sasmal et al. (2012b)
DIO (strain and gender unknown)	7	14	Souers et al. (2007)
DIO (strain and gender unknown)	23	14	Vasudevan et al. (2005a)
DIO (strain and gender unknown)	15	14	Souers et al. (2005a)
DIO (strain and gender unknown)	17	14	Souers et al. (2005b)
DIO AKR/J (gender unknown)	10	15	Carpenter et al. (2006)
DIO AKR/J (gender unknown)	10	21	Tavares et al. (2006b)
DIO AKR/J (gender unknown)	15	26	Tavares et al. (2006a)
DIO (strain and gender unknown)	31	28	Kym et al. (2005)
DIO C57BL/6NCrl:BR male	16	28	Kowalski et al. (2006)
DIO C57BL/6J (gender unknown)	9	137	Mihalic et al. (2012)
DIO female (strain unknown)	33	238	Mihalic et al. (2012)
REDUCED BODY WEIGHT IN RATS			
DIO Long Evans (gender unknown)	15	14	Gehlert et al. (2009)
DIO Sprague-Dawley male	15	14	Dyck et al. (2006)
DIO Wistar female	17	28	Semple et al. (2009)

**Data shown for the most potent analog in the cited reference at the highest dose tested.*

antagonist (Chen et al., 2012). Compound 38 is a potent (Ki 13 nM) and selective MCHR2 antagonist with good oral bioavailability and pharmacokinetics suitable for *in vivo* studies (Chen et al., 2012). However, no *in vivo* data have been reported with this compound.

CLINICAL STUDIES WITH MCHR1 ANTAGONISTS

The intense interest in MCHR1 antagonists has resulted in more than 80 publications and 100 patent applications describing various unique antagonists (Johansson, 2011). Five compounds have reached testing in human subjects, but none has proceeded into advanced Phase II studies to rigorously test their efficacy in causing chronic weight loss (**Figure 2**). A major issue with many lead compounds is increased cardiovascular risk due to high-affinity hERG binding and drug-induced QTc prolongation (Mendez-Andino and Wos, 2007).

The Amgen MCHR1 antagonist AMG 076 entered Phase I safety and tolerability testing in 2004, but there have been no subsequent reports of its status since 2005. GlaxoSmithKline MCHR1 antagonist GW-856464 also entered Phase I studies in 2004 (Cheon,

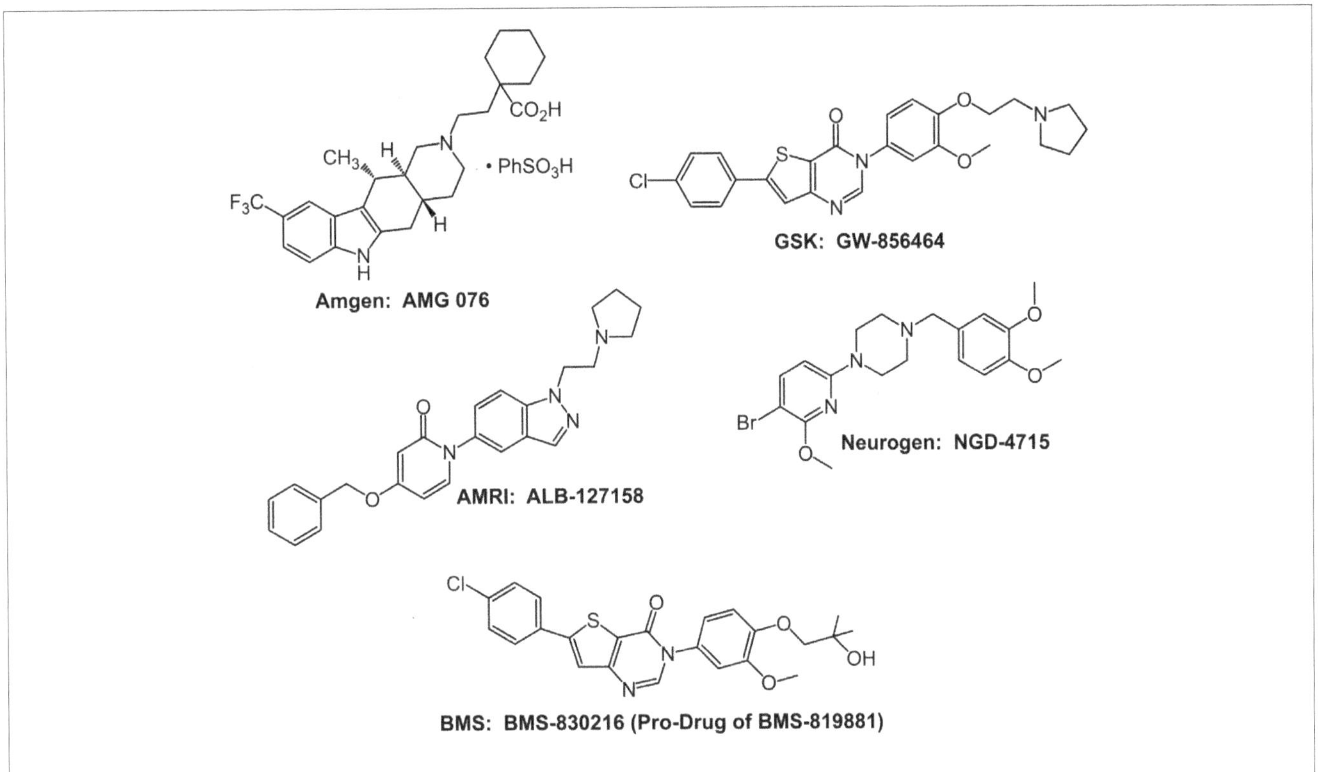

FIGURE 2 | Structures of the five MCHR1 antagonists that have been evaluated in Phase I safety and tolerability studies.

2012). However, on August 24, 2010, Carmen Drahl reported via Twitter that "low bioavailability precluded further development."

NGD-4715 is a selective MCHR1 antagonist developed by Neurogen. In a May 2, 2007 press release, Neurogen announced that NGD-4715 was safe and well-tolerated in a Phase I clinical trial. Neurogen was acquired by Ligand Pharmaceuticals in 2009; as of February 22, 2013, the Wikipedia entry for NGD-4715 quotes an e-mail from Ligand that there are "no plans for further development on the compound." In a May 31, 2011 press release, AMRI announced that its MCHR1 antagonist, ALB-127158(a), was well-tolerated in a Phase I single ascending-dose study and 14-day multiple ascending-dose safety and tolerability study. An encouraging result reported by some subjects was loss of appetite. Despite the reported tolerability and suggestion of efficacy, in a subsequent press release dated October 4, 2011, AMRI announced that development was terminated before the initiation of Phase II studies.

Bristol–Myers Squibb (BMS) conducted the longest clinical trial with an MCHR1 antagonist. As of February 22, 2013, the BMS website indicates BMS-830216 was evaluated in a 28-day Phase I study to assess the safety, tolerability, and effect on body weight and other obesity-related factors of different doses of BMS-830216. A summary of the clinical results with BMS-830216 is available on the NIH website (http://www.ncats.nih.gov/files/BMS-830216.pdf), which indicates that BMS-830216 is a prodrug of the antagonist BMS-819881 and a potent ($K_i = 10$ nM) and selective MCHR1 antagonist. BMS-830216 was generally safe and well-tolerated at all doses in the Phase I study for up to 28 days. However, no indications of weight loss or reduced food intake were observed, and the compound did not proceed to Phase II studies.

FUTURE PROSPECTS

A rich literature of rodent genetics and rodent pharmacology demonstrates a significant role for MCH, acting via the MCHR1 within the hypothalamus, in maintaining energy homeostasis. This knowledge has stimulated more than 20 companies to seek MCHR1 selective compounds for the treatment of obesity. Five companies are known to have succeeded in identifying development candidates that proceeded through preclinical safety studies and enabled Phase I clinical safety and tolerability testing. Three of the compounds, NGD-4715, ALB-127158(a), and BMS-830216 (**Figure 1**), were found generally safe and well-tolerated in the Phase I studies. However, BMS-830216, which was tested for 28 days in obese subjects, failed to show any significant weight loss efficacy. No compounds have proceeded into Phase II studies in which chronic efficacy could be evaluated.

After almost 15 years of research, studies have failed to detect anti-obesity efficacy with MCHR1 antagonists in the clinic. There are multiple reasons that might account for this disconnect between rodent and human studies. First, compounds tested in the clinic may not have had the appropriate properties to sufficiently block the MCHR1 receptor and achieve an effect of energy balance. For instance, the MCHR1 antagonists may not have reached the hypothalamic sites of MCH action. Since there have been no reported studies measuring the level of receptor occupancy of the clinical compounds, it is possible that the compounds failed to sufficiently penetrate the brain: blood barrier resulting in low and insufficient receptor occupancy. Second, studies utilizing a positron emission tomography (PET) ligand demonstrated that an NPY5R antagonist must achieve >90% receptor occupancy sustained over 24 h to cause weight loss (Erondu et al., 2006). Similarly, in DIO mouse studies, maximum weight loss was observed only when an MCHR1 antagonist blocked >90% of the MCHR1 receptors for 24 h (unpublished data by the author). Clearly, a MCHR1 PET ligand could guide compound dose selection to assure 24 h of high receptor blockade (Erondu et al., 2006; Philippe et al., 2012). Third, since humans also express MCHR2 in the hypothalamus (Sailer et al., 2001), MCH signaling in humans may involve both MCHR1 and MCHR2, such that blockade of the MCHR1 alone may not be sufficient to achieve efficacy in obesity. Fourth, the role of MCH in human energy homeostasis may not be as significant as its role in rodents, consequently, blockade of MCHR1 would be inherently ineffective as a treatment for obesity.

In the author's opinion, there is, at best, only a modest probability that an MCHR1 antagonist will be developed as a treatment for obesity. Following the failure of five Phase I compounds to progress to Phase II efficacy studies, the enthusiasm for MCHR1 antagonists has clearly dimmed. Moreover, after more than a decade of drug discovery effort by more than 20 companies, there are currently no known MCHR1 antagonists in the clinic for obesity. Should any company continue to seek MCHR1 antagonists, the author suggests that they should proceed only with the aid of a PET ligand, perhaps [^{11}C]SNAP-7941, or another on-target biomarker to assess receptor occupancy (Philippe et al., 2012). Companies might also consider focusing their chemistry efforts on identifying a dual MCHR1 and MCHR2 antagonist, to assure that all MCH-mediated signaling involved in energy homeostasis is effectively blocked. Finally, an effective MCH antagonist therapy for obesity must not only achieve meaningful weight loss, but it must also be well-tolerated. Although not discussed in this review, there is significant rodent genetic and pharmacologic data indicating that MCH participates in other CNS behaviors (Saito and Nagasaki, 2008; Yumiko and Nagasaki, 2008; Antal-Zimanyi and Khawaja, 2009; Torterolo et al., 2009; Chung et al., 2011). In particular, studies in multiple rodent models suggest blockade of MCH signaling may be anxiolytic (Antal-Zimanyi and Khawaja, 2009; Chung et al., 2011). Tolerability may be a substantial hurdle for an effective MCH receptor antagonist to overcome.

ACKNOWLEDGMENTS

I thank Tanya MacNeil for reviewing and editing the manuscript and Michele McColgan for preparing the figures. Current information about the structure and function of the MCH receptors can be found at the IUPHAR database (IUPHAR-DB): http://www.iuphar-db.org/DATABASE/FamilyMenuForward?familyId$=$37.

REFERENCES

Abbott, C. R., Kennedy, A. R., Wren, A. M., Rossi, M., Murphy, K. G., Seal, L. J., et al. (2003). Identification of hypothalamic nuclei involved in the orexigenic effect of melanin-concentrating hormone. *Endocrinology* 144, 3943–3949.

Able, S. L., Ivarsson, M., Fish, R. L., Clarke, T. L., McCourt, C., Duckworth, J. M., et al. (2009). Localisation of melanin-concentrating hormone receptor 1 in rat brain and evidence that sleep parameters are not altered despite high central receptor occupancy. *Eur. J. Pharmacol.* 616, 101–106.

Ahnaou, A., Dautzenberg, F. M., Huysmans, H., Steckler, T., and Drinkenburg, W. H. I. M. (2011). Contribution of melanin-concentrating hormone (MCH1) receptor to thermoregulation and sleep stabilization: evidence from MCH1 (-/-) mice. *Behav. Brain Res.* 218, 42–50.

Alon, T., and Friedman, J. M. (2006). Late-onset leanness in mice with targeted ablation of melanin concentrating hormone neurons. *J. Neurosci.* 26, 389–397.

An, S., Cutler, G., Zhao, J. J., Huang, S. G., Tian, H., Li, W., et al. (2001). Identification and characterization of a melanin-concentrating hormone receptor. *Proc. Natl. Acad. Sci. U.S.A.* 98, 7576–7581.

Antal-Zimanyi, I., and Khawaja, X. (2009). The role of melanin-concentrating hormone in energy homeostasis and mood disorders. *J. Mol. Neurosci.* 39, 86–98.

Asakawa, A., Inui, A., Goto, K., Yuzuriha, H., Takimoto, Y., Inui, T., et al. (2002). Effects of agouti-related protein, orexin and melanin-concentrating hormone on oxygen consumption in mice. *Int. J. Mol. Med.* 10, 523–525.

Astrand, A., Bohlooly, Y., Larsdotter, S., Mahlapuu, M., Andersen, H., Tornell, J., et al. (2004). Mice lacking melanin-concentrating hormone receptor 1 demonstrate increased heart rate associated with altered autonomic activity. *Am. J. Physiol. Regul. Integr. Comp. Physiol.* 287, R749–R758.

Audinot, V., Zuana, O. D., Fabry, N., Ouvry, C., Nosjean, O., Henlin, J. M., et al. (2009). S38151 [p-guanidinobenzoyl-[Des-Gly(10)]-MCH(7-17)] is a potent and selective antagonist at the MCH(1) receptor and has anti-feeding properties in vivo. *Peptides* 30, 1997–2007.

Baird, J. P., Rios, C., Gray, N. E., Walsh, C. E., Fischer, S. G., and Pecora, A. L. (2006). Effects of melanin-concentrating hormone on licking microstructure and brief-access taste responses. *Am. J. Physiol. Regul. Integr. Comp. Physiol.* 291, 1265–1274.

Baird, J. P., Rios, C., Loveland, J. L., Beck, J., Tran, A., and Mahoney, C. E. (2007). Effects of hindbrain melanin-concentrating hormone and neuropeptide Y administration on licking for water, saccharin, and sucrose solutions. *Am. J. Physiol. Regul. Integr. Comp. Physiol.* 294, 329–343.

Balavoine, F., Malabre, P., Alleaume, T., Rey, A., Cherfils, V., Jeanneton, O., et al. (2007). Design and synthesis of novel hydantoin-containing melanin-concentrating hormone receptor antagonists. *Bioorg. Med. Chem. Lett.* 17, 3754–3759.

Bednarek, M. A. (2007). Peptide ligands for the melanin-concentrating hormone (MCH) receptor 1. *Curr. Top. Med. Chem.* 7, 1425–1432.

Bednarek, M. A., Hreniuk, D. L., Tan, C., Palyha, O. C., MacNeil, D. J., Van der Ploeg, L. H., et al. (2002). Synthesis and biological evaluation in vitro of selective, high affinity peptide antagonists of human melanin-concentrating hormone action at human melanin-concentrating hormone receptor 1. *Biochemistry* 41, 6383–6390.

Bell, C. G., Meyre, D., Samson, C., Boyle, C., Lecoeur, C., Tauber, M., et al. (2005). Association of melanin-concentrating hormone receptor 1 5' polymorphism with early-onset extreme obesity. *Diabetes* 54, 3049–3055.

Bittencourt, J. C. (2011). Anatomical organization of the melanin-concentrating hormone peptide family in the mammalian brain. *Gen. Comp. Endocrinol.* 172, 185–197.

Bjursell, M., Gerdin, A. K., Ploj, K., Svensson, D., Svensson, L., Oscarsson, J., et al. (2006). Melanin-concentrating hormone receptor 1 deficiency increases insulin sensitivity in obese leptin-deficient mice without affecting body weight. *Diabetes* 55, 725–733.

Borowsky, B., Durkin, M. M., Ogozalek, K., Marzabadi, M. R., DeLeon, J., Lagu, B., et al. (2002). Antidepressant, anxiolytic and anorectic effects of a melanin-concentrating hormone-1 receptor antagonist. *Nat. Med.* 8, 825–830.

Bradley, R. L., Mansfield, J. P., Maratos-Flier, E., and Cheatham, B. (2002). Melanin-concentrating hormone activates signaling pathways in 3T3-L1 adipocytes. *Am. J. Physiol. Endocrinol. Metab.* 283, E584–E592.

Carpenter, A. J., Al Barazanji, K. A., Barvian, K. K., Bishop, M. J., Britt, C. S., Cooper, J. P., et al. (2006). Novel benzimidazole-based MCH R1 antagonists. *Diabetes* 16, 4994–5000.

Casatti, C. A., Elias, C. F., Sita, L. V., Frigo, L., Furlani, V. C., Bauer, J. A., et al. (2002). Distribution of melanin-concentrating hormone neurons projecting to the medial mammillary nucleus. *Neuroscience* 115, 899–915.

Chagnon, Y. C., Bureau, A., Gendron, D., Bouchard, R. H., Merette, C., Roy, M. A., et al. (2007). Possible association of the pro-melanin-concentrating hormone gene with a greater body mass index as a side effect of the antipsychotic olanzapine. *Am. J. Med. Genet. B Neuropsychiatr. Genet.* 144B, 1063–1069.

Chen, X., Mihalic, J., Fan, P., Liang, L., Lindstrom, M., Wong, S., et al. (2012). Discovery and characterization of a potent and selective antagonist of melanin-concentrating hormone receptor 2. *Bioorg. Med. Chem. Lett.* 22, 363–366.

Chen, Y., Hu, C., Hsu, C. K., Zhang, Q., Bi, C., Asnicar, M., et al. (2002). Targeted disruption of the melanin-concentrating hormone receptor-1 results in hyperphagia and resistance to diet-induced obesity. *Endocrinology* 143, 2469–2477.

Cheon, H. G. (2012). "Antiobesity effects of melanin-concentrating hormone receptor 1 (MCH-R1) antagonists," in *Appetite Control, Handbook of Experimental Pharmacology*, ed. H.-G. Joost (Heidelberg: Springer), 209.

Chung, S., Parks, G. S., Lee, C., and Civelli, O. (2011). Recent updates on the melanin-concentrating hormone (MCH) and its receptor system: lessons from MCH1R antagonists. *J. Mol. Neurosci.* 43, 115–121.

Della-Zuana, O., Audinot, V., Levenez, V., Ktorza, A., Presse, F., Nahon, J. L., et al. (2012). Peripheral injections of melanin-concentrating hormone receptor 1 antagonist S38151 decrease food intake and body weight in rodent obesity models. *Front. Endocrinol. (Lausanne)* 3:160. doi:10.3389/fendo.2012.00160

Della-Zuana, O., Presse, F., Ortola, C., Duhault, J., Nahon, J. L., and Levens, N. (2002). Acute and chronic administration of melanin-concentrating hormone enhances food intake and body weight in Wistar and Sprague-Dawley rats. *Int. J. Obes.* 26, 1289–1295.

Dyck, B., Markison, S., Zhao, L., Tamiya, J., Grey, J., Rowbottom, M. W., et al. (2006). A thienopyridazinone-based melanin-concentrating hormone receptor 1 antagonist with potent in vivo anorectic properties. *J. Med. Chem.* 49, 3753–3756.

Elias, C. F., Sita, L. V., Zambon, B. K., Oliveira, E. R., Vasconcelos, L. A., and Bittencourt, J. C. (2008). Melanin-concentrating hormone projections to areas involved in somatomotor responses. *J. Chem. Neuroanat.* 35, 188–201.

Erondu, N., Gantz, I., Musser, B., Suryawanshi, S., Mallick, M., Addy, C., et al. (2006). Neuropeptide Y5 receptor antagonism does not induce clinically meaningful weight loss in overweight and obese adults. *Cell Metab.* 4, 275–282.

Gao, X. B. (2009). Electrophysiological effects of MCH on neurons in the hypothalamus. *Peptides* 30, 2025–2030.

Gehlert, D. R., Rasmussen, K., Shaw, J., Li, X., Ardayfio, P., Craft, L., et al. (2009). Preclinical evaluation of melanin-concentrating hormone receptor 1 antagonism for the treatment of obesity and depression. *J. Pharmacol. Exp. Ther.* 329, 429–438.

Georgescu, D., Sears, R. M., Hommel, J. D., Barrot, M., Bolanos, C. A., Marsh, D. J., et al. (2005). The hypothalamic neuropeptide melanin-concentrating hormone acts in the nucleus accumbens to modulate feeding behavior and forced-swim performance. *J. Neurosci.* 25, 2933–2940.

Ghoussaini, M., Vatin, V., Lecoeur, C., Abkevich, V., Younus, A., Samson, C., et al. (2007). Genetic study of the melanin-concentrating hormone receptor 2 in childhood and adulthood severe obesity. *J. Clin. Endocrinol. Metab.* 92, 4403–4409.

Gibson, W. T., Pissios, P., Trombly, D. J., Luan, J., Keogh, J., Wareham, N. J., et al. (2004). Melanin-concentrating hormone receptor mutations and human obesity: functional analysis. *Obes. Res.* 12, 743–749.

Glick, M., Segal-Lieberman, G., Cohen, R., and Kronfeld-Schor, N. (2009). Chronic MCH infusion causes a decrease in energy expenditure and body temperature, and an increase in serum IGF-1 levels in mice. *Endocrine* 36, 479–485.

Goldstein, C., Schroeder, J. C., Fortin, J. P., Goss, J. M., Schaus, S. E., Beinborn, M., et al. (2010). Two naturally occurring mutations in the type 1 melanin-concentrating hormone receptor abolish agonist-induced signaling. *J. Pharmacol. Exp. Ther.* 335, 799–806.

Gomori, A., Ishihara, A., Ito, M., Mashiko, S., Matsushita, H., Yumoto, M., et al. (2003). Chronic intracerebroventricular infusion of MCH causes obesity in mice. *Am. J. Physiol. Endocrinol. Metab.* 284, E583–E588.

Gomori, A., Ishihara, A., Ito, M., Matsushita, H., Ito, M., Mashiko, S., et al. (2007). Blockade of MCH1 receptor signalling ameliorates obesity and related hepatic steatosis in ovariectomized mice. *Br. J. Pharmacol.* 151, 900–908.

Guesdon, B., Paradis, E., Samson, P., and Richard, D. (2008). Effects of intracerebroventricular and intra-accumbens melanin-concentrating hormone agonism on food intake and energy expenditure. *Am. J. Physiol. Regul. Integr. Comp. Physiol.* 296, 469–475.

Guyon, A., Conductier, G., Rovere, C., Enfissi, A., and Nahon, J. L. (2009). Melanin-concentrating hormone producing neurons: activities and modulations. *Peptides* 30, 2031–2039.

Hadden, M., Deering, D. M., Henderson, A. J., Surman, M. D., Luche, M., Khmelnitsky, Y., et al. (2010). Synthesis and SAR of 4-aryl-1-(indazol-5-yl)pyridin-2(1H)ones as MCH-1 antagonists for the treatment of obesity. *Bioorg. Med. Chem. Lett.* 20, 7020–7023.

Haga, Y., Mizutani, S., Naya, A., Kishino, H., Iwaasa, H., Ito, M., et al. (2011). Discovery of novel phenylpyridone derivatives as potent and selective MCH1R antagonists. *Bioorg. Med. Chem.* 19, 883–893.

Hawes, B. E., Kil, E., Green, B., O'Neill, K., Fried, S., and Graziano, M. P. (2000). The melanin-concentrating hormone receptor couples to multiple G proteins to activate diverse intracellular signaling pathways. *Endocrinology* 141, 4524–4532.

Hertzog, D. L., Al Barazanji, K. A., Bigham, E. C., Bishop, M. J., Britt, C. S., Carlton, D. L., et al. (2006). The discovery and optimization of pyrimidinone-containing MCH R1 antagonists. *Bioorg. Med. Chem. Lett.* 16, 4723–4727.

Hervieu, G. J. (2006). Further insights into the neurobiology of melanin-concentrating hormone in energy and mood balances. *Expert Opin. Ther. Targets* 10, 211–229.

Hervieu, G. J., Cluderay, J. E., Harrison, D., Meakin, J., Maycox, P., Nasir, S., et al. (2000). The distribution of the mRNA and protein products of the melanin-concentrating hormone (MCH) receptor gene, slc-1, in the central nervous system of the rat. *Eur. J. Neurosci.* 12, 1194–1216.

Hervieu, G. J., Maulon-Feraille, L., Chambers, J. K., Cluderay, J. E., Wilson, S., Presse, F., et al. (2003). "The melanin-concentrating hormone," in *Handbook of Chemical Neuroanatomy; Vol. 20 Peptide Receptors*, Part II, eds A. Bjorklund and T. Hokfelt (Amsterdam: Elsevier), 31–101.

Hill, J., Duckworth, M., Murdock, P., Rennie, G., Sabido-David, C., Ames, R. S., et al. (2001). Molecular cloning and functional characterization of MCH2, a novel human MCH receptor. *J. Biol. Chem.* 276, 20125–20129.

Huang, C. Q., Baker, T., Schwarz, D., Fan, J., Heise, C. E., Zhang, M., et al. (2005). 1-(4-Amino-phenyl)-pyrrolidin-3-yl-amine and 6-(3-amino-pyrrolidin-1-yl)-pyridin-3-yl-amine derivatives as melanin-concentrating hormone receptor-1 antagonists. *Bioorg. Med. Chem. Lett.* 15, 3701–3706.

Ito, M., Gomori, A., Ishihara, A., Oda, Z., Mashiko, S., Matsushita, H., et al. (2003). Characterization of MCH-mediated obesity in mice. *Am. J. Physiol. Endocrinol. Metab.* 284, 940–945.

Ito, M., Gomori, A., Suzuki, J., Tsujioka, S., Sasaki, M., Matsuda, M., et al. (2008). Antagonism of central melanin-concentrating hormone 1 receptor alleviates steatohepatitis in mice. *J. Endocrinol.* 198, 309–315.

Ito, M., Ishihara, A., Gomori, A., Egashira, S., Matsushita, H., Mashiko, S., et al. (2009). Melanin-concentrating hormone 1-receptor antagonist suppresses body-weight gain correlated with high receptor occupancy levels in diet-induced obesity mice. *Eur. J. Pharmacol.* 624, 77–83.

Jeon, J. Y., Bradley, R. L., Kokkotou, E. G., Marino, F. E., Wang, X., Pissios, P., et al. (2006). MCH-/- mice are resistant to aging-associated increases in body weight and insulin resistance. *Diabetes* 55, 428–434.

Johansson, A. (2011). Recent progress in the discovery of melanin-concentrating hormone 1-receptor antagonists. *Expert Opin. Ther. Pat.* 21, 905–925.

Kamata, M., Yamashita, T., Imaeda, T., Tanaka, T., Terauchi, J., Miyamoto, M., et al. (2011). Discovery, synthesis, and structure-activity relationship of 6-aminomethyl-7,8-dihydronaphthalenes as human melanin-concentrating hormone receptor 1 antagonists. *Bioorg. Med. Chem.* 19, 5539–5552.

Kasai, S., Kamata, M., Masada, S., Kunitomo, J., Kamaura, M., Okawa, T., et al. (2012). Synthesis, structure-activity relationship, and pharmacological studies of novel melanin-concentrating hormone receptor 1 antagonists 3-aminomethylquinolines: reducing human ether-a-go-go-related gene (hERG) associated liabilities. *J. Med. Chem.* 55, 4336–4351.

Kasai, S., Kamaura, M., Kamata, M., Aso, K., Ogino, H., Nakano, Y., et al. (2011). Melanin-concentrating hormone receptor 1 antagonists: synthesis, structure-activity relationship, docking studies, and biological evaluation of 2,3,4,5-tetrahydro-1H-3-benzazepine derivatives. *Bioorg. Med. Chem.* 19, 6261–6273.

Kennedy, A. R., Todd, J. F., Stanley, S. A., Abbott, C. R., Small, C. J., Ghatei, M. A., et al. (2001). Melanin-concentrating hormone (MCH) suppresses thyroid stimulating hormone (TSH) release, in vivo and in vitro, via the hypothalamus and the pituitary. *Endocrinology* 142, 3265–3268.

Kokkotou, E., Jeon, J. Y., Wang, X., Marino, F. E., Carlson, M., Trombly, D. J., et al. (2005). Mice with MCH ablation resist diet-induced obesity through strain-specific mechanisms. *Am. J. Physiol. Regul. Integr. Comp. Physiol.* 289, R117–R124.

Kokkotou, E., Moss, A. C., Torres, D., Karagiannides, I., Cheifetz, A., Liu, S., et al. (2008). Melanin-concentrating hormone as a mediator of intestinal inflammation. *Proc. Natl. Acad. Sci. U.S.A.* 105, 10613–10618.

Kolakowski, L. F. Jr., Jung, B. P., Nguyen, T., Johnson, M. P., Lynch, K. R., Cheng, R., et al. (1996). Characterization of a human gene related to genes encoding somatostatin receptors. *FEBS Lett.* 398, 253–258.

Kowalski, T. J., and Sasikumar, T. (2007). Melanin-concentrating hormone receptor-1 antagonists as antiobesity therapeutics: current status. *Biodrugs* 21, 311–321.

Kowalski, T. J., Spar, B. D., Weig, B., Farley, C., Cook, J., Ghibaudi, L., et al. (2006). Effects of a selective melanin-concentrating hormone 1 receptor antagonist on food intake and energy homeostasis in diet-induced obese mice. *Eur. J. Pharmacol.* 535, 182–191.

Kym, P. R., Iyengar, R., Souers, A. J., Lynch, J. K., Judd, A. S., Gao, J., et al. (2005). Discovery and characterization of aminopiperidinecoumarin melanin concentrating hormone receptor 1 antagonists. *J. Med. Chem.* 48, 5888–5891.

Lakaye, B., Minet, A., Zorzi, W., and Grisar, T. (1998). Cloning of the rat brain cDNA encoding for the SLC-1 G protein-coupled receptor reveals the presence of an intron in the gene. *Biochim. Biophys. Acta* 1401, 216–220.

Ludwig, D. S., Tritos, N. A., Mastaitis, J. W., Kulkarni, R., Kokkotou, E., Elmquist, J., et al. (2001). Melanin-concentrating hormone overexpression in transgenic mice leads to obesity and insulin resistance. *J. Clin. Invest.* 107, 379–386.

MacNeil, D. J., and Bednarek, M. A. (2009). MCH receptor peptide agonists and antagonists. *Peptides* 30, 2008–2013.

Marsh, D. J., Weingarth, D. T., Novi, D. E., Chen, H. Y., Trumbauer, M. E., Chen, A. S., et al. (2002). Melanin-concentrating hormone 1 receptor-deficient mice are lean, hyperactive, and hyperphagic and have altered metabolism. *Proc. Natl. Acad. Sci. U.S.A.* 99, 3240–3245.

Mashiko, S., Ishihara, A., Gomori, A., Moriya, R., Ito, M., Iwaasa, H., et al. (2005). Antiobesity effect of a melanin-concentrating hormone 1 receptor antagonist in diet-induced obese mice. *Endocrinology* 146, 3080–3086.

Maulon-Feraille, L., Della-Zuana, O., Suply, T., Rovere-Jovene, C., Audinot, V., Levens, N., et al. (2002). Appetite-boosting property of pro-melanin-concentrating hormone131-165 (neuropeptide-glutamic acid-isoleucine) is associated with proteolytic resistance. *J. Pharmacol. Exp. Ther.* 302, 766–773.

McBriar, M. D., Guzik, H., Shapiro, S., Paruchova, J., Xu, R., Palani, A., et al. (2006). Discovery of orally efficacious melanin-concentrating hormone receptor-1 antagonists as antiobesity agents. Synthesis, SAR, and biological evaluation of bicyclo[3.1.0]hexyl ureas. *J. Med. Chem.* 49, 2294–2310.

Mendez-Andino, J. L., Colson, A. O., Meyers, K. M., Mitchell, M. C., Hodge, K., Howard, J. M., et al. (2007). The efficacy and cardiac evaluation of aminomethyl tetrahydronaphthalene ketopiperazines: a novel class of potent MCH-R1 antagonists. *Bioorg. Med. Chem.* 15, 2092–2105.

Mendez-Andino, J. L., and Wos, J. A. (2007). MCH-R1 antagonists: what is keeping most research programs away from the clinic? *Drug Discov. Today* 12, 972–979.

Mihalic, J. T., Fan, P., Chen, X., Chen, X., Fu, Y., Motani, A., et al. (2012). Discovery of a novel melanin concentrating hormone receptor 1 (MCHR1) antagonist with reduced hERG inhibition. *Bioorg. Med. Chem. Lett.* 22, 3781–3785.

Mitra, A., Klockars, A., Gosnell, B. A., Le Greves, M., Olszewski, P. K., Levine, A. S., et al. (2012). Expression levels of genes encoding melanin concentrating hormone (MCH) and MCH receptor change in taste aversion, but MCH injections do not alleviate aversive responses. *Pharmacol. Biochem. Behav.* 100, 581–586.

Mori, M., Harada, M., Terao, Y., Sugo, T., Watanabe, T., Shimomura, Y., et al. (2001). Cloning of a novel G protein-coupled receptor, SLT, a subtype of the melanin-concentrating hormone receptor. *Biochem. Biophys. Res. Commun.* 283, 1013–1018.

Moriya, M., Kishino, H., Sakuraba, S., Sakamoto, T., Suga, T., Takahashi, H., et al. (2009). Identification of 2-aminobenzimidazoles as potent melanin-concentrating hormone 1-receptor (MCH1R) antagonists. *Bioorg. Med. Chem. Lett.* 19, 3568–3572.

Mul, J. D., la Fleur, S. E., Toonen, P. W., Afrasiab-Middelman, A., Binnekade, R., and Verheij, M. M. (2011). Chronic loss of melanin-concentrating hormone affects motivational aspects of feeding in the rat. *PLoS ONE* 6:e19600. doi:10.1371/journal.pone.0019600

Nagasaki, H., Chung, S., Dooley, C. T., Wang, Z., Li, C., Saito, Y., et al. (2009). The pharmacological properties of a novel MCH(1) receptor antagonist isolated from combinatorial libraries. *Eur. J. Pharmacol.* 602, 194–202.

Nahon, J. L., Presse, F., Bittencourt, J. C., Sawchenko, P. E., and Vale, W. (1989). The rat melanin-concentrating hormone messenger ribonucleic acid encodes multiple putative neuropeptides coexpressed in the dorsolateral hypothalamus. *Endocrinology* 125, 2056–2065.

Palani, A., Shapiro, S., McBriar, M. D., Clader, J. W., Greenlee, W. J., Spar, B., et al. (2005). Biaryl ureas as potent and orally efficacious melanin concentrating hormone receptor 1 antagonists for the treatment of obesity. *J. Med. Chem.* 48, 4746–4749.

Pereira-da-Silva, M., De Souza, C. T., Gasparetti, A. L., Saad, M. J. A., and Velloso, L. A. (2005). Melanin-concentrating hormone induces insulin resistance through a mechanism independent of body weight gain. *J. Endocrinol.* 186, 193–201.

Philippe, C., Schirmer, E., Mitterhauser, M., Shanab, K., Lanzenberger, R., Karanikas, G., et al. (2012). Radiosynthesis of [(11)C]SNAP-7941-the first PET-tracer for the melanin concentrating hormone receptor 1 (MCHR1). *Appl. Radiat. Isot.* 70, 2287–2294.

Pissios, P., Bradley, R. L., and Maratos-Flier, E. (2006). Expanding the scales: the multiple roles of MCH in regulating energy balance and other biological functions. *Endocr. Rev.* 27, 606–620.

Pissios, P., and Maratos-Flier, E. (2003). Melanin-concentrating hormone: from fish skin to skinny mammals. *Trends Endocrinol. Metab* 14, 243–248.

Pissios, P., Ozcan, U., Kokkotou, E., Okada, T., Liew, C. W., Liu, S., et al. (2007). Melanin concentrating hormone is a novel regulator of islet function and growth. *Diabetes* 56, 311–319.

Pissios, P., Trombly, D. J., Tzameli, I., and Maratos-Flier, E. (2003). Melanin-concentrating hormone receptor 1 activates extracellular signal-regulated kinase and synergizes with G(s)-coupled pathways. *Endocrinology* 144, 3514–3523.

Qu, D., Ludwig, D. S., Gammeltoft, S., Piper, M., Pelleymounter, M. A., Cullen, M. J., et al. (1996). A role for melanin-concentrating hormone in the central regulation of feeding behaviour. *Nature* 380, 243–247.

Rodriguez, M., Beauverger, P., Naime, I., Rique, H., Ouvry, C., Souchaud, S., et al. (2001). Cloning and molecular characterization of the novel human melanin-concentrating hormone receptor MCH2. *Mol. Pharmacol.* 60, 632–639.

Rondini, T. A., Rodrigues, B. C., de Oliveira, A. P., Bittencourt, J. C., and Elias, C. F. (2007). Melanin-concentrating hormone is expressed in the laterodorsal tegmental nucleus only in female rats. *Brain Res. Bull.* 74, 21–28.

Sailer, A. W., Sano, H., Zeng, Z., McDonald, T. P., Pan, J., Pong, S. S., et al. (2001). Identification and characterization of a second melanin-concentrating hormone receptor, MCH-2R. *Proc. Natl. Acad. Sci. U.S.A.* 98, 7564–7569.

Saito, Y., and Nagasaki, H. (2008). The melanin-concentrating hormone system and its physiological functions. *Results Probl. Cell Differ.* 46, 159–179.

Saito, Y., Nothacker, H. P., Wang, Z., Lin, S. H., Leslie, F., and Civelli,

O. (1999). Molecular characterization of the melanin-concentrating-hormone receptor. *Nature* 400, 265–269.

Sakamaki, R., Uemoto, M., Inui, A., Asakawa, A., Ueno, N., Ishibashi, C., et al. (2005). Melanin-concentrating hormone enhances sucrose intake. *Int. J. Mol. Med.* 15, 1033–1039.

Sasikumar, T. K., Qiang, L., Burnett, D. A., Greenlee, W. J., Hawes, B. E., Kowalski, T. J., et al. (2006). Novel aminobenzimidazoles as selective MCH-R1 antagonists for the treatment of metabolic diseases. *Bioorg. Med. Chem. Lett.* 16, 5427–5431.

Sasmal, S., Balaji, G., Kanna Reddy, H. R., Balasubrahmanyam, D., Srinivas, G., Kyasa, S., et al. (2012a). Design and optimization of quinazoline derivatives as melanin concentrating hormone receptor 1 (MCHR1) antagonists. *Bioorg. Med. Chem. Lett.* 22, 3157–3162.

Sasmal, S., Balasubrahmanyam, D., Kanna Reddy, H. R., Balaji, G., Srinivas, G., Cheera, S., et al. (2012b). Design and optimization of quinazoline derivatives as melanin concentrating hormone receptor 1 (MCHR1) antagonists: part 2. *Bioorg. Med. Chem. Lett.* 22, 3163–3167.

Sears, R. M., Liu, R. J., Narayanan, N. S., Sharf, R., Yeckel, M. F., Laubach, M., et al. (2010). Regulation of nucleus accumbens activity by the hypothalamic neuropeptide melanin-concentrating hormone. *J. Neurosci.* 30, 8263–8273.

Segal-Lieberman, G., Bradley, R. L., Kokkotou, E., Carlson, M., Trombly, D. J., Wang, X., et al. (2003). Melanin-concentrating hormone is a critical mediator of the leptin-deficient phenotype. *Proc. Natl. Acad. Sci. U.S.A.* 100, 10085–10090.

Semjonous, N. M., Smith, K. L., Parkinson, J. R., Gunner, D. J., Liu, Y. L., Murphy, K. G., et al. (2009). Coordinated changes in energy intake and expenditure following hypothalamic administration of neuropeptides involved in energy balance. *Int. J. Obes. (Lond.)* 33, 775–785.

Semple, G., Tran, T. A., Kramer, B., Hsu, D., Han, S., Choi, J., et al. (2009). Pyrimidine-based antagonists of h-MCH-R1 derived from ATC0175: in vitro profiling and in vivo evaluation. *Bioorg. Med. Chem. Lett.* 19, 6166–6171.

Shearman, L. P., Camacho, R. E., Sloan, S. D., Zhou, D., Bednarek, M. A., Hreniuk, D. L., et al. (2003). Chronic MCH-1 receptor modulation alters appetite, body weight and adiposity in rats. *Eur. J. Pharmacol.* 475, 37–47.

Shimada, M., Tritos, N. A., Lowell, B. B., Flier, J. S., and Maratos-Flier, E. (1998). Mice lacking melanin-concentrating hormone are hypophagic and lean. *Nature* 396, 670–674.

Souers, A. J., Gao, J., Brune, M., Bush, E., Wodka, D., Vasudevan, A., et al. (2005a). Identification of 2-(4-benzyloxyphenyl)-N-[1-(2-pyrrolidin-1-yl-ethyl)-1H-indazol-6-yl]acetamide, an orally efficacious melanin-concentrating hormone receptor 1 antagonist for the treatment of obesity. *J. Med. Chem.* 48, 1318–1321.

Souers, A. J., Gao, J., Wodka, D., Judd, A. S., Mulhern, M. M., Napier, J. J., et al. (2005b). Synthesis and evaluation of urea-based indazoles as melanin-concentrating hormone receptor 1 antagonists for the treatment of obesity. *Bioorg. Med. Chem. Lett.* 15, 2752–2757.

Souers, A. J., Iyengar, R. R., Judd, A. S., Beno, D. W., Gao, J., Zhao, G., et al. (2007). Constrained 7-fluorocarboxychromone-4-aminopiperidine based Melanin-concentrating hormone receptor 1 antagonists: the effects of chirality on substituted indan-1-ylamines. *Bioorg. Med. Chem. Lett.* 17, 884–889.

Suply, T., Della-Zuana, O., Audinot, V., Rodriguez, M., Beauverger, P., Duhault, J., et al. (2001). SLC-1 receptor mediates effect of melanin-concentrating hormone on feeding behavior in rat: a structure-activity study. *J. Pharmacol. Exp. Ther.* 299, 137–146.

Surman, M. D., Freeman, E. E., Grabowski, J. F., Hadden, M., Henderson, A. J., Jiang, G. W., et al. (2010). 5-(Pyridinon-1-yl)indazoles and 5-(furopyridinon-5-yl) indazoles as MCH-1 antagonists. *Bioorg. Med. Chem. Lett.* 20, 7015–7019.

Suzuki, T., Kameda, M., Ando, M., Miyazoe, H., Sekino, E., Ito, S., et al. (2009). Discovery of novel diarylketoxime derivatives as selective and orally active melanin-concentrating hormone 1 receptor antagonists. *Bioorg. Med. Chem. Lett.* 19, 5339–5345.

Takekawa, S., Asami, A., Ishihara, Y., Terauchi, J., Kato, K., Shimomura, Y., et al. (2002). T-226296: a novel, orally active and selective melanin-concentrating hormone receptor antagonist. *Eur. J. Pharmacol.* 438, 129–135.

Tan, C. P., Sano, H., Iwaasa, H., Pan, J., Sailer, A. W., Hreniuk, D. L., et al. (2002). Melanin-concentrating hormone receptor subtypes 1 and 2: species-specific gene expression. *Genomics* 79, 785–792.

Tavares, F. X., Al Barazanji, K. A., Bigham, E. C., Bishop, M. J., Britt, C. S., Carlton, D. L., et al. (2006a). Potent, selective, and orally efficacious antagonists of melanin-concentrating hormone receptor 1. *J. Med. Chem.* 49, 7095–7107.

Tavares, F. X., Al Barazanji, K. A., Bishop, M. J., Britt, C. S., Carlton, D. L., Cooper, J. P., et al. (2006b). 6-(4-chlorophenyl)-3-substituted-thieno[3,2-d]pyrimidin-4(3H)-one-based melanin-concentrating hormone receptor 1 antagonist. *J. Med. Chem.* 49, 7108–7118.

Torterolo, P., Sampogna, S., and Chase, M. H. (2009). MCHergic projections to the nucleus pontis oralis participate in the control of active (REM) sleep. *Brain Res.* 1268, 76–87.

Vasudevan, A., Souers, A. J., Freeman, J. C., Verzal, M. K., Gao, J., Mulhern, M. M., et al. (2005a). Aminopiperidine indazoles as orally efficacious melanin concentrating hormone receptor-1 antagonists. *Bioorg. Med. Chem. Lett.* 15, 5293–5297.

Vasudevan, A., Verzal, M. K., Wodka, D., Souers, A. J., Blackburn, C., Che, J. L., et al. (2005b). Identification of aminopiperidine benzamides as MCHr1 antagonists. *Bioorg. Med. Chem. Lett.* 15, 3412–3416.

Vaughan, J. M., Fischer, W. H., Hoeger, C., Rivier, J., and Vale, W. (1989). Characterization of melanin-concentrating hormone from rat hypothalamus. *Endocrinology* 125, 1660–1665.

Wermter, A. K., Reichwald, K., Buch, T., Geller, F., Platzer, C., Huse, K., et al. (2005). Mutation analysis of the MCHR1 gene in human obesity. *Eur. J. Endocrinol.* 152, 851–862.

Whitlock, B. K., Daniel, J. A., McMahon, C. D., Buonomo, F. C., Wagner, C. G., Steele, B., et al. (2005). Intracerebroventricular melanin-concentrating hormone stimulates food intake in sheep. *Domest. Anim. Endocrinol.* 28, 224–232.

Xu, R., Li, S., Paruchova, J., McBriar, M. D., Guzik, H., Palani, A., et al. (2006). Bicyclic[4.1.0]heptanes as phenyl replacements for melanin concentrating hormone receptor antagonists. *Bioorg. Med. Chem.* 14, 3285–3299.

Yao, Y., Fu, L. Y., Zhang, X., and van den Pol, A. N. (2012). Vasopressin and oxytocin excite MCH neurons, but not other lateral hypothalamic GABA neurons. *Am. J. Physiol. Regul. Integr. Comp. Physiol.* 302, R815–R824.

Yumiko, S., and Nagasaki, H. (2008). "The melanin-concentrating hormone system and its physiological functions," in *Orphan G Protein-Coupled Receptors and Novel Neuropeptides*, eds O. Civelli and Q.-Y. Zhou (Berlin: Springer), 159–179.

Zheng, H., Patterson, L. M., Morrison, C., Banfield, B. W., Randall, J. A., Browning, K. N., et al. (2005). Melanin concentrating hormone innervation of caudal brainstem areas involved in gastrointestinal functions and energy balance. *Neuroscience* 135, 611–625.

Zhou, D., Shen, Z., Strack, A. M., Marsh, D. J., and Shearman, L. P. (2005). Enhanced running wheel activity of both *Mch1r*- and *Pmch*-deficient mice. *Regul. Pept.* 124, 53–63.

15

Functional significance of GnRH and kisspeptin, and their cognate receptors in teleost reproduction

Renjitha Gopurappilly†, Satoshi Ogawa and Ishwar S. Parhar*

Brain Research Institute, School of Medicine and Health Sciences, Monash University Sunway Campus, Selangor, Malaysia

Edited by:
Hubert Vaudry, University of Rouen, France

Reviewed by:
Vincent Prevot, INSERM, France
Jae Young Seong, Korea University, South Korea

***Correspondence:**
Ishwar S. Parhar, Brain Research Institute, School of Medicine and Health Sciences, Monash University Sunway Campus, Petaling Jaya 46150, Selangor, Malaysia.
e-mail: ishwar@monash.edu

Guanine nucleotide binding protein (G-protein)-coupled receptors (GPCRs) are eukaryotic transmembrane proteins found in all living organisms. Their versatility and roles in several physiological processes make them the single largest family of drug targets. Comparative genomic studies using various model organisms have provided useful information about target receptors. The similarity of the genetic makeup of teleosts to that of humans and other vertebrates aligns with the study of GPCRs. Gonadotropin-releasing hormone (GnRH) represents a critical step in the reproductive process through its cognate GnRH receptors (GnRHRs). Kisspeptin (Kiss1) and its cognate GPCR, GPR54 (=kisspeptin receptor, Kiss-R), have recently been identified as a critical signaling system in the control of reproduction. The Kiss1/Kiss-R system regulates GnRH release, which is vital to pubertal development and vertebrate reproduction. This review highlights the physiological role of kisspeptin-Kiss-R signaling in the reproductive neuroendocrine axis in teleosts through the modulation of GnRH release. Moreover, we also review the recent developments in GnRHR and Kiss-R with respect to their structural variants, signaling mechanisms, ligand interactions, and functional significance. Finally, we discuss the recent progress in identifying many teleost GnRH-GnRHR and kisspeptin-Kiss-R systems and consider their physiological significance in the control of reproduction.

Keywords: GnRH receptor, kisspeptin receptor, GPR54, reproduction, teleost fish

INTRODUCTION

Guanine nucleotide binding protein (G-protein)-coupled receptors (GPCRs) play a pivotal role in various physiological processes (Marinissen and Gutkind, 2001), and GPCRs are now recognized as major pharmaceutical drug targets (Shoichet and Kobilka, 2012). GPCR sequencing in model organisms has proven vital for identifying novel GPCRs and their ligands with potential therapeutic value (Metpally and Sowdhamini, 2005). Evolutionary comparisons of GPCR sequences may allow for the identification of conserved motifs and the recognition of key functional residues (Attwood, 2001; Bjarnadottir et al., 2005). As research models, fish have been used largely to exploit their aquaculture potential. However, in recent years, there has been a trend toward using them in biomedical research as models of human disease. Because fish are phylogenetically diverse, they can be used to understand the fundamental principles of vertebrate evolution and disease processes. Therefore, the teleost genome provides an additional model to study the evolution and function of GPCRs (Metpally and Sowdhamini, 2005).

The hypothalamic-pituitary-gonadal (HPG) axis regulates puberty in vertebrates, primarily through the hypothalamic secretion of gonadotropin-releasing hormone (GnRH). This decapeptide hormone stimulates the release of the following gonadotropins from the anterior pituitary: follicle-stimulating hormone (FSH) for gamete growth and luteinizing hormone (LH) for gamete maturation and release (Ankley and Johnson, 2004; Weltzien et al., 2004). Recently, kisspeptin, a novel neuropeptide encoded by the metastasis suppressor gene, Kiss1/KISS1 (rodents/human), and its cognate GPCR, kisspeptin receptor (Kiss-R) (=GPR54), have been identified as potent regulators of reproduction, particularly for the onset of puberty (de Roux et al., 2003; Seminara et al., 2003). The kisspeptin-GPR54 system is vital to the onset of puberty, as it is critical to the activation of GnRH neurons. In 2004, we were the first to report the expression of GPR54 mRNA in GnRH neurons in a cichlid fish, tilapia, which strongly supports this concept (Parhar et al., 2004). Following this discovery, the presence of GPR54 in GnRH neurons has been demonstrated in several mammalian and non-mammalian species (Irwig et al., 2004; Han et al., 2005; Messager et al., 2005; Grone et al., 2010). Moreover, the innervation of kisspeptin fibers to GnRH neurons has been illustrated in several vertebrates (Clarkson and Herbison, 2006; Ramaswamy et al., 2008; Servili et al., 2011). The HPG axis is regulated by a number of GPCRs that play important roles in reproduction and sex hormone-dependent diseases (Heitman and Ijzerman, 2008). These receptors are therefore referred to as "reproductive" GPCRs. Numerous GPCRs with roles in reproduction have been discovered in recent years (Millar and Newton, 2010). In this review, we focus on the GnRH receptor (GnRHR), the recently deorphanized Kiss-R, and the regulation of GnRH secretion by an intricate interplay between the two in the teleosts.

GnRH RECEPTOR TYPES

STRUCTURAL VARIANTS

Gonadotropin-releasing hormone is the hypothalamic decapeptide, which is mainly responsible for reproductive function. It is secreted from the hypothalamus into the hypophyseal portal circulation via the median eminence, which binds and activates the GnRHR that is expressed on the surface of the pituitary gonadotrope cells in mammals (Neill, 2002). In teleosts, the equivalent of the median eminence is incorporated into the rostral neurohypophysis of the pituitary (Batten and Ingleton, 1987). GnRH fibers have been observed to directly innervate the neurohypophysis in the pituitary (Kah et al., 1986; Parhar et al., 2002). In the pituitary, GnRH interacts with high-affinity GnRHRs in cell membranes of gonadotrophs, leading to biosynthesis and secretion of LH and FSH (Karges et al., 2003). To date, more than 20 forms of GnRH and the corresponding genes have been identified (Tsai, 2006; Chen and Fernald, 2008; Okubo and Nagahama, 2008; Roch et al., 2011; Tostivint, 2011; Kochman, 2012). These have a broad range of functions, including neuroendocrine, neurotransmitter/neuromodulatory, paracrine and autocrine functions (Millar et al., 2004), and each GnRH type is capable of serving all these roles. Structural and phylogenetic analysis of the GnRH genes classifies GnRH types into three forms (White and Fernald, 1998). Most vertebrate species possess at least two or three GnRH forms (Sherwood, 1987; Sherwood et al., 1993; Sealfon et al., 1997; Millar, 2003). GnRH-II (=GnRH2) is ubiquitously found in the most vertebrates, which was first isolated from the chicken (cGnRH-II) (Miyamoto et al., 1984). Because GnRH2 structure is highly conserved in the vertebrate species, it most likely serves critical functions and evolved the earliest (Millar et al., 2004). The hypothalamic form is designated GnRH type I (GnRH1) (Troskie et al., 1998), which is the species-specific form and regulates pituitary LH release (Parhar, 2002), and most of which have been identified in fish (Okubo and Nagahama, 2008). A third GnRH type (salmon GnRH-III = GnRH3) is only exhibited in the forebrain of teleost fish. A recent gene synteny analysis of the genomic regions comprising fish GnRH3 has found similar arrangement of GnRH3 gene cluster in the tetrapod genomes (Roch et al., 2011), which indicates that tetrapod GnRH3 was lost after divergence of fish and tetrapod lineages (Kim et al., 2011; Tostivint, 2011). Lamprey GnRH-I and -III, have recently been categorized as GnRH type IV (GnRH4), exclusive to the jawless fish (Roch et al., 2011).

GnRH receptor gene sequence was first identified from the mouse αT3 gonadotrope cell line (Tsutsumi et al., 1992; Millar et al., 2004). The ligand binding pocket of the GnRHR is formed by residues in the extracellular loops and the interior of transmembrane helices, indicating that GnRH partially enters the transmembrane core (Forfar and Lu, 2011). Mammalian GnRHR homologs have been isolated from non-mammalian species such as reptile, amphibians, birds, teleosts, and invertebrate species (Millar, 2003). The first teleost GnRHR was isolated from the African catfish (Tensen et al., 1997), and piscine GnRHR homologous sequences have been isolated from various teleosts such as the goldfish (Illing et al., 1999), Japanese eel (Okubo et al., 2000), trout (Madigou et al., 2000), striped bass (Alok et al., 2000), cichlid (Robison et al., 2001; Parhar et al., 2005a), medaka (Okubo et al., 2001), salmon (Jodo et al., 2003), fugu (Moncaut et al., 2005), and cobia (Mohamed et al., 2007). In some teleosts, there are four or five GnRHR isoforms (Jodo et al., 2003; Moncaut et al., 2005). Recent phylogenetic analyses based on amino acid sequence identity have classified teleosts GnRHR isoforms into three major groups (Mollusk et al., 2011; Roch et al., 2011). Furthermore, a recent classification based on genome synteny analysis has also revealed three major lineages of fish GnRHR types that further subdivide into five classes: non-mammalian type I (GnRHRn1 and GnRHRn1b), non-mammalian type II (GnRHRn2), and non-mammalian type III (GnRHRn3 and GnRHRn3b) (Kim et al., 2011) (**Table 1**). The genome synteny-based classification has clearly demonstrated high conservation of neighboring genes of GnRHR types, which are also found in tetrapod GnRHR containing genome fragments (Kim et al., 2011). The neighboring gene sets of fish GnRHRn1, found in GnRHRn1b are probably generated by the teleost-specific third round genome duplication (Kim et al., 2011).

LOCALIZATION AND FUNCTION OF GnRHR TYPES

Localization of the various GnRHRs may provide some insight into their role in the physiology of reproduction. Five teleost GnRHR types (GnRHRn1, GnRHRn1b, GnRHRn2, GnRHRn3, and GnRHRn3b) have been localized in various reproductive organs including the gonads, brain, and pituitary (Lethimonier et al., 2004). In the European sea bass, five GnRHR genes show differential expression in various tissues, in which GnRHR1A (GnRHRn3b) and GnRHR (GnRHRn2) are widely distributed in reproductive and non-reproductive tissues including the eye, kidney, gills, gut, and liver, whereas GnRHRII (GnRHRn3), GnRHR2B (GnRHRn1), and GnRHR2C (GnRHRn1b) are more restricted to the central nervous system (Moncaut et al., 2005). This finding suggests multiple neuroendocrine and neuromodulatory roles of GnRH types throughout the body of teleosts (Jodo et al., 2003).

In the brain, the distribution of GnRHR types has been studied by RT-PCR, *in situ* hybridization and immunohistochemical approaches (**Table 1**). *In situ* hybridization studies in the European seabass have demonstrated the expression of GnRHR (GnRHRn2) in the forebrain, and the midbrain (Gonzalez-Martinez et al., 2004). In *Astatotilapia burtoni*, GnRHR1 (classified as GnRHRn1 based on sequence homology) is expressed in restricted brain regions including the telencephalon, preoptic area, ventral hypothalamus, and thalamus, whereas GnRH-R2 (GnRHRn3) is expressed in many more brain areas (Chen and Fernald, 2006). In the tilapia, GnRHR1 (GenBank accession number: XM_003437572) and/or GnRHR3 (XM_003437677) (both are classified as GnRHRn1) immunoreactive cells have been shown in the forebrain and midbrain (Soga et al., 2005). Most GnRHR types are found in brain areas involved in reproductive functions (Volkoff and Peter, 1999), and several GnRHR types are also found in the brain region that is known to be involved in appetite control, feeding, and stress responses (Chandroo et al., 2004; Volkoff et al., 2005).

In situ hybridization studies have demonstrated the expression offish GnRHR in the pituitary: GnRHRn1 [*A. burtoni* GnRHR1, striped seabass GnRHR (AF218841)], GnRHRn1b (European seabass GnRHR2C), GnRHRn2 (European seabass GnRHR, African catfish GnRHR1), GnRHRn3 (*A. burtoni* GnRH-R2, European seabass GnRHRII), and GnRHRn3b [European seabass GnRHR1A, Rainbow Trout GnRHR (NP_001117823), African catfish GnRHR1 (X97497), Goldfish GnRHRA, and Goldfish

Table 1 | GnRH receptors in teleosts.

Type	Species	Original name	Accession number/ ensembl ID	Ligand selectivity	Localization		Reference
					Brain	Pituitary	
GnRHRn1	Medaka	GnRHR3	NP_001098393	GnRH2 = GnRH3 > GnRH1	+	+	Okubo et al. (2003)
	Zebrafish	GnRHR4	NP_001091663	ND	ND	ND	
	Green pufferfish	GnRHR1/III-3	BAE45698	ND	ND	ND	
	Fugu	GnRHR-II-like	XP_003967097	ND	ND	ND	
	Stickleback	GnRHR	ENSGACP00000014249	ND	ND	ND	
	European seabass	GnRHR2B	CAE54807	ND	+	−	Moncaut et al. (2005)
	Platyfish	GnRHR	ENSXMAP00000002818	ND	ND	ND	
	Cod	GnRHR	ENSGMOP00000013942	ND	ND	ND	
	Tilapia	GnRHR-II-like	XP_003440455	ND	+	+	Soga et al. (2005)
	Coelacanth	GnRHR	ENSLACP00000020711	ND	ND	ND	
	Astatotilapia	GnRHR1	AAK29745	GnRH2 > GnRH3 > GnRH1	+	+	Robison et al. (2001)
GnRHRn1b	Medaka	GnRHR1	NP_001098352	GnRH2 ≥ GnRH3 = GnRH1	ND	ND	Okubo et al. (2001)
	Green pufferfish	GnRHR1/III-1	BAE45694	ND	ND	ND	
	Fugu	GnRHR	ENSTRUP00000018665	ND	ND	ND	
	Stickleback	GnRHR	ENSGACP00000019583	ND	ND	ND	
	European seabass	GnRHR2C	CAE54805	ND	+	+	Moncaut et al. (2005)
	Platyfish	GnRHR	ENSXMAP00000011787	ND	ND	ND	
GnRHRn2	Zebrafish	GnRH-R2	NP_001138451	ND	ND	ND	
	Medaka	GnRHR	ENSORLP00000015859	ND	ND	ND	
	Green pufferfish	GnRHR1/III-2	BAE45696	ND	ND	ND	
	Fugu	GnRHR	ENSTRUP00000014430	ND	ND	ND	
	Stickleback	GnRHR	ENSGACP00000021774	ND	ND	ND	
	European seabass	GnRHR	CAD11992	ND	+	+	Madigou et al. (2000)
	Cod	GnRHR	ENSGMOP00000000888	ND	ND	ND	
	Platyfish	GnRHR	ENSXMAP00000018201	ND	ND	ND	
GnRHRn3	Zebrafish	GnRHR3	NP_001170921	ND	ND	ND	
	Medaka	GnRH-R2	NP_001098392	GnRH2 > GnRH3 > GnRH1	ND	ND	Okubo et al. (2001)
	Green pufferfish	GnRH-R2/nml-2	BAE45702	ND	ND	ND	
	Fugu	GnRHR	ENSTRUP00000014399	ND	ND	ND	
	Stickleback	GnRHR	ENSGACP00000004101	ND	ND	ND	
	European seabass	GnRHRII	AAS49921	ND	+	+	Moncaut et al. (2005)
	Coelacanth	GnRHR	ENSLACP00000018841	ND	ND	ND	
	Tilapia	GnRHR	ENSONIP00000001826	ND	ND	ND	
	Astatotilapia	GnRH-R2	AAU89433	ND	+	+	Chen and Fernald (2006)
GnRHRn3b	Zebrafish	GnRHR1	NP_001138452	ND	ND	ND	
	Green pufferfish	GnRH-R2/nml-1	BAE45702	ND	ND	ND	
	Fugu	GnRHR	ENSTRUP00000014399	ND	ND	ND	
	Stickleback	GnRHR	ENSGACP00000000651	ND	ND	ND	
	European seabass	GnRHR1A	CAE54804	ND	+	+	Moncaut et al. (2005)
	Cod	GnRH-R1b	ADD92008	ND	ND	ND	
	Goldfish	GnRHRA	AAD20001	GnRH2 > GnRH3 > mGnRH1	+	+	Illing et al. (1999)
	Goldfish	GnRHRB	AAD20002	GnRH2 > GnRH3 > mGnRH1	+	+	Illing et al. (1999)

ND, not determined.

GnRHRB] (Illing et al., 1999; Alok et al., 2000; Madigou et al., 2000; Gonzalez-Martinez et al., 2004; Moncaut et al., 2005; Chen and Fernald, 2006) (**Figure 1A**). Within the pituitary cells, most GnRHR types have mainly been localized in the proximal pars distal is of the pituitary where the gonadotrophs (LH and FSH) are exist, which includes GnRHRn1: Tilapia GnRHR1/R3, *A. burtoni* GnRHR1; GnRHRn2: European seabass GnRHR; GnRHRn3/3b: *A. burtoni* GnRH-R2, Rainbow trout GnRHR, Goldfish GnRHRA

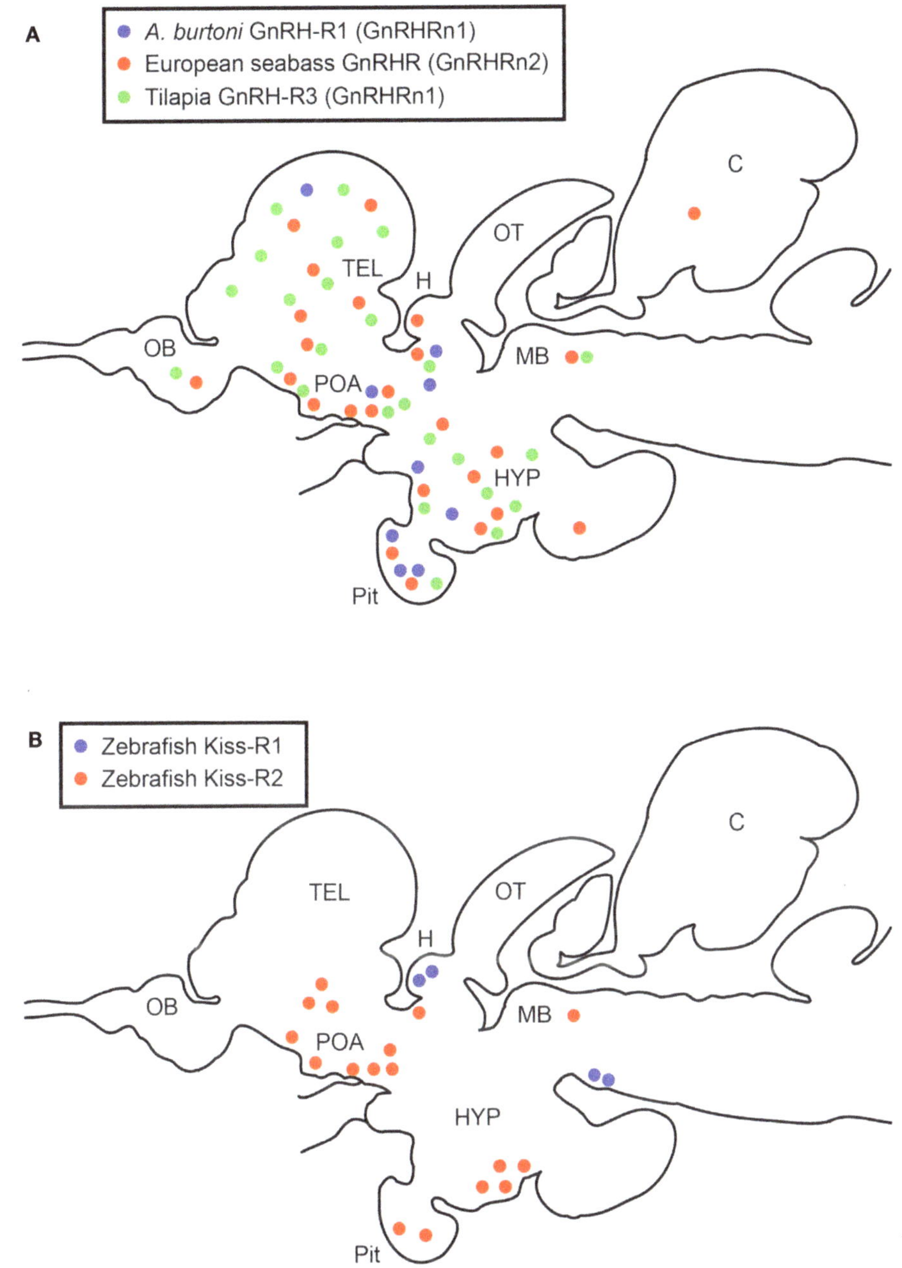

FIGURE 1 | Schematic diagrams showing distribution of GnRHRs (A) and Kiss-Rs (B)-expressing cells in the brain and pituitary of teleosts. (A) Expression patterns of three GnRHR types expressing cells in three cichlid species, European seabass, *Astatotilapia burtoni*, and Nile tilapia (Gonzalez-Martinez et al., 2004; Soga et al., 2005; Chen and Fernald, 2006). *A. burtoni* GnRHR1 (GnRHRn1), blue; European seabass GnRHR (GnRHRn2), red; Tilapia GnRHR3 (GnRHRn1), green circles. **(B)** Expression patterns of two Kiss-R types expressing cells in the zebrafish brain (Servili et al., 2011; Ogawa et al., 2012a). Kiss-R1 (GPR54b), blue; Kiss-R2 (GPR54a), red circles. OB, olfactory bulb; TEL, telencephalon; POA, preoptic area; H, habenula; OT, optic tectum; HYP, hypothalamus; C, cerebellum; pit, pituitary; MB, midbrain.

and GnRHRB (Madigou et al., 2000; Parhar et al., 2002; Gonzalez-Martinez et al., 2004). In some teleosts, the presence of multiple GnRHR types have also been demonstrated in other pituitary cell types such as lactotropes, somatotropes, thyrotropes, melanotropes, corticotropes, and somatolactin cells (Illing et al., 1999; Parhar et al., 2002).

GnRHR SIGNALING, CYCLING, AND DESENSITIZATION

A recent review by Levavi-Sivan and Avitan (2005) elegantly describes the GnRHR signaling pathway in gonadotrophs (**Figure 2A**). Mammalian and non-mammalian GnRHRs promote a conformational change in the GnRH peptide structure, which is essential for G-protein coupling and signal transduction

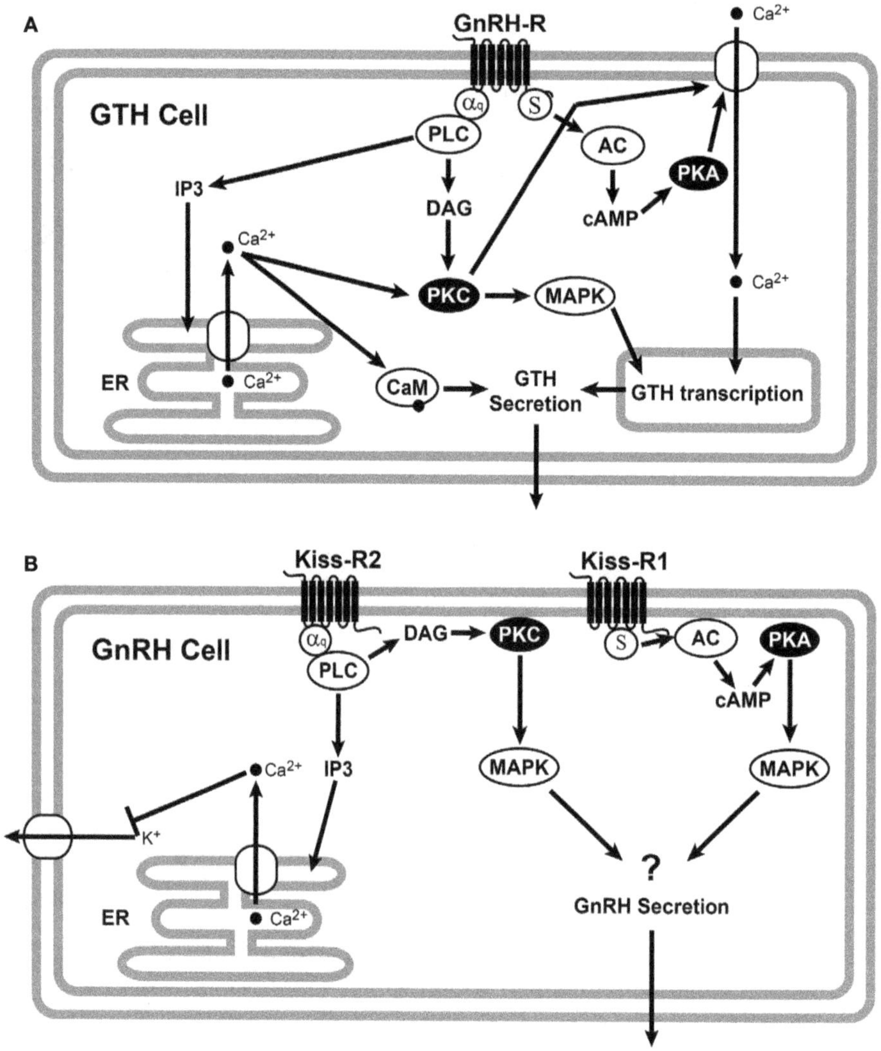

FIGURE 2 | Schematic representation of GnRHR (A) and Kiss-R (B) signaling. (A) GnRH binds to the Gq/11-coupled membrane receptors. Activation of Gq/11 proteins stimulates phospholipase C (PLC) activity to generate inositol triphosphate (IP3) and diacylglycerol (DAG). Increases of these signal messengers lead to the activation of protein kinase C (PKC) and an increase in intracellular Ca^{2+} concentration from the endoplasmic reticulum (ER). The PKC and Ca^{2+} pathways are involved in the GnRH regulation of GTH subunit gene expression, while GTH secretion is mainly mediated by the GnRH-induced increase in intracellular calcium through the calmodulin (CaM). It has also been proposed that GnRH caused GTP loading on Gs and increased intracellular cAMP via activation of adenylyl cyclase (AC), which elevates GnRH release via the cAMP-dependent protein kinase (PKA) (Liu et al., 2002). **(B)** Binding of kisspeptin to teleosts Kiss-R2 activates the Gq/11 and PLC to generate IP3 and DAG. IP3 causes intracellular Ca^{2+} release from the ER, which activates PKC and mitogen-activated protein kinase (MAPK) cascade. However, teleosts Kiss-R could be activated by the cAMP/PKA pathway probably through Gs. All the figures were adopted from Ando et al. (2001), Krsmanovic et al. (2003), Oakley et al. (2009), d'Anglemont de Tassigny and Colledge (2010), Rønnekleiv et al. (2010).

(Illing et al., 1999; Cheung and Hearn, 2002; Levavi-Sivan and Avitan, 2005), suggesting similar receptor activation mechanisms. Ligand binding to GnRHR activates phospholipase C to generate inositol (Levavi-Sivan and Avitan, 2005), which mobilizes intracellular Ca^{2+} stores and activates protein kinase C. In teleosts, the cAMP signaling pathway is involved in GnRH release (Yaron et al., 2003; Levavi-Sivan and Avitan, 2005). In the tilapia, GnRH regulates glycoprotein hormone α and LHβ transcription through the PKC and PKA pathways and regulates FSHβ transcription through the PKC and PAPK-independent pathways (Gur et al., 2002). GnRHRs and GPCRs typically undergo desensitization and internalization including receptor phosphorylation, after being activated (McArdle et al., 2002). This phosphorylation stabilizes the association of GPCRs with β-arrestin, which prevents effector activation and acts as an adapter, targeting desensitized GPCRs for internalization (Ferguson, 2001) by endocytosis. Different GnRHR type may have different rates of desensitization and internalization and may also have different repertoire of signaling possibilities (McArdle et al., 2002).

REGULATION OF FISH GnRHR

GnRH receptor is known to be regulated by several factors. In the tilapia, GnRHR3 has been shown to be up-regulated by its own ligand in the pituitary (Levavi-Sivan et al., 2004). A dopamine-agonist suppressed tilapia GnRHR3 mRNA levels, which indicates an inhibitory effect of dopamine on GnRHR3 synthesis (Levavi-Sivan et al., 2004). Furthermore, tilapia GnRHR3 mRNA levels are higher in vitellogenic females than in maturing males, which could be due to the effect of higher estradiol-17β levels in females on tilapia GnRHR3 mRNA levels (Levavi-Sivan et al., 2004). In female *A. burtoni*, GnRH-R2 mRNA levels are elevated in mouth-brooding female brain compared to fed condition, which could be due to low androgens and estrogens levels (Grone et al., 2012). In rare minnow *Gobiocypris rarus*, bisphenol A, an endocrine disrupting chemical has been recently reported to affect gene expression of GnRHR1A gene in the brains of females (Qin et al., 2013). Although not many studies on promoter analysis of a fish GnRHR have been done, fish GnRHR gene seems to be sensitive to sex steroids as reported in mammals (Hapgood et al., 2005). In the Atlantic cod, pituitary GnRH-R2a but not GnRH-R1b gene expression increases in late-vitellogenic and running females. Continuous light inhibits the increase of pituitary GnRH-R2a expression seen during the normal spawning period (Hildahl et al., 2013). These results suggest that GnRHR is also influenced by nutrition and environmental factors most probably via steroid hormone levels.

GPR54

Kisspeptin, encoded by the KISS1/Kiss1 gene, is an endogenous ligand for GPR54 (thus called Kiss-R) and promotes GnRH secretion (Kotani et al., 2001; Kaiser and Kuohung, 2005; Dungan et al., 2006). Kiss-R is widely expressed in many reproductive tissues. Mounting evidence suggests the critical role of kisspeptin in the modulation of GnRH secretion in the central nervous system (Irwig et al., 2004; Han et al., 2005; Messager et al., 2005). The kisspeptin-Kiss-R signaling system in various vertebrate species has been described in terms of distribution and physiology (Oakley et al., 2009). This signaling pathway is significant in the reproductive axis in vertebrates, although the location, developmental timing, and expression patterns differ. The anatomy and physiology of piscine kisspeptin-Kiss-R signaling has been extensively reviewed (Elizur, 2009; Zohar et al., 2010; Ogawa and Parhar, 2013). Current knowledge on the gene expression, distribution, and physiological function of piscine kisspeptin and Kiss-R is as follows.

KISSPEPTIN RECEPTOR TYPES IN TELEOSTS

Kisspeptin receptor was first identified as an orphan GPCR (Lee et al., 1999). Mammalian Kiss-R is weakly homologous to galanin receptors (44–45%) but does not bind to either galanin or galanin-like peptides (Lee et al., 1999). We have previously reported a non-mammalian GPR54 for the first time in the tilapia (Parhar et al., 2004). Since then, many groups have identified Kiss-R in several non-mammalian vertebrates. In fish, there are two Kiss-R types (Kiss1Ra/GPR54-1 and Kiss1Rb/GPR54-2 in zebrafish, GPR54a and GPR54b in goldfish) (Lee et al., 2009; Li et al., 2009), while *Xenopus* have three Kiss-R types (GPR54-1a, GPR54-1b, and GPR54-2) (Lee et al., 2009). Genome and cDNA analyses has revealed that the Kiss-R genes contain five exons, although medaka Kiss-R1 and sea bass Kiss-R2 have six exons (Tena-Sempere et al., 2012). Our recent *in silico* study has identified four Kiss-R homologous sequences in an early sarcopterygian, Coelacanth *Latimeria chalumnae* genome, which leads to further clarification of molecular evolution of Kiss-R in vertebrates (describe in below).

Two Kiss-R types have been identified in the Senegalese sole (Mechaly et al., 2009), goldfish (Li et al., 2009), zebrafish (Biran et al., 2008), medaka (Lee et al., 2009), striped bass (Zmora et al., 2012), and sea bass (Tena-Sempere et al., 2012). In Perciform teleosts, the Southern Bluefin Tuna, and the Yellowtail Kingfish, two mRNA transcript variants of Kiss-R2 have been identified (Nocillado et al., 2012). With two different Kiss-R genes, two kisspeptin types (Kiss1 and Kiss2) have been identified in several teleosts such as zebrafish, medaka (Kanda et al., 2008; van Aerle et al., 2008; Kitahashi et al., 2009), goldfish (Li et al., 2009), sea bass (Felip et al., 2009), chub mackerel (Selvaraj et al., 2010), and striped bass (Zmora et al., 2012). Two kisspeptin types have also been identified in *Xenopus* and elephant shark (Lee et al., 2009), which suggests that the kisspeptin-Kiss-R systems function independently, especially in controlling teleost reproduction. Some teleosts possess only one kisspeptin type (Kiss2) or/and its receptor (Kiss-R2) (Tena-Sempere et al., 2012). Previous genome synteny analyses (Um et al., 2010; Tena-Sempere et al., 2012) have suggested that the Kiss-R genes previously identified from tilapia (Parhar et al., 2004), a cichlid *A. burtoni* (Grone et al., 2010), gray mullet (Nocillado et al., 2007), cobia (Mohamed et al., 2007), fathead minnow (Filby et al., 2008), Atlantic croaker (Mechaly et al., 2009), Senegalese sole (Mechaly et al., 2011), Atlantic halibut (Mechaly et al., 2010), and European eel (Pasquier et al., 2011) belong to the Kiss-R2 subfamily. Therefore, in teleosts, Kiss2-Kiss-R2 is evolutionarily highly conserved and may be functionally equivalent to mammalian Kiss1-Kiss-R.

The nomenclature for two Kiss-R types has been classified based on phylogenetic analysis (Um et al., 2010). Recent genome synteny-based classification studies have clearly demonstrated high conservation of neighboring genes of four fish Kiss-R types (Lee et al., 2009). The fish Kiss1Ra-containing genome fragments have a large array of common neighboring genes, which include ATP6V0B, RABL5, ODF2L, CYR61, C1QL3, GPT, FUZ, CCDC24, and B4GALT2, while the fish Kiss1Rb-containing genome fragments have conserved PSAT1, ZCCHC6, and ISCA1. Ligand-receptor binding assays have shown that while Kiss1 peptide (Kiss1–10) activates Kiss1Rb (GPR54-2) more efficiently than Kiss2 peptide (Kiss2-10) in zebrafish (Lee et al., 2009) and sea bass (Tena-Sempere et al., 2012), Kiss2–10 performs more efficiently in goldfish (Li et al., 2009). Kiss1Ra (GPR54-1) is activated by Kiss1–10 in goldfish (Li et al., 2009) and activated by Kiss1–10 and Kiss2–10 in zebrafish and sea bass (Lee et al., 2009; Tena-Sempere et al., 2012). Interestingly, human Kiss1–10 was an effective homolog in activating Kiss-R2 in the orange spotted grouper (which ordinarily has only Kiss2/Kiss-R2 pair) (Shi et al., 2010). Therefore, in the following sections, fish Kiss1Ra and Kiss1Rb are designated as Kiss-R2 and Kiss-R1, respectively.

DISTRIBUTION

Two Kiss-R genes are highly expressed in various reproductive tissues including the brain, pituitary, and gonads and partially in other peripheral tissues (Nocillado et al., 2007; Biran et al., 2008; Filby et al., 2008; van Aerle et al., 2008; Li et al., 2009; Mechaly et al., 2009; Tena-Sempere et al., 2012) (**Table 2**). Kiss-R gene expression has been described in specific parts and throughout the teleost brain (Biran et al., 2008; Filby et al., 2008; Martinez-Chavez et al., 2008; van Aerle et al., 2008; Shahjahan et al., 2010). In the Senegalese sole, the two Kiss-R isoforms (Kiss1r_v1 and Kiss1r_v2) exhibit differential patterns in the brain (Mechaly et al., 2009). In the brain of fathead minnow, *Pimephales promelas*, *kiss1r* (homologous to Kiss-R2) gene expression is largely seen in various brain regions including the olfactory bulbs, the dorsal and ventral telencephalon, the hypothalamic nuclei, the midbrain, and the hindbrain (Filby et al., 2008). In the zebrafish, *in situ* hybridization has shown that most *kiss-r1* (GPR54-2) mRNA is expressed in the habenula (Ogawa et al., 2010, 2012a; Servili et al., 2011), whereas *kiss-r2* (GPR54-1) mRNA is widely expressed in the fish brain, especially in the olfactory bulb, telencephalon, preoptic area, midbrain, hypothalamic nuclei, cerebellum, and spinal cord (Grone et al., 2010; Servili et al., 2011; Ogawa et al., 2012a) (**Figure 1B**).

The distinct expression patterns of two Kiss-R types indicate their specific roles in reproductive and non-reproductive functions in fish. The habenula, a conserved structure in the brain of vertebrates has been shown to play important roles in various brain functions and behaviors, which include circadian rhythmicity, feeding, stress, sleep, affective states, and maternal and sexual behaviors (Teitelbaum and Epstein, 1962; Modianos et al., 1974; Corodimas et al., 1992; Matthews-Felton et al., 1995; Klemm, 2004; Zhao and Rusak, 2005). In mammals, the habenula expresses neuropeptides such as substance P (SP) and neuropeptide Y (NPY) (Neckers et al., 1979; Smith et al., 1985). In rats, GnRH-immunoreactive non-neuronal mast cells have been observed in the habenula (Khalil et al., 2003), which have also been noted in GFP-GnRH transgenic rats (Parhar et al., 2005b). Similarly in the habenula of teleosts, there are groups of cells immunoreactive to neuropeptides such as SP and corticotropin-releasing factor,(Villani et al., 1991; Mousa and Mousa, 2006), and expression of *tac2a*/*tac3a* gene (encoding neurokinin B) has been recently identified in the habenula of zebrafish (Biran et al., 2012; Ogawa et al., 2012b). These neuropeptide containing cells in the habenula may co-express Kiss-R to regulate a variety of neuroendocrine functions. As Kiss-R2 are widely expressed in the preoptic-hypothalamic regions in fish, Kiss-R2 could also be expressed in other neuronal populations in addition to GnRH neurons, which could play a key role in the control of reproduction, as has been suggested in mice (Herbison et al., 2010; Hanchate et al., 2012).

In some teleosts, Kiss-R is also expressed in the pituitary (Filby et al., 2008; Martinez-Chavez et al., 2008; Shahjahan et al.,

Table 2 | Kisspeptin receptors in teleosts.

Type	Species	Original name	Accession number/ ensembl ID	Ligand selectivity	Localization		Reference
					Brain	Pituitary	
Kiss-R1a	Coelacanth	Kiss-R1a	ENSLACP00000018620	ND	ND		
Kiss-R1b	Goldfish	GRP54b	ACK77793	Kiss1 > Kiss2 (SRE)	+	+	Li et al. (2009)
	Zebrafish	GPR54-2/Kiss1Rb	EU047918/ ENSDARP00000088021	Kiss1 > Kiss2	+	+	Lee et al. (2009), Servili et al. (2011), Ogawa et al. (2012a)
	Medaka	GPR54-1/Kiss1Rb	ENSORLP00000002102	ND	ND		Lee et al. (2009)
	Coelacanth	Kiss-R1b	ENSLACP00000000327	ND	ND		
Kiss-R2a	Goldfish	GPR54a	ACK77792	Kiss2 > Kiss1 (CRE)	+	+	Li et al. (2009)
	Zebrafish	GPR54-1/Kiss1Ra	EU047917/ ENSDARP00000011859	Kiss1 = Kiss2	+	−	Lee et al. (2009), Servili et al. (2011), Ogawa et al. (2012a)
	Cod	Kiss1R	ENSGMOP00000011986	ND	ND		
	Coelacanth	Kiss-R2a	ENSLACP00000019382	ND	ND		
	Fugu	Kiss1R	ENSTRUP00000035136	ND	ND		
	Stickleback	Kiss-R	ENSGACP00000022743	ND	ND		
	Tetraodon	Kiss1R	ENSTNIP00000017204	ND	ND		
	Tilapia	Kiss1R	ENSONIP00000011710	ND	ND		
	Medaka	GPR54-2/Kiss1Ra	ENSORLP00000022191	ND	ND		Lee et al. (2009)
	Platyfish	Kiss1R	ENSXMAP00000017086	ND	ND		
Kiss-R2b	Coelacanth	Kiss-R2b	ENSLACP00000001512	ND	ND		
	Green anole	GPR54-like	XP_003217188	ND	ND		
	Platypus	GPR54b	XP_001507133	ND	ND		

ND, not determined. SRE, binding response shown with serum response element; CRE, binding response shown with cAMP response element.

2010) (**Table 2**). In the pituitary of goldfish, Kiss-R2 (GPR54a) is expressed in the gonadotrophs, somatotrophs, and lactotrophs (Yang et al., 2010), which corresponds with the existence of fiber innervation of Kiss2-immunoreactive fibers in the pituitary of zebrafish (Servili et al., 2011). In mammals, kisspeptin appears to directly stimulate the secretion of LH, growth hormone, and prolactin secretion (Gutiérrez-Pascual et al., 2007; Kadokawa et al., 2008a,b). These results suggest that the hypothalamic kisspeptin-Kiss-R system regulates the reproductive functions at the level of the brain as well as at the level of the pituitary.

EXPRESSION OF KISS-R IN GnRH NEURONS

Our group (Parhar et al., 2004) was the first to report Kiss-R (Kiss-R2) and GnRH co-localization in tilapia using single-cell gene profiling coupled with laser-captured microdissection. This finding has established the concept that kisspeptin directly regulates GnRH neurons. We demonstrated expression of Kiss-R2 mRNA transcripts in all three GnRH neuronal types in tilapia (Parhar et al., 2004), which has also been confirmed in another cichlid by *in situ* hybridization (Grone et al., 2010). A close association between Kiss2 fibers and GnRH neurons have been established by a recent immunohistochemical study in zebrafish (Servili et al., 2011). In the mullet, Kiss-R2 gene expression positively correlates with GnRH2 and GnRH3 (Nocillado et al., 2007). In the early larval and juvenile cobia brain, Kiss-R (homologous to Kiss-R2) expression and all three GnRH mRNAs remains remarkably similar (Mohamed et al., 2007). These results suggest that Kiss-R2 and GnRH have coordinated roles at early pubertal stages in fish. In zebrafish, *kiss1*, *kiss2*, GnRH2, and GnRH3 mRNA levels are increased at the start of the pubertal phase (Kitahashi et al., 2009), indicating its role in controlling the onset of puberty. A very recent study in the *Morone* species has demonstrated that Kiss-R2 is co-localized in GnRH1 neurons in the preoptic area, while Kiss-R1 is expressed in cells attached to GnRH1 fibers, indicating two different GnRH1 regulatory methods (Zmora et al., 2012). These findings also indicate potential relationships between Kiss-Rs and multiple GnRHs, implicating kisspeptin-Kiss-R in the development and maturation of the piscine reproductive system.

KISS-R SIGNALING IN TELEOSTS

The ligand specificity of the piscine Kiss/Kiss-R system has previously been demonstrated by analyzing PKC-MAPK activation in several teleosts species (Biran et al., 2008; Lee et al., 2009; Tena-Sempere et al., 2012) (**Figure 2B**). All piscine Kiss-Rs tested successfully activated luciferase expression with the help of an SRE promoter, indicating the significance of PKC-MAPKs as a signaling pathway (similar to mammals) (Tena-Sempere et al., 2012). However, variances in kisspeptin length and receptor-ligand combinations have resulted in observable differentiation. Mammalian Kiss-Rs require a core sequence of kisspeptin (Kiss-10) to optimally activate Kiss-R (Kotani et al., 2001). All available fish Kiss2 sequences show a conserved Arg (position 13), indicating a putative mature Kiss2–12 peptide, while Kiss1 sequencing revealed a mature Kiss1–15 peptide due to the presence of a conserved N-terminal Gln (Tena-Sempere et al., 2012), which has further been supported by more active kisspeptin results from pyroglutamylation of the N-terminal Gln (Lee et al., 2009). Only zebrafish and sea bass have served in the testing of longer kisspeptins (Kiss1–15 and Kiss2–12) (Lee et al., 2009; Zmora et al., 2012). In all cases, the longer peptides have activated Kiss-Rs more effectively than their respective shorter peptide form with some exceptions (Lee et al., 2009; Tena-Sempere et al., 2012).

The cAMP/PKA pathway is activated more potently by Kiss-R1 than Kiss-R2 in zebrafish, goldfish, and sea bass (Tena-Sempere et al., 2012). Maximum activation of Kiss-R1 in goldfish is achieved with Kiss2–10 (Li et al., 2009), while it is most potently activated by Kiss1–15 in sea bass (Tena-Sempere et al., 2012). The single-ligand test using Kiss1–10 in zebrafish found that the cAMP/PKA pathway could be activated through Kiss-R1 (but not Kiss-R2) activation (Biran et al., 2008). In the orange spotted grouper, where the Kiss-R2 was solely studied, there was no observable PKA signaling pathway (Shi et al., 2010), which is consistent with previous piscine observations that Kiss-R2s have compromised signaling through this pathway. In some species, GPR54 duplicates have exhibited differentiation in signaling. However, further analysis of fish species is required to specify defined signaling patterns (Tena-Sempere et al., 2012).

INDEPENDENT FUNCTION OF TWO KISSPEPTIN-KISS-R SYSTEMS

In several teleost species, the onset of puberty marks a significant increase in Kiss-R mRNA expression (Biran et al., 2008; Filby et al., 2008; Martinez-Chavez et al., 2008). GPR54 is only induced in the mullet brain during the pubertal stages, leading to speculation that it also plays a role in reproductive development (Nocillado et al., 2007). In the brain of the fathead minnow, the highest expression of Kiss-R1 mRNA coincides with higher levels of GnRH gene expression in sexually mature females compared to prepubertal females (Filby et al., 2008). Although kisspeptin is considered to be a potent regulator of reproductive function, the specific function of two kisspeptin-Kiss-R systems has not been well understood due to poor ligand selectivity of two Kiss-R types for Kiss1 and Kiss2 peptides (Um et al., 2010). Physiological studies in some teleosts have suggested that Kiss2 exhibits higher potency in reproductive regulation compared to Kiss1 (Felip et al., 2009; Kitahashi et al., 2009; Li et al., 2009; Akazome et al., 2010; Shahjahan et al., 2010). Conversely, in the medaka, Kiss1 but not Kiss2 neurons in the hypothalamus exhibit estrogen sensitivity (Mitani et al., 2010), which suggests that Kiss1 but not Kiss2 plays a role in central reproductive regulation in the medaka (Oka, 2009). In the *Morone* species, Kiss1 is more potent in inducing LH release, with Kiss2 downregulating GnRH1 and Kiss-R2 gene expression during recrudescence (Zmora et al., 2012). These highly diverse observations suggest that the kisspeptin-Kiss-R pathway plays important roles in piscine reproduction; however, given the diversity of reproduction strategies, environmental niches and the timing of sexual maturation, and inconsistency in experimental approaches, it is difficult to establish a unifying theme (Oakley et al., 2009).

A recent study in zebrafish has managed to demonstrate an independent function of two kisspeptin-Kiss-R systems (Ogawa et al., 2012a). In zebrafish, Kiss1 neurons are solely present in the habenula, whereas Kiss2 neurons are only expressed in the preoptic-hypothalamic nuclei (Kitahashi et al., 2009; Servili et al.,

2011). Similarly in zebrafish, Kiss-R1 mRNA expression occurs mainly in the habenula, whereas Kiss-R2 mRNA expression occurs widely around the brain (Kitahashi et al., 2009; Servili et al., 2011). This anatomical correspondence between kisspeptin and Kiss-R types clearly indicates that their ligand-receptor pairs functionally represent the key-keyhole interaction in zebrafish. Therefore, zebrafish is an attractive model system to study independent functions of two kisspeptin-Kiss-R systems in vertebrates. We have recently revealed that the Kiss1 neurons in the habenula that project into the interpeduncular nucleus (IPN) could modulate the serotonergic system through an autocrine mechanism (Ogawa et al., 2012a). However, the precise mechanism that underlies this finding and its role in serotonin regulation remains unknown.

EVOLUTIONARY SIGNIFICANCE OF THE KISSPEPTIN-KISS-R SYSTEM

The fishes provide excellent animal models to study the principles that underlie the vertebrate kisspeptin and Kiss-R systems from an evolutionary viewpoint (Akazome et al., 2010). The conserved genomic organization and gene synteny of the *kiss* and *kiss-r* genes indicates that they originated from a common ancestral gene (Akazome et al., 2010; Um et al., 2010). The vertebrate lineage exhibits this conserved genome organization, spanning mammalian, and non-mammalian species (Tena-Sempere et al., 2012). Our genome synteny analysis found four predicted Kiss-R homologous types in the Coelacanth genome (Kiss-R1a, Kiss-R1b, Kiss-R2a, and Kiss-R2b) (**Table 2**). Genes surrounding Coelacanth Kiss-R1a gene are also found in the genomic region of *Xenopus* GPR54-1a and mammalian Kiss-R genes but absent in fish Kiss-R types. Coelacanth Kiss-R1b is close to fish Kiss1Rb and *Xenopus* GPR54-1b. Neighboring genes of Coelacanth Kiss-R2a were found in a region surrounding *Xenopus* GPR54-2 and fish Kiss1Ra but were absent in the human Kiss-R. Coelacanth Kiss-R2b is close to Platypus GPR54b and Green anole (*Anolis carolinensis*) GPR54-like sequence. Based on the phylogenetic analysis, it can be hypothesized that the two ancestral Kiss-R lineages (Kiss-R1 and Kiss-R2) were first duplicated into four Kiss-R lineages during chromosome duplication in ancestral fish (**Figure 3**). Among the four lineages, Kiss-R1a and Kiss-R2b lineages have been lost in bony fish, Kiss-R2b lineage could have been lost in amphibian but may exist in reptile and platypus, and only Kiss-R1a lineage is preserved in human. However, in the Coelacanth genome, all four Kiss-R lineages are still conserved. These results correspond with the concept of molecular evolutional history of vertebrate Kiss-R genes that has been previously proposed (Lee et al., 2009; Zohar et al., 2010).

The alternating actions and importance of both Kiss1 and Kiss2 were very recently demonstrated in the *Morone* species (Zmora et al., 2012). They concluded that the organization of the kisspeptin system suggests a transitional evolutionary state between early to late evolving vertebrates. The evolutionary transition between multiple forms of kisspeptin, present in evolutionarily older vertebrates such as frogs and some fish, to a single form, as evident in higher vertebrates, is exemplified in the kisspeptin systems of the various fish species studied thus far (Um et al., 2010; Zmora et al., 2012). In the Coelacanth genome, only one kisspeptin-homologous sequence (ENSLACP00000010201, FNFNPFGLRF) was identified, which is close to fish Kiss2. Genes surrounding the Coelacanth Kiss1 (LDHB, GYS2, SLC25A3, STRAP, and GOLT1B) were found in the Stickleback Kiss2, *Xenopus* Kiss2, and Zebrafish Kiss2, but not in the human Kiss1. Therefore, in the Coelacanth, Kiss1 lineage could have been lost, although genes rounding the human Kiss1 such as REN, ETNK2, and SNRPE are still conserved in the Coelacanth genome. The complete disappearance of Kiss1 and its functional relocation in different fish species clearly shows its evolutionary transition (Zmora et al., 2012). However, the physiological significance of two or loss of one Kiss system in fish species still remains unknown. The evolution of kisspeptin-Kiss-R system may be closely related to the evolution of reproductive traits. It is hence crucial to examine kisspeptin-Kiss-R system in fish species with one-Kiss and those with two-Kiss systems from the viewpoint of diversity of reproductive physiology, i.e., single- or multiple-spawner, seasonal breeder, social or non-social species, viviparous or non-viviparous fish, lifespan, and sex changing fish.

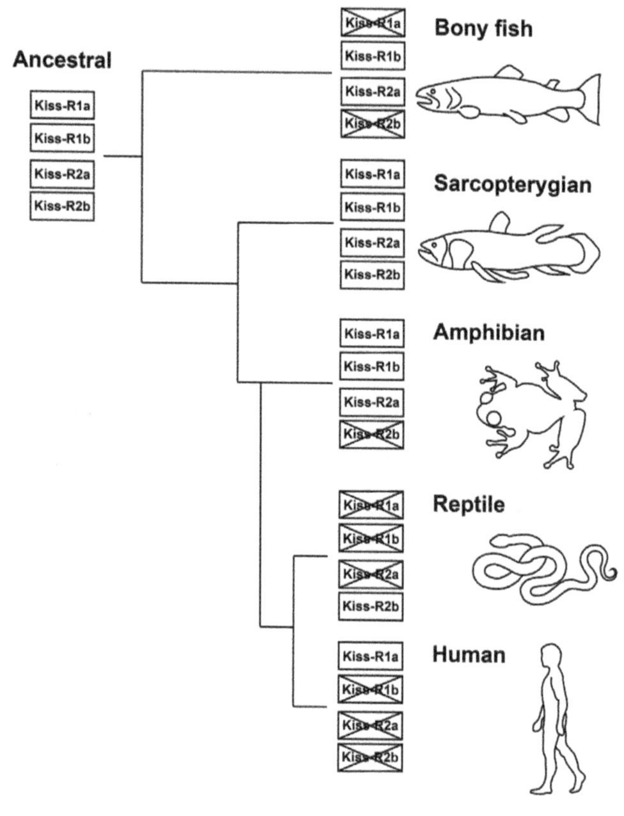

FIGURE 3 | Proposed molecular evolutionary history of the Kiss-R genes. Four Kiss-R types originated from two common ancestral Kiss-R genes (Kiss-R1 and Kiss-R2), diversified through gene or chromosome duplication and gene modification and deletion. Four Kiss-R types are still conserved in the Coelacanth genome.

CONCLUDING REMARKS

The hypothalamic GnRH system has been well studied, and the specific functional roles of the various receptor-ligand pairs have been delineated for both mammalian and non-mammalian vertebrates. However, research on the kisspeptin/GnRH relationship in non-mammalian vertebrates, including fish, is still in its infancy. Studies have so far shown in fish that kisspeptins directly regulate GnRH neurons and GnRH release via interactions with Kiss-Rs. However, there are numerous unknown or unconfirmed (confirmed in mammals but not in fish) matters regarding the GPCRs in fish reproduction. Understanding the precise mechanism of endocrine regulation of fish reproduction based on GPCRs is necessary to determine the precise physiological roles of kisspeptin-GnRH pathways.

ACKNOWLEDGMENTS

We thank Dr. Takashi Kitahashi for his contractive comments. This work was supported by grants from Malaysian Ministry of Higher Education, FRGS/2/2010/ST/MUSM/03/2 (to Satoshi Ogawa and Ishwar S. Parhar), Malaysian Ministry of Science, Technology, and Innovation, 02-02-10-SF0044 (to Ishwar S. Parhar and Satoshi Ogawa), and Monash University Sunway Campus, M-2-2-06 and M-2-07 (to Satoshi Ogawa), MM-2-5-06 and MM-7-07 (to Ishwar S. Parhar) and Neuroscience Research Strength grant (to Ishwar S. Parhar).

REFERENCES

Akazome, Y., Kanda, S., Okubo, K., and Oka, Y. (2010). Functional and evolutionary insights into vertebrate kisspeptin systems from studies of fish brain. *J. Fish Biol.* 76, 161–182.

Alok, D., Hassin, S., Sampath, K. R., Trant, J. M., Yu, K., and Zohar, Y. (2000). Characterization of a pituitary GnRH-receptor from a perciform fish, *Morone saxatilis*: functional expression in a fish cell line. *Mol. Cell. Endocrinol.* 168, 65–75.

Ando, H., Hew, C. L., and Urano, A. (2001). Signal transduction pathways and transcription factors involved in the gonadotropin-releasing hormone-stimulated gonadotropin subunit gene expression. *Comp. Biochem. Physiol. B Biochem. Mol. Biol.* 129, 525–532.

Ankley, G. T., and Johnson, R. D. (2004). Small fish models for identifying and assessing the effects of endocrine-disrupting chemicals. *ILAR J.* 45, 469–483.

Attwood, T. K. (2001). A compendium of specific motifs for diagnosing GPCR subtypes. *Trends Pharmacol. Sci.* 22, 162–165.

Batten, T. F. C., and Ingleton, P. M. (1987). "The structure and function of the hypothalamus and pituitary gland," in *Fundamentals of Comparative Vertebrate Endocrinology*, eds I. Chester-Jones, P. M. Ingleton, and J. G. Phillips (New York: Plenum Press), 285–409.

Biran, J., Ben-Dor, S., and Levavi-Sivan, B. (2008). Molecular identification and functional characterization of the kisspeptin/kisspeptin receptor system in lower vertebrates. *Biol. Reprod.* 79, 776–786.

Biran, J., Palevitch, O., Ben-Dor, S., and Levavi-Sivan, B. (2012). Neurokinin Bs and neurokinin B receptors in zebrafish-potential role in controlling fish reproduction. *Proc. Natl. Acad. Sci. U.S.A.* 109, 10269–10274.

Bjarnadottir, T. K., Schioth, H. B., and Fredriksson, R. (2005). The phylogenetic relationship of the glutamate and pheromone G-protein-coupled receptors in different vertebrate species. *Ann. N. Y. Acad. Sci.* 1040, 230–233.

Chandroo, K. P., Duncan, I. J. H., and Moccia, R. D. (2004). Can fish suffer? Perspectives on sentience, pain, fear and stress. *Appl. Anim. Behav. Sci.* 86, 225–250.

Chen, C. C., and Fernald, R. D. (2006). Distributions of two gonadotropin-releasing hormone receptor types in a cichlid fish suggest functional specialization. *J. Comp. Neurol.* 495, 314–323.

Chen, C. C., and Fernald, R. D. (2008). GnRH and GnRH receptors: distribution, function and evolution. *J. Fish Biol.* 73, 1099–1120.

Cheung, T. C., and Hearn, J. P. (2002). Molecular cloning and tissue expression of the gonadotropin-releasing hormone receptor in the tammar wallaby (*Macropus eugenii*). *Reprod. Fertil. Dev.* 14, 157–164.

Clarkson, J., and Herbison, A. E. (2006). Postnatal development of kisspeptin neurons in mouse hypothalamus; sexual dimorphism and projections to gonadotropin-releasing hormone neurons. *Endocrinology* 147, 5817–5825.

Corodimas, K. P., Rosenblatt, J. S., and Morrell, J. I. (1992). The habenular complex mediates hormonal stimulation of maternal behavior in rats. *Behav. Neurosci.* 106, 853–865.

d'Anglemont de Tassigny, X., and Colledge, W. H. (2010). The role of kisspeptin signaling in reproduction. *Physiology (Bethesda)* 25, 207–217.

de Roux, N., Genin, E., Carel, J. C., Matsuda, F., Chaussain, J. L., and Milgrom, E. (2003). Hypogonadotropic hypogonadism due to loss of function of the KiSS1-derived peptide receptor GPR54. *Proc. Natl. Acad. Sci. U.S.A.* 100, 10972–10976.

Dungan, H. M., Clifton, D. K., and Steiner, R. A. (2006). Minireview: kisspeptin neurons as central processors in the regulation of gonadotropin-releasing hormone secretion. *Endocrinology* 147, 1154–1158.

Elizur, A. (2009). The KiSS1/GPR54 system in fish. *Peptides* 30, 164–170.

Felip, A., Zanuy, S., Pineda, R., Pinilla, L., Carrillo, M., Tena-Sempere, M., et al. (2009). Evidence for two distinct KiSS genes in non-placental vertebrates that encode kisspeptins with different gonadotropin-releasing activities in fish and mammals. *Mol. Cell. Endocrinol.* 312, 61–71.

Ferguson, S. S. (2001). Evolving concepts in G protein-coupled receptor endocytosis: the role in receptor desensitization and signaling. *Pharmacol. Rev.* 53, 1–24.

Filby, A. L., Aerle, R. V., Duitman, J., and Tyler, C. R. (2008). The kisspeptin/gonadotropin-releasing hormone pathway and molecular signaling of puberty in fish. *Biol. Reprod.* 78, 278–289.

Forfar, R., and Lu, Z.-L. (2011). Role of the transmembrane domain 4/extracellular loop 2 junction of the human gonadotropin-releasing hormone receptor in ligand binding and receptor conformational selection. *J. Biol. Chem.* 286, 34617–34626.

Gonzalez-Martinez, D., Madigou, T., Mananos, E., Cerda-Reverter, J. M., Zanuy, S., Kah, O., et al. (2004). Cloning and expression of gonadotropin-releasing hormone receptor in the brain and pituitary of the European sea bass: an in situ hybridization study. *Biol. Reprod.* 70, 1380–1391.

Grone, B. P., Carpenter, R. E., Lee, M., Maruska, K. P., and Fernald, R. D. (2012). Food deprivation explains effects of mouthbrooding on ovaries and steroid hormones, but not brain neuropeptide and receptor mRNAs, in an African cichlid fish. *Horm. Behav.* 62, 18–26.

Grone, B. P., Maruska, K. P., Korzan, W. J., and Fernald, R. D. (2010). Social status regulates kisspeptin receptor mRNA in the brain of *Astatotilapia burtoni*. *Gen. Comp. Endocrinol.* 169, 98–107.

Gur, G., Bonfil, D., Safarian, H., Naor, Z., and Yaron, Z. (2002). GnRH signaling pathways regulate differentially the tilapia gonadotropin subunit genes. *Mol. Cell. Endocrinol.* 189, 125–134.

Gutiérrez-Pascual, E., Martínez-Fuentes, A. J., Pinilla, L., Tena-Sempere, M., Malagón, M. M., and Castaño, J. P. (2007). Direct pituitary effects of kisspeptin: activation of gonadotrophs and somatotrophs and stimulation of luteinising hormone and growth hormone secretion. *J. Neuroendocrinol.* 19, 521–530.

Han, S. K., Gottsch, M. L., Lee, K. J., Popa, S. M., Smith, J. T., Jakawich, S. K., et al. (2005). Activation of gonadotropin-releasing hormone neurons by kisspeptin as a neuroendocrine switch for the onset of puberty. *J. Neurosci.* 25, 11349–11356.

Hanchate, N. K., Parkash, J., Bellefontaine, N., Mazur, D., Colledge, W. H., d'Anglemont de Tassigny, X., et al. (2012). Kisspeptin-GPR54 signaling in mouse NO-synthesizing neurons participates in the hypothalamic control of ovulation. *J. Neurosci.* 32, 932–945.

Hapgood, J. P., Sadie, H., Van Biljon, W., and Ronacher, K. (2005). Regulation of expression of mammalian gonadotropin-releasing hormone receptor genes. *J. Neuroendocrinol.* 17, 619–638.

Heitman, L. H., and Ijzerman, A. P. (2008). G protein-coupled receptors of the hypothalamic-pituitary-gonadal axis: a case for Gnrh, LH, FSH, and GPR54 receptor ligands. *Med. Res. Rev.* 28, 975–1011.

Herbison, A. E., d'Anglemont de Tassigny, X., Doran, J., and Colledge, W. H. (2010). Distribution and postnatal development of Gpr54 gene expression in mouse brain and gonadotropin-releasing hormone neurons. *Endocrinology* 151, 312–321.

Hildahl, J., Taranger, G. L., Norberg, B., Haug, T. M., and Weltzien, F.-A. (2013). Differential regulation of GnRH ligand and receptor genes in the brain and pituitary of Atlantic cod exposed to different photoperiod. *Gen. Comp. Endocrinol.* 180, 7–14.

Illing, N., Troskie, B. E., Nahorniak, C. S., Hapgood, J. P., Peter, R. E., and Millar, R. P. (1999). Two gonadotropin-releasing hormone receptor subtypes with distinct ligand selectivity and differential distribution in brain and pituitary in the goldfish (*Carassius auratus*). *Proc. Natl. Acad. Sci. U.S.A.* 96, 2526–2531.

Irwig, M. S., Fraley, G. S., Smith, J. T., Acohido, B. V., Popa, S. M., Cunningham, M. J., et al. (2004). Kisspeptin activation of gonadotropin releasing hormone neurons and regulation of KiSS-1 mRNA in the male rat. *Neuroendocrinology* 80, 264–272.

Jodo, A., Ando, H., and Urano, A. (2003). Five different types of putative GnRH receptor gene are expressed in the brain of masu salmon (*Oncorhynchus masou*). *Zool. Sci.* 20, 1117–1125.

Kadokawa, H., Matsui, M., Hayashi, K., Matsunaga, N., Kawashima, C., Shimizu, T., et al. (2008a). Peripheral administration of kisspeptin-10 increases plasma concentrations of GH as well as LH in prepubertal Holstein heifers. *J. Endocrinol.* 196, 331–334.

Kadokawa, H., Suzuki, S., and Hashizume, T. (2008b). Kisspeptin-10 stimulates the secretion of growth hormone and prolactin directly from cultured bovine anterior pituitary cells. *Anim. Reprod. Sci.* 105, 404–408.

Kah, O., Breton, B., and Dulka, J. G. (1986). A reinvestigation of the Gn-RH (gonadotropin-releasing hormone) systems in the goldfish brain using antibodies to salmon Gn-RH. *Cell Tissue Res.* 244, 327–337.

Kaiser, U. B., and Kuohung, W. (2005). KiSS-1 and GPR54 as new players in gonadotropin regulation and puberty. *Endocrine* 26, 277–284.

Kanda, S., Akazome, Y., Matsunaga, T., Yamamoto, N., Yamada, S., Tsukamura, H., et al. (2008). Identification of KiSS-1 product kisspeptin and steroid-sensitive sexually dimorphic kisspeptin neurons in medaka (*Oryzias latipes*). *Endocrinology* 149, 2467–2476.

Karges, B., Karges, W., and De Roux, N. (2003). Clinical and molecular genetics of the human GnRH receptor. *Hum. Reprod. Update* 9, 523–530.

Khalil, M. H., Silverman, A.-J., and Silver, R. (2003). Mast cells in the rat brain synthesize gonadotropin-releasing hormone. *J. Neurobiol.* 56, 113–124.

Kim, D.-K., Cho, E. B., Moon, M. J., Park, S., Hwang, J.-I., Kah, O., et al. (2011). Revisiting the evolution of gonadotropin-releasing hormones and their receptors in vertebrates: secrets hidden in genomes. *Gen. Comp. Endocrinol.* 170, 68–78.

Kitahashi, T., Ogawa, S., and Parhar, I. S. (2009). Cloning and expression of kiss2 in the zebrafish and medaka. *Endocrinology* 150, 821–831.

Klemm, W. R. (2004). Habenular and interpeduncularis nuclei: shared components in multiple-function networks. *Med. Sci. Monit.* 10, RA261–RA273.

Kochman, K. (2012). Evolution of gonadotropin-releasing hormone (GnRH) structure and its receptor. *J. Anim. Feed Sci.* 21, 3–30.

Kotani, M., Detheux, M., Vandenbogaerde, A., Communi, D., Vanderwinden, J. M., Le Poul, E., et al. (2001). The metastasis suppressor gene KiSS-1 encodes kisspeptins, the natural ligands of the orphan G protein-coupled receptor GPR54. *J. Biol. Chem.* 276, 34631–34636.

Krsmanovic, L. Z., Mores, N., Navarro, C. E., Arora, K. K., and Catt, K. J. (2003). An agonist-induced switch in G protein coupling of the gonadotropin-releasing hormone receptor regulates pulsatile neuropeptide secretion. *Proc. Natl. Acad. Sci. U.S.A.* 100, 2969–2974.

Lee, D. K., Nguyen, T., O'Neill, G. P., Cheng, R., Liu, Y., Howard, A. D., et al. (1999). Discovery of a receptor related to the galanin receptors. *FEBS Lett.* 446, 103–107.

Lee, Y. R., Tsunekawa, K., Moon, M. J., Um, H. N., Hwang, J. I., Osugi, T., et al. (2009). Molecular evolution of multiple forms of kisspeptins and GPR54 receptors in vertebrates. *Endocrinology* 150, 2837–2846.

Lethimonier, C., Madigou, T., Munoz-Cueto, J. A., Lareyre, J. J., and Kah, O. (2004). Evolutionary aspects of GnRHs, GnRH neuronal systems and GnRH receptors in teleost fish. *Gen. Comp. Endocrinol.* 135, 1–16.

Levavi-Sivan, B., and Avitan, A. (2005). Sequence analysis, endocrine regulation, and signal transduction of GnRH receptors in teleost fish. *Gen. Comp. Endocrinol.* 142, 67–73.

Levavi-Sivan, B., Safarian, H., Rosenfeld, H., Elizur, A., and Avitan, A. (2004). Regulation of gonadotropin-releasing hormone (GnRH)-receptor gene expression in tilapia: effect of GnRH and dopamine. *Biol. Reprod.* 70, 1545–1551.

Li, S., Zhang, Y., Liu, Y., Huang, X., Huang, W., Lu, D., et al. (2009). Structural and functional multiplicity of the kisspeptin/GPR54 system in goldfish (*Carassius auratus*). *J. Endocrinol.* 201, 407–418.

Liu, F., Usui, I., Evans, L. G., Austin, D. A., Mellon, P. L., Olefsky, J. M., et al. (2002). Involvement of both Gq/11 and Gs proteins in gonadotropin-releasing hormone receptor-mediated signaling in LβT2 Cells. *J. Biol. Chem.* 277, 32099–32108.

Madigou, T., Mananos-Sanchez, E., Hulshof, S., Anglade, I., Zanuy, S., and Kah, O. (2000). Cloning, tissue distribution, and central expression of the gonadotropin-releasing hormone receptor in the rainbow trout (*Oncorhynchus mykiss*). *Biol. Reprod.* 63, 1857–1866.

Marinissen, M. J., and Gutkind, J. S. (2001). G-protein-coupled receptors and signaling networks: emerging paradigms. *Trends Pharmacol. Sci.* 22, 368–376.

Martinez-Chavez, C. C., Minghetti, M., and Migaud, H. (2008). GPR54 and rGnRH I gene expression during the onset of puberty in Nile tilapia. *Gen. Comp. Endocrinol.* 156, 224–233.

Matthews-Felton, T., Corodimas, K. P., Rosenblatt, J. S., and Morrell, J. I. (1995). Lateral habenula neurons are necessary for the hormonal onset of maternal behavior and for the display of postpartum estrus in naturally parturient female rats. *Behav. Neurosci.* 109, 1172–1188.

McArdle, C. A., Franklin, J., Green, L., and Hislop, J. N. (2002). Signalling, cycling and desensitisation of gonadotropin-releasing hormone receptors. *J. Endocrinol.* 173, 1–11.

Mechaly, A. S., Vinas, J., Murphy, C., Reith, M., and Piferrer, F. (2010). Gene structure of the Kiss1 receptor-2 (Kiss1r-2) in the Atlantic halibut: insights into the evolution and regulation of Kiss1r genes. *Mol. Cell. Endocrinol.* 317, 78–89.

Mechaly, A. S., Vinas, J., and Piferrer, F. (2009). Identification of two isoforms of the kisspeptin-1 receptor (kiss1r) generated by alternative splicing in a modern teleost, the Senegalese sole (*Solea senegalensis*). *Biol. Reprod.* 80, 60–69.

Mechaly, A. S., Vinas, J., and Piferrer, F. (2011). Gene structure analysis of kisspeptin-2 (Kiss2) in the Senegalese sole (*Solea senegalensis*): characterization of two splice variants of Kiss2, and novel evidence for metabolic regulation of kisspeptin signaling in non-mammalian species. *Mol. Cell. Endocrinol.* 339, 14–24.

Messager, S., Chatzidaki, E. E., Ma, D., Hendrick, A. G., Zahn, D., Dixon, J., et al. (2005). Kisspeptin directly stimulates gonadotropin-releasing hormone release via G protein-coupled receptor 54. *Proc. Natl. Acad. Sci. U.S.A.* 102, 1761–1766.

Metpally, R. P., and Sowdhamini, R. (2005). Genome wide survey of G protein-coupled receptors in *Tetraodon nigroviridis*. *BMC Evol. Biol.* 5:41. doi:10.1186/1471-2148-5-41

Millar, R. P. (2003). GnRH II and type II GnRH receptors. *Trends Endocrinol. Metab.* 14, 35–43.

Millar, R. P., Lu, Z. L., Pawson, A. J., Flanagan, C. A., Morgan, K., and Maudsley, S. R. (2004). Gonadotropin-releasing hormone receptors. *Endocr. Rev.* 25, 235–275.

Millar, R. P., and Newton, C. L. (2010). The year in G protein-coupled receptor research. *Mol. Endocrinol.* 24, 261–274.

Mitani, Y., Kanda, S., Akazome, Y., Zempo, B., and Oka, Y. (2010). Hypothalamic Kiss1 but not Kiss2 neurons are involved in estrogen feedback in medaka (*Oryzias latipes*). *Endocrinology* 151, 1751–1759.

Miyamoto, K., Hasegawa, Y., Nomura, M., Igarashi, M., Kangawa, K., and Matsuo, H. (1984). Identification of the second gonadotropin-releasing hormone in chicken hypothalamus: evidence that gonadotropin secretion is probably controlled by two distinct gonadotropin-releasing hormones in avian species. *Proc. Natl. Acad. Sci. U.S.A.* 81, 3874–3878.

Modianos, D. T., Hitt, J. C., and Flexman, J. (1974). Habenular lesions produce decrements in feminine, but not masculine, sexual behavior in rats. *Behav. Biol.* 10, 75–87.

Mohamed, J. S., Benninghoff, A. D., Holt, G. J., and Khan, I. A. (2007). Developmental expression of the G protein-coupled receptor 54 and three GnRH mRNAs in the teleost fish cobia. *J. Mol. Endocrinol.* 38, 235–244.

Mollusk, A., Nematode, A. A., Echinoderm, G., Hemichordate, G., Mollusk, G., Arthropod, A. C. R., et al. (2011). "GnRHR superfamily: vertebrates and invertebrates," in *Handbook of Neuroendocrinology*, eds G. Fink, D. W. Pfaff, and J. Levine (Amsterdam/Boston: Elsevier/Academic Press), 81.

Moncaut, N., Somoza, G., Power, D. M., and Canario, A. V. (2005). Five gonadotropin-releasing hormone receptors in a teleost fish: isolation, tissue distribution and phylogenetic relationships. *J. Mol. Endocrinol.* 34, 767–779.

Mousa, S. A., and Mousa, M. A. (2006). Involvement of corticotropin-releasing factor and adrenocorticotropic hormone in the ovarian maturation, seawater acclimation, and induced spawning of *Liza ramada*. *Gen. Comp. Endocrinol.* 146, 167–179.

Neckers, L. M., Schwartz, J., Wyatt, R. J., and Speciale, S. G. (1979). Substance P afferents from the habenula innervate the dorsal raphe nucleus. *Exp. Brain Res.* 37, 619–623.

Neill, J. D. (2002). Minireview: GnRH and GnRH receptor genes in the human genome. *Endocrinology* 143, 737–743.

Nocillado, J. N., Biran, J., Lee, Y. Y., Levavi-Sivan, B., Mechaly, A. S., Zohar, Y., et al. (2012). The Kiss2 receptor (Kiss2r) gene in Southern Bluefin Tuna, *Thunnus maccoyii* and in Yellowtail Kingfish, *Seriola lalandi* – functional analysis and isolation of transcript variants. *Mol. Cell. Endocrinol.* 362, 211–220.

Nocillado, J. N., Levavi-Sivan, B., Carrick, F., and Elizur, A. (2007). Temporal expression of G-protein-coupled receptor 54 (GPR54), gonadotropin-releasing hormones (GnRH), and dopamine receptor D2 (drd2) in pubertal female grey mullet, *Mugil cephalus*. *Gen. Comp. Endocrinol.* 150, 278–287.

Oakley, A. E., Clifton, D. K., and Steiner, R. A. (2009). Kisspeptin signaling in the brain. *Endocr. Rev.* 30, 713–743.

Ogawa, S., Kitahashi, T., Ng, K. W., and Parhar, I. S. (2010). "Autocrine regulation of kiss1 in the habenula of the zebrafish," in *Proceedings of the 7th International Congress of Neuroendocrinology*, abstr., Rouen, P2–P20.

Ogawa, S., Ng, K. W., Ramadasan, P. N., Nathan, F. M., and Parhar, I. S. (2012a). Habenular Kiss1 neurons modulate the serotonergic system in the brain of zebrafish. *Endocrinology* 153, 2398–2407.

Ogawa, S., Ramadasan, P. N., Goschorska, M., Anantharajah, A., We Ng, K., and Parhar, I. S. (2012b). Cloning and expression of tachykinins and their association with kisspeptins in the brains of zebrafish. *J. Comp. Neurol.* 520, 2991–3012.

Ogawa, S., and Parhar, I. S. (2013). Anatomy of the kisspeptin systems in teleosts. *Gen. Comp. Endocrinol.* 181, 169–174.

Oka, Y. (2009). Three types of gonadotropin-releasing hormone neurones and steroid-sensitive sexually dimorphic kisspeptin neurones in teleosts. *J. Neuroendocrinol.* 21, 334–338.

Okubo, K., Ishii, S., Ishida, J., Mitani, H., Naruse, K., Kondo, M., et al. (2003). A novel third gonadotropin-releasing hormone receptor in the medaka *Oryzias latipes*: evolutionary and functional implications. *Gene* 314, 121–131.

Okubo, K., and Nagahama, Y. (2008). Structural and functional evolution of gonadotropin-releasing hormone in vertebrates. *Acta Physiol. (Oxf.)* 193, 3–15.

Okubo, K., Nagata, S., Ko, R., Kataoka, H., Yoshiura, Y., Mitani, H., et al. (2001). Identification and characterization of two distinct GnRH receptor subtypes in a teleost, the medaka *Oryzias latipes*. *Endocrinology* 142, 4729–4739.

Okubo, K., Suetake, H., Usami, T., and Aida, K. (2000). Molecular cloning and tissue-specific expression of a gonadotrophin-releasing hormone receptor in the Japanese eel. *Gen. Comp. Endocrinol.* 119, 181–192.

Parhar, I. S. (2002). Cell migration and evolutionary significance of GnRH subtypes. *Prog. Brain Res.* 141, 3–17.

Parhar, I. S., Ogawa, S., and Sakuma, Y. (2004). Laser-captured single digoxigenin-labeled neurons of gonadotropin-releasing hormone types reveal a novel G protein-coupled receptor (Gpr54) during maturation in cichlid fish. *Endocrinology* 145, 3613–3618.

Parhar, I. S., Ogawa, S., and Sakuma, Y. (2005a). Three GnRH receptor types in laser-captured single cells of the cichlid pituitary display cellular and functional heterogeneity. *Proc. Natl. Acad. Sci. U.S.A.* 102, 2204–2209.

Parhar, I. S., Soga, T., Ogawa, S., Ogawa, S., Pfaff, D. W., and Sakuma, Y. (2005b). Nonmammalian gonadotropin-releasing hormone molecules in the brain of promoter transgenic rats. *Proc. Natl. Acad. Sci. U.S.A.* 102, 5880–5885.

Parhar, I. S., Soga, T., Sakuma, Y., and Millar, R. P. (2002). Spatio-temporal expression of gonadotropin-releasing hormone receptor subtypes in gonadotropes, somatotropes and lactotropes in the cichlid fish. *J. Neuroendocrinol.* 14, 657–665.

Pasquier, J., Lafont, A. G., Leprince, J., Vaudry, H., Rousseau, K., and Dufour, S. (2011). First evidence for a direct inhibitory effect of kisspeptins on LH expression in the eel, *Anguilla anguilla*. *Gen. Comp. Endocrinol.* 173, 216–225.

Qin, F., Wang, L., Wang, X., Liu, S., Xu, P., Wang, H., et al. (2013). Bisphenol A affects gene expression of gonadotropin-releasing hormones and type I GnRH receptors in brains of adult rare minnow *Gobiocypris rarus*. *Comp. Biochem. Physiol. C Toxicol. Pharmacol.* 157, 192–202.

Ramaswamy, S., Guerriero, K. A., Gibbs, R. B., and Plant, T. M. (2008). Structural interactions between kisspeptin and GnRH neurons in the mediobasal hypothalamus of the male rhesus monkey (*Macaca mulatta*) as revealed by double immunofluorescence and confocal microscopy. *Endocrinology* 149, 4387–4395.

Robison, R. R., White, R. B., Illing, N., Troskie, B. E., Morley, M., Millar, R. P., et al. (2001). Gonadotropin-releasing hormone receptor in the teleost *Haplochromis burtoni*: structure, location, and function. *Endocrinology* 142, 1737–1743.

Roch, G. J., Busby, E. R., and Sherwood, N. M. (2011). Evolution of GnRH: diving deeper. *Gen. Comp. Endocrinol.* 171, 1–16.

Rønnekleiv, O. K., Bosch, M. A., and Zhang, C. (2010). Regulation of endogenous conductances in GnRH neurons by estrogens. *Brain Res.* 1364, 25–34.

Sealfon, S. C., Weinstein, H., and Millar, R. P. (1997). Molecular mechanisms of ligand interaction with the gonadotropin-releasing hormone receptor. *Endocr. Rev.* 18, 180–205.

Selvaraj, S., Kitano, H., Fujinaga, Y., Ohga, H., Yoneda, M., Yamaguchi, A., et al. (2010). Molecular characterization, tissue distribution, and mRNA expression profiles of two Kiss genes in the adult male and female chub mackerel (*Scomber japonicus*) during different gonadal stages. *Gen. Comp. Endocrinol.* 169, 28–38.

Seminara, S. B., Messager, S., Chatzidaki, E. E., Thresher, R. R., Acierno, J. S. Jr., Shagoury, J. K., et al. (2003). The GPR54 gene as a regulator of puberty. *N. Engl. J. Med.* 349, 1614–1627.

Servili, A., Le Page, Y., Leprince, J., Caraty, A., Escobar, S., Parhar, I. S., et al. (2011). Organization of two independent kisspeptin systems derived from evolutionary-ancient kiss genes in the brain of zebrafish. *Endocrinology* 152, 1527–1540.

Shahjahan, M., Motohashi, E., Doi, H., and Ando, H. (2010). Elevation of Kiss2 and its receptor gene expression in the brain and pituitary of grass puffer during the spawning season. *Gen. Comp. Endocrinol.* 169, 48–57.

Sherwood, N. (1987). The GnRH family of peptides. *Trends Neurosci.* 10, 129–132.

Sherwood, N. M., Lovejoy, D. A., and Coe, I. R. (1993). Origin of mammalian gonadotropin-releasing hormones. *Endocr. Rev.* 14, 241–254.

Shi, Y., Zhang, Y., Li, S., Liu, Q., Lu, D., Liu, M., et al. (2010). Molecular identification of the Kiss2/Kiss1ra system and its potential function during 17alpha-methyltestosterone-induced sex reversal in the orange-spotted grouper, *Epinephelus coioides*. *Biol. Reprod.* 83, 63–74.

Shoichet, B. K., and Kobilka, B. K. (2012). Structure-based drug screening for G-protein-coupled receptors. *Trends Pharmacol. Sci.* 33, 268–272.

Smith, Y., Parent, A., Kerkérian, L., and Pelletier, G. (1985). Distribution of neuropeptide Y immunoreactivity in the basal forebrain and upper brainstem of the squirrel monkey (*Saimiri sciureus*). *J. Comp. Neurol.* 236, 71–89.

Soga, T., Ogawa, S., Millar, R. P., Sakuma, Y., and Parhar, I. S. (2005). Localization of the three GnRH types and GnRH receptors in the brain of a cichlid fish: insights into their neuroendocrine and neuromodulator functions. *J. Comp. Neurol.* 487, 28–41.

Teitelbaum, P., and Epstein, A. N. (1962). The lateral hypothalamic syndrome: recovery of feeding and drinking after lateral hypothalamic lesions. *Psychol. Rev.* 69, 74–90.

Tena-Sempere, M., Felip, A., Gomez, A., Zanuy, S., and Carrillo, M. (2012). Comparative insights of the kisspeptin/kisspeptin receptor system: lessons from non-mammalian vertebrates. *Gen. Comp. Endocrinol.* 175, 234–243.

Tensen, C., Okuzawa, K., Blomenrohr, M., Rebers, F., Leurs, R., Bogerd, J., et al. (1997). Distinct efficacies for two endogenous ligands on a single cognate gonadoliberin receptor. *Eur. J. Biochem.* 243, 134–140.

Tostivint, H. (2011). Evolution of the gonadotropin-releasing hormone (GnRH) gene family in relation to vertebrate tetraploidizations. *Gen. Comp. Endocrinol.* 170, 575–581.

Troskie, B., Illing, N., Rumbak, E., Sun, Y. M., Hapgood, J., Sealfon, S., et al. (1998). Identification of three putative GnRH receptor subtypes in vertebrates. *Gen. Comp. Endocrinol.* 112, 296–302.

Tsai, P. S. (2006). Gonadotropin-releasing hormone in invertebrates: structure, function, and evolution. *Gen. Comp. Endocrinol.* 148, 48–53.

Tsutsumi, M., Zhou, W., Millar, R. P., Mellon, P. L., Roberts, J. L., Flanagan, C. A., et al. (1992). Cloning and functional expression of a mouse gonadotropin-releasing hormone receptor. *Mol. Endocrinol.* 6, 1163–1169.

Um, H. N., Han, J. M., Hwang, J. I., Hong, S. I., Vaudry, H., and Seong, J. Y. (2010). Molecular coevolution of kisspeptins and their receptors from fish to mammals. *Ann. N. Y. Acad. Sci.* 1200, 67–74.

van Aerle, R., Kille, P., Lange, A., and Tyler, C. R. (2008). Evidence for the existence of a functional Kiss1/Kiss1 receptor pathway in fish. *Peptides* 29, 57–64.

Villani, L., Guarnieri, T., Salsi, U., and Bollini, D. (1991). Substance P in the habenulo-interpeduncular system of the goldfish. *Brain Res. Bull.* 26, 225–228.

Volkoff, H., Canosa, L. F., Unniappan, S., Cerda-Reverter, J. M., Bernier, N. J., Kelly, S. P., et al. (2005). Neuropeptides and the control of food intake in fish. *Gen. Comp. Endocrinol.* 142, 3–19.

Volkoff, H., and Peter, R. E. (1999). Actions of two forms of gonadotropin releasing hormone and a GnRH antagonist on spawning behavior of the goldfish *Carassius auratus. Gen. Comp. Endocrinol.* 116, 347–355.

Weltzien, F. A., Andersson, E., Andersen, O., Shalchian-Tabrizi, K., and Norberg, B. (2004). The brain-pituitary-gonad axis in male teleosts, with special emphasis on flatfish (Pleuronectiformes). *Comp. Biochem. Physiol. A Mol Integr. Physiol.* 137, 447–477.

White, R. B., and Fernald, R. D. (1998). Genomic structure and expression sites of three gonadotropin-releasing hormone genes in one species. *Gen. Comp. Endocrinol.* 112, 17–25.

Yang, B., Jiang, Q., Chan, T., Ko, W. K., and Wong, A. O. (2010). Goldfish kisspeptin: molecular cloning, tissue distribution of transcript expression, and stimulatory effects on prolactin, growth hormone and luteinizing hormone secretion and gene expression via direct actions at the pituitary level. *Gen. Comp. Endocrinol.* 165, 60–71.

Yaron, Z., Gur, G., Melamed, P., Rosenfeld, H., Elizur, A., and Levavi-Sivan, B. (2003). Regulation of fish gonadotropins. *Int. Rev. Cytol.* 225, 131–185.

Zhao, H., and Rusak, B. (2005). Circadian firing-rate rhythms and light responses of rat habenular nucleus neurons in vivo and in vitro. *Neuroscience* 132, 519–528.

Zmora, N., Stubblefield, J., Zulperi, Z., Biran, J., Levavi-Sivan, B., Muñoz-Cueto, J.-A., et al. (2012). Differential and gonad stage-dependent roles of kisspeptin1 and kisspeptin2 in reproduction in the modern teleosts, morone species. *Biol. Reprod.* 86, 177.

Zohar, Y., Munoz-Cueto, J. A., Elizur, A., and Kah, O. (2010). Neuroendocrinology of reproduction in teleost fish. *Gen. Comp. Endocrinol.* 165, 438–455.

16

Peripheral injections of melanin-concentrating hormone receptor 1 antagonist S38151 decrease food intake and body weight in rodent obesity models

Odile Della-Zuana*[1]*, Valérie Audinot*[2]*, Viviane Levenez*[1]*, Alain Ktorza*[1]*, Françoise Presse*[3,4]*, Jean-Louis Nahon*[3,4] *and Jean A. Boutin*[2]**

[1] *Maladies Métaboliques, Institut de Recherches SERVIER, Suresnes, France*
[2] *Biotechnologie, Pharmacologie Moléculaire et Cellulaire, Institut de Recherches SERVIER, Croissy-sur-Seine, France*
[3] *Genomics and Evolution in Neuroendocrinology, Institut de Pharmacologie Moléculaire et Cellulaire, UMR7275, Centre National de la Recherche Scientifique, Valbonne, France*
[4] *Genomics and Evolution in Neuroendocrinology, Université de Nice Sophia Antipolis, Nice, France*

Edited by:
Hubert Vaudry, University of Rouen, France

Reviewed by:
Berta Levavi-Sivan, The Hebrew University, Israel
James A. Carr, Texas Tech University, USA

****Correspondence:***
Jean A. Boutin, Biotechnologie, Pharmacologie Moléculaire et Cellulaire, Institut de Recherches SERVIER, 125 chemin de Ronde, 78290 Croissy-sur-Seine, France.
e-mail: jean.boutin@fr.netgrs.com

The compound S38151 is a nanomolar antagonist that acts at the melanin-concentrating hormone receptor 1 (MCH_1). S38151 is more stable than its purely peptide counterpart, essentially because of the blockade of its N-terminus. Therefore, its action on various models of obesity was studied. Acute intra-cerebroventricular (i.c.v.) administration of S38151 in wild-type rats counteracted the effect of the stable precursor of melanin-concentrating hormone (MCH), NEI-MCH, in a dose-dependent manner (from 0.5 to 50 nmol/kg). In genetically obese Zucker *fa/fa* rats, daily i.c.v. administration of S38151 induced dose-dependent (5, 10, and 20 nmol/kg) inhibition of food intake, water intake, and body weight gain, as well as increased motility (maximal effect observed at 20 nmol/kg). In Zucker *fa/fa* rats, intraperitoneal injection of S38151 (30 mg/kg) induced complete inhibition of food consumption within 1 h. Daily intraperitoneal injection of S38151 (10 and 30 mg/kg) into genetically obese *ob/ob* mice or diet-induced obese mice is able to limit body weight gain. Furthermore, S38151 administration (10 and 30 mg/kg) does not affect food intake, water intake, or body weight gain in MCHR1-deleted mice, demonstrating that its effects are linked to its interaction with MCH_1. These results validate MCH_1 as a target of interest in obesity. S38151 cannot progress to the clinical phase because it is still too poorly stable *in vivo*.

Keywords: melanin-concentrating hormone, receptors, peptide antagonists, feeding behavior, rat, mice, obesity models

INTRODUCTION

Melanin-concentrating hormone (MCH) is a 17-amino-acid, cyclic pseudopeptide that is responsible for the bleaching of skin in teleost fishes (Kawauchi et al., 1983). In mammals, MCH is a 19-amino-acid cyclic peptide (Vaughan et al., 1989). Its actions are not linked to pigmentation, but to a variety of properties, originally centered on appetite regulation and obesity (Qu et al., 1996; Pissios et al., 2006). MCH acts in several processes, including sleep/arousal (Hervieu, 2006; Peyron et al., 2009), emotionality (Hervieu, 2006), and memory (Adamantidis and de Lecea, 2009). MCH is encoded as a pre-pro-hormone, and also gives rise to two other neuropeptides after proteo-cleavage: (1) neuropeptide N-G (NGE), the function of which is elusive, and (2) neuropeptide E-I (NEI) (Nahon et al., 1989), which displays various functions (Maulon-Feraille et al., 2002; Bittencourt and Celis, 2008). NEI-MCH is more potent than MCH in stimulating feeding in rats, for proteolytic-protective reasons (Maulon-Feraille et al., 2002). MCH is mainly synthesized in cell bodies of the lateral hypothalamus and sub-*zona incerta* in the central nervous system (Bittencourt et al., 1992). MCH is also synthesized in peripheral organs, such as the gut, arteries, testes, thymus, and pancreatic β-cells (Hervieu and Nahon, 1995).

Two MCH receptors (MCH_1 and MCH_2) were identified a decade ago. MCH_1 was known for quite some time as SLC-1, an orphan receptor in humans (Lakaye et al., 1998). It was established as a genuine MCH receptor in 1999 by at least three different groups (Bachner et al., 1999; Chambers et al., 1999; Saito et al., 1999). The subsequent search for analogs of the protein led to the cloning of a second receptor, MCH_2 (Mori et al., 2001; Rodriguez et al., 2001; Sailer et al., 2001; Wang et al., 2001). This second receptor is expressed in humans, dogs, and ferrets, but not in rodents. In mammalian species, the highest expression levels of both receptors are found in the frontal cortex, amygdala, and nucleus accumbens; however, they are also expressed in hypothalamic areas regulating energy balance, such as the arcuate nucleus and the ventral medial hypothalamus. MHCRs are also moderately expressed in peripheral organs. In rodents, MCH acts through MCH_1, which implicates MCH_1 in obesity and energy homeostasis.

Several genetically engineered strains of mice have been reported. MCH_1-knockout (MCH_1-KO) mice (mice do not express a functional $MCHR_2$ protein) exhibit a phenotype of leanness and resistance to diet-induced obesity, characterized by hyperphagia, hyperactivity, and hypermetabolism

(Chen et al., 2002; Marsh et al., 2002; Pissios, 2009). This phenotype is attributed to increased energy expenditure, resulting from increased locomotor activity and increased resting energy expenditure. Paradoxically, these mice exhibit significant hyperphagia.

The molecular pharmacology of MCH_1 has been studied in some detail. After the centrally important works of teams at Takeda and Synaptic/Lundbeck (Borowsky et al., 2002; Takekawa et al., 2002), many non-peptide compounds were screened and found active at MCHR1. Most of these small molecules inhibit MCH-mediated feeding behavior; however, they may also affect energy expenditure. Interestingly, MCH_1 antagonists of different chemical classes exhibit anxiolytic and anti-depressant effects, a finding that would likely contribute to the success of these molecules in obese populations that might also have depression and anxiety. However, cardiovascular risk associated with human ether-a-go-go-related gene (hERG)-binding activity of biaryl-containing compounds has plagued many of these non-peptide MCH_1 antagonist programs (Mendez-Andino and Wos, 2007; Meyers et al., 2007; Johansson, 2011).

Alternatively, several dozen MCH analogs have been synthesized and tested by binding, leading to the discovery of peptide super-agonists and mild antagonists. Some of these have been tested on MCH_2, and present major selectivity to MCH_1. Structure activity relationship is now well-established concerning the peptide ligands. Although small molecules had been synthesized as potent and moderately selective MCH_1 antagonists, there was still an interest in finding new peptides with antagonistic activities. Pioneering works by Bednarek's group described such interesting compounds. In agreement with our initial search for better agonists (Audinot et al., 2001a,b), we explored the possibility of designing natural peptides or pseudopeptides [pseudopeptides are peptides including one or more exotic aminoacid(s) in their sequence] with good MCH_1 antagonism and fair *in vivo* stability. We succeeded in describing S38151 (Audinot et al., 2009), a potent peptide at MCH_1 with antagonistic activity in the nanomolar range. The aim of the present study was to evaluate the possible inhibition of S38151 on food and water intakes, body weight, and motility after one-time or repeated daily peripheral administration in different rodent models of obesity. Confirmation of the MCH_1-mediated actions of S38151 was tested in mice with genetic ablation of the receptor. Mice with genetic ablation of MCH_1 were used to confirm that the transient inhibition of S38151 onto the bodyweight was mediated by MCH_1.

MATERIALS AND METHODS

PEPTIDES

MCH and S38151 (Audinot et al., 2009) were obtained from Polypeptide Laboratories (Illkirch, France) and/or from Genepep (Saint Jean de Védas, France). They were of purity exceeding 97%. S38151 is a pseudopeptide, the sequence of which is: [p-guanidinobenzoyl-(Des-Gly10)-MCH (7–17)], or pGua-Cys-Met-Leu-Arg-Val-Tyr-Arg-Pro-Cys; both cysteines are linked together with a disulfide bridge. The molecular weight of S38151 is 1485 g/L. All of the various lots were systematically analyzed using mass spectrometry.

S38151 STABILITY STUDIES

First, S38151 was incubated for 16 h at 4°C and 37°C in mouse plasma or in TRIS buffer (pH 7.4). Next, plasma proteins were precipitated with two volumes of acetonitrile. After centrifugation and dilution with a water/acetonitrile mixture (50/50 v/v), the supernatant was injected onto a triple quadripole mass spectrometer (Ultima, Micromass WATERS Corporation, Milford, USA). The liquid chromatographic system consisted of an Agilent 1100 analytic pump (Agilent, Santa Clara, USA) equipped with an Alpha Mos CTC autosampler (Alpha Mos, Toulouse, France). Mass detection was performed using the m/z transition 743.5 > 163, in positive electrospray. A second stability study was performed at a lower concentration (1 μM) and for 4 h, with the following sampling times: 0, 15, 45, 90, and 240 min. At each sampling time, 50 μL of plasma were precipitated with two volumes of acetonitrile, and after centrifugation were directly injected onto the LC-MS/MS system. The same treatment was used for the buffer samples. Although brains from S38151-treated animals were analyzed to determine the amount of compound detectable in the brain, none was detected (data not shown).

ANIMALS

These experiments were conducted with male Wistar and Zucker *fa/fa* rats (10–13 weeks of age, weighing 325–350 g) together with C57BL/6J mice, *ob/ob* mice, and MCH_1-KO mice (14 weeks of age, weighing 25, 45, and 25 g, respectively) (Iffa Credo and Charles River, L'Arbresle, France). The animals were housed individually in a room with a 12-h light/dark cycle (lights on at 07:30 and off at 19:30), at 22 ± 3°C and 55% relative humidity. Normal food and tap water were available *ad libitum* unless otherwise stated. All animal procedures described in this study comply with French laws regulating animal experimentation (Decree No 87-848 19th October 1987 and the ministerial Decree of 10 April 1988) and were approved by the animal ethics committee of the Servier Research Institute.

INTRA-CEREBROVENTRICULAR CANNULA IMPLANTATION

Acute i.c.v. injections in rats

Wistar and Zucker *fa/fa* rats were anesthetized with Forène (Abbott Laboratories, Queenborough, UK), and a stainless steel guide cannula (Plastic Products Co, Roanoke, Va, USA) was stereotaxically implanted into the right lateral ventricle at the following coordinates relative to the bregma: AP −0.8 mm, $L = -1.2$ mm, and $V = -3.5$ mm. After a 7-day recovery period, during which the animals were handled each day to minimize non-specific stress, they were lightly anesthetized with Forène. Human/mouse/rat MCH (1 μg in a volume of 2.5 μL, Bachem, Voisins-le-Bretonneux, France) or an equivalent volume of artificial cerebrospinal fluid (CSF) was then injected through the intraventricular cannula. Immediately after injection, the animals quickly recovered and were returned to their home cages. Only those animals responding within 2 h with a robust increase in food intake, indicating correct cannula placement, were used in the experiments described below. Two days after MCH injection, the rats were randomly assigned to different groups and studied in one of the following protocols.

Acute central peptide administration and feeding studies in Wistar rats

Wistar rats were habituated for at least 2 weeks before experiment to a diet of food pellets (6 mm diameter) of the following composition: 67.5% food flour, 26.5% sucrose, 5% gum tragacanth, and 1.25% magnesium stearate (A03 UAR, Orge, France). The food pellets were present in a metal food hopper attached to the inside of each cage. At 09:00 on the day of study, the animals were lightly anesthetized with Forene® (Abbott, France). Thereafter, rats were injected intra-cerebroventricular (i.c.v.) with vehicle (artificial CSF) or with S38151 [0.5, 5, 10, 20, 30, or 50 nmol/kg (0.7, 1.4, 14, 28, 42, or 70 μg/kg, respectively)] in a volume of 2.5 μL, 20 min prior to the injection of human/rat NEI-MCH [5 nmol/kg (18.7 μg/kg) in a volume of 2.5 μL].

Food intake was measured at different times after peptide injection. Food spillage was carefully quantified during each time period, and intake measurements were corrected for this loss. At the end of the experiments, the animals were euthanized and the positions of the cannulae were assessed by the injection of 100 μL Evans blue dye (2 mg/mL) followed by the visual examination of brain slices. Only data obtained from animals with correctly positioned cannulae were included in the final data analysis.

Daily central peptide administration and feeding studies in Zucker rats

The TSE Drinking and Feeding Monitor system was used to analyze ingestive behavior in these experiments (TSE Technical & Scientific Equipment GmbH, Bad Homburg, Germany). The rats' motility was also determined in these experiments using the MoTil® system (TSE). Zucker *fa/fa* rats were placed individually into plastic cages to which were attached both a feeding and a drinking sensor. The animals were habituated to normal food (A03 UAR, Orge, France) and water for at least 2 weeks before experimentation. One hour prior to the beginning of the dark phase, Zucker *fa/fa* rats were injected i.c.v. with different doses of S38151 [5, 10, or 20 nmol/kg (3.5, 14, or 28 μg/kg, respectively)] or with an equivalent volume of artificial CSF vehicle (10 μL). The injections were repeated daily for a total of 7 days. After 7 days, the injections were stopped and each measured parameter was followed during a 5-day washout period.

ACUTE PERIPHERAL PEPTIDE ADMINISTRATION AND FEEDING STUDIES IN ZUCKER RATS

Zucker fa/fa rats were habituated in the same conditions as Wistar rats (described in section "Acute Central Peptide Administration and Feeding Studies in Wistar Rats"). At 09:00 on the day of study, after fasting for 24 h, either vehicle (normal saline) or S38151 [30 mg/kg (20 μmol/kg)] was administered intraperitoneally (i.p.).

CONDITIONED TASTE AVERSION

These experiments were performed according to previously described methods (Criscione et al., 1998; Welzl et al., 2001). In brief, Wistar rats were individually housed in plastic cages with free access to normal food and water. During a 7-day habituation period, the water bottle was removed from the cages overnight (from 16:00 to 10:00). At 10:00, water was made available to the animals from 250-mL plastic bottles to which a normal drinking spout was attached. The bottles were weighed before and after presentation to the animals to determine the quantity of water ingested during this period. After 4 days of this treatment regime, which served to habituate the animals to the experimental protocol and to randomize the animals, 0.2% saccharine was presented instead of water. Twenty minutes after the test period, the animals were injected i.p. with lithium chloride (75 mg/kg) or i.c.v. with S38151 [20 nmol/kg (28 μg/kg)] or vehicle (artificial CSF). Four, 7, 11, and 14 days later, the consumption of saccharine was determined. Considerable care was taken in these experiments to first prevent and then quantify any leakage of saccharine solution during the presentations.

PICA

These experiments were performed with modifications to previously described methods (Madden et al., 1999). Rats were individually housed in wire-bottomed plastic cages with free access to both food pellets (6 mm diameter A03 UAR) and kaolin powder. The food pellets were presented in a small porcelain bowl on the floor of the cage. The kaolin powder was presented in a metal feeding dish attached to the inside of the cage. After a 2-week habituation period to these conditions, the animals were randomized into five treatment groups based on the quantity of food eaten during the stabilization period. In addition, those rats that consistently spilled the kaolin powder were eliminated from the study. One day after randomization, the animals were injected just before the beginning of the dark phase with either cyclophosphamide (100 mg/kg, i.p.), or S38151 [20 nmol/kg (28 μg/kg) i.c.v.] or vehicle [(artificial CSF) i.c.v.]. After injection, the quantity of kaolin and food ingested during the following 24-h period was determined. Food or kaolin spilled by the animals was collected at the end of the experiment, and total food and kaolin intake measurements were corrected for this loss.

CONSTRUCTION OF MCHr1$^{-/-}$ MICE

Construction of the targeting vector

The MCHR1$^{-/-}$ mouse model was custom-constructed by genOway (Lyon, France). The construction of the targeting vector and knock-in strategy were designed and performed by genOway (Lyon, France). A genomic clone containing the murine Mchr1 locus was isolated from a C57BL/6J RPCI-24 BAC genomic library by using a probe corresponding to the murine Mchr1 exon 2: one BAC clone (544N15) containing the Mchr1 locus. The genomic organization of the targeted locus was determined by subcloning the XhoI-SpeI genomic fragment into the pZErO™-2 vector (Invitrogen, Carlsbad, California). The 7.4-kb XhoI-SpeI genomic insert was sequenced and the Mchr1 sequence was generated. The genomic clone (containing the entire gene) was used to construct the targeting vector. Briefly, a 5.1-kb XhoI/ApaI fragment comprising Mchr1 exons 1 and 2 and a 1.1-kb ApaI/BglII fragment located downstream of Mchr1 exon 2 were used to flank a NEO cassette (FRT-PGK promoter-Neo^R cDNA-FRT-LoxP) (**Figure 1A**); a negative (DTA) selection cassette was introduced at the 5′ end of the long arm of homology.

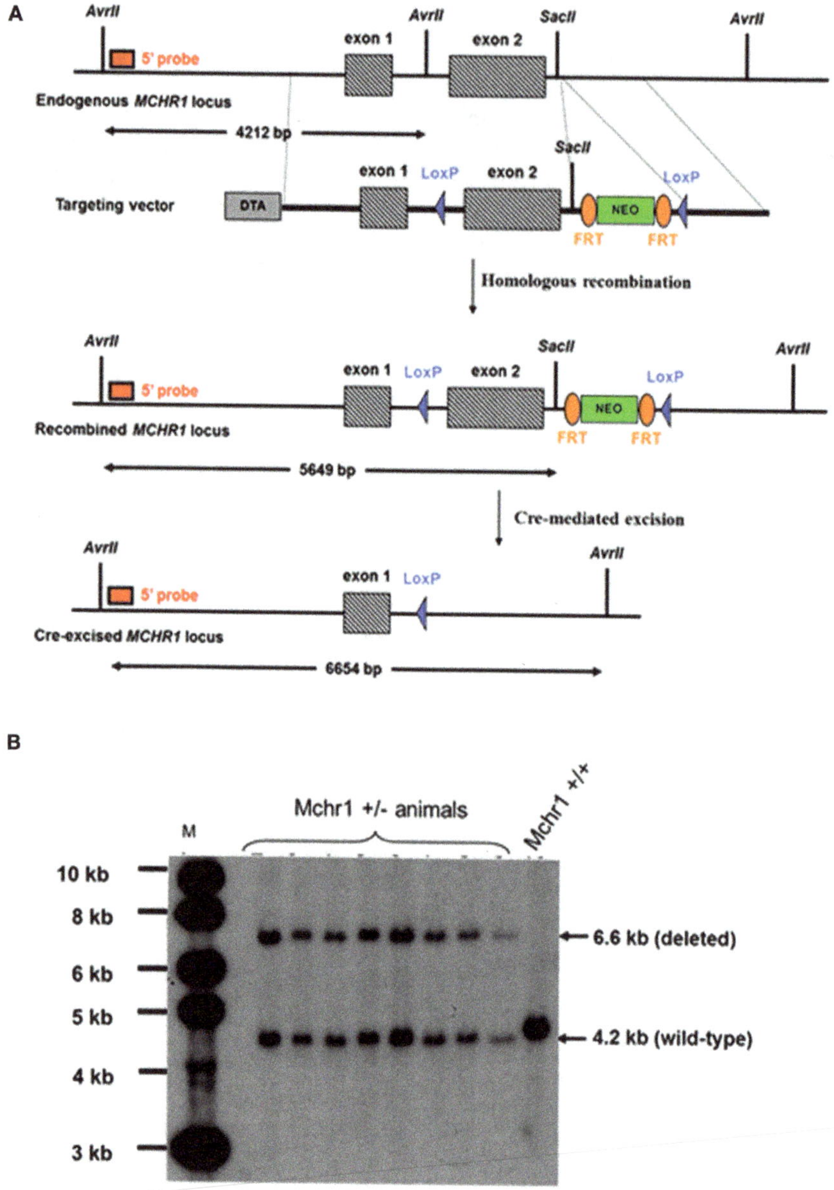

FIGURE 1 | Construction of MCHR1$^{-/-}$ mice. (A) Strategy for the construction of MCHR1$^{-/-}$ mice. The *Mchr1* locus (containing exons 1–2) and the targeting construct [containing the neomycin (PGK-Neo) cassette with flanking segments homologous to the locus] are shown. The probe used in all Southern blot analyses was a 0.65-kb fragment located in a region upstream of exon 1. **(B)** Southern blot analysis of the offspring of MchR1-deleted mice, compared with C57BL/6J mice. Digestion of tail DNA with AvrII/SacII resulted in the following diagnostic fragments: a wild-type band (4.2 kb), and a deleted allele band (6.6 kb).

Screening of Mchr1-recombined ES cell clones

NotI-linearized targeting vector was transfected into 129SvPas ES cells (genOway, Lyon, France) according to genOway's modified electroporation procedures (i.e., 10^8 ES cells in the presence of 100 μg of linearized plasmid, 800 V, 300 μF). Positive selection was started 48 h after electroporation, by adding 200 μg/mL of G418 (150 μg/mL of active component, Life Technologies, Inc.). A total of 333 resistant clones were isolated and amplified in 96-well plates, and duplicates were made of the 96-well plates. The set of plates containing ES cell clones amplified on gelatin was screened by PCR and further confirmed by Southern blotting.

5′ PCR screening conditions were: GW676 primer specific for a region upstream of *Mchr1* exon 1 (5′-GATATCAATTCGGGACACATGG-3′) and GW681 primer specific for the Neo^R selection cassette (5′-TCTCGGCAGGAGCAAGGTGAGATGACAG-3′). PCR conditions were 94°C/2 min, and 35 cycles of (94°C/30 s, 59°C/30 s, and 68°C/6 min) followed by 68°C/10 min, resulting in a 6509-bp mutated allele. 3′ PCR screening conditions were: GW668 primer specific for the Neo® selection cassette (5′-ATCA

GGACATAGCGTTGGCTAC-3′) and GW669 primer to hybridize the region downstream of the *Mchr1* gene (5′-ATGAGAAGTG ACCAGCAAGAGC-3′). PCR conditions were 94°C/2 min, and 35 cycles of (94°C/30 s, 61°C/30 s, and 68°C/2 min), followed by 68°C/10 min, resulting in a 1609-bp recombined allele. Both PCR reactions were performed using Long Expand High Fidelity polymerase (Roche®) and reaction buffer 3. PCR products were then digested with PmeI to confirm the integration of the distal *loxP* site within the recombined allele. Briefly, for Southern blot analysis, genomic DNA was digested with AvrII/SacII and then hybridized with a 0.65-kb probe; *Mchr1* ± clones gave rise to a 4.2-kb wild-type signal and 5.6-kb recombined signal.

In vitro Cre-mediated deletion of Mchr1-recombined ES cell clones

Two recombined ES cell clones were used to perform Cre-mediated deletion of the floxed *Mchr1* region. Supercoiled Cre-expressing plasmid was transfected into *Mchr1*-recombined ES cells (genOway, Lyon, France) according to genOway standard procedures. No selection was applied. One hundred ES cell clones were isolated and amplified in 96-well plates, and duplicates were made of the 96-well plates. The set of plates containing ES cell clones amplified on gelatin was screened by PCR and further confirmed by Southern blotting. The PCR screening conditions were: GW787 primer specific for *Mchr1* exon 1 (5′-AGCTCTGAAGGAGAAGGGAATG-3′) and GW669 primer to hybridize the region downstream of the *Mchr1* gene (5′-ATGAGAAGTGACCAGCAAGAGC-3′). The PCR conditions were 94°C/2 min, and 35 cycles of (94°C/30 s, 59°C/30 s, and 68°C/6 min), followed by 68°C/10 min, resulting in a 4481-bp recombined allele and a 1564-bp deleted allele. The PCR reaction was performed using Long Expand High Fidelity polymerase (Roche®) and reaction buffer 3. Briefly, for Southern blot analysis, genomic DNA was digested with AvrII/SacII and then hybridized with a 0.65-kb probe. The *Mchr1* wild-type allele gave rise to a 4.2-kb signal, the *Mchr1*-recombined allele gave rise to a 5.6-kb signal, and the *Mchr1* deleted allele gave rise to a 6.6-kb signal.

Generation of chimeric mice and breeding scheme

One floxed mutated *Mchr1* ES cell clone (clone #2A9-2A10) was microinjected into C57BL/6J blastocysts, and gave rise to male chimeras with a significant ES cell contribution (as determined by Agouti coat color). After mating with C57BL/6J females, germline transmission was confirmed by the genotyping of tail DNA from offspring using PCR and Southern blot analysis. Knock-out heterozygous animals were screened as described in section "Screening of Mchr1-Recombined ES Cell Clones." PCR screening conditions were: GW787 primer specific for *Mchr1* exon 1 (5′-AGCTCTGAAGGAGAAGGGAATG-3′) and GW669 primer to hybridize the region downstream of the *Mchr1* gene (5′-ATGAGAAGTGACCAGCAAGAGC-3′). PCR conditions were 94°C/2 min, and 35 cycles of (94°C/30 s, 59°C/30 s, and 68°C/6 min), followed by 68°C/10 min, resulting in a 3.1-kb signal for the wild-type allele and 1.6-kb signal for the deleted allele. The PCR reaction was performed using Long Expand High Fidelity polymerase (Roche®) and reaction buffer 3. Briefly, for Southern blot analysis, genomic DNA was digested with AvrII/SacII and then hybridized with a 0.65-kb probe. The wild-type *Mchr1* allele gave rise to a 4.2-kb signal and the deleted *Mchr1* allele gave rise to a 6.6-kb signal (**Figure 1B**). F1 male and female heterozygous animals were interbred to obtain *Mchr1*-null mice, and offspring were also screened by PCR and Southern blot analysis as described in this section.

FOOD INTAKE IN C57BL/6J AND ob/ob MICE

For the MCH daily repeated i.c.v. injection studies, 13-week-old female C57BL/6J and *ob/ob* mice were used (Harlan, Gannat, France).

FOOD INTAKE INDUCED OBESITY IN C57BL/6J, ob/ob, AND MCHr1-KO MICE

In these studies, 13-week-old female C57BL/6J, ob/ob, and MCH_1-KO mice were used. The mice were maintained on a 12-h light/dark cycle (lights on at 07:30 and off at 19:30) at 22 ± 3°C, and supplied with food pellets (6 mm diameter A03, UAR Laboratory chow, Epinay Villemuisson France) and tap water *ad libitum*. To induce obesity in C57BL/6J (creating diet-induced obese, or DIO, mice), mice were fed a high-fat diet (60 kcal% fat, 20 kcal% protein, 20 kcal% carbohydrate, ref D12492 from Research Diets, New Brunswick, NJ08901, USA) for 8 weeks starting at 4 weeks of age. In these experiments, DIO mice, ob/ob mice, and $MCH_1^{-/-}$ mice were individually housed in a modular chamber that was placed on an activity platform to concurrently measure the food intake, water intake, and activity of the mice (ADDENFI, Les Cordeliers, Paris, France). For at least 2 weeks before experimentation, mice were habituated to a diet of 6 mm diameter food pellets of the following composition: 67.5% food flour, 26.5% sucrose, 5% gum tragacanth, 1.25% magnesium stearate (A03 UAR, Orge, France), and to i.p. injection. After this habituation period, food intake, drink intake, and body weight were measured for 3 consecutive days. The mice were randomized into three groups based on their food and water intake over the three preceding 24-h periods, and on their body weight. Next, the quantity of food eaten over each 24-h period during the 5 days of i.p. treatment with S38151 [10 and 30 mg/kg/day (7 and 20 μmol/kg/day)] or vehicle was determined and corrected for spillage.

DATA AND STATISTICAL ANALYSIS

Data were grouped together and presented as mean ± standard error (SEM). The individual statistical tests that were used in these studies are described in detail in the figure legends. In each case, *P*-values less than 0.05 were considered statistically significant.

RESULTS

S38151 CHARACTERISTICS AND SERUM STABILITY

S38151 was synthesized during a process that was attempting to find peptides or pseudopeptides with affinity at MCH_1 receptor that also had greater stability in biological media. This pseudopeptide is derived from another, very similar agonist, pGua (MCH7-17) (Audinot et al., 2001a, 2009). In Chinese hamster ovary cells over-expressing MCH_1, S38151 exhibited a K_i of 80 nM in a $[^{125}I]$-S36057 binding assay and was a potent and full antagonist ($KB = 4.3$ nM in a GTPγS binding assay, and $KB = 210$ nM in a calcium flux assay) (Audinot et al., 2009). This activity was specific to MCH_1, since it has no activity with respect to MCHR2 at concentrations of less than 10 μM. This compound was also evaluated on a series of 70 targets, comprising monoaminergic and peptidergic receptors as well as enzymes, ionic channels, and transporters. S38151 did not display any activity regarding these targets at concentrations of less than 10 μM (data not shown). The peptide was incubated either in a buffered solution (pH 7.4) or in mouse plasma for 16 h, at either 4°C or 37°C. **Figure 2** clearly shows that at 37°C, a minimal portion of S38151 is detectable, suggesting that it has limited stability in plasma.

THE EFFECT OF A SINGLE i.c.v. INJECTION OF S38151 ON NEI-MCH-INDUCED FOOD INTAKE IN WISTAR RATS

The acute effects of a single i.c.v. injection of S38151 on NEI-MCH-induced food intake in Wistar rats are summarized in **Figure 3**. During the first 2 h after its injection, NEI-MCH produced a significant increase in food intake above the corresponding values observed in vehicle-injected control animals (T1h: 3.18 g ± 1.09 vs. 0.45 g ± 0.19; T2h: 2.73 g ± 0.89 vs. 1.25 g ± 0.38). Relative to control values, the increase in food intake induced by NEI-MCH became progressively greater during the following 4-h period (from T1 h to T4 h). During the first and second hours, the MCHR1 antagonist S38151 produced a statistically significant dose-related inhibition of the increase in food intake produced by NEI-MCH. Nearly complete inhibition of NEI-MCH-induced food intake was observed at the dose of 50 nmol/kg S38151. Thereafter, for each dose of S38151, food intake increased essentially in parallel with the food increase in the NEI-MCH-treated group. Food intake during the entire 24-h period in the control group was not significantly altered by NEI-MCH, or by any combination of NEI-MCH and S38151.

THE EFFECTS OF DAILY S38151 i.c.v. INJECTIONS ON FOOD INTAKE, BODY WEIGHT, AND MOTILITY IN ZUCKER fa/fa RATS

The effects of daily S38151 i.c.v. injection on the measured parameters are depicted in **Figure 4**. During the 7-day experimental period, injection of 28 μg/kg (5 nmol/rat) S38151 1 h before the dark phase resulted in dose-dependent inhibition of food intake. However, the change in food intake only reached statistical significance at the dose of 20 nmol/kg (28 μg/kg) S38151. Immediately after the injections were terminated, food intake returned to control levels for the duration of the washout period.

In contrast to food intake, water consumption appeared to be more sensitive to inhibition of MCHR1; water intake was significantly inhibited in response to all injected doses of S38151 except for the 5 nmol/rat dose. Immediately after the injections were terminated, water intake returned to control levels during the washout period. In a manner similar to water intake, motility also appeared to be more sensitive to the effects of MCH_1 blockade; motility was significantly increased at both the 10 nmol/kg and 20 nmol/kg doses of S38151. Notably, the increase in motility was not terminated after the S38151 injections were stopped. This finding was most marked during the washout period after administration of the 20 nmol/kg dose of S38151, during which motility remained significantly elevated. During the 7-day experimental period, S38151 produced a dose-dependent reduction in body weight gain compared with control rats at the 10 and 20 nmol/kg doses. After the injections were stopped, body weight gain exhibited a tendency to return to control values. However, body weight gain remained significantly less than control values during the washout period after injection of 10 nmol/kg S38151.

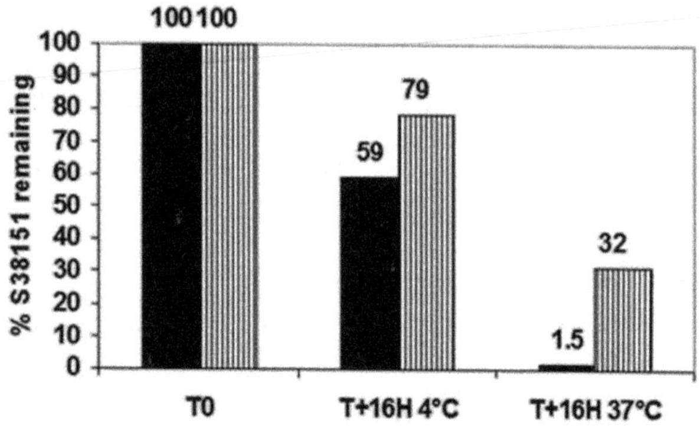

FIGURE 2 | Studies regarding the stability of S38151. A solution of S38151 (40 μM) was incubated with either Tris buffer, pH 7.4 (hatched bars), or mouse plasma samples (dark bars) for 16 h at 4°C or 37°C. The samples were analyzed using liquid chromatography coupled to mass spectrometry. Experiments were repeated three times. The chart presented is representative of the experimental results.

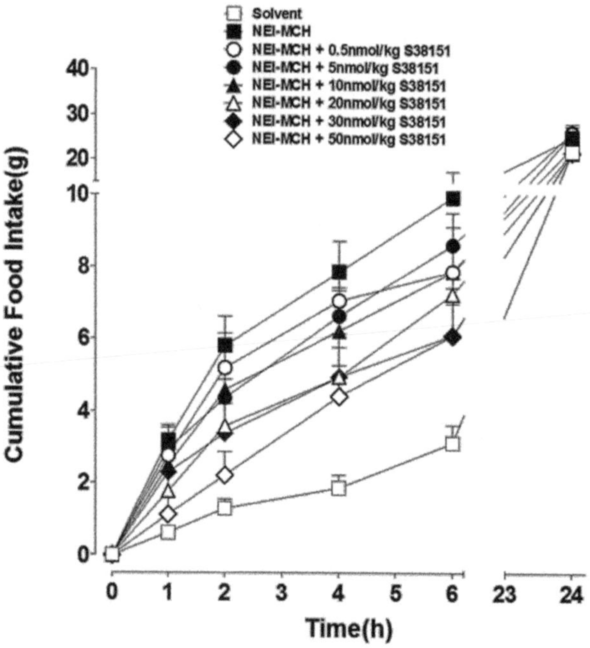

FIGURE 3 | The effect of S38151 on NEI-MCH-induced food intake in Wistar rats after acute central administration. Satiated rats were injected (i.c.v.) at the beginning of the light phase with 5 μg NEI-MCH, 5 μg NEI-MCH + differing doses of S38151 (0.5–50 nmol/kg), or an equivalent volume of artificial cereblospinal fluid vehicle (5 μL). Cumulative food intake was measured at 1, 2, 4, 6, and 24 h post-injection. Results are expressed as mean ± SEM (n = 10–11 rats per group). Repeated measures Two-Way ANOVA (treatment × time) was followed by *post hoc* Student-Neuman-Keuls analysis to compare all groups of animals.

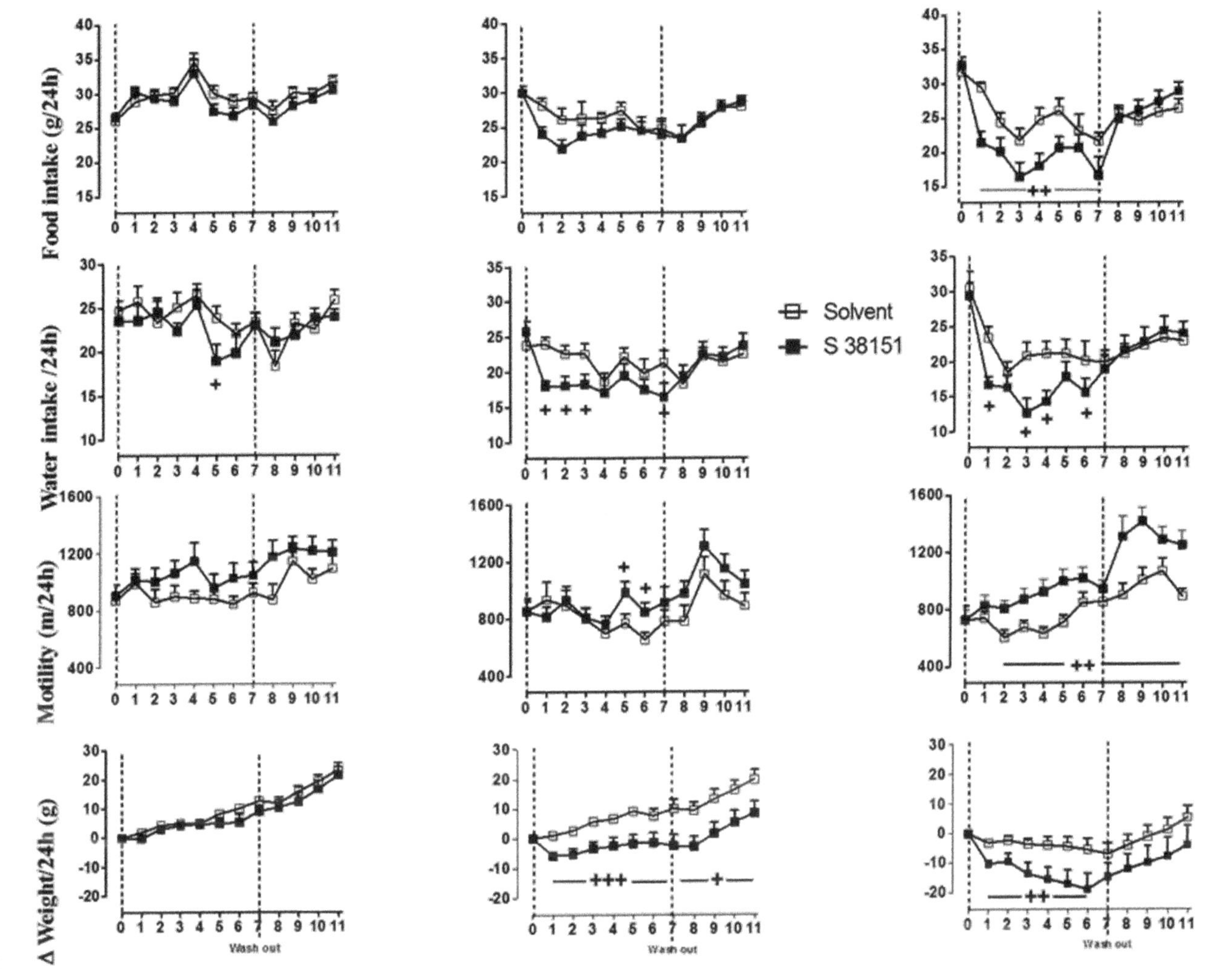

FIGURE 4 | The effects of repeated daily central administration of S38151 on food intake, water intake, body weight, and motility in Zucker *fa/fa* rats. One hour prior the beginning of the dark phase, different doses of S38151 (5, 10, or 20 nmol/kg) or vehicle were injected (i.c.v.) once daily for 7 days, followed by a washout period of 5 days. Results are expressed as mean ± SEM ($n = 8$ rats per group). Repeated measures Two-Way ANOVA (treatment × time) was performed with a repeated measure of the factor "time." Significant treatment and interaction effects are shown on the graph. $^{+}P < 0.05$; $^{++}P < 0.01$; $^{+++}P < 0.001$.

THE EFFECTS OF S38151 ON CONDITIONED TASTE AVERSION AND PICA IN ZUCKER fa/fa RATS

The results of the conditioned taste aversion test are shown in **Figure 5A**. The consumption of 0.2% saccharine during the first exposure (test day 0) before treatment was well matched between the three groups. Subsequent injection of lithium chloride resulted in a significant reduction in 0.2% saccharine consumption during test days 4, 7, 11, and 14 compared with the control group. In contrast, S38151 injection did not affect 0.2% saccharine consumption.

In the Pica test, vehicle-injected control animals ate 27 ± 1 g of normal food and very little kaolin (0.05 ± 0.01 g) during the 24-h experimental period (**Figure 5B**). Cyclophosphamide (i.p. injection) resulted in the nearly complete suppression of spontaneous food intake, which was accompanied by a significant increase in kaolin intake. In contrast, i.c.v. injection of S38151 [20 nmol/kg (28 μg/kg)] significantly reduced food intake but did not significantly alter kaolin intake compared with control values.

THE EFFECT OF A SINGLE i.p. INJECTION OF S38151 ON FOOD INTAKE IN FASTED ZUCKER fa/fa RATS

The acute effect of i.p.-injected S38151 on food intake in Zucker fa/fa rats is summarized in **Figure 6**. After a 24-h period of food restriction, rats ate 3.6 ± 0.4 g during the first hour after the food pellets were put back. S38151 (i.p. injection) at the dose of 30 mg/kg (approximately 60 nmol/rat) 1 h before re-feeding induced a dramatic fall in food intake from the first hour (0.09 ± 0.06 g) to 6 h compared with the control group. This decrease maintained statistical significance up to 24 h after drug administration.

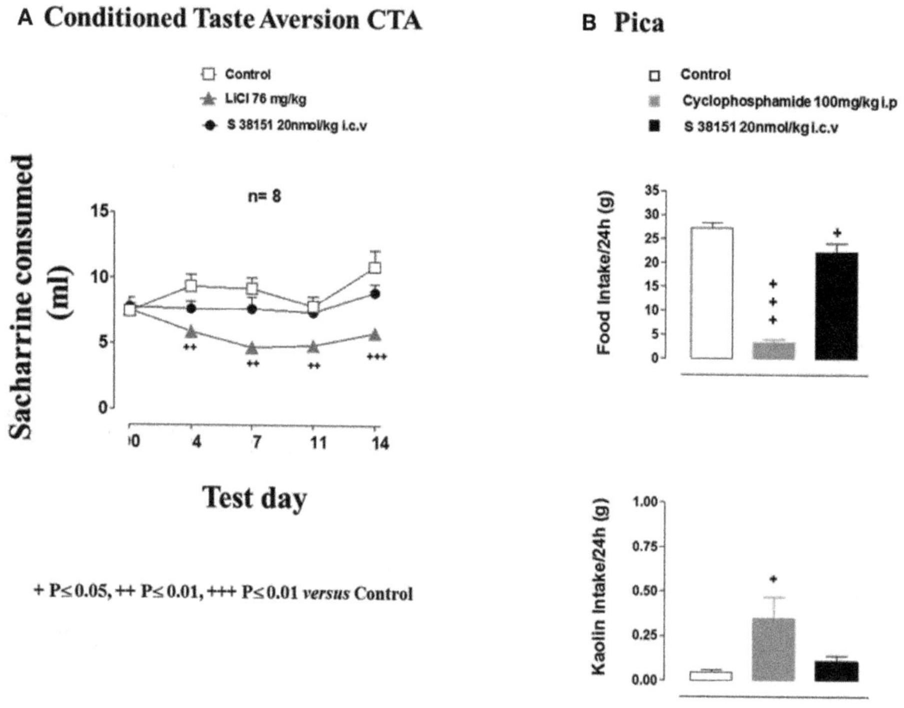

FIGURE 5 | The effects of S38151 on conditioned taste aversion and pica in Zucker *fa/fa* rats. (A) In the conditioned taste aversion test, after a period of habituation of the animals to the experimental protocol, Zucker *fa/fa* rats were presented with 0.2% saccharine for 20 min after drinking water was removed from their cages for 18 h (test day 0). Animals were then injected (i.p.) with vehicle or lithium chloride, or with S38151 (20 nmol/kg, i.c.v). On test days 4, 7, 11, and 14, rats were presented with 0.2% saccharine, and the quantity consumed during a 20-min period was determined. Results are expressed as mean ± SEM ($n = 10$–11 rats per group). Repeated measures Two-Way ANOVA (treatment × time) was followed by *post hoc* Student-Neuman-Keuls analysis to compare all groups of animals. $^{++}P < 0.01$, $^{+++}P < 0.001$. **(B)** In the pica test, Zucker *fa/fa* rats were injected (i.c.v.) with 20 nmol/kg S38151, or an equivalent volume of artificial cerebrospinal fluid vehicle. Food and kaolin intake during the following 24-h period were each measured. Results are expressed as mean ± SEM ($n = 8$ rats per group). One-Way ANOVA was followed by Dunnett's test, which compared the treated group with the control group. $^{+}P < 0.05$, $^{+++}P < 0.001$.

THE EFFECTS OF DAILY i.c.v. INJECTION OF MCH ON FOOD INTAKE AND BODY WEIGHT IN ob/ob MICE

Food intake

Food intake in vehicle-infused C57BL/6J mice ranged from 3 to 4 g/day during the 5-day experimental period (**Figure 7A**). Infusion of MCH at 5 μg/mouse/day (100 nmol/kg/day) resulted in a sustained and significant increase in food intake above the values observed in vehicle-infused mice on day 5 ($\Delta = +1.3$ g vs. controls). Food intake in ob/ob mice (**Figure 7C**) ranged from 3.5 to 5 g/day during the experimental period, and was significantly greater than that observed in C57BL/6J mice. Infusion of MCH at 5 μg/mouse/day in ob/ob mice significantly increased food intake above the values obtained in vehicle-infused control animals. The increase in food intake produced by MCH infusion in ob/ob mice on day 5 was significantly greater than that observed in lean mice ($\Delta = +3.2$ g vs. controls).

Body weight

In C57BL/6J mice, body weight remained stable during the 5-day experimental period (**Figure 7B**). Infusion of MCH resulted in a significant increase in body weight on day 5 ($\Delta = +1.3$ g vs. controls). Body weight tended to decrease slightly during the experimental period in vehicle-infused ob/ob mice (**Figure 7D**). However, infusion of MCH reversed this trend, and body weight had increased significantly above control levels after 5 days of treatment ($\Delta = +2.1$ g vs. controls). The increase in body weight in MCH-infused ob/ob mice on day 5 was significantly greater than that observed in either group of lean mice.

THE EFFECTS OF DAILY S38151 i.p. INJECTION ON FOOD AND WATER INTAKE, BODY WEIGHT, AND MOTILITY IN ob/ob MICE

The effects of daily i.p. injection of S38151 on the measured parameters are depicted in **Figure 8**. During the 6-day experimental period, i.p. injection of S38151 1 h before the dark phase produced a dose-dependent inhibition of food intake that reached significance starting on day 3 only at the highest dose of 30 mg/kg (20 μmol/kg/day). Water intake presented the same profile, but did not reach statistical significance because of the greater variability in water consumption among mice. During the 6-day experimental period, S38151 produced a dose-dependent reduction in body weight compared with control mice, with the 30 mg/kg dose reaching statistical significance at days 1, 4, 5, and 6. In contrast, motility appeared to be similar among all groups. On day 6, an improvement of metabolic parameters (significant reductions in glycemia and insulinemia) was observed at a dose of 30 mg/kg (data not shown).

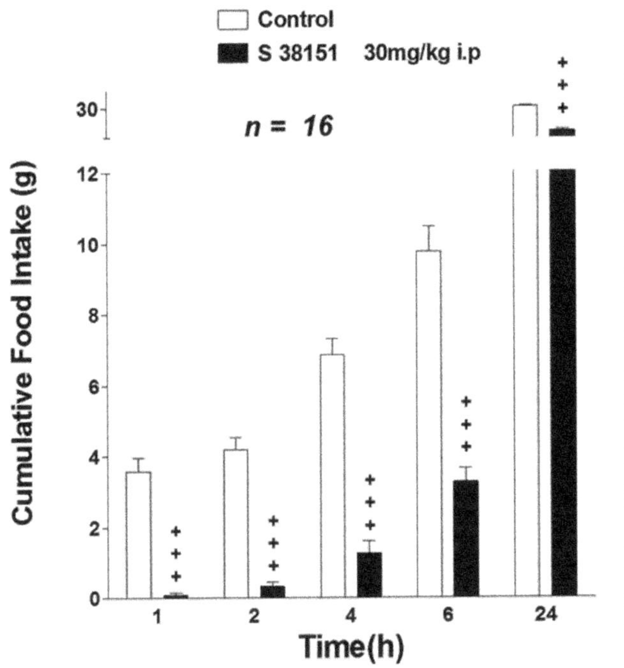

FIGURE 6 | The effect of S38151 on food intake in Zucker *fa/fa* rats after acute peripheral administration. Rats were fasted for 24 h, and then injected (i.p.) at the beginning of the light phase with vehicle (normal saline) or 30 mg/kg S38151. Cumulative food intake was measured 1, 2, 4, 6, and 24 h after injection. Results are expressed as mean ± SEM ($n = 16$ rats per group). Repeated measures Two-Way ANOVA (treatment × time) was followed by *post hoc* Student-Neuman-Keuls analysis to compare all groups of animals. $^{+}P < 0.05$.

THE EFFECTS OF DAILY i.p. INJECTION OF S38151 ON FOOD INTAKE, BODY WEIGHT, AND MOTILITY IN DIO MICE

The effects of daily i.p. injection of S38151 on the measured parameters are depicted in **Figure 9**. During the 5-day experimental period, i.p. injection of S38151 1 h before the dark phase produced a dose-dependent inhibition of food and drink intake that reached significance beginning on day 2 only at the 30 mg/kg dose. A reduction in body weight gain was observed at the 10 and 30 mg/kg doses (7 and 20 μmol/kg/day, respectively), which reached statistical significance at day 3 and day 1, respectively, compared with control mice. S38151 induced a similar significant reduction in motility at the two tested doses from day 3 to day 5. At day 6, an improvement of metabolic parameters (significant reductions in glycemia and insulinemia) was observed at a dose of 30 mg/kg (data not shown). In another experiment, daily i.p. administration of 30 mg/kg S38151 for 16 days induced a significant reduction of body weight gain that was accompanied by reduced glycemia and insulinemia, as well as a significant reduction of triglycerides, free fatty acids, and fat mass (data not shown).

THE EFFECTS OF DAILY i.p. INJECTION OF S38151 ON FOOD INTAKE, BODY WEIGHT, AND MOTILITY IN MCH_1-KO MICE

During the 5-day experimental period, i.p. injection of S38151 1 h before the dark phase did not induce any significant effects on the food intake, drink intake, or body weight of MHCR1-KO mice; however, a significant reduction in motility was observed at the highest dose of 30 mg/kg (20 μmol/kg/day) (**Figure 10**).

DISCUSSION

In the present study, we have investigated the effects of a selective MCH_1 peptide antagonist, S38151 (Audinot et al., 2001a, 2009), on food intake, drinking, body weight, and/or motility in lean rats and mice, as well as in Zucker *fa/fa* rats, *ob/ob* mice, and DIO mice. Central acute administration of S38151 inhibited proMCH131-165 (MCH-NEI peptide)-induced feeding in lean animals in a dose-dependent manner. This effect lasted for over 6 h, in agreement with the estimated concentration of compound still present in plasma. In several obese rodent models (7-day treatment in Zucker *fa/fa* rats, 6-day treatment in *ob/ob* mice, and 5-day treatment in DIO mice), S38151 produced a robust and dose-dependent reduction in food intake and body weight gain. Drinking behavior was also inhibited in Zucker *fa/fa* rats and DIO mice. However, the cessation of S38151 injections resulted in a rapid resumption of feeding and drinking behaviors in Zucker *fa/fa* rats, a transitory action that greatly contrasted with the persistent weight loss. Repeated daily blockade of MCH_1 receptors with S38151 reduced food intake and body weight with attenuated magnitude in leptin-deficient *ob/ob* mice relative to that observed in DIO mice. This observation was also reported with another MCH_1 antagonist (Kowalski et al., 2006), presumably owing to the emergence of multiple alterations in leptin-responsive neuronal pathways implicated in the feeding behavior of *ob/ob* mice.

To clearly establish the involvement of MCH_1 in the mode of action of S38151 on feeding and weight controls, its effects were evaluated in MCH_1-KO mice. Consistent with direct MCH_1 antagonism, S38151 did not produce any significant effect on feeding, drinking, or body weight gain in MCH_1-KO mice treated for 5 days. Combined with the growing literature on MCH_1 antagonists (see reviews Mendez-Andino and Wos, 2007; Johansson, 2011), these data strengthen the validation of MCH_1 as a strong candidate for developing anti-obesity drugs.

Intriguingly, repeated daily MCH_1 antagonism by S38151 induced persistent hypermobility in Zucker *fa/fa* rats, but did not affect locomotor activity in *ob/ob* mice, and even reduced motility in DIO mice. The differential response may result from differences in species (rat vs. mouse) or genetic background (*ob/ob* vs. C57BL/6J), or may be related to an off-target mechanism. When treated with S38151 for 5 days, MCH_1-KO mice exhibited a reduction in motility similar to that noted in DIO mice. Therefore, the observed disparity in motor activity likely arose from off-target (i.e., MCH_1-independent) effects of S38151.

In recent years, MCH_1 antagonists have been described as central to the regulation of energy expenditure and food intake. However, unlike for neuropeptide Y receptor 5 antagonists [see Block et al. (2002) and references therein], data suggest that small molecule antagonists of MCH_1 would have much broader activity, especially regarding mood regulation (and more generally, depression). Vast programs of drug synthesis and testing have been published in the literature. One of the surprising key features of those programs is that it appeared to be difficult to find

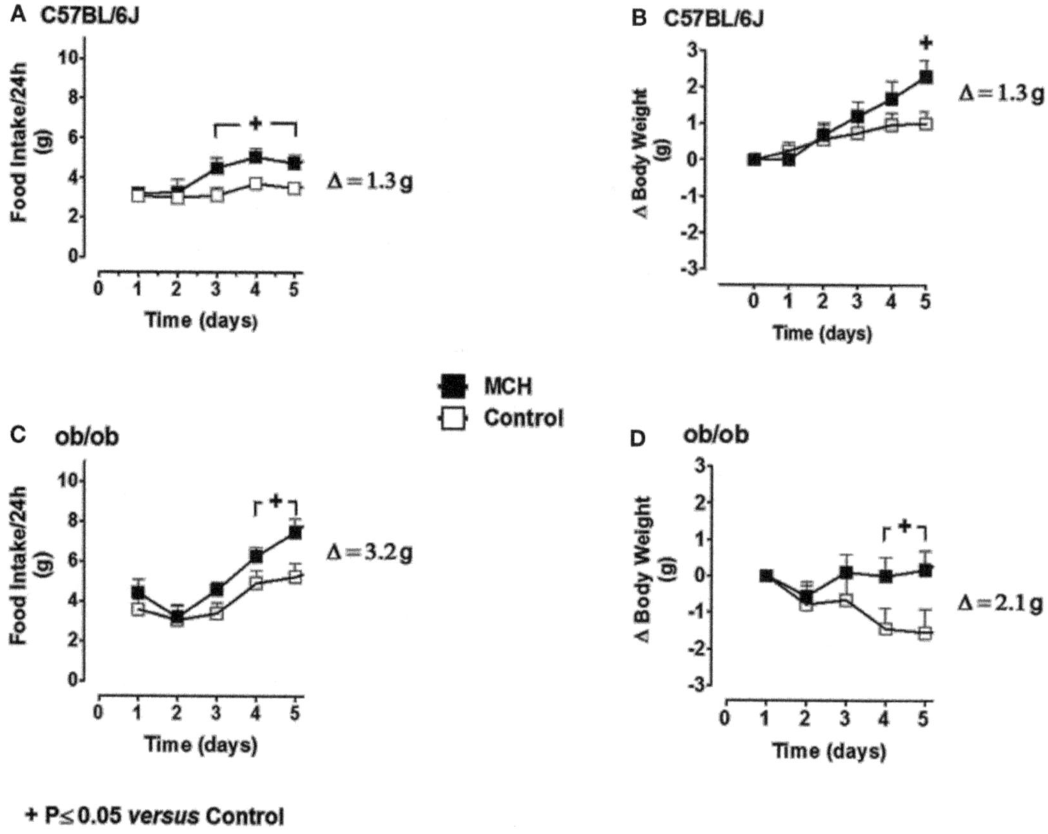

FIGURE 7 | The effect of repeated daily central administration of MCH to lean (C57BL/6J) and obese (*ob/ob*) mice. C57BL/6J (**A** and **B**) and *ob/ob* (**C** and **D**) mice were administered MCH (5 μg/mouse/day) or artificial cerebrospinal fluid vehicle through i.c.v. injections for 5 consecutive days. Results are expressed as mean ± SEM ($n = 10$ mice per group). Repeated measures Two-Way ANOVA (treatment × time) was followed by complementary analysis of the treatment's effect at a fixed level of time to compare all groups of mice with the control group. $^{+}P < 0.05$.

compounds with potent antagonists against MCH_1 that lacked activity regarding the hERG channel [see Mendez-Andino and Wos for a complete review (Mendez-Andino and Wos, 2007)].

Regarding the onset of obesity, it is well-known that the adipocyte has a central role, so it seemed interesting to find a way to act directly upon this cell type. MCH_1 is expressed in adipocytes, suggesting that fat cells may be targets of MCH antagonists under physiological conditions (Bradley et al., 2000). This hypothesis was confirmed by our study using DIO mice treated with daily S38151 injections for 16 days, in which a reduction in fat mass was observed concomitant with improvements in glucose and lipid profiles. Indeed, acting through the central control of appetite has often failed, particularly for two reasons: (1) the number of "rescue" systems in the brain circuits is so important that inhibiting one pathway would lead to the "takeover" of one or several alternate pathways (Nair and Ren, 2009); (2) in some cases acting on a central system, such as the MCH-ergic system, to control appetite has promoted adverse effects, and particularly pro-depressive effects (Roy et al., 2007; Lagos et al., 2011; Garcia-Fuster et al., 2012). Therefore, it was interesting to observe whether a potent (in the nM range) MCH_1 antagonist that was theoretically incapable of penetrating the blood/brain barrier and fairly specific (as a derivative of the natural MCH_1 agonist MCH) would have an effect *in vivo*, as it was already known to be active i.c.v. (Audinot et al., 2009). S38151 appears to fulfill the task. Indeed, despite a longer stability than unmodified peptides, its stability in blood remains too low to expect further reasonable activity in humans. However, it remains interesting to note that the blockade of the N-terminus of the peptide with a *para*-guanidinobenzoyl moiety may enhance its stability in biological media.

Furthermore, we were unable to detect traces of this pseudopeptide in the brains of i.p.-injected animals. Similarly, its effect could not be correlated with aversion owing to a bad test. Finally, S38151 significantly reduced weight gain in rodent obesity models, and (most importantly) was inactive in our MCH_1-KO mouse model, strongly suggesting not only the nature of its target but also its potency and selectivity.

The process through which S38151 induces weight loss remains poorly understood at the molecular level. We hypothesize that it acts locally at the adipocyte level. Indeed, in their paper on a small, non-peptide antagonist (SCH-A) of MCH_1 activity, Kowalski et al. (2006) performed a careful and complete study to describe the mechanism of action of this compound at the adipocyte level. To our knowledge, few peptide MCH agonists or antagonists have been used *in vivo*. Indeed, as reviewed by

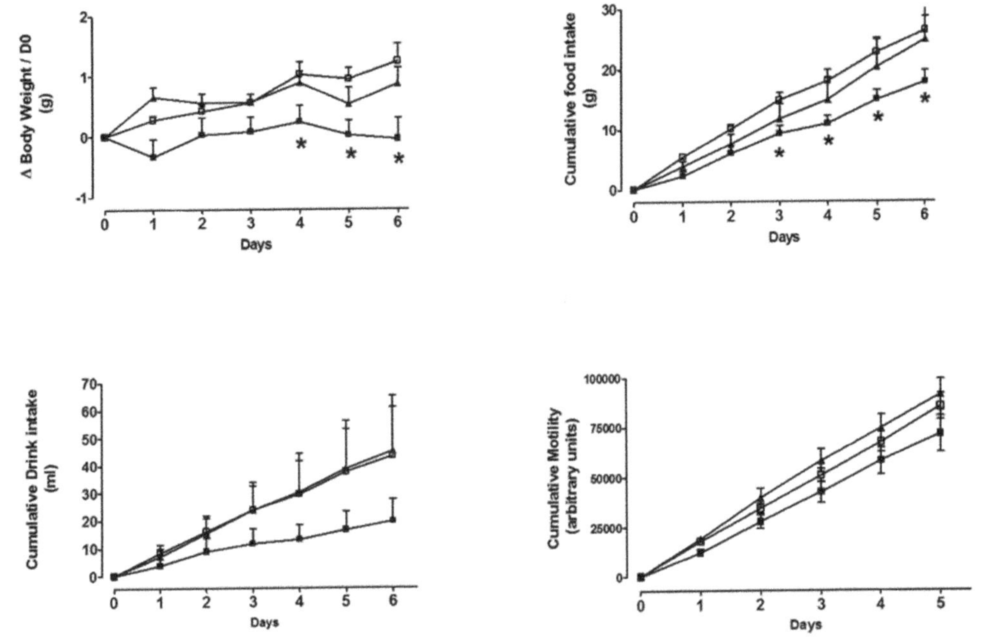

FIGURE 8 | The effects of repeated daily S38151 injection on food and water intake, body weight, and motility in *ob/ob* mice. Genetically modified *ob/ob* mice were administered S38151 (10 and 30 mg/kg, i.p.) or vehicle (normal saline i.p.) for 6 consecutive days. Results are expressed as mean ± SEM ($n = 8$ mice per group). White squares for controls, dark squares for 10 mg/kg, and dark triangles for 30 mg/kg. Repeated measures Two-Way ANOVA (treatment × time) was followed by complementary analysis of each treatment's effect at a fixed level of time to compare all groups of mice with the control group. $^{*}P < 0.05$.

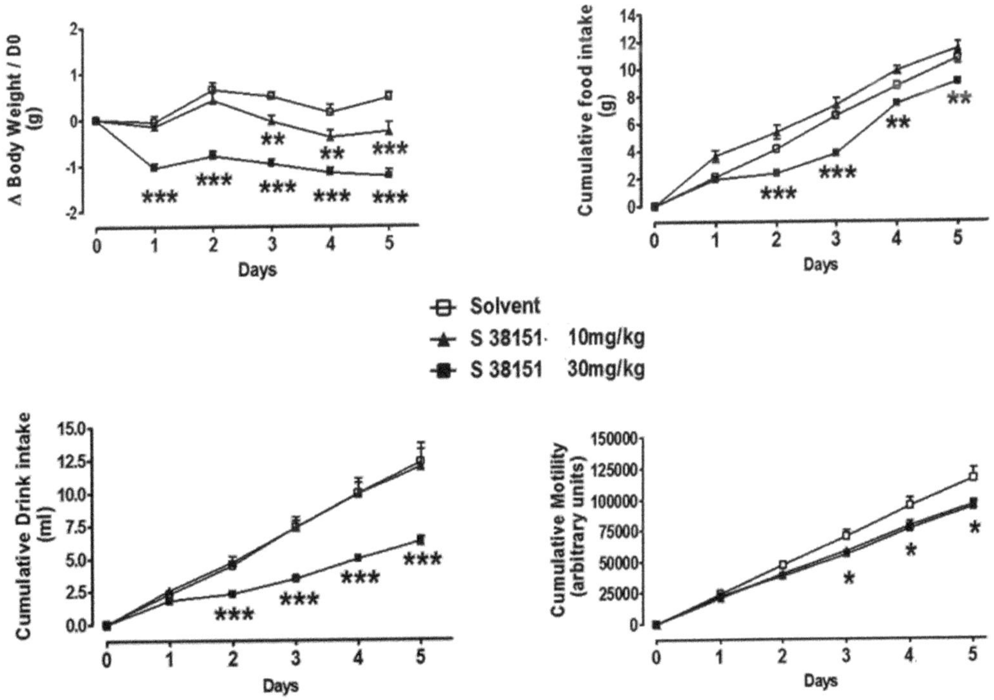

FIGURE 9 | The effects of repeated daily S38151 injection on food and water intake, body weight, and motility in diet-induced obese (DIO) mice. DIO mice were administered S38151 (10 and 30 mg/kg, i.p.) or vehicle (normal saline i.p.) for 5 consecutive days. Results are expressed as mean ± SEM ($n = 8$ mice per group). Repeated measures Two-Way ANOVA (treatment × time) was followed by complementary analysis of each treatment's effect at a fixed level of time to compare all groups of mice with the control group. $^{*}P < 0.05$, $^{**}P < 0.01$, $^{***}P < 0.001$.

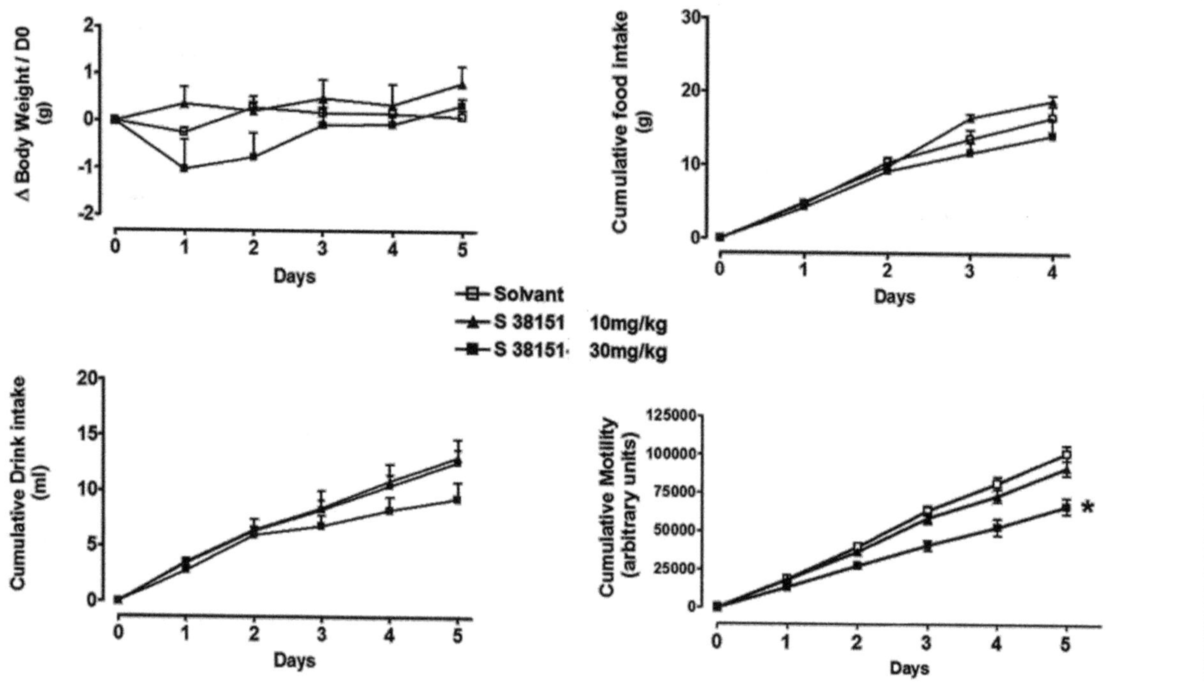

FIGURE 10 | The effects of repeated daily S38151 injection on food and water intake, body weight, and motility in MCHR1-KO mice. MCH_1-KO mice were administered S38151 (10 and 30 mg/kg, i.p.) or vehicle (normal saline i.p.) for 5 consecutive days. Results are expressed as mean ± SEM ($n = 8$ mice per group). Repeated measures Two-Way ANOVA (treatment × time) was followed by complementary analysis of each treatment's effect at a fixed level of time to compare all groups of mice with the control group. $*P < 0.05$.

Bednarek (2007), peptide ligands at MCH_1 were used *in vivo* by Mashiko et al. (2005) and Shearman et al. (2003) to demonstrate the effects of peptide MCH_1 antagonists on diet-induced obesity. Both compounds were administered through i.c.v. injection. To our knowledge, none of the reported agonists or antagonists was administered through i.p. injection. The validation of the agonistic nature of MCH, MCH derivatives, or peptides derived from them, has been reported on several occasions regarding feeding behavior, and has always involved administration through i.c.v. injection (Suply et al., 2001) or on their other effects (Chung et al., 2009; Lagos et al., 2009). All of these data have been reviewed by MacNeil and Bednarek (2009).

ACKNOWLEDGMENTS

The authors would like to thank Marc Bertrand and his team (TES, Orléans, France) for their work on S38151 stability.

REFERENCES

Adamantidis, A., and de Lecea, L. (2009). A role for Melanin-Concentrating Hormone in learning and memory. *Peptides* 30, 2066–2070.

Audinot, V., Beauverger, P., Lahaye, C., Suply, T., Rodriguez, M., Ouvry, C., et al. (2001a). Structure-activity relationship studies of melanin-concentrating hormone (MCH)-related peptide ligands at SLC-1, the human MCH receptor. *J. Biol. Chem.* 276, 13554–13562.

Audinot, V., Lahaye, C., Suply, T., Beauverger, P., Rodriguez, M., Galizzi, J. P., et al. (2001b). [125I]-S36057: a new and highly potent radioligand for the melanin-concentrating hormone receptor. *Br. J. Pharmacol.* 133, 371–378.

Audinot, V., Della Zuana, O., Fabry, N., Ouvry, C., Nosjean, O., Henlin, J. M., et al. (2009). S38151 [p-guanidinobenzoyl-[Des-Gly(10)]-MCH(7-17)] is a potent and selective antagonist at the MCH(1) receptor and has anti-feeding properties *in vivo*. *Peptides* 30, 1997–2007.

Bachner, D., Kreienkamp, H., Weise, C., Buck, F., and Richter, D. (1999). Identification of melanin concentrating hormone (MCH) as the natural ligand for the orphan somatostatin-like receptor 1 (SLC-1). *FEBS Lett.* 457, 522–524.

Bednarek, M. A. (2007). Peptide ligands for the melanin-concentrating hormone (MCH) receptor 1. *Curr. Top. Med. Chem.* 7, 1425–1432.

Bittencourt, J., and Celis, M. E. (2008). Anatomy, function and regulation of neuropeptide EI (NEI). *Peptides* 29, 1441–1450.

Bittencourt, J. C., Presse, F., Arias, C., Peto, C., Vaughan, J., Nahon, J. L., et al. (1992). The melanin-concentrating hormone system of the rat brain: an immuno- and hybridization histochemical characterization. *J. Comp. Neurol.* 319, 218–245.

Block, M. H., Boyer, S., Brailsford, W., Brittain, D. R., Carroll, D., Chapman, S., et al. (2002). Discovery and optimization of a series of carbazole ureas as NPY5 antagonists for the treatment of obesity. *J. Med. Chem.* 45, 3509–3523.

Borowsky, B., Durkin, M. M., Ogozalek, K., Marzabadi, M. R., DeLeon, J., Lagu, B., et al. (2002). Antidepressant, anxiolytic and anorectic effects of a melanin-concentrating hormone-1 receptor antagonist. *Nat. Med.* 8, 825–830.

Bradley, R. L., Kokkotou, E. G., Maratos-Flier, E., and Cheatham, B. (2000). Melanin-concentrating hormone regulates leptin synthesis and secretion in rat adipocytes. *Diabetes* 49, 1073–1077.

Chambers, J., Ames, R. S., Bergsma, D., Muir, A., Fitzgerald, L. R., Hervieu, G., et al. (1999). Melanin-concentrating hormone is the cognate ligand for the orphan G-protein-coupled receptor SLC-1. *Nature* 400, 261–265.

Chen, Y., Hu, C., Hsu, C. K., Zhang, Q., Bi, C., Asnicar, M., et al. (2002). Targeted disruption of the melanin-concentrating hormone receptor-1 results in hyperphagia and resistance to diet-induced obesity. *Endocrinology* 143, 2469–2477.

Chung, S., Hopf, F. W., Nagasaki, H., Li, C. Y., Belluzzi, J. D., Bonci, A., et al. (2009). The melanin-concentrating hormone system modulates cocaine reward. *Proc. Natl. Acad. Sci. U.S.A.* 106, 6772–6777.

Criscione, L., Rigollier, P., Batzl-Hartmann, C., Rueger, H., Stricker-Krongrad, A., Wyss, P., et al. (1998). Food intake in free-feeding and energy-deprived lean rats is mediated by the neuropeptide Y5 receptor. *J. Clin. Invest.* 102, 2136–2145.

Garcia-Fuster, M. J., Parks, G. S., Clinton, S. M., Watson, S. J., Akil, H., and Civelli, O. (2012). The melanin-concentrating hormone (MCH) system in an animal model of depression-like behavior. *Eur. Neuropsychopharmacol.* 22, 607–613.

Hervieu, G., and Nahon, J. L. (1995). Pro-melanin concentrating hormone messenger ribonucleic acid and peptides expression in peripheral tissues of the rat. *Neuroendocrinology* 61, 348–364.

Hervieu, G. J. (2006). Further insights into the neurobiology of melanin-concentrating hormone in energy and mood balances. *Expert Opin. Ther. Targets* 10, 211–229.

Johansson, A. (2011). Recent progress in the discovery of melanin-concentrating hormone 1-receptor antagonists. *Expert Opin. Ther. Pat.* 21, 905–925.

Kawauchi, H., Kawazoe, I., Tsubokawa, M., Kishida, M., and Baker, B. I. (1983). Characterization of melanin-concentrating hormone in chum salmon pituitaries. *Nature* 305, 321–323.

Kowalski, T. J., Spar, B. D., Weig, B., Farley, C., Cook, J., Ghibaudi, L., et al. (2006). Effects of a selective melanin-concentrating hormone 1 receptor antagonist on food intake and energy homeostasis in diet-induced obese mice. *Eur. J. Pharmacol.* 535, 182–191.

Lagos, P., Torterolo, P., Jantos, H., Chase, M. H., and Monti, J. M. (2009). Effects on sleep of melanin-concentrating hormone (MCH) microinjections into the dorsal raphe nucleus. *Brain Res.* 1265, 103–110.

Lagos, P., Urbanavicius, J., Scorza, M. C., Miraballes, R., and Torterolo, P. (2011). Depressive-like profile induced by MCH microinjections into the dorsal raphe nucleus evaluated in the forced swim test. *Behav. Brain Res.* 218, 259–266.

Lakaye, B., Minet, A., Zorzi, W., and Grisar, T. (1998). Cloning of the rat brain cDNA encoding for the SLC-1 G protein-coupled receptor reveals the presence of an intron in the gene. *Biochim. Biophys. Acta* 1401, 216–220.

MacNeil, D. J., and Bednarek, M. A. (2009). MCH receptor peptide agonists and antagonists. *Peptides* 30, 2008–2013.

Madden, L. J., Seeley, R. J., and Woods, S. C. (1999). Intraventricular neuropeptide Y decreases need-induced sodium appetite and increases pica in rats. *Behav. Neurosci.* 113, 826–832.

Marsh, D. J., Weingarth, D. T., Novi, D. E., Chen, H. Y., Trumbauer, M. E., Chen, A. S., et al. (2002). Melanin-concentrating hormone 1 receptor-deficient mice are lean, hyperactive, and hyperphagic and have altered metabolism. *Proc. Natl. Acad. Sci. U.S.A.* 99, 3240–3245.

Mashiko, S., Ishihara, A., Gomori, A., Moriya, R., Ito, M., Iwaasa, H., et al. (2005). Antiobesity effect of a melanin-concentrating hormone 1 receptor antagonist in diet-induced obese mice. *Endocrinology* 146, 3080–3086.

Maulon-Feraille, L., Della-Zuana, O., Suply, T., Rovere-Jovene, C., Audinot, V., Levens, N., et al. (2002). Appetite-boosting property of pro-melanin-concentrating hormone(131-165) (neuropeptide-glutamic acid-isoleucine) is associated with proteolytic resistance. *J. Pharmacol. Exp. Ther.* 302, 766–773.

Mendez-Andino, J. L., and Wos, J. A. (2007). MCH-R1 antagonists: what is keeping most research programs away from the clinic? *Drug Discov. Today* 12, 972–979.

Meyers, K. M., Mendez-Andino, J. L., Colson, A. O., Warshakoon, N. C., Wos, J. A., Mitchell, M. C., et al. (2007). Aminomethyl tetrahydronaphthalene ketopiperazine MCH-R1 antagonists–Increasing selectivity over hERG. *Bioorg. Med. Chem. Lett.* 17, 819–822.

Mori, M., Harada, M., Terao, Y., Sugo, T., Watanabe, T., Shimomura, Y., et al. (2001). Cloning of a novel G protein-coupled receptor, SLT, a subtype of the melanin-concentrating hormone receptor. *Biochem. Biophys. Res. Commun.* 283, 1013–1018.

Nahon, J. L., Presse, F., Bittencourt, J. C., Sawchenko, P. E., and Vale, W. (1989). The rat melanin-concentrating hormone messenger ribonucleic acid encodes multiple putative neuropeptides coexpressed in the dorsolateral hypothalamus. *Endocrinology* 125, 2056–2065.

Nair, R. P., and Ren, J. (2009). Pharmacotherapy of obesity – benefit, bias and hyperbole. *Curr. Med. Chem.* 16, 1888–1897.

Peyron, C., Sapin, E., Leger, L., Luppi, P. H., and Fort, P. (2009). Role of the melanin-concentrating hormone neuropeptide in sleep regulation. *Peptides* 30, 2052–2059.

Pissios, P. (2009). Animals models of MCH function and what they can tell us about its role in energy balance. *Peptides* 30, 2040–2044.

Pissios, P., Bradley, R. L., and Maratos-Flier, E. (2006). Expanding the scales: the multiple roles of MCH in regulating energy balance and other biological functions. *Endocr. Rev.* 27, 606–620.

Qu, D., Ludwig, D. S., Gammeltoft, S., Piper, M., Pelleymounter, M. A., Cullen, M. J., et al. (1996). A role for melanin-concentrating hormone in the central regulation of feeding behaviour. *Nature* 380, 243–247.

Rodriguez, M., Beauverger, P., Naime, I., Rique, H., Ouvry, C., Souchaud, S., et al. (2001). Cloning and molecular characterization of the novel human melanin-concentrating hormone receptor MCH2. *Mol. Pharmacol.* 60, 632–639.

Roy, M., David, N., Cueva, M., and Giorgetti, M. (2007). A study of the involvement of melanin-concentrating hormone receptor 1 (MCHR1) in murine models of depression. *Biol. Psychiatry* 61, 174–180.

Sailer, A. W., Sano, H., Zeng, Z., McDonald, T. P., Pan, J., Pong, S. S., et al. (2001). Identification and characterization of a second melanin-concentrating hormone receptor, MCH-2R. *Proc. Natl. Acad. Sci. U.S.A.* 98, 7564–7569.

Saito, Y., Nothacker, H. P., Wang, Z., Lin, S. H., Leslie, F., and Civelli, O. (1999). Molecular characterization of the melanin-concentrating-hormone receptor. *Nature* 400, 265–269.

Shearman, L. P., Camacho, R. E., Sloan, S. D., Zhou, D., Bednarek, M. A., Hreniuk, D. L., et al. (2003). Chronic MCH-1 receptor modulation alters appetite, body weight and adiposity in rats. *Eur. J. Pharmacol.* 475, 37–47.

Suply, T., Della, Z. O., Audinot, V., Rodriguez, M., Beauverger, P., Duhault, J., et al. (2001). SLC-1 receptor mediates effect of melanin-concentrating hormone on feeding behavior in rat: a structure-activity study. *J. Pharmacol. Exp. Ther.* 299, 137–146.

Takekawa, S., Asami, A., Ishihara, Y., Terauchi, J., Kato, K., Shimomura, Y., et al. (2002). T-226296: a novel, orally active and selective melanin-concentrating hormone receptor antagonist. *Eur. J. Pharmacol.* 438, 129–135.

Vaughan, J. M., Fischer, W. H., Hoeger, C., Rivier, J., and Vale, W. (1989). Characterization of melanin-concentrating hormone from rat hypothalamus. *Endocrinology* 125, 1660–1665.

Wang, S., Behan, J., O'Neill, K., Weig, B., Fried, S., Laz, T., et al. (2001). Identification and pharmacological characterization of a novel human melanin-concentrating hormone receptor, mch-r2. *J. Biol. Chem.* 276, 34664–34670.

Welzl, H., D'Adamo, P., and Lipp, H. P. (2001). Conditioned taste aversion as a learning and memory paradigm. *Behav. Brain Res.* 125, 205–213.

17

Central urocortin 3 and type 2 corticotropin-releasing factor receptor in the regulation of energy homeostasis: critical involvement of the ventromedial hypothalamus

Peilin Chen[1†], Christine Van Hover[2†], Daniel Lindberg[1] and Chien Li[1]*

[1] Department of Pharmacology, University of Virginia Health System, Charlottesville, VA, USA
[2] Department of Neuroscience, University of Virginia Health System, Charlottesville, VA, USA

Edited by:
Hubert Vaudry, University of Rouen, France

Reviewed by:
Tamás Kozicz, Radboud University Nijmegen, Netherlands
Eric Zorrilla, The Scripps Research Institute, USA

***Correspondence:**
Chien Li, Department of Pharmacology, University of Virginia Health System, P.O. Box 800735, 1300 Jefferson Park Avenue, Charlottesville, VA 22908, USA.
e-mail: cl4xd@virginia.edu

† Peilin Chen and Christine Van Hover have contributed equally to this work.

The vital role of the corticotropin-releasing factor (CRF) peptide family in the brain in coordinating response to stress has been extensively documented. The effects of CRF are mediated by two G-protein-coupled receptors, type 1 and type 2 CRF receptors (CRF_1 and CRF_2). While the functional role of CRF_1 in hormonal and behavioral adaptation to stress is well-known, the physiological significance of CRF_2 remains to be fully appreciated. Accumulating evidence has indicated that CRF_2 and its selective ligands including urocortin 3 (Ucn 3) are important molecular mediators in regulating energy balance. Ucn 3 is the latest addition of the CRF family of peptides and is highly selective for CRF_2. Recent studies have shown that central Ucn 3 is important in a number of homeostatic functions including suppression of feeding, regulation of blood glucose levels, and thermoregulation, thus reinforcing the functional role of central CRF_2 in metabolic regulation. The brain loci that mediate the central effects of Ucn 3 remain to be fully determined. Anatomical and functional evidence has suggested that the ventromedial hypothalamus (VMH), where CRF_2 is prominently expressed, appears to be instrumental in mediating the effects of Ucn 3 on energy balance, permitting Ucn 3-mediated modulation of feeding and glycemic control. Thus, the Ucn 3-VMH CRF_2 system is an important neural pathway in the regulation of energy homeostasis and potentially plays a critical role in energy adaptation in response to metabolic perturbations and stress to maintain energy balance.

Keywords: CRF, Ucn 3, VMH, energy balance, feeding, glucose

INTRODUCTION

Corticotropin-releasing factor (CRF) was discovered in 1981 by Vale and colleagues at the Salk Institute (Vale et al., 1981). Its existence had been hypothesized for many years prior to the 1981 paper characterizing the amino acid sequence of the peptide. Since then, the importance of CRF family of peptides and receptors in stress has steadily emerged. Extensive investigation has demonstrated that CRF is critical in regulating the hypothalamic-pituitary-adrenal (HPA) axis and in integrating endocrine, autonomic, and behavioral responses to stressors (Perrin and Vale, 1999).

In addition to CRF, additional members of the CRF peptide family including urocortins (Ucns) 1, 2, and 3 have been identified in mammals, including humans (Vaughan et al., 1995; Hsu and Hsueh, 2001; Lewis et al., 2001; Reyes et al., 2001). Accumulating evidence suggests that the central actions of Ucn peptides may account for some stress-related effects originally attributed to CRF (Bale and Vale, 2004; Hashimoto et al., 2004; Venihaki et al., 2004; Jamieson et al., 2006; Kuperman et al., 2010). For example, Ucn 1 appears to be involved in the later stage of the stress response and adaptation to stress, while Ucns 2 and 3 may be involved in attenuating the stress response (Ryabinin et al., 2012).

Additionally, the Ucns have been shown to be involved in various physiological regulations including energy balance, cardiovascular function, and behavioral modulation. Ucn 1, 2, and 3 all suppress feeding (Spina et al., 1996; Hashimoto et al., 2004; Fekete et al., 2007), and deficiency in Ucn 2 improves glucose and insulin homeostasis (Chen et al., 2006). Ucn 1 and 2 decrease cardiac output and heart rate, and may be protective against ischemia (Latchman, 2002; Bale et al., 2004; Hashimoto et al., 2004). Behaviorally, Ucn 1 plays a critical role in anxiety-like and depressive behavior, and may be involved in the predisposition of alcohol consumption (Vetter et al., 2002; Ryabinin et al., 2012). Ucn 2 may be linked to depression but not anxiety (Ryabinin et al., 2012). Ucn 2 appears to influence social behavior, including aggression (Breu et al., 2012), as mice deficient in Ucn 2 are less aggressive and prefer passive social interaction. Finally, Ucn 1 and CRF receptors have been found in the auditory system (Graham et al., 2010) and the peptide appears to be involved in the development and maintenance of hearing (Vetter et al., 2002).

Urocortin 3 is the latest addition of the CRF family of peptides, initially identified in the brains of humans and rodents (Hsu and Hsueh, 2001; Lewis et al., 2001). Sequence analyses show that Ucn 3 is more closely related to Ucn 2 than Ucn 1 or CRF. Human and mouse Ucn 3 share 40% homology with human and mouse Ucn 2, but only 21 and 18%, respectively, with human and mouse Ucn 1 and 32 and 26% with CRF (Lewis et al., 2001). Accumulating evidence, as discussed below, has suggested that Ucn 3 is a critical regulator in energy homeostasis.

CORTICOTROPHIN-RELEASING FACTOR RECEPTORS

Two receptors have been identified for CRF: type 1 and type 2 CRF receptors (CRF_1 and CRF_2), and amino acid sequence analysis has shown that the two receptors share approximately 70% homology (Perrin and Vale, 1999; Bale and Vale, 2004). Both CRF_1 and CRF_2 are G-protein-coupled receptors with seven transmembrane domains. These receptors signal predominantly through increased cAMP production, but additional signaling pathways including Ca^{2+}, mitogen-activated protein kinase (MAPK), phospholipase C, protein kinase B, and ion channels have also been shown to couple to CRFRs (Kiang, 1997; Grammatopoulos, 2000; Brar et al., 2002). The two receptors differ significantly in their binding affinity for CRF peptides and anatomical distribution within the central nervous system (Chalmers et al., 1995; Van Pett et al., 2000; Hsu and Hsueh, 2001; Lewis et al., 2001). Biochemical studies have shown that CRF binds CRF_1 with high affinity while showing modest affinity for CRF_2 (Bale and Vale, 2004). Ucn 1 binds both CRF_1 and CRF_2 with equally high affinity while Ucn 2 and Ucn 3 demonstrate preferential specificity for CRF_2. However, while Ucn 2 may bind and stimulate CRF_1 at high, pharmacological concentrations (Reyes et al., 2001), Ucn 3 is highly selective to CRF_2 and displays minimal affinity for CRF_1 (Hsu and Hsueh, 2001; Lewis et al., 2001).

A circulating protein has been identified that binds CRF. It has been suggested that the function of CRF binding protein (CRFBP) is mainly to sequester CRF to reduce its HPA axis stimulation. Levels of CRFBP are elevated in pregnancy to dampen the negative effect of stress responses on the developing fetus (Goland, 1986). In addition to CRFBP, a splice variant of CRF_2 has been identified that contains only the extracellular domain of the receptor and shown to circulate, bind, and sequester CRF as well (Bon et al., 1997; Chen et al., 2005). This splice variant also binds Ucn 1 but has very low affinity for Ucn 2 and 3 (Chen et al., 2005).

Anatomical mapping studies have demonstrated that CRF_1 and CRF_2 have distinct distributions in the brain. CRF_1 has a wide distribution throughout the brain with high density in the medial septal area, amygdala, and cerebellum (Chalmers et al., 1995; Van Pett et al., 2000). CRF_2 has three major variants that differ in their N-terminal domains: $CRF_{2(a)}$, $CRF_{2(b)}$, and $CRF_{2(c)}$. In murine brains, $CRF_{2(a)}$ is predominantly expressed in the hypothalamus, lateral septum (LS), and dorsal raphe (Chalmers et al., 1995; Van Pett et al., 2000). $CRF_{2(b)}$ is found predominantly in the periphery, including in skeletal muscle, the gastrointestinal tract, and the heart (Kanno, 1999; Wiley and Davenport, 2004; Porcher et al., 2005; Tache and Bonaz, 2007). $CRF_{2(c)}$ is found only in the human brain (Kostich et al., 1998).

The function of CRF_1 has been closely associated with the stress response, including the release of adrenocorticotropic hormone (ACTH) from the anterior pituitary and behavioral adaptation to stressors (Bale and Vale, 2004). The physiological role of CRF_2, however, is less defined. Functional studies have shown this receptor is involved in an array of homeostatic regulations, with most of its actions regulating energy balance by modulating feeding, blood glucose levels, and energy expenditure. This review will focus on recent advances in the understanding of the physiological role of CRF_2 and Ucn 3 in the brain, particularly in the hypothalamus, in the regulation of energy balance.

CRF_2 IN ENERGY HOMEOSTASIS

Loss-of-function studies with CRF_2 null mice and pharmacological studies with CRF_2 agonists both suggest that endogenous CRF_2 plays a physiological role in energy balance. Evidence from several studies that examined ingestive behavior of CRF_2 null mice showed that endogenous CRF_2 is required for the anorectic effect of CRF peptide and is involved in control of the meal size during active phase of eating and following acute exposure to the stress (Bale et al., 2000; Coste et al., 2000; Pelleymounter et al., 2000; Tabarin et al., 2007). Similarly, infusion of antisense oligonucleotides to CRF_2 mRNA attenuates both CRF and Ucn 1-induced hypophagia and corticosterone secretion (Smagin et al., 1998). Furthermore, CRF_2 deletion protects mice from high-fat diet-induced insulin resistance and glucose intolerance (Bale et al., 2003). Taken together, it is clear that CRF_2 is responsible for mediating the effect of CRF family peptides on the suppression of feeding and is involved in corticosterone secretion and glucose homeostasis.

In addition to feeding, CRF_2 is involved in regulating energy expenditure. CRF_2 knockout (KO) mice have more active metabolism and lose heat faster than wildtype (WT) mice (Carlin et al., 2006), suggesting an exaggerated level of sympathetic activity. Moreover, CRF_2 KO mice have higher brown adipose tissue (BAT) temperature and, when given a choice between room temperature and warm areas, prefer warmer areas more than WT mice (Carlin et al., 2006). The KO mice also have higher oxygen consumption and carbon dioxide production and reduced respiratory exchange rate (Carlin et al., 2006), indicating a preference in fatty acid oxidation over carbohydrate utilization in the KO mice. It was suggested that a lack of functional CRF_2 leads to elevated CRF_1 activity, which consequently increases sympathetic nervous system (SNS) activity to promote lipolysis (Carlin et al., 2006). This hypothesis appears to disagree with pharmacological studies, as activation of central CRF_2 (discussed below), in most cases, results in increased SNS activity. This apparent discrepancy may result from a number of possibilities including compensatory mechanisms due to total body KO of the receptor as compared to acute, local stimulation of the receptor in the brain. Obviously more studies are needed to further elucidate this issue.

Leptin, a hormone secreted by adipocytes, is a potent appetite suppressant (Uehara et al., 1998; Zigman, 2003). A number of studies suggest that its effect on feeding may involve the CRF receptor system. Though leptin treatment greatly decreases food intake, when co-administered with a non-selective CRF receptor antagonist, food intake remains at a nearly normal level (Gardner et al., 1998), suggesting the CRF system is a downstream target of leptin in the brain. However, this notion was recently challenged by a study (Harris, 2010) demonstrating that CRF_2 is not essential for the effects of leptin on energy balance, including feeding and body weight regulation. Again this discrepancy may be due to the nature of global CRF_2 KO, which potentially results in functional compensation such as exaggerated CRF_1 activity in these mice (Carlin et al., 2006). Therefore, central or specific brain area deletions of CRF_2 may be necessary to further evaluate the interaction of leptin and the CRF system in the brain.

UROCORTIN 3

ANATOMICAL LOCATION OF Ucn 3

Urocortin 3 is found both in the periphery and in the brain. In the periphery, it is expressed in the digestive tract, muscle, thyroid and adrenal glands, pancreas, heart, spleen, and skin (Hsu and Hsueh, 2001; Lewis et al., 2001). In the brain, neurons expressing Ucn 3 are concentrated in the medial amygdala (MeA) and hypothalamus (Lewis et al., 2001; Li et al., 2002). In the hypothalamus, the major Ucn 3 cell population is near the rostral perifornical hypothalamic area (rPFA; Li et al., 2002). Specifically, Ucn 3-positive cells are gathered around the fornix lateral to the paraventricular nucleus of the hypothalamus (PVH). This group extends rostrally and stays close to the fornix into the posterior part of the bed nucleus of the stria terminalis (pBNST) and medially into the anterior parvicellular part of the PVH (PVHap). A recent study has elucidated anatomical heterogeneity within this hypothalamic Ucn 3 cell population, as neurons of the rostral part (PVHap/pBNST) project to the ventromedial hypothalamus (VMH), and those of the caudal part, residing in the rostral perifornical hypothalamus (rPFH), projects to the LS (Chen et al., 2011). A second group of Ucn 3-positive cells is found in the median preoptic nucleus (MnPO; Li et al., 2002). In the forebrain, prominent Ucn 3 nerve fibers and terminals are found in the VMH, LS, MeA, and BNST (Li et al., 2002). These areas also express high levels of CRF_2 (Chalmers et al., 1995; Van Pett et al., 2000). This overlap of Ucn 3 and CRF_2 distribution and the high affinity of the peptide for the receptor strongly suggest that Ucn 3 is an endogenous ligand for CRF_2 in these brain areas.

METABOLIC EFFECTS OF Ucn 3

All 3 Ucns bind CRF_2 and may each be responsible for some of the receptor's energy homeostatic effects. However, Ucn 3 alone has myriad metabolic effects.

Feeding

Central administration, KO, and overexpression studies reveal a role of Ucn 3 in the regulation of feeding. When directly infused into the lateral ventricles, Ucn 3 decreases nocturnal food and water intake in a dose dependent manner, primarily due to decreased meal frequency, and this effect was eliminated with concomitant CRF_2 antagonist treatment (Fekete et al., 2007). The anorectic effect of Ucn 3 is not due to distaste for food, as no concurrent taste aversion develops (Fekete et al., 2007). Consistent with pharmacological evidence, genetic Ucn 3 deficiency appears to lead to overeating. Though Ucn 3 KO mice have similar body weights to WT animals, KO mice eat more and have increased accumulated food intake. Similar to CRF_2 null mice, Ucn 3 KO mice exhibit elevated nocturnal feeding, when greatest spontaneous food intake naturally occurs (Chao et al., 2012). Taken together, it is clear that Ucn 3 in the brain functions as a potent anorectic agent. However, a study that used genetic overexpression of Ucn 3 challenged this notion. Under regular chow-fed condition, mice with overexpression of Ucn 3 (*Ucn3+*) have higher body mass-adjusted food intake than WT and are heavier than WT controls due to increased lean body mass (Jamieson et al., 2011). On the other hand, *Ucn3+* mice do not gain as much weight as WT mice when fed with a high-fat diet (Jamieson et al., 2011). This result seems to be in line with the notion of Ucn 3 as an anorectic agent. The discrepancy between different mouse models can be due to a number of possibilities including the ramification of Ucn 3 overexpression both in the brain as well as in the periphery.

A temporally and spatially controlled viral approach to overexpress Ucn 3 in the rPFH shows that Ucn 3 in the rPFH does not modulate food intake (Kuperman et al., 2010), as mice with Ucn 3 overexpression in the rPFH ingest consume similar amount of food as control mice (Kuperman et al., 2010). The rPFH-specific Ucn 3-overexpressing mice show a trend toward being heavier, but retain the same fat–lean mass percentages as control mice (Kuperman et al., 2010). As mentioned above, Ucn 3 cells in the rPFH project mainly to the LS with minimal projection to the VMH. Therefore, it is reasonable to assume that CRF_2 in the LS will be overstimulated in this mouse model. Interestingly, a number of studies have shown that CRF_2 in the LS is involved in suppression of food intake (Wang and Kotz, 2002; Bakshi et al., 2007). Currently, it is unclear as to why overexpression of Ucn 3 in the rPFH fails to suppress feeding. The expression of CRF receptor has been shown to be subject to ligand-induced receptor down-regulation (Rabadan-Diehl et al., 1996; Eghbal-Ahmadi et al., 1997). It is conceivable that chronic elevated Ucn 3 input to the LS in Ucn 3 rPFH overexpression mice may lead to alteration in CRF_2 expression and consequently reduced response to Ucn 3 stimulation in the LS. Thus, it is possible that acute stimulation of CRF_2 in the LS suppresses feeding, but chronic stimulation of CRF_2 in the LS in mice with Ucn 3 overexpression in the rPFH may lead to negative feedback to balance the effect of CRF_2 in feeding. Clearly, more studies are needed to elucidate the effect of Ucn 3 overexpression in the regulation of food intake. In addition to Ucn 3, Ucn 1 neurons in the midbrain Edinger–Westphal nucleus have been shown to innervate the LS (Kozicz et al., 1998; Bittencourt et al., 1999). Therefore, both Ucn 1 and 3 may contribute to the effect of CRF_2 on feeding in the LS.

The mechanism of Ucn 3-induced anorexia has not been directly studied. Central administration of CRF_2 agonists, including Ucn 3, have been shown to inhibit gastric emptying (Martinez et al., 2004; Stengel and Tache, 2009), and elevate blood glucose levels (Jamieson et al., 2006; Chen et al., 2010). Both reduced gut motility and hyperglycemia have been shown to induce satiation and reduce feeding (Ritter, 2004; Cummings and Overduin, 2007; Wolfgang et al., 2007; Cha et al., 2008). Therefore, multiple mechanisms are potentially involved in mediating the anorectic effect of Ucn 3 in the brain.

Energy homeostasis

Similarly to CRF_2, Ucn 3 is also involved in energy expenditure. Central administration of Ucn 3 increases motor activity (Ohata and Shibasaki, 2004). Similarly, transgenic Ucn 3 overexpression mice (*Ucn3+*) have an increased respiratory exchange ratio and increased motor activity in their home cages (Jamieson et al., 2011). Furthermore, mice with Ucn 3 overexpressed in the rPFH had an increased respiratory exchange ratio and elevated heat production (Kuperman et al., 2010). This is consistent with the notion that Ucn 3 is involved in SNS activity and energy homeostasis. Ucn 3 KO mice, on the other hand, do not show the same pattern; there are no differences in oxygen consumption, heat production, or activity levels (Chao et al., 2012). Therefore, KO of Ucn 3 in specific brain areas may provide better insight into the role of specific populations of Ucn 3 cells in the brain in energy expenditure.

Glucose homeostasis

Several studies have revealed a complex role of Ucn 3 in glucose homeostasis. Though adult Ucn 3 KO mice fed a chow diet show no differences in glucose tolerance and insulin sensitivity compared to WT mice (Li et al., 2007), Ucn 3 KOs have lower basal insulin levels and show a greater rebound in blood glucose levels after the initial hypoglycemia during an insulin tolerance test (Li et al., 2007; Chao et al., 2012). Furthermore, under high-fat diet feeding, adult KO mice are more metabolically resilient. The Ucn 3 KO mice have lower plasma insulin and blood glucose concentrations than WT mice, remain sensitive to insulin and do not develop glucose intolerance and liver steatosis with the same frequency of WT mice (Li et al., 2007). Moreover, aged KO mice show better glucose homeostasis than age-matched WT mice (Li et al., 2007). Overall, Ucn 3 deficiency appears to protect the mice from metabolic disorders caused by high-fat feeding. It is noteworthy that Ucn 3 is expressed in pancreatic β cells and has been shown to play a critical role as a local regulator in insulin secretion (Li et al., 2003). Thus, it is likely that Ucn 3 in both the brain and in the periphery, especially in the pancreas, contribute to the phenotypes observed in Ucn 3 null mice.

On the other hand, *Ucn3+* transgenic mice also appear to be protected against excessive metabolic challenge, having decreased fed and fasting blood glucose levels and increased tolerance to glucose when challenged in a glucose tolerance test (Jamieson et al., 2011). Fasting insulin levels in *Ucn3+* mice are also lower than that in WT mice, though an insulin tolerance test shows no differences in insulin sensitivity (Jamieson et al., 2011). When challenged with a high-fat diet, *Ucn3+* mice fare better than the WT littermates, maintaining normal body weight and low blood glucose levels, but display comparable insulin sensitivity to the WT control mice (Jamieson et al., 2011). Though *Ucn3+* mice show improved glucose homeostasis and insulin sensitivity, overexpression of Ucn 3 in the rPFH produces the opposite effect; rPFH Ucn 3-overexpressing mice show reduced insulin sensitivity and increases basal insulin levels, however they show no difference in glucose tolerance (Kuperman et al., 2010).

While genetic KO of Ucn 3 appears to have metabolic protective qualities, the effect of Ucn 3 overexpression is unclear. Full body overexpression of Ucn 3 seems protective, while targeted overexpression within the rPFH appears metabolically detrimental. Interestingly, *Ucn3+* mice have lower fasting blood glucose levels and higher energy intake under basal conditions (Jamieson et al., 2011). As stated earlier, CRF_2 is expressed abundantly in a number of peripheral tissues including skeletal muscle (Perrin et al., 1995; Stenzel et al., 1995; Wiley and Davenport, 2004; Porcher et al., 2005; Kuperman et al., 2011). Stimulation of muscle CRF_2 has been shown to promote thermogenesis (Solinas et al., 2006). Moreover, muscle CRF_2 is involved in regulating skeletal muscle mass (Hinkle et al., 2003) and consistent with this notion, *Ucn3+* mice have increased muscle mass (Jamieson et al., 2011). Thus, it is conceivable that the improved glucose homeostasis of *Ucn3+* mice is due, at least in part, to stimulation of muscle CRF_2 by ectopic overexpression of Ucn 3 in the periphery.

Thermoregulation

Functional studies have shown that Ucn 3 is involved in thermoregulation, potentially acting on brown fat. It was found that Ucn 3 induced a significant increase in body temperature, from 37.2 to 38.6°C (99.0 to 101.5°F), when injected into the lateral ventricles of rats (Telegdy et al., 2006). Temperature gradually decreased after peaking 2 h after Ucn 3 administration, but remained significantly elevated for a total of 4 h (Telegdy et al., 2006). Moreover, pretreating animals with CRF_2 but not CRF_1 antagonists completely blocked Ucn 3-induced hyperthermia, indicating that the pyrogenic action of Ucn 3 is mediated by CRF_2 (Telegdy and Adamik, 2008). Noraminophenazone, a cyclooxygenase inhibitor, simultaneously applied with Ucn 3 also prevented the temperature increase and also attenuated the increase when administered 30 min after Ucn 3 treatment (Telegdy et al., 2006). This indicates that the arachidonic acid cascade forming prostaglandin is a downstream target of central Ucn 3 and CRF_2 system in thermoregulation. Currently, the brain loci that may mediate the effect of Ucn 3 in body temperature remain elusive. The MnPO is known to be a center for thermoregulation and expresses high concentrations of the prostaglandin receptor EP3 (Morrison et al., 2008). It has been shown that prostaglandins play an important role in the MnPO through EP3 to regulate body temperature (Morrison et al., 2008). Furthermore, the presence of a group of Ucn 3 cells in the MnPO (Li et al., 2002) suggests that Ucn 3 might be involved in MnPO mediates pyrogenic effects.

REGULATION OF Ucn 3 EXPRESSION IN THE BRAIN

The expression of Ucn 3 in the brain has been determined in a number of stress paradigms and metabolic challenges. It was found that restraint stress rapidly elevates Ucn 3 gene expression in the MeA and that the elevated Ucn 3 mRNA levels return to basal levels 4 h after the stress (Jamieson et al., 2006). Restraint stress also increases Ucn 3 mRNA levels in the rPFA but with a slower time course compared to that of the MeA (Venihaki et al., 2004; Jamieson et al., 2006). Adrenalectomy greatly elevates Ucn 3 expression in the rPFA, while corticosterone replacement returns the expression to a basal level (Jamieson et al., 2006). This result indicates that corticosterone may be involved in stress-mediated Ucn 3 gene expression in the rPFA. Hemorrhage decreases Ucn 3 expression in the MeA after 30 min, and 48 h of food deprivation also decreases Ucn 3 expression in the MeA (Jamieson et al., 2006).

The expression of Ucn 3 has also been examined in genetically obese rodent models. Food deprivation increases Ucn 3 mRNA expression in the dorsal part of the medial amygdala (MeD) in obese Fa/Fa Zuker rats and has no effect on Ucn 3 expression in the rPFH (Poulin et al., 2012). In contrast, lean Fa/? rats show increased Ucn 3 expression in the rPFH but not the MeD after food deprivation (Poulin et al., 2012). Ucn 3 mRNA expression returns to normal after 24 h of refeeding (Poulin et al., 2012). In ob/ob obese mice, Ucn 3 expression is significantly reduced in the MeA (**Figure 1**; Li and Vale, 2002), and leptin treatment reverses Ucn 3 expression in this area. Interestingly, pair-feeding in ob/ob mice

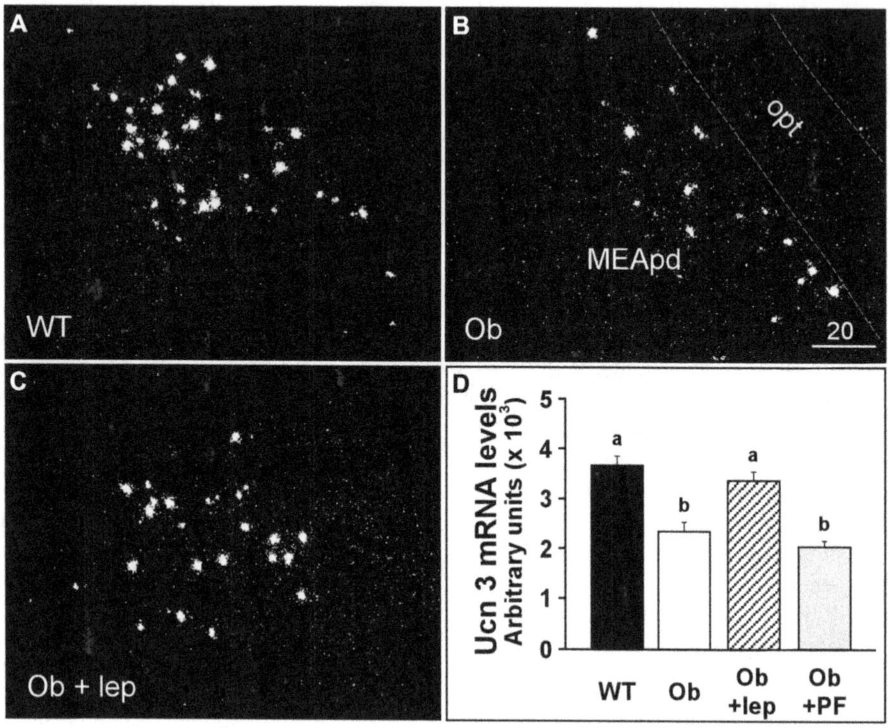

FIGURE 1 | Representative darkfield photomicrographs showing Ucn 3 mRNA expression (white clusters) in a wildtype mouse (A), an ob/ob obese mouse (B), and an ob/ob mouse treated with leptin (0.1 mg/kg/day for 2 days) (C). (D) Summary of Ucn 3 mRNA levels in the MeA of WT and Ob/ob obese mice treated with vehicle or leptin. The Ucn 3 mRNA levels in an additional group of Ob/ob mice that was paired-fed were also determined. Different letters represent statistical significance: $p < 0.05$. MeApd, medial nucleus of amygdala, posterodorsal part; opt, optic tract. Scale bar = 20 μm.

failed to modulate Ucn 3 expression in the MeA. These results indicate that Ucn 3 expression in the MeA is regulated by leptin. Taken together, these studies further support the notion that endogenous Ucn 3 in the brain is sensitive to metabolic signals and energy status and potentially plays an important role in regulating energy homeostasis.

THE VENTROMEDIAL HYPOTHALAMUS

The anatomical distribution of CRF_2 in the brain has provided important insight into possible areas that mediate the effects of CRF_2 in energy balance. The VMH has received significant attention due to its abundant expression of CRF_2 and well-known role in regulating energy homeostasis, feeding, and blood glucose levels.

The VMH is parceled on cytoarchitectonic grounds into three major divisions: dorsomedial (VMHdm), central, and the ventrolateral (VMHvl) parts (Gurdjian, 1927). The VMH volume is larger in males compared with females, and this difference is largely accounted for by the VMHvl, which in females is significantly smaller than that in males (Dugger et al., 2007). Further, VMHvl in female rats express higher levels of estrogen receptors than that in males, and has been shown to play a critical role in regulating lordosis behavior in females (Flanagan-Cato, 2011) and aggressiveness in males (Lin et al., 2011).

The VMH has long been considered a critical brain area in the regulation of energy homeostasis. Lesion of the VMH results in hyperphagia, hyperinsulinemia, reduction of SNS activity, increase of fat mass, and reduction of energy expenditure that ultimately leads to storage of excess of energy and obesity (Bernardis and Frohman, 1971; Inoue et al., 1977; Cox and Powley, 1981; Niijima et al., 1984; Sakaguchi et al., 1988; Ruffin and Nicolaidis, 1999; King, 2006). Conversely, stimulation of the VMH results in predominately opposite phenotypes including induction of satiety, increase in SNS activity, lipolysis, and thermogenesis (King, 2006). In recent years, the importance of the VMH in energy homeostasis has been further ascertained with the aid of improved molecular tools and mouse genetics (Sternson et al., 2005; King, 2006; Chao et al., 2012). For example, mice with VMH-specific deletion of a number of genes including the leptin receptor (Dhillon et al., 2006; Bingham et al., 2008), estrogen receptor α (Musatov et al., 2006, 2007), and vesicular glutamate transporter-2 (VGLUT2; Tong et al., 2007) result in a number of abnormalities such as increased feeding, reduced energy expenditure, impaired glucose homeostatic regulation, and obesity. Moreover, mice bearing a deletion of steroidogenic factor 1 (SF1), a transcription factor involved in steroidogenesis that is highly enriched in the VMH, show similar phenotypes in energy homeostasis and are obese (Luo et al., 1994; Sadovsky et al., 1995; Shinoda et al., 1995).

EXPRESSION OF CRF_2 IN THE VMH

The VMH is one of the brain areas with prominent CRF_2 expression (Chalmers et al., 1995; Van Pett et al., 2000). The expression is concentrated in the dorsomedial part of the nucleus with decreasing density toward the ventrolateral division of the VMH. The expression of CRF_2 in the VMH has been shown to be sensitive to energy status and stress. For example, leptin injection increases and fasting decreases CRF_2 expression in the VMH and ob/ob mice or Fa/Fa Zucker rats have lower CRF_2 in the VMH compared to WT controls (Richard et al., 1996; Makino et al., 1998, 1999; Nishiyama et al., 1999). Furthermore, restraint stress and glucocorticoids increase CRF_2 levels in the VMH (Makino et al., 1998, 1999). Thus, these data support the notion that CRF_2 in the VMH is important in regulating energy balance.

Currently, detailed neurochemical phenotypes of CRF_2-positive cells within the VMH remain unclear. Several proteins have been found to be expressed in the VMH including SF1, pituitary adenylate cyclase-activating polypeptide, the leptin receptor, and VGLUT2 (Fei et al., 1997; Elmquist et al., 1998; Ziegler et al., 2002; Segal et al., 2005; Kurrasch et al., 2007). It has been shown that CRF_2 extensively colocalizes with VGLUT2 in the VMH (Chen et al., 2010). VGLUT2 mediates glutamate uptake into synaptic vesicles of excitatory neurons (Fremeau et al., 2001; Herzog et al., 2001; Takamori et al., 2001) and has been used extensively as a marker for excitatory glutamatergic neurons. The colocalization of CRF_2 and VGLUT2 suggests that CRF_2 is expressed predominately in excitatory neurons in the VMH. As mentioned above, SF1 is a nuclear receptor that regulates the transcription of key genes involved in sexual development and reproduction (Parker et al., 2002). In adults, SF1 expression is specifically confined to the VMH (Parker et al., 2002). In SF1 null mice, CRF_2 mRNA expression is nearly undetectable in the VMH (Luo et al., 1994; Sadovsky et al., 1995; Shinoda et al., 1995), suggesting CRF_2 is expressed in SF1 cells in the VMH. Consistent with this notion, it was found that more than 90% of CRF_2 neurons in the dorsomedial part of the nucleus are also SF1-positive (**Figure 2**) with less colocalization of these two materials in the VMHvl (Digruccio et al., 2007).

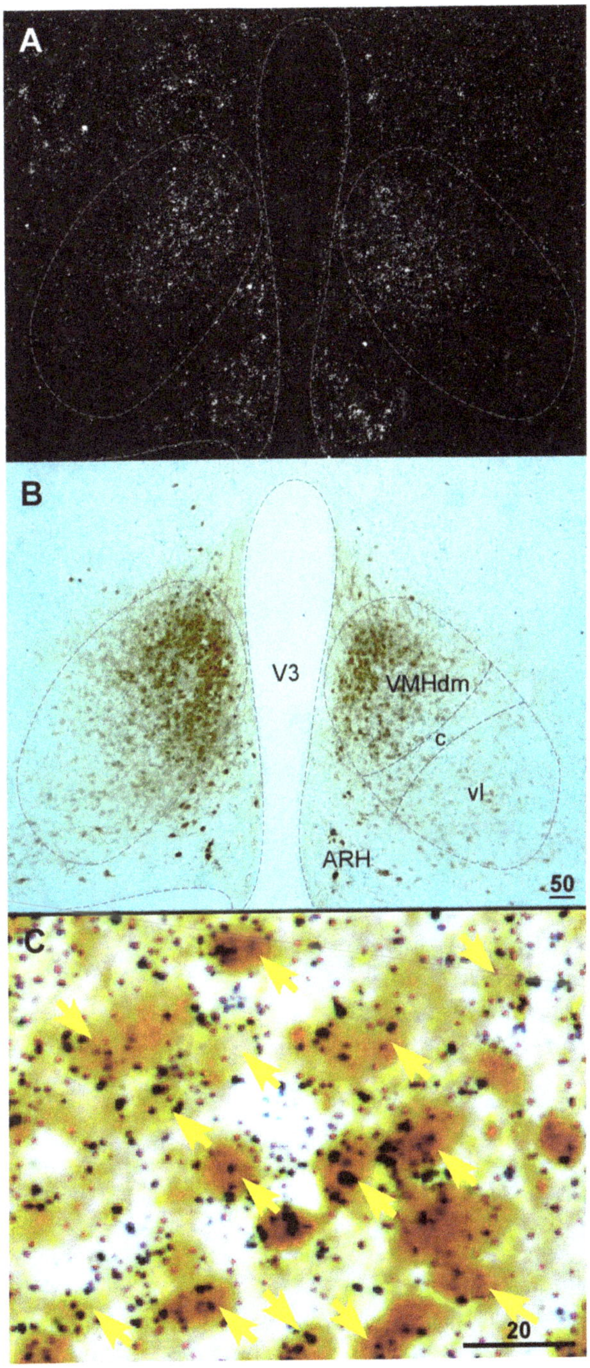

FIGURE 2 | (A) Darkfield photomicrograph showing CRFR2 mRNA signal revealed by *in situ* hybridization in the basal hypothalamic area of a transgenic mouse expressing Cre recombinase (Cre) and enhanced yellow fluorescent protein (EYFP) in SF1-positive cells. Note that CRFR2 mRNA hybridization signal (white clusters) was abundant in the dorsomedial part of the VMH (VMHdm). **(B)** Bright field photomicrograph of the same area in **(A)** showing SF1-positive cells, revealed by immunostaining with anti-green fluorescent protein antibody (darkbrown precipitates) in the VMH. **(C)** High magnification of boxed area in **(A)** showing colocalization of CRFR2 (black dot clusters) and SF1 (brown precipitates) in the VMH. ARH, arcuate nucleus of hypothalamus; V3, third ventricle; VMHc, central part of the VMH; VMHdm, dorsomedial part of the VMH; VMHvl, ventrolateral part of the VMH. Scale bar = 50 μm **(B)**, 20 μm **(C)**.

CRF LIGANDS INPUT INTO THE VMH

The anatomical distribution of a number of the CRF family peptides has been determined, and it was found that CRF and Ucn 1-expressing neurons provide minor innervation to the VMH (Swanson et al., 1983; Kozicz et al., 1998; Bittencourt et al., 1999). Interestingly, low levels of Ucn 1-immunoreactivity have been detected in cells in the VMH (Kozicz et al., 1998), suggesting Ucn 1 may be a local factor in the nucleus. Although Ucn 2 fiber distribution has not been determined, Ucn 2-positive cells have been found in a number of brain areas including the magnocellular part of the PVH, locus ceruleus, and facial motor nucleus (Reyes et al., 2001), and none of these areas provide extensive projection into the VMH (McBride and Sutin, 1977; Luiten and Room, 1980; Berk and Finkelstein, 1981; Kita and Oomura, 1982; Zaborszky, 1982; Fahrbach et al., 1989; Chen et al., 2011). Compared to other CRF innervations, Ucn 3 neuronal fibers abundantly innervate the VMH (Li et al., 2002). Similar to the expression of CRF_2 in the VMH, Ucn 3-positive axonal fibers and terminals concentrate in the dorsomedial part of the VMH with reduced density toward the ventrolateral part of the nucleus (Li et al., 2002). As stated above, Ucn 3 neurons in the PVHap provide the major Ucn 3 afferent input into the VMH and Ucn 3 cells in the pBNST and the MeA comparatively provide moderate input into the nucleus (Chen et al., 2011). Interestingly, Ucn 3 cells in the rPFH, immediately caudal and adjacent to the PVHap, provide minimal Ucn 3 afferent input into the VMH and instead send strong innervation into the LS.

Neural inputs into the PVHap and MeA have been studied (Sawchenko and Swanson, 1983; Swanson and Petrovich, 1998; Uehara et al., 1998; Maras and Petrulis, 2010; Carrillo et al., 2011; Northcutt and Lonstein, 2011; Radley and Sawchenko, 2011; Van Hover et al., 2011). In general, the two brain areas receive similar afferent input from a number of brain regions including the septal nuclei and amygdala. However, a few subtle but significant exceptions should be noted. The PVHap receives prominent inputs from the hypothalamus, cortex, and brainstem, whereas the MeA receives strong inputs from the bed nucleus of the accessory olfactory tract and nucleus of stria medullaris. These findings suggest Ucn 3 cells in the PVHap receive inputs that transmit visceral and autonomic information while the Ucn 3 cell group in the MeA receives afferents that relay olfactory information. Thus, it is conceivable that central Ucn 3 may serve as a common peptide neurotransmitter in the various neural pathways that convey information from assorted neural signals into the VMH to coordinate the regulation of energy homeostasis.

FUNCTION OF CRF_2 IN THE VMH

When the function of CRF_2 in the VMH was first assessed by injecting Ucn 1 into the VMH, it was found that the peptide potently suppresses food intake (Ohata et al., 2000). However, because CRF_1 has been suggested to be expressed in the VMH (Cheng et al., 2007) and Ucn 1 has equally high affinity for both CRF_1 and CRF_2 (Vaughan et al., 1995), it remains possible that CRF_1 may also contribute to the anorectic effect of Ucn 1 in the VMH. More recently, when the CRF_2-selective ligand Ucn 3 was identified (Lewis et al., 2001), the function of CRF_2 in the VMH was re-examined by site-specific injection of Ucn 3 into the VMH (Fekete et al., 2007; Chen et al., 2010). Consistent with the Ucn 1 injection study, stimulation of CRF_2 by Ucn 3 in the VMH significantly suppresses feeding. Moreover, stimulation of CRF_2 in other regions including the PVH, amygdala, and the lateral hypothalamus fails to modulate feeding (Ohata et al., 2000; Fekete et al., 2007; Chen et al., 2010), reinforcing the notion that VMH CRF_2 plays a critical role in mediating the effect of CRF peptides in suppressing food intake.

In addition to appetite suppression, activation of CRF_2 in the VMH results in rapid elevation of blood glucose levels (Chen et al., 2010). This is consistent with the function of VMH neurons in glucose homeostasis, as VMH neurons have been suggested to play an important role in regulating glucose levels via glucose sensing, and modulating glucose production in peripheral tissues (Kang et al., 2004; Levin et al., 2004). On the other hand, it has been shown that stimulation of CRF_2 in the VMH suppresses insulin-induced release of glucagon and epinephrine (McCrimmon et al., 2006), indicating that VMH CRF_2 exerts a negative control over the counterregulatory response (CRR). Taken together, it is possible that the functional role of CRF_2 in the VMH in glucose homeostasis is context dependent. When blood glucose is low as a result of hyperinsulinemia, CRF_2 in the VMH negatively regulates the CRR response. On the other hand, under normoglycemia, CRF_2 induces acute hyperglycemia to facilitate fuel mobilization perhaps in response to stress. We have also found that CRF_2-positive neurons in the VMH are sensitive to glucose, as high glucose inhibits and low glucose stimulates the neuronal activity (Digruccio et al., 2007).

Type 2 CRF receptor has been shown to modulate the HPA axis. For example, CRF_2 KO mice display altered HPA hormonal secretion, and central Ucn 3 injection facilitates stress-induced ACTH secretion (Jamieson et al., 2006). On the other hand, activation of CRF_2 in the VMH fails to modulate HPA hormone secretion (Chen et al., 2010), indicating that the receptor in the VMH is not essential for central Ucn 3-induced HPA activation. Thus, CRF_2-positive brain loci that are important for modulation of the HPA axis remain to be determined.

PHYSIOLOGICAL ROLE OF CRF_2 IN THE VMH

To probe the physiological role of endogenous CRF_2 in the VMH, VMH-specific CRF_2 knockdown mice were generated by injection of a lentiviral vector expressing CRF_2 small hairpin RNA (shRNA; Chao et al., 2012). Mice injected with CRF_2 shRNA displayed significantly reduced CRF_2 mRNA levels and gain more weight, mostly in white fat, than control mice. Furthermore, similar to Ucn 3 null mice, mice with reduced CRFR2 in the VMH exhibited elevated basal food intake and ate more than the control mice after overnight fasting. This result indicates that CRF_2 in the VMH serves as a brake to facilitate the cessation of feeding. This study suggests that CRF_2 in the VMH plays a critical role in mediating the effect of central Ucn 3 in energy balance.

In addition to elevated feeding, mice with decreased expression of CRF_2 in the VMH display reduced lipolysis and increased adiposity in white fat (Chao et al., 2012). This is likely due to reduced SNS activity, as the VMH has been shown to regulate lipolysis via sympathetic outflow (Kumon et al., 1976; Takahashi and Shimazu, 1981; Ruffin and Nicolaidis, 1999). Interestingly, CRF_2 knockdown in the VMH has no major impact in heat production or uncoupling protein 1 expression in BAT, suggesting that CRF_2 in the VMH does not significantly modulate thermogenesis in BAT. This result appears to disagree with earlier reports that VMH is involved in regulating thermogenesis in BAT (Perkins et al., 1981; Kim et al., 2011). Anatomical studies have demonstrated a compartment-specific organization of innervation of different peripheral organs, as abdominal fat and subcutaneous fat are innervated by different neural pathways (Kreier et al., 2002, 2006). It is possible that CRF_2-positive neurons are a subpopulation of cells in the VMH that regulate SNS outflow to white fat without significant functional impact on BAT. Heterogeneity of VMH neurons has been reported as overlapping but distinct subpopulation of neurons in the VMHvl that are critical in regulating fighting and mating (Lin et al., 2011).

Consistent with the function of CRF_2 in regulating blood glucose levels, mice with reduced CRF_2 expression in the VMH show improved glucose homeostasis compared to control mice (Chao et al., 2012). Moreover, mice with CRF_2 knocked down in the VMH exhibit an exaggerated rebound in blood glucose levels compared to control mice after the initial hypoglycemic response to insulin challenge. This result agrees with the study by McCrimmon et al.

(2006), who found that injection of Ucn 3 into the VMH suppresses the hypoglycemia-induced CRR response. Taken together, these studies strongly argue that CRF_2 is a critical molecular mediator in VMH regulation of glucose homeostasis.

NEUROCIRCUITS UNDERLYING THE EFFECT OF VMH

To understand how VMH CRF_2 neurons regulate output functions and to describe an anatomical link between these neurons and the SNS, it is necessary to determine their axonal projections to identify downstream targets in the brain. A number of anterograde tracing studies utilizing different tracers have been performed to evaluate the projections of VMH neurons. Generally, it was found that VMH neurons project extensively to neighboring hypothalamic nuclei including the anterior and paraventricular nucleus, BNST, and periaqueductal gray (PAG; Saper et al., 1976; Canteras et al., 1994). These anatomical studies raise an interesting dilemma. Although it is clear that VMH activity modulates SNS activity, these studies failed to observe direct VMH efferents within well-known autonomic centers in the brainstem. Thus, it was concluded that the VMH likely modulates SNS activity indirectly by first projecting to a relay center such as the PAG.

Recently, using a conditional viral tracing approach, we have found that VMH neurons project to a number of important brainstem autonomic centers including the parabrachial nucleus, C1 catecholaminergic cell group in the rostral ventrolateral medulla, and the nucleus of solitary tract (Lindberg et al., 2011). Moreover, we have used the same approach to find that CRF_2-positive cells in the VMH show similar axonal projections to these brainstem areas (**Figure 3**; Lindberg et al., 2011). These studies demonstrate that VMH neurons, including cells that express CRF_2, can potentially modulate SNS activity by direct projections to brainstem autonomic centers.

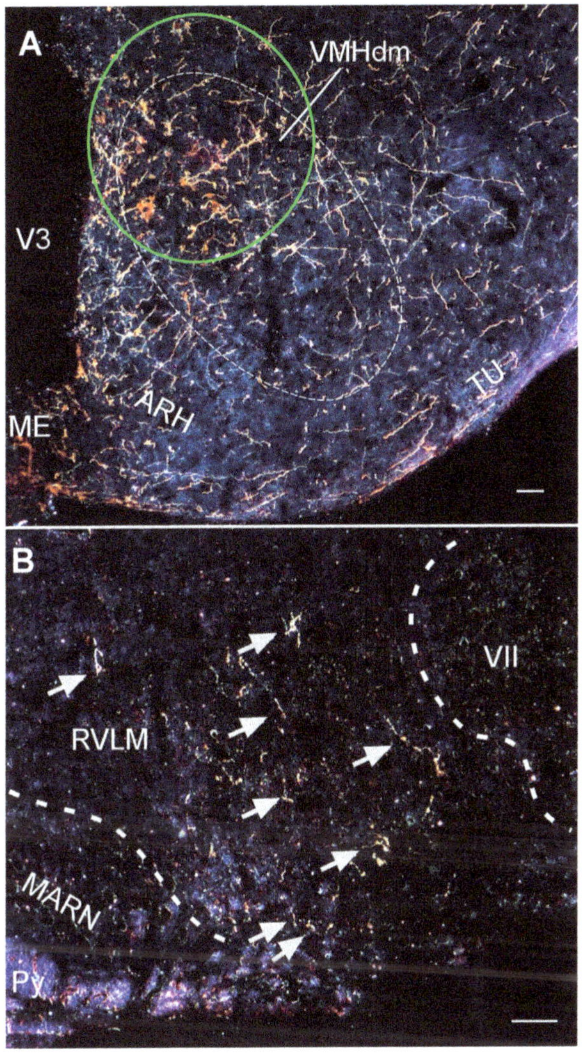

FIGURE 3 | (A) Darkfield photomicrograph showing the injection site (green circle) of an adenoviral vector encoding Cre-regulated expression of farnesylated green fluorescent protein (GFP_f) delivered into the VMH of a CRFR2-Cre mouse. The expression of GFP_f is normally silenced due to a Cre-regulated transcription block sequence inserted upstream of GFP_f reporter cassette. In the presence of Cre, the transcription block sequence is removed to allow GFP_f to be expressed in Cre-positive cells. **(B)** Darkfield photomicrograph depicting the distribution of VMH CRFR2-positive fibers (golden staining) within the rostral ventrolateral medulla (RVLM). ARH, arcuate nucleus of hypothalamus; MARN, magnocellular reticular nucleus; ME, median eminence; Py, pyramidal tract; Tu, tuberal nucleus; V3, third ventricle; VII, facial nucleus; VMHdn, dorsomedial part of the ventromedial nucleus of hypothalamus. Scale bar = 50 μm.

CONCLUSION

The function of CRF peptides and their receptors in coordinating hormonal, neuronal, and behavioral responses to stress is well recognized. Pharmacological studies have determined that the CRF_2 receptors are involved in the regulation of energy homeostasis. Recent studies using various genetic mouse models and molecular tools have further ascertained the critical role of CRF_2 and its selective ligands, including Ucn 3, in feeding, blood glucose regulation, SNS output, and peripheral metabolism. Moreover, CRF_2 in the VMH mediates most, if not all, of the effects of central Ucn 3 on energy homeostasis.

It is clear that conflicting results have been observed between whole body and region- or tissue-specific KO or overexpression mouse models. Furthermore, several studies have demonstrated that anatomical or even functional heterogeneity exists within a seemingly single Ucn 3 cell population in the hypothalamus. Thus, a more detailed understanding of the physiological function of CRF_2 and its selective ligands in the brain will be aided by brain region-specific transgenic animal models permitting manipulation of ligand or receptor expression. Study of such models will provide insight into the specific roles of CRF_2 in modulating metabolic functions.

Regulation of energy balance under diverse challenges including stress, starvation, or high-fat diet requires numerous adaptive mechanisms in both central and peripheral tissues. It is now clear that central CRF_2 and Ucn 3 are involved in this regulation, as the expression of the receptor and ligands are closely regulated under these challenges. It is thus conceivable that dysregulated CRF_2 or ligand function potentially cause or exacerbate metabolic perturbations. This hypothesis can be easily tested with the above mentioned rodent models to determine the functional role of the CRF_2 system in metabolic diseases. Moreover, a better understanding of the molecular mechanisms by which various stressors or metabolic signals regulate the expression and/or function of CRF_2 and its ligand will provide significant insight into the potential role of the CRF family and its receptors in the pathophysiology of metabolic disorders including obesity and diabetes.

ACKNOWLEDGMENTS

We thank Dr. Ruth Stornetta for providing comments on the manuscript. This work was supported by the National Institute of Diabetes and Digestive and Kidney Diseases Grant R01 DK-078049 (to Chien Li).

REFERENCES

Bakshi, V. P., Newman, S. M., Smith-Roe, S., Jochman, K. A., and Kalin, N. H. (2007). Stimulation of lateral septum CRF2 receptors promotes anorexia and stress-like behaviors: functional homology to CRF1 receptors in basolateral amygdala. *J. Neurosci.* 27, 10568–10577.

Bale, T. L., Anderson, K. R., Roberts, A. J., Lee, K. F., Nagy, T. R., and Vale, W. (2003). Corticotropin-Releasing factor receptor-2-deficient mice display abnormal homeostatic responses to challenges of increased dietary fat and cold. *Endocrinology* 144, 2580–2587.

Bale, T. L., Contarino, A., Smith, G. W., Chan, R. K. W., Gold, L. H., Sawchenko, P. E., et al. (2000). Mice deficient for corticotropin-releasing hormone receptor-2 display anxiety-like behavior and are hypersensitive to stress. *Nat. Genet.* 24, 410–414.

Bale, T. L., Hoshijima, M., Gu, Y., Dalton, N., Anderson, K. R., Lee, K. F., et al. (2004). The cardiovascular physiologic actions of urocortin II: acute effects in murine heart failure. *Proc. Natl. Acad. Sci. U.S.A.* 101, 3697–3702.

Bale, T. L., and Vale, W. W. (2004). CRF and CRF receptors: role in stress responsivity and other behaviors. *Annu. Rev. Pharmacol. Toxicol.* 44, 525–557.

Berk, M. L., and Finkelstein, J. A. (1981). Afferent projections to the preoptic area and hypothalamic regions in the rat brain. *Neuroscience* 6, 1601–1624.

Bernardis, L. L., and Frohman, L. A. (1971). Effects of hypothalamic lesions at different loci on development of hyperinsulinemia and obesity in the weanling rat. *J. Comp. Neurol.* 141, 107–115.

Bingham, N. C., Anderson, K. K., Reuter, A. L., Stallings, N. R., and Parker, K. L. (2008). Selective loss of leptin receptors in the ventromedial hypothalamic nucleus results in increased adiposity and a metabolic syndrome. *Endocrinology* 149, 2138–2148.

Bittencourt, J. C., Vaughan, J., Arias, C., Rissman, R. A., Vale, W. W., and Sawchenko, P. E. (1999). Urocortin expression in rat brain: evidence against a pervasive relationship of urocortin-containing projections with targets bearing type 2 CRF receptors. *J. Comp. Neurol.* 415, 285–312.

Bon, K., Lanteri-Minet, M., De Pommery, J., Michiels, J. F., and Menetrey, D. (1997). Cyclophosphamide cystitis as a model of visceral pain in rats: minor effects at mesodiencephalic levels as revealed by the expression of c-fos, with a note on Krox-24. *Exp. Brain Res.* 113, 249–264.

Brar, B. K., Stephanou, A., Knight, R., and Latchman, D. S. (2002). Activation of protein kinase B/Akt by urocortin is essential for its ability to protect cardiac cells against hypoxia/reoxygenation-induced cell death. *J. Mol. Cell. Cardiol.* 34, 483–492.

Breu, J., Touma, C., Hölter, S. M., Knapman, A., Wurst, W., and Deussing, J. M. (2012). Urocortin 2 modulates aspects of social behaviour in mice. *Behav. Brain Res.* 233, 331–336.

Canteras, N. S., Simerly, R. B., and Swanson, L. W. (1994). Organization of projections from the ventromedial nucleus of the hypothalamus: a Phaseolus vulgaris-leucoagglutinin study in the rat. *J. Comp. Neurol.* 348, 41–79.

Carlin, K. M., Vale, W. W., and Bale, T. L. (2006). Vital functions of corticotropin-releasing factor (CRF) pathways in maintenance and regulation of energy homeostasis. *Proc. Natl. Acad. Sci. U.S.A.* 103, 3462–3467.

Carrillo, M., Ricci, L. A., and Melloni, R. H. (2011). Glutamate and the aggression neural circuit in adolescent anabolic steroid-treated Syrian hamsters (*Mesocricetus auratus*). *Behav. Neurosci.* 125, 753–763.

Cha, S. H., Wolfgang, M., Tokutake, Y., Chohnan, S., and Lane, M. D. (2008). Differential effects of central fructose and glucose on hypothalamic malonyl-CoA and food intake. *Proc. Natl. Acad. Sci. U.S.A.* 105, 16871–16875.

Chalmers, D. T., Lovenberg, T. W., and De Souza, E. B. (1995). Localization of novel corticotropin-releasing factor receptor (CRF2) mRNA expression to specific subcortical nuclei in rat brain: comparison with CRF1 receptor mRNA expression. *J. Neurosci.* 15, 6340–6350.

Chao, H., Digruccio, M., Chen, P., and Li, C. (2012). Type 2 corticotropin-releasing factor receptor in the ventromedial nucleus of hypothalamus is critical in regulating feeding and lipid metabolism in white adipose tissue. *Endocrinology* 153, 166–176.

Chen, A., Brar, B., Choi, C. S., Rousso, D., Vaughan, J., Kuperman, Y., et al. (2006). Urocortin 2 modulates glucose utilization and insulin sensitivity in skeletal muscle. *Proc. Natl. Acad. Sci. U.S.A.* 103, 16580–16585.

Chen, A. M., Perrin, M. H., Digruccio, M. R., Vaughan, J. M., Brar, B. K., Arias, C. M., et al. (2005). A soluble mouse brain splice variant of type 2alpha corticotropin-releasing factor (CRF) receptor binds ligands and modulates their activity. *Proc. Natl. Acad. Sci. U.S.A.* 102, 2620–2625.

Chen, P., Lin, D., Giesler, J., and Li, C. (2011). Identification of urocortin 3 afferent projection to the ventromedial nucleus of the hypothalamus in rat brain. *J. Comp. Neurol.* 519, 2023–2042.

Chen, P., Vaughan, J., Donaldson, C., Vale, W. W., and Li, C. (2010). Injection of Urocortin 3 into the ventromedial hypothalamus modulates feeding, blood glucose levels and hypothalamic POMC gene expression but not the HPA axis. *Am. J. Physiol. Endocrinol. Metab.* 298, E337–E345.

Cheng, H., Zhou, L., Zhu, W., Wang, A., Tang, C., Chan, O., et al. (2007). Type 1 corticotropin-releasing factor receptors in the ventromedial hypothalamus promote hypoglycemia-induced hormonal counterregulation. *Am. J. Physiol. Endocrinol. Metab.* 293, E705–E712.

Coste, S. C., Kesterson, R. A., Heldwein, K. A., Stevens, S. L., Heard, A. D., Hollis, J. H., et al. (2000). Abnormal adaptations to stress and impaired cardiovascular function in mice lacking corticotropin-releasing hormone receptor-2. *Nat. Genet.* 24, 403–409.

Cox, J. E., and Powley, T. L. (1981). Prior vagotomy blocks VMH obesity in pair-fed rats. *Am. J. Physiol.* 240, E573–E583.

Cummings, D. E., and Overduin, J. (2007). Gastrointestinal regulation of food intake. *J. Clin. Invest.* 117, 13–23.

Dhillon, H., Zigman, J. M., Ye, C., Lee, C. E., Mcgovern, R. A., Tang, V., et al. (2006). Leptin directly activates SF1 neurons in the VMH, and this action by leptin is required for normal body-weight homeostasis. *Neuron* 49, 191–203.

Digruccio, M., Chen, P., Cheng, J., Moenter, S., and Li, C. (2007). Generation of transgenic mice expression Cre recombinase in type 2 corticotropin-releasing factor receptor (CRFR2) neurons in the brain. *Soc. Neurosci. Abstr.* 198, 111.

Dugger, B. N., Morris, J. A., Jordan, C. L., and Breedlove, S. M. (2007). Androgen receptors are required for full masculinization of the ventromedial hypothalamus (VMH) in rats. *Horm. Behav.* 51, 195–201.

Eghbal-Ahmadi, M., Hatalski, C. G., Avishai-Eliner, S., and Baram, T. Z. (1997). Corticotropin releasing factor receptor type II (CRF2) messenger ribonucleic acid levels in the hypothalamic ventromedial nucleus of the infant rat are reduced by maternal deprivation. *Endocrinology* 138, 5048–5051.

Elmquist, J. K., Bjorbaek, C., Ahima, R. S., Flier, J. S., and Saper, C. B. (1998). Distributions of leptin receptor mRNA isoforms in the rat brain. *J. Comp. Neurol.* 395, 535–547.

Fahrbach, S. E., Morrell, J. I., and Pfaff, D. W. (1989). Studies of ventromedial hypothalamic afferents in the rat using three methods of HRP application. *Exp. Brain Res.* 77, 221–233.

Fei, H., Okano, H. J., Li, C., Lee, G. H., Zhao, C., Darnell, R., et al. (1997). Anatomic localization of alternatively spliced leptin receptors (Ob-R) in mouse brain and other tissues. *Proc. Natl. Acad. Sci. U.S.A.* 94, 7001–7005.

Fekete, E. M., Inoue, K., Zhao, Y., Rivier, J. E., Vale, W. W., Szucs, A., et al. (2007). Delayed satiety-like actions and altered feeding microstructure by a selective type 2 corticotropin-releasing factor agonist in rats: intra-hypothalamic urocortin 3 administration reduces food intake by prolonging the post-meal interval. *Neuropsychopharmacology* 32, 1052–1068.

Flanagan-Cato, L. M. (2011). Sex differences in the neural circuit that mediates female sexual receptivity. *Front. Neuroendocrinol.* 32, 124–136.

Fremeau, R. T. Jr., Troyer, M. D., Pahner, I., Nygaard, G. O., Tran, C. H., Reimer, R. J., et al. (2001).

The expression of vesicular glutamate transporters defines two classes of excitatory synapse. *Neuron* 31, 247–260.

Gardner, J. D., Rothwell, N. J., and Luheshi, G. N. (1998). Leptin affects food intake via CRF-receptor-mediated pathways. *Nat. Neurosci.* 1, 103.

Goland, R. S. (1986). High Levels of Corticotropin-Releasing Hormone Immunoactivity in Maternal and Fetal Plasma during Pregnancy. *J. Clin. Endocrinol. Metab.* 63, 1199–1203.

Graham, C. E., Basappa, J., and Vetter, D. E. (2010). A corticotropin-releasing factor system expressed in the cochlea modulates hearing sensitivity and protects against noise-induced hearing loss. *Neurobiol. Dis.* 38, 246–258.

Grammatopoulos, D. K. (2000). Urocortin, but not corticotropin-releasing hormone (CRH), activates the mitogen-activated protein kinase signal transduction pathway in human pregnant myometrium: an effect mediated via R1 and R2 CRH receptor subtypes and stimulation of Gq-proteins. *Mol. Endocrinol.* 14, 2076–2091.

Gurdjian, E. S. (1927). The diencephalon of the albino rat. Studies on the brain of the rat. No. 2. *J. Comp. Neurol.* 43, 1–114.

Harris, R. B. (2010). Leptin responsiveness of mice deficient in corticotrophin-releasing hormone receptor type 2. *Neuroendocrinology* 92, 198–206.

Hashimoto, K., Nishiyama, M., Tanaka, Y., Noguchi, T., Asaba, K., Hossein, P. N., et al. (2004). Urocortins and corticotropin releasing factor type 2 receptors in the hypothalamus and the cardiovascular system. *Peptides* 25, 1711–1721.

Herzog, E., Bellenchi, G. C., Gras, C., Bernard, V., Ravassard, P., Bedet, C., et al. (2001). The existence of a second vesicular glutamate transporter specifies subpopulations of glutamatergic neurons. *J. Neurosci.* 21, RC181.

Hinkle, R. T., Donnelly, E., Cody, D. B., Samuelsson, S., Lange, J. S., Bauer, M. B., et al. (2003). Activation of the CRF 2 receptor modulates skeletal muscle mass under physiological and pathological conditions. *Am. J. Physiol. Endocrinol. Metab.* 285, E889–E898.

Hsu, S. Y., and Hsueh, A. J. (2001). Human stresscopin and stresscopin-related peptide are selective ligands for the type 2 corticotropin-releasing hormone receptor. *Nat. Med.* 7, 605–611.

Inoue, S., Campfield, L. A., and Bray, G. A. (1977). Comparison of metabolic alterations in hypothalamic and high fat diet-induced obesity. *Am. J. Physiol.* 233, R162–R168.

Jamieson, P. M., Cleasby, M. E., Kuperman, Y., Morton, N. M., Kelly, P. A., Brownstein, D. G., et al. (2011). Urocortin 3 transgenic mice exhibit a metabolically favourable phenotype resisting obesity and hyperglycaemia on a high-fat diet. *Diabetologia* 54, 2392–2403.

Jamieson, P. M., Li, C., Kukura, C., Vaughan, J., and Vale, W. (2006). Urocortin 3 modulates the neuroendocrine stress response and is regulated in rat amygdala and hypothalamus by stress and glucocorticoids. *Endocrinology* 147, 4578–4588.

Kang, L., Routh, V. H., Kuzhikandathil, E. V., Gaspers, L. D., and Levin, B. E. (2004). Physiological and molecular characteristics of rat hypothalamic ventromedial nucleus glucosensing neurons. *Diabetes* 53, 549–559.

Kanno, T. (1999). Corticotropin-releasing factor modulation of Ca^{2+} influx in rat pancreatic beta-cells. *Diabetes* 48, 1741–1746.

Kiang, J. G. (1997). Corticotropin-releasing factor-like peptides increase cytosolic Ca^{2+} in human epidermoid A-431 cells. *Eur. J. Pharmacol.* 329, 237–244.

Kim, K. W., Zhao, L., Donato, J. Jr., Kohno, D., Xu, Y., Elias, C. F., et al. (2011). Steroidogenic factor 1 directs programs regulating diet-induced thermogenesis and leptin action in the ventral medial hypothalamic nucleus. *Proc. Natl. Acad. Sci. U.S.A.* 108, 10673–10678.

King, B. M. (2006). The rise, fall, and resurrection of the ventromedial hypothalamus in the regulation of feeding behavior and body weight. *Physiol. Behav.* 87, 221–244.

Kita, H., and Oomura, Y. (1982). An HRP study of the afferent connections to rat medial hypothalamic region. *Brain Res. Bull.* 8, 53–62.

Kostich, W. A., Chen, A., Sperle, K., and Largent, B. L. (1998). Molecular identification and analysis of a novel human corticotropin-releasing factor (CRF) receptor: the CRF2γ receptor. *Mol. Endocrinol.* 12, 1077–1085.

Kozicz, T., Yanaihara, H., and Arimura, A. (1998). Distribution of urocortin-like immunoreactivity in the central nervous system of the rat. *J Comp. Neurol.* 391, 1–10.

Kreier, F., Fliers, E., Voshol, P. J., Van Eden, C. G., Havekes, L. M., Kalsbeek, A., et al. (2002). Selective parasympathetic innervation of subcutaneous and intra-abdominal fat – functional implications. *J. Clin. Invest.* 110, 1243–1250.

Kreier, F., Kap, Y. S., Mettenleiter, T. C., Van Heijningen, C., Van Der Vliet, J., Kalsbeek, A., et al. (2006). Tracing from fat tissue, liver, and pancreas: a neuroanatomical framework for the role of the brain in type 2 diabetes. *Endocrinology* 147, 1140–1147.

Kumon, A., Takahashi, A., Hara, T., and Shimazu, T. (1976). Mechanism of lipolysis induced by electrical stimulation of the hypothalamus in the rabbit. *J. Lipid Res.* 17, 551–558.

Kuperman, Y., Issler, O., Regev, L., Musseri, I., Navon, I., Neufeld-Cohen, A., et al. (2010). Perifornical Urocortin-3 mediates the link between stress-induced anxiety and energy homeostasis. *Proc. Natl. Acad. Sci. U.S.A.* 107, 8393–8398.

Kuperman, Y., Issler, O., Vaughan, J., Bilezikjian, L., Vale, W., and Chen, A. (2011). Expression and regulation of corticotropin-releasing factor receptor type 2beta in developing and mature mouse skeletal muscle. *Mol. Endocrinol.* 25, 157–169.

Kurrasch, D. M., Cheung, C. C., Lee, F. Y., Tran, P. V., Hata, K., and Ingraham, H. A. (2007). The neonatal ventromedial hypothalamus transcriptome reveals novel markers with spatially distinct patterning. *J. Neurosci.* 27, 13624–13634.

Latchman, D. S. (2002). Urocortin. *Int. J. Biochem. Cell Biol.* 34, 907–910.

Levin, B. E., Routh, V. H., Kang, L., Sanders, N. M., and Dunn-Meynell, A. A. (2004). Neuronal glucosensing: what do we know after 50 years? *Diabetes* 53, 2521–2528.

Lewis, K., Li, C., Perrin, M. H., Blount, A., Kunitake, K., Donaldson, C., et al. (2001). Identification of urocortin III, an additional member of the corticotropin-releasing factor (CRF) family with high affinity for the CRF2 receptor. *Proc. Natl. Acad. Sci. U.S.A.* 98, 7570–7575.

Li, C., Chen, P., Vaughan, J., Blount, A., Chen, A., Jamieson, P. M., et al. (2003). Urocortin III is expressed in pancreatic beta-cells and stimulates insulin and glucagon secretion. *Endocrinology* 144, 3216–3224.

Li, C., Chen, P., Vaughan, J., Lee, K. F., and Vale, W. (2007). Urocortin 3 regulates glucose-stimulated insulin secretion and energy homeostasis. *Proc. Natl. Acad. Sci. U.S.A.* 104, 4206–4211.

Li, C., and Vale, W. (2002). Regulation of Urocortin III mRNA expression in the ob/ob obese mouse: involvement of leptin. *Endocr. Soc. Abstr.* 84, 198.

Li, C., Vaughan, J., Sawchenko, P. E., and Vale, W. W. (2002). Urocortin III-immunoreactive projections in rat brain: partial overlap with sites of type 2 corticotrophin-releasingFfactor receptor expression. *J. Neurosci.* 22, 991–1001.

Lin, D., Boyle, M. P., Dollar, P., Lee, H., Lein, E. S., Perona, P., et al. (2011). Functional identification of an aggression locus in the mouse hypothalamus. *Nature* 470, 221–226.

Lindberg, D. R., Chen, P., and Li, C. (2011). Mapping the efferent projections of urocortin-3 sensitive neurons of the ventromedial hypothalamic nucleus. *Soc. Neurosci. Abstr.* 601.16, SS17.

Luiten, P. G., and Room, P. (1980). Interrelations between lateral, dorsomedial and ventromedial hypothalamic nuclei in the rat. An HRP study. *Brain Res.* 190, 321–332.

Luo, X., Ikeda, Y., and Parker, K. L. (1994). A cell-specific nuclear receptor is essential for adrenal and gonadal development and sexual differentiation. *Cell* 77, 481–490.

Makino, S., Asaba, K., Nishiyama, M., and Hashimoto, K. (1999). Decreased type 2 corticotropin-releasing hormone receptor mRNA expression in the ventromedial hypothalamus during repeated immobilization stress. *Neuroendocrinology* 70, 160–167.

Makino, S., Nishiyama, M., Asaba, K., Gold, P. W., and Hashimoto, K. (1998). Altered expression of type 2 CRH receptor mRNA in the VMH by glucocorticoids and starvation. *Am. J. Physiol.* 275, R1138–R1145.

Maras, P. M., and Petrulis, A. (2010). Anatomical connections between the anterior and posterodorsal subregions of the medial amygdala: integration of odor and hormone signals. *Neuroscience* 170, 610–622.

Martinez, V., Wang, L., Million, M., Rivier, J., and Tache, Y. (2004). Urocortins and the regulation of gastrointestinal motor function and visceral pain. *Peptides* 25, 1733–1744.

McBride, R. L., and Sutin, J. (1977). Amygdaloid and pontine projections to the ventromedial nucleus of the hypothalamus. *J. Comp. Neurol.* 174, 377–396.

McCrimmon, R. J., Song, Z., Cheng, H., Mcnay, E. C., Weikart-Yeckel, C., Fan, X., et al. (2006). Corticotrophin-releasing factor receptors within the ventromedial hypothalamus regulate hypoglycemia-induced hormonal counterregulation. *J. Clin. Invest.* 116, 1723–1730.

Morrison, S. F., Nakamura, K., and Madden, C. J. (2008). Central control of thermogenesis in mammals. *Exp. Physiol.* 93, 773–797.

Musatov, S., Chen, W., Pfaff, D. W., Kaplitt, M. G., and Ogawa, S. (2006). RNAi-mediated silencing of estrogen receptor {alpha} in the ventromedial nucleus of hypothalamus abolishes female sexual behaviors. *Proc. Natl. Acad. Sci. U.S.A.* 103, 10456–10460.

Musatov, S., Chen, W., Pfaff, D. W., Mobbs, C. V., Yang, X. J., Clegg, D. J., et al. (2007). Silencing of estrogen receptor alpha in the ventromedial nucleus of hypothalamus leads to metabolic syndrome. *Proc. Natl. Acad. Sci. U.S.A.* 104, 2501–2506.

Niijima, A., Rohner-Jeanrenaud, F., and Jeanrenaud, B. (1984). Role of ventromedial hypothalamus on sympathetic efferents of brown adipose tissue. *Am. J. Physiol.* 247, R650–R654.

Nishiyama, M., Makino, S., Asaba, K., and Hashimoto, K. (1999). Leptin effects on the expression of type-2 CRH receptor mRNA in the ventromedial hypothalamus in the rat. *J. Neuroendocrinol.* 11, 307–314.

Northcutt, K. V., and Lonstein, J. S. (2011). Neuroanatomical projections of the species-specific tyrosine hydroxylase-immunoreactive cells of the male prairie vole bed nucleus of the stria terminalis and medial amygdala. *Brain Behav. Evol.* 77, 176–192.

Ohata, H., and Shibasaki, T. (2004). Effects of urocortin 2 and 3 on motor activity and food intake in rats. *Peptides* 25, 1703–1709.

Ohata, H., Suzuki, K., Oki, Y., and Shibasaki, T. (2000). Urocortin in the ventromedial hypothalamic nucleus acts as an inhibitor of feeding behavior in rats. *Brain Res.* 861, 1–7.

Parker, K. L., Rice, D. A., Lala, D. S., Ikeda, Y., Luo, X., Wong, M., et al. (2002). Steroidogenic factor 1: an essential mediator of endocrine development. *Recent Prog. Horm. Res.* 57, 19–36.

Pelleymounter, M. A., Joppa, M., Carmouche, M., Cullen, M. J., Brown, B., Murphy, B., et al. (2000). Role of corticotropin-releasing factor (CRF) receptors in the anorexic syndrome induced by CRF. *J. Pharmacol. Exp. Ther.* 293, 799–806.

Perkins, M. N., Rothwell, N. J., Stock, M. J., and Stone, T. W. (1981). Activation of brown adipose tissue thermogenesis by the ventromedial hypothalamus. *Nature* 289, 401–402.

Perrin, M., Donaldson, C., Chen, R., Blount, A., Berggren, T., Bilezikjian, L., et al. (1995). Identification of a second corticotropin-releasing factor receptor gene and characterization of a cDNA expressed in heart. *Proc. Natl. Acad. Sci. U.S.A.* 92, 2969–2973.

Perrin, M. H., and Vale, W. W. (1999). Corticotropin releasing factor receptors and their ligand family. *Ann. N. Y. Acad. Sci.* 885, 312–328.

Porcher, C., Juhem, A., Peinnequin, A., Sinniger, V., and Bonaz, B. (2005). Expression and effects of metabotropic CRF1 and CRF2 receptors in rat small intestine. *Am. J. Physiol. Gastrointest. Liver Physiol.* 288, G1091–G1103.

Poulin, A.-M., Lenglos, C., Mitra, A., and Timofeeva, E. (2012). Hypothalamic expression of urocortin 3 and the type 2 corticotropin-releasing factor receptor is regulated according to feeding state in lean but not obese Zucker rats. *Neuropharmacology* 63, 147–153.

Rabadan-Diehl, C., Kiss, A., Camacho, C., and Aguilera, G. (1996). Regulation of messenger ribonucleic acid for corticotropin releasing hormone receptor in the pituitary during stress. *Endocrinology* 137, 3808–3814.

Radley, J. J., and Sawchenko, P. E. (2011). A common substrate for prefrontal and hippocampal inhibition of the neuroendocrine stress response. *J. Neurosci.* 31, 9683–9695.

Reyes, T. M., Lewis, K., Perrin, M. H., Kunitake, K. S., Vaughan, J., Arias, C. A., et al. (2001). Urocortin II: A member of the corticotropin-releasing factor (CRF) neuropeptide family that is selectively bound by type 2 CRF receptors. *Proc. Natl. Acad. Sci. U.S.A.* 98, 2843–2848.

Richard, D., Rivest, R., Naimi, N., Timofeeva, E., and Rivest, S. (1996). Expression of corticotropin-releasing factor and its receptors in the brain of lean and obese Zucker rats. *Endocrinology* 137, 4786–4795.

Ritter, R. C. (2004). Gastrointestinal mechanisms of satiation for food. *Physiol. Behav.* 81, 249–273.

Ruffin, M., and Nicolaidis, S. (1999). Electrical stimulation of the ventromedial hypothalamus enhances both fat utilization and metabolic rate that precede and parallel the inhibition of feeding behavior. *Brain Res.* 846, 23–29.

Ryabinin, A. E., Tsoory, M. M., Kozicz, T., Thiele, T. E., Neufeld-Cohen, A., Chen, A., et al. (2012). Urocortins: CRF's siblings and their potential role in anxiety, depression and alcohol drinking behavior. *Alcohol* 46, 349–357.

Sadovsky, Y., Crawford, P. A., Woodson, K. G., Polish, J. A., Clements, M. A., Tourtellotte, L. M., et al. (1995). Mice deficient in the orphan receptor steroidogenic factor 1 lack adrenal glands and gonads but express P450 side-chain-cleavage enzyme in the placenta and have normal embryonic serum levels of corticosteroids. *Proc. Natl. Acad. Sci. U.S.A.* 92, 10939–10943.

Sakaguchi, T., Takahashi, M., and Bray, G. A. (1988). Diurnal changes in sympathetic activity. Relation to food intake and to insulin injected into the ventromedial or suprachiasmatic nucleus. *J. Clin. Invest.* 82, 282–286.

Saper, C. B., Swanson, L. W., and Cowan, W. M. (1976). The efferent connections of the ventromedial nucleus of the hypothalamus of the rat. *J. Comp. Neurol.* 169, 409–442.

Sawchenko, P. E., and Swanson, L. W. (1983). The organization of forebrain afferents to the paraventricular and supraoptic nuclei of the rat. *J. Comp. Neurol.* 218, 121–144.

Segal, J. P., Stallings, N. R., Lee, C. E., Zhao, L., Socci, N., Viale, A., et al. (2005). Use of laser-capture microdissection for the identification of marker genes for the ventromedial hypothalamic nucleus. *J. Neurosci.* 25, 4181–4188.

Shinoda, K., Lei, H., Yoshii, H., Nomura, M., Nagano, M., Shiba, H., et al. (1995). Developmental defects of the ventromedial hypothalamic nucleus and pituitary gonadotroph in the Ftz-F1 disrupted mice. *Dev. Dyn.* 204, 22–29.

Smagin, G. N., Howell, L. A., Ryan, D. H., De Souza, E. B., and Harris, R. B. (1998). The role of CRF2 receptors in corticotropin-releasing factor- and urocortin-induced anorexia. *Neuroreport* 11, 1601–1606.

Solinas, G., Summermatter, S., Mainieri, D., Gubler, M., Montani, J. P., Seydoux, J., et al. (2006). Corticotropin-releasing hormone directly stimulates thermogenesis in skeletal muscle possibly through substrate cycling between de novo lipogenesis and lipid oxidation. *Endocrinology* 147, 31–38.

Spina, M., Merlo-Pich, E., Basso, A. M., Rivier, J., Vale, W., and Koob, G. F. (1996). Appetite-suppressing effects of urocortin, a CRF-related neuropeptide. *Science* 273, 1561–1564.

Stengel, A., and Tache, Y. (2009). Neuroendocrine control of the gut during stress: corticotropin-releasing factor signaling pathways in the spotlight. *Annu. Rev. Physiol.* 71, 219–239.

Stenzel, P., Kesterson, R., Yeung, W., Cone, R. D., Rittenberg, M. B., and Stenzel-Poore, M. P. (1995). Identification of a novel murine receptor for corticotropin-releasing hormone expressed in the heart. *Mol. Endocrinol.* 9, 637–645.

Sternson, S. M., Shepherd, G. M. G., and Friedman, J. M. (2005). Topographic mapping of VMH –> arcuate nucleus microcircuits and their reorganization by fasting. *Nat. Neurosci.* 8, 1356–1363.

Swanson, L. W., and Petrovich, G. D. (1998). What is the amygdala? *Trends Neurosci.* 21, 323–331.

Swanson, L. W., Sawchenko, P. E., Rivier, J., and Vale, W. W. (1983). Organization of ovine corticotropin-releasing factor immunoreactive cells and fibers in the rat brain: an immunohistochemical study. *Neuroendocrinology* 36, 165–186.

Tabarin, A., Diz-Chaves, Y., Consoli, D., Monsaingeon, M., Bale, T. L., Culler, M. D., et al. (2007). Role of the corticotropin-releasing factor receptor type 2 in the control of food intake in mice: a meal pattern analysis. *Eur. J. Neurosci.* 26, 2303–2314.

Tache, Y., and Bonaz, B. (2007). Corticotropin-releasing factor receptors and stress-related alterations of gut motor function. *J. Clin. Invest.* 117, 33–40.

Takahashi, A., and Shimazu, T. (1981). Hypothalamic regulation of lipid metabolism in the rat: effect of hypothalamic stimulation on lipolysis. *J. Auton. Nerv. Syst.* 4, 195–205.

Takamori, S., Rhee, J. S., Rosenmund, C., and Jahn, R. (2001). Identification of differentiation-associated brain-specific phosphate transporter as a second vesicular glutamate transporter (VGLUT2). *J. Neurosci.* 21, RC182.

Telegdy, G., and Adamik, A. (2008). Involvement of CRH receptors in urocortin-induced hyperthermia. *Peptides* 29, 1937–1942.

Telegdy, G., Adamik, A., and Tóth, G. (2006). The action of urocortins on body temperature in rats. *Peptides* 27, 2289–2294.

Tong, Q., Ye, C., Mccrimmon, R. J., Dhillon, H., Choi, B., Kramer, M. D., et al. (2007). Synaptic glutamate release by ventromedial hypothalamic neurons is part of the neurocircuitry that prevents hypoglycemia. *Cell Metab.* 5, 383–393.

Uehara, Y., Shimizu, H., Ohtani, K., Sato, N., and Mori, M. (1998). Hypothalamic corticotropin-releasing hormone is a mediator of the anorexigenic effect of leptin. *Diabetes* 47, 890–893.

Vale, W., Spiess, J., Rivier, C., and Rivier, J. (1981). Characterization of a 41 residue ovine hypothalamic peptide that stimulates the secretion of corticotropin and β-endorphin. *Science* 213, 1394–1397.

Van Hover, C., Chen, P., and Li, C. (2011). Stress-activated afferent inputs into the medial amygdala: Implication of neuropathways mediating stress-activation of Urocortin 3 neurons in the amygdala. *Soc. Neurosci. Abstr.* 191.14, UU27.

Van Pett, K., Viau, V., Bittencourt, J. C., Chan, R. K. W., Li, H.-Y., Arias, C., et al. (2000). Distribution of mRNAs encoding CRF receptors in brain and pituitary of rat and mouse. *J. Comp. Neurol.* 428, 191–212.

Vaughan, J. M., Donaldson, C., Bittencourt, J., Perrin, M. H., Lewis, K., Sutton, S., et al. (1995). Urocortin, a mammalian neuropeptide related to fish urotensin I and to corticotropin-releasing factor. *Nature* 378, 287–292.

Venihaki, M., Sakihara, S., Subramanian, S., Dikkes, P., Weninger, S. C., Liapakis, G., et al. (2004). Urocortin III, a brain neuropeptide of the corticotropin-releasing hormone family: modulation by stress and attenuation of some anxiety-like behaviours. *J. Neuroendocrinol.* 16, 411–422.

Vetter, D. E., Li, C., Zhao, L., Contarino, A., Liberman, M. C., Smith, G. W., et al. (2002). Urocortin-deficient mice show hearing impairment and increased anxiety-like behavior. *Nat. Genet.* 31, 363–369.

Wang, C., and Kotz, C. (2002). Urocortin in the lateral septal area modulates feeding induced by orexin A in the lateral hypothalamus. *Am. J. Physiol. Regul. Integr. Comp. Physiol.* 283, R358–R367.

Wiley, K. E., and Davenport, A. P. (2004). CRF2 receptors are highly expressed in the human cardiovascular system and their cognate ligands urocortins 2 and 3 are potent vasodilators. *Br. J. Pharmacol.* 143, 508–514.

Wolfgang, M. J., Cha, S. H., Sidhaye, A., Chohnan, S., Cline, G., Shulman, G. I., et al. (2007). Regulation of hypothalamic malonyl-CoA by central glucose and leptin. *Proc. Natl. Acad. Sci. U.S.A.* 104, 19285–19290.

Zaborszky, L. (1982). Afferent connections of the medial basal hypothalamus. *Adv. Anat. Embryol. Cell Biol.* 69, 1–107.

Ziegler, D. R., Cullinan, W. E., and Herman, J. P. (2002). Distribution of vesicular glutamate transporter mRNA in rat hypothalamus. *J. Comp. Neurol.* 448, 217–229.

18

Physiological roles of GPR10 and PrRP signaling

Garron T. Dodd and Simon M. Luckman*

Faculty of Life Sciences, AV Hill Building, University of Manchester, Manchester, UK

Edited by:
Hubert Vaudry, University of Rouen, France

Reviewed by:
Günter K. Stalla, Max-Planck-Institute of Psychiatry, Germany
Tatsushi Onaka, Jichi Medical University, Japan

***Correspondence:**
Simon M. Luckman, Faculty of Life Sciences, AV Hill Building, The University of Manchester, Oxford Road, Manchester M13 9PT, UK.
e-mail: simon.luckman@manchester.ac.uk

Prolactin-releasing peptide (PrRP) was first isolated from bovine hypothalamus, and was found to act as an endogenous ligand at the G-protein-coupled receptor 10 (GPR10 or hGR3). Although originally named as it can affect the secretion of prolactin from anterior pituitary cells, the potential functions for this peptide have been greatly expanded over the past decade. Anatomical, pharmacological, and physiological studies indicate that PrRP, signaling via the GPR10 receptor, may have a wide range of roles in neuroendocrinology; such as in energy homeostasis, stress responses, cardiovascular regulation, and circadian function. This review will provide the current knowledge of the PrRP and GPR10 signaling system, its putative functions, implications for therapy, and future perspectives.

Keywords: PrRP, GPR10, energy intake, stress, dorsomedial hypothalamic nucleus, nucleus tractus solitarius, energy metabolism

INTRODUCTION

Seven-transmembrane-domain receptors (7TMRs) make up a receptor superfamily related by common signaling features and a structure that spans the cell membrane seven times. All 7TMRs are coupled to guanine nucleotide binding proteins (G-proteins) and, as such, are more commonly referred to as G-protein-coupled receptors (GPCRs; Probst et al., 1992). In the human genome, over 800 GPCRs have been annotated (>4% of the genome), many of which since have been implicated in diverse physiological roles from photoreception to olfaction, and from mood to appetite (Fredriksson et al., 2003). This diverse functionality infers immense therapeutic potential for the treatment of disease and, in fact, as many as half of the currently marketed drugs target GPCRs (Flower, 1999). Advances in genomics over the last century, that have allowed genome-wide homology analysis, have facilitated the discovery of so many new GPCRs. Currently the GenBank/EMBL database has over 1000 clones of eukaryotic GPCRs recorded, and many of the predicted receptors have no known ligand. These are termed "orphan" GPCRs. Although many of the GPCR genes probably correspond to homologs of sensory olfactory receptors, which are predicted to exist in considerable number in the genome, the remainder could encode for diverse unknown receptors, which may play important physiological roles (Buck and Axel, 1991). Due to the undoubted therapeutic potential for the treatment of different pathologies, the discovery of ligands by the "de-orphanization" of GPCRs and an understanding of their physiological function is the focus of an intense research effort that has far reaching implications for both frontier and translational science.

One of the first GPCRs to be de-orphanized was G-protein-coupled receptor 10 (GPR10; also known as hGR3 or UHR-1). GPR10 was originally cloned in hypothalamic tissue using low stringency PCR primers designed against to the highly conserved GPCR transmembrane domains 2 and 6 (Welch et al., 1995). The cloned receptor showed sequence similarity to the neuropeptide Y (NPY) receptor (31% overall and 46% in the transmembrane regions), however, it could not be activated by either NPY or pancreatic polypeptide (Marchese et al., 1995). This presented the scientific community with a novel problem, in that this represented the first GPCR for which its discovery preceded that of its endogenous ligand. Initial GPR10 localization studies indicated high mRNA expression in the anterior pituitary (Fujii et al., 1999). As hypothalamus derived factors frequently play important roles in regulating anterior pituitary function, it seemed intuitive that the natural ligand for GPR10 might exist in the hypothalamus. Using this insight, GPR10 was finally de-orphanized by Hinuma et al. (1998), using a novel reverse pharmacology approach. For reasons described below, the receptor ligand was termed prolactin-releasing peptide (PrRP). Later studies, using other *in vitro* heterologous expression systems, demonstrated that PrRP shows some promiscuous binding to another RFamide peptide family receptor, neuropeptide FF receptor 2 (NPFF-2R) (Engstrom et al., 2003; Ma et al., 2009). However, to date, PrRP is the only ligand known to have significant affinity for GPR10.

Initial studies showed that PrRP could stimulate prolactin secretion from dispersed anterior pituitary cells; hence, the peptide's name (Hinuma et al., 1998). However since its discovery, the importance of PrRP in the physiological regulation of

Abbreviations: 7TMR, seven-transmembrane-domain receptors; ACTH, adrenocorticotropic hormone; AP, area postrema; BL, basolateral amygdaloid nucleus; BNST, bed nucleus of the stria terminalis; CCK, cholecystokinin-8; Ce, central amygdaloid nucleus; DMN, dorsomedial hypothalamic nucleus; GABA, γ-aminobutyric acid; GPCR, G-protein-coupled receptors; GPR10, G-protein-coupled receptor 10; LH, lateral hypothalamic area; MCPO, magnocellular preoptic nucleus; MD, mediodorsal thalamic nucleus; MPO, medial preoptic nucleus; ox, optic chiasm; NPFF-R2, neuropeptide FF receptor 2; NPY, neuropeptide Y; NTS, nucleus of the tractus solitarius; OLETF, Otsuka Long-Evans Tokushima Fatty; Pe, periventricular hypothalamic nucleus; PrRP, prolactin-releasing peptide; PT, paratenial thalamic nucleus; PVN, paraventricular hypothalamic nucleus; Rt, reticular nucleus of the thalamus; SM, nucleus of the stria medullaris; SO, supraoptic hypothalamic nucleus; SpVe, spinal vestibular nucleus; TH, tyrosine hydroxylase; VLH, ventrolateral hypothalamic nucleus; VLM, ventrolateral medulla.

prolactin secretion has been put in doubt (see below). Instead, the PrRP-GPR10 signaling pathway has been implicated in a range of other physiological systems. For example, central administration of PrRP inhibits food intake and increases energy expenditure in rats and mice (Lawrence et al., 2000, 2004), suggesting that PrRP plays roles in the regulation of energy balance. It also elevates circulating plasma levels of adrenocorticotropic hormone (ACTH) level, suggesting an association of PrRP with stress responses (Takayanagi and Onaka, 2010). Moreover, PrRP also can affect the cardiovascular system (Samson et al., 2000) and circadian cyclicity (Zhang et al., 2000, 2001; Lin et al., 2002a). This article aims to review the current understanding of the physiological roles for PrRP and GPR10 signaling in the mammalian system, and to highlight future directions for research.

PrRP AND GPR10 EXPRESSION

Determining the expression patterns of both receptor and ligand gives key insight into physiological function. *In situ* hybridization histology, RT-PCR, and immunohistochemical studies indicate that PrRP is expressed in neurons of the nucleus tractus solitarius (NTS), the ventrolateral medulla (VLM), and in the caudal portion of the dorsomedial hypothalamic nucleus (DMN) (**Figure 1**) (Chen et al., 1999; Maruyama et al., 1999; Ibata et al., 2000; Lee et al., 2000). PrRP mRNA has also been found in a number of peripheral tissues, including the adrenal gland, pancreas, placenta, and testis (Fujii et al., 1999; Matsumoto et al., 1999a; Kalliomaki et al., 2004).

The co-localization of PrRP with tyrosine hydroxylase (TH) in the caudal NTS and VLM, suggests that these PrRP cells are a subset of A2 and A1 noradrenergic neurons, respectively (Chen et al., 1999). The highest numbers of PrRP cell bodies are found within the NTS, and interestingly as the hypothalamus shows the highest levels of PrRP fiber immunoreactivity, this suggested the possible projection of PrRP from the brainstem to the hypothalamus (Hinuma et al., 1998; Fujii et al., 1999; Matsumoto et al., 1999a). PrRP-immunoreactive fibers are visible in many areas of the brain, such as the DMN, area postrema (AP), pontine parabrachial area, preoptic areas, bed nucleus of the stria terminalis (BNST), amygdala, mediodorsal nucleus of the thalamus, septal nucleus, and ependymal linings of the ventricles and blood vessels (Lin, 2008). One of the major projection sites is the paraventricular hypothalamus (PVN), where PrRP neurons appear to synapse directly on corticotrophin-releasing hormone (CRH) (Matsumoto et al., 1999a) and oxytocin neurons (Maruyama et al., 1999). Cell-specific connections also have been identified on magnocellular oxytocin/vasopressin neurons of the hypothalamic supraoptic nucleus (Maruyama et al., 1999), somatostatin neurons in the hypothalamic periventricular nucleus (Iijima et al., 2001), and on catecholaminergic cells of the adrenal medulla (Fujiwara et al., 2005).

Distribution of the GPR10 receptor has been investigated using autoradiography, *in situ* hybridization, and RT-PCR (Fujii et al., 1999; Roland et al., 1999; Ibata et al., 2000). The relative level of expression is high in the anterior pituitary, reticular nucleus of the thalamus (Rt), periventricular hypothalamus, DMN, AP, and NTS; with moderate expression in the BNST, PVN, medial preoptic area and nucleus, ventrolateral hypothalamus, stomach, femur, and adrenal gland (Roland et al., 1999).

There is good complementarity in the localization of GPR10 receptor immunoreactive PrRP fiber staining in many brain areas (BNST, supraoptic nucleus, PVN, DMN, and NTS). However, it is interesting to note discrepancies in localization, which might be surprising if GPR10 is the only receptor for PrRP. In fact, many peptide systems have significant mismatches between the distribution of the ligand and their respective cognate receptors. Much of this mismatch might be explained by redundancy in function, that is a receptor will not respond if it is not in contact with the ligand. It may be energetically convenient not to lose the expression of a receptor if there is no evolutionary pressure to do so. Furthermore, peptides often have permissive actions and may not function as classical transmitters at tightly regulated synaptic junctions. For instance, PrRP may be released from neuronal fibers terminating at the ventricular zones, and may enter and diffuse within the cerebral spinal fluid (Iijima et al., 1999); or as seen with substance P, PrRP may diffuse through the neuronal tissue to reach distant receptor sites (Duggan et al., 1990). Although GPR10 is considered to be the cognate receptor for PrRP, others (perhaps currently unknown) may exist. For example, PrRP has significant affinity at neuropeptide FF receptor 2 (NPFF-R2) in *in vitro* studies, and there is potential for overlap between the presence of PrRP and NPFF-R2 particular in the hypothalamus and adrenal gland (Gouarderes et al., 2004). Nevertheless, the diverse distribution profile of receptors and ligand may underlie the diverse physiological roles played by PrRP-GPR10 signaling, and each function needs careful investigation. In the absence of receptor-selective antagonists, this is probably best achieved in receptor knockout mice.

ROLE OF PrRP IN PROLACTIN SECRETION

As high expression of GPR10 is seen in the anterior pituitary, initial studies investigating the physiological action of PrRP focused on hypophysiotropic secretion (Hinuma et al., 1998; Lin et al., 2002b). Preliminary *in vitro* studies, which gave rise to the name of the peptide, described an action of PrRP on prolactin secretion from anterior pituitary tumor cell lines and primary cell cultures (Hinuma et al., 1998). Subsequent studies investigating the relevance of PrRP *in vivo* as a central mediator of prolactin release were controversial, with positive results being reliant on high intravenous PrRP doses administered during specific phases of female rat estrous cycle (Matsumoto et al., 1999b). Other studies demonstrated no prolactin release following central administration of PrRP (Matsumoto et al., 2000; Seal et al., 2002). Moreover, as no PrRP immunoreactivity is found in the median eminence or in hypophysiotropic cells of the hypothalamus (Matsumoto et al., 1999a; Maruyama et al., 2001), classically associated with the secretion of pituitary hormones, the question remains how does PrRP access the pituitary? PrRP may act upon the anterior pituitary as a hormone secreted from peripheral tissues (adrenal, pancreas, testis, placenta), or by an indirect central mechanism possibly via hypophysiotropic neurons (Morales and Sawchenko, 2003). This is a strong possibility, since central administration of PrRP can affect a number of anterior pituitary hormones (Seal et al., 2002). Interestingly, in fish and amphibians, PrRP fibers project to and

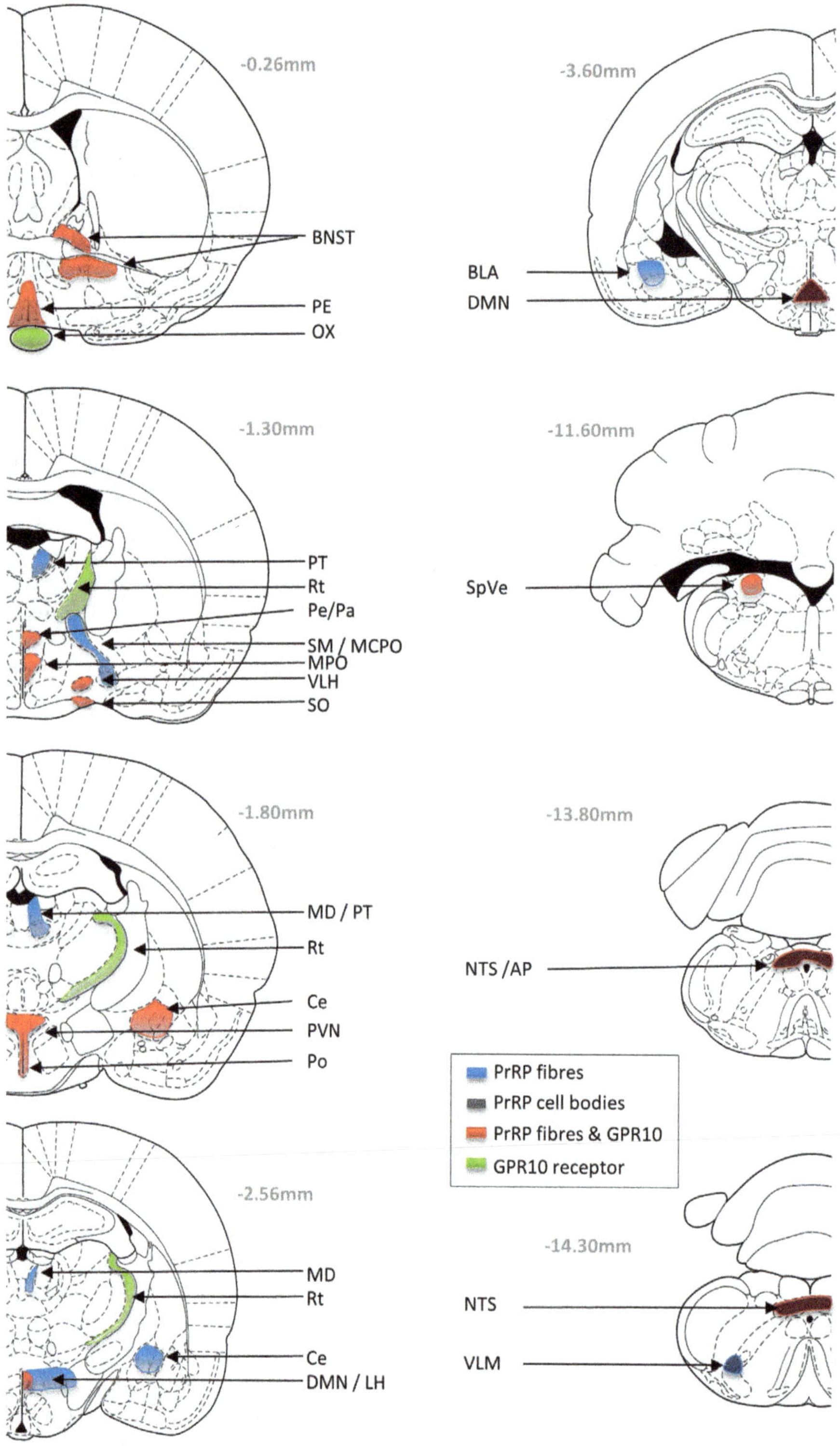

FIGURE 1 | Schematic drawings showing the neuronal distribution of PrRP and GPR10 receptor in the Paxions and Watson rat brain atlas (Paxinos and Watson, 1998; Sun et al., 2005). Blue areas represent PrRP-immunopositive nerve fibers; black checkers represent PrRP cells bodies; green areas represent GPR10 expression; and red areas represent overlap of PrRP and GPR10 expression. AP, area postrema; BL, basolateral amygdaloid nucleus; BNST, bed nucleus of the stria terminalis; Ce, central amygdaloid nucleus; DMN, dorsomedial hypothalamic nucleus; LH, lateral hypothalamic area; MCPO, magnocellular preoptic nucleus; MD, mediodorsal thalamic nucleus; MPO, medial preoptic nucleus; ox, optic chiasm; PVN, paraventricular hypothalamic nucleus; Pe, periventricular hypothalamic nucleus; PT, paratenial thalamic nucleus; Rt, reticular thalamic nucleus; SM, nucleus of the stria medullaris; SO, supraoptic hypothalamic nucleus; NTS, nucleus of the tractus solitarius; SpVe, spinal vestibular nucleus; VLH, ventrolateral hypothalamic nucleus.

terminate on prolactin-producing cells of the pituitary and systemic injection of PrRP into rainbow trout causes a release in prolactin and somatolactin (Moriyama et al., 2002; Seale et al., 2002; Sakamoto et al., 2006). PrRP may, therefore, represent an ancient factor for the direct regulation of prolactin secretion that is now evolutionary redundant in this function in higher mammals. Thus, the name, PrRP, may represent a misnomer, as research over the past decade has implicated this signaling pathway in alternative physiological systems.

CONSERVED FUNCTION OF PrRP AND GPR10 SIGNALING IN FEEDING BEHAVIOR

Prolactin-releasing peptide belongs to the RFamide neuropeptide family (Osugi et al., 2006). Although this family impacts on a diverse range of physiological functions, almost all have been shown to modulate food intake (Bechtold and Luckman, 2007). This involvement of the RFamides in feeding behavior has been demonstrated across most animal taxa, including coelenterates, mollusks, amphibians, birds, and mammals, suggesting an evolutionary conserved role in energy homeostasis (Dockray, 2004).

Numerous studies suggest a pivotal role of PrRP in the homeostatic regulation of feeding and energy balance. Evidence from our group has shown that central administration of PrRP decreases feeding and body weight gain in rats and mice without causing adverse effects (Lawrence et al., 2000, 2002; Bechtold and Luckman, 2006), and that PrRP mRNA in the DMN, NTS, and VLM is downregulated in states of negative energy balance (Lawrence et al., 2000). Importantly, these central anorexic actions of PrRP are not present in mice (Bechtold and Luckman, 2006) or rats (Watanabe et al., 2005) that lack functional expression of GPR10, highlighting the significance of endogenous PrRP-GPR10 signaling in food intake. The significance of this system to energy homeostasis generally is validated further by the obese and hyperphagic phenotypes of both PrRP$^{-/-}$ and GPR10$^{-/-}$null mice (Gu et al., 2004; Takayanagi et al., 2008).

As PrRP induces hypophagia without evoking a conditioned taste aversion or disrupting the normal behavioral satiety sequence (Lawrence et al., 2002), it seems likely that PrRP-GPR10 signaling plays an integral part of the brain's endogenous appetitive neurochemistry. In fact, PrRP induces a significant temporal advancement in the behavioral satiety sequence, an affect associated with natural satiety factors like cholecystokinin-8 (CCK) (Lawrence et al., 2002). Furthermore, experiments with PrRP$^{-/-}$mice or PrRP-neutralizing antibodies, in the laboratory of Tatsushi Onaka, show that PrRP regulates meal size rather than meal frequency, indicating that PrRP may mediate appetite by direct actions on satiation (Takayanagi et al., 2008). As the brainstem medulla oblongata and, in particular, the NTS receives extensive gastrointestinal vagal inputs, these PrRP neurons are an obvious candidate for a role in gut-brain signaling. CCK is released from enteroendocrine cells in response to a meal, and acts via the CCK$_1$ receptor on vagal afferent neurons which terminate in the NTS (Saper, 2004). PrRP neurons localized in both the NTS and the VLM show strong functional activation in response to anorexic doses of CCK (Lawrence et al., 2002). Central administration of PrRP elicits a similar pattern of neuronal c-Fos protein expression as that observed following intraperitoneal administration of CCK (Luckman, 1992; Lawrence et al., 2002; Bechtold and Luckman, 2006), and the anorexic effects of CCK are impaired in both PrRP $^{-/-}$ and GPR10$^{-/-}$null mice (Bechtold and Luckman, 2006; Takayanagi et al., 2008).

The downstream actions of PrRP neurons within the brainstem remain to be clarified. However, PrRP receptor is present in the dorsal vagal complex (Roland et al., 1999; Ibata et al., 2000) and PrRP can act pre-synaptically to affect the firing of preganglionic vagal efferents involved in regulating gut function (Morales and Sawchenko, 2003). Thus, although not proven, it is likely that PrRP-GPR10 signaling within the dorsal vagal complex may mediate the effects of CCK on the parasympathetic regulation of gut motility and secretion. The sensation of satiety, and integration with descending motor pathways to regulate feeding, requires integration with higher brain centers. PrRP-immunoreactive fibers and GPR10 mRNA expression have been demonstrated in a number of hypothalamic nuclei (Fujii et al., 1999; Maruyama et al., 1999; Roland et al., 1999; Ibata et al., 2000; Lee et al., 2000). In particular, PrRP-containing neurons in the NTS project directly to the PVN (Onaka, 2004), where neurons containing CRH or oxytocin possess PrRP receptor (Lin et al., 2002a; Takayanagi and Onaka, 2010). Though anorexic doses of PrRP activate neurons expressing CRH or oxytocin in the PVN (Bechtold and Luckman, 2006; Mera et al., 2006), it is difficult to relate this specifically to satiety signaling, as these neurons may equally be involved in responses to stress (see below). However, PrRP-induced anorexia is attenuated by CRH receptor antagonists (Bechtold and Luckman, 2006), while oxytocin receptor antagonists attenuate the anorexic actions of both PrRP and CCK (Olson et al., 1991; Blevins et al., 2003). Further work will be required to dissect the relative importance of ascending PrRP pathways on satiety and stress-related stimuli. Additional consideration for the role of DMN PrRP neurons in the regulation of feeding behavior is needed also. However, our working model is that PrRP-GPR10 signaling mediates the CCK-vagal regulation of gut function following a meal at the level of the dorsal vagal complex in the brainstem. Further integration with higher brain centers is achieved through the projection of PrRP neurons to the hypothalamus. This may include CRH and oxytocin neurons of the PVN, the latter, at least, having an accepted role in the descending fine regulation of the dorsal vagal complex and feeding control (Samson et al., 2000; Yamada et al., 2009; Onaka et al., 2010).

ENERGY HOMEOSTASIS

Though the evidence for PrRP-GPR10 functioning in satiation is strong, this does not infer a role in overall energy balance, and an interaction with other metabolic regulators might be expected. We have shown that the expression of PrRP is down regulated in situation where the animal is in real (e.g., fasting or lactation) or in perceived (e.g., Zucker rat) negative energy balance (Ellacott et al., 2002). That is, situations which correlate with reduced leptin signaling. Leptin is an adipose-derived hormone, that signals levels of peripheral fat storage to the brain to regulate long-term metabolism (Denver et al., 2011). Immunohistochemical studies have suggested that PrRP neurons (and TH-positive cells) in the brainstem and hypothalamus of the rat express leptin receptors and, thus, that there is a direct cellular effect of the hormone (Hay-Schmidt et al., 2001; Ellacott et al., 2002). However, a more recent paper failed to co-localize leptin receptor in brainstem PrRP neurons of the mouse (Garfield et al., 2012). Leptin induces the expression of phosphorylated signal transducer and activator of transcription protein 3 (pSTAT3) in PrRP neurons, especially those in the DMH (Takayanagi et al., 2008). Central co-administration of PrRP and leptin results in augmented hypophagia and body weight loss (Ellacott et al., 2002), and the hypophagic effects of leptin are impaired in $PrRP^{-/-}$ (Takayanagi et al., 2008) and $GPR10^{-/-}$ null mice (our unpublished results). PrRP-GPR10 clearly has a role in the response to leptin, but whether this is due to a direct or indirect effect of leptin on PrRP neurons remains to be determined.

The maintenance of energy homeostasis involves the balance of both energy intake and energy expenditure. Interestingly pair-feeding studies indicate that the reduced weight gain measured in rats treated with PrRP is not accounted for solely by a reduction in food intake, suggesting that PrRP also affects energy expenditure (Lawrence et al., 2000, 2004). PrRP administration acutely increases body temperature, O_2 consumption, and UCP-1 expression of brown adipose tissue in rats (long before any effect on body weight), suggesting direct modulation by PrRP of energy expenditure (Lawrence et al., 2004). Furthermore, $GPR10^{-/-}$ knockout mice exhibit a much lower basal metabolic rate, when compared with wild-type mice (our unpublished data), which likely contributes to the obese phenotype of these animals (Gu et al., 2004). Thus, PrRP-GPR10 signaling can induce energy expenditure and thermogenesis, which is interesting considering the known role of the DMN in thermoregulation (Willette et al., 1984; Aicher et al., 1995; Horiuchi et al., 2002). In addition, PrRP may play a role in mediating energy consumption under stressful conditions, as the increase oxygen consumption seen in response to stressful stimuli is attenuated in $PrRP^{-/-}$ mice (Onaka et al., 2010).

ROLES OF PrRP AND GPR10 SIGNALING IN THE CONTROL OF STRESS RESPONSES

Brain nuclei expressing PrRP and GPR10, such as in the medulla oblongata and the hypothalamus, have been implicated in mediating stress responses (Onaka, 2004). PrRP neurons within these regions respond to a variety of stressful stimuli including body restraint, fear conditioning (Zhu and Onaka, 2003), footstock, hemorrhage (Uchida et al., 2010), and inflammatory stress (Mera et al., 2006). PrRP neurons may, therefore, play an important role in the neuroendocrine response to stress.

Retro-grade tracing of the PrRP neurons innervating the PVN indicates that the fibers originate within the VLM and NTS, where they co-localizes with noradrenaline in the A1 and A2 neuronal populations, respectively (Chen et al., 1999; Minami et al., 1999; Roland et al., 1999; Morales et al., 2000; Maruyama et al., 2001). These noradrenergic neurons are well known mediators of stress in the central nervous system. Models of emotional stress, including conditioned fear stimulation and water immersion/restraint activate medullary PrRP neurons and increases PrRP mRNA expression (Maruyama et al., 2001; Morales and Sawchenko, 2003; Zhu and Onaka, 2003). Interestingly, PrRP and noradrenaline, which co-localize in A1/A2 cells, act synergistically to induce systemic ACTH release (Maruyama et al., 2001).

One way in which PrRP may influence stress response is by the dense network of PrRP clustered on CRH and oxytocin neurons in the PVN and BNST (Iijima et al., 1999; Maruyama et al., 1999; Ibata et al., 2000). Central administration of PrRP dramatically increases c-Fos expression in CRH neurons in the PVN, an effect that results in the concomitant release of ACTH, oxytocin, and corticosterone into the systemic circulation (Matsumoto et al., 2000; Seal et al., 2002). Importantly, blockade of endogenous PrRP signaling by administration of PrRP neutralizing antibodies attenuates stress induced activation of PVN neurons and reduces systemic oxytocin release (Zhu and Onaka, 2003; Mera et al., 2006).

Although contacts are seen between PrRP fibers and CRH neurons in the PVN (Matsumoto et al., 2000), their relative paucity suggests that these synapses are unlikely to be responsible for the entire modulation of CRH neurons in the PVN. Double *in situ* hybridization shows that the majority of cells expressing GPR10 in the PVN are in fact CRH-negative, whereas GPR10 is co-expressed extensively with CRH in the BNST (Lin et al., 2002b). The BNST not only receives extensive PrRP nerve fibers (Maruyama et al., 1999), it is involved with stress responses via a direct modulation of the PVN (Palkovits et al., 1980; Lin et al., 2002b). It, therefore, seems possible that PrRP may also regulate CRH neurons in the PVN indirectly via the BNST. These results suggest that whether directly or indirectly, PrRP is a potent stimulator of CRH neurons in the PVN, inferring access to the hypothalamic–pituitary–adrenal axial control of stress.

Stressful stimuli affect food intake and energy expenditure, while food intake and energy expenditure affect stress responses (Kawakami et al., 2008). For instance $PrRP^{-/-}$ mice show a reduced increase in oxygen consumption following stressful stimuli (Onaka et al., 2010). It seems tempting to suggest that PrRP may modulate food intake in times of stress. Although only speculative further examination of this hypothesis using conditional transgenic mice for PrRP and GPR10 could help shed light on this theory.

EFFECTS OF PrRP AND GPR10 ON BLOOD PRESSURE

Central injection of PrRP results in a significant increase in blood pressure and cardiovascular output in conscious, unrestrained rats (Samson et al., 2000). Numerous studies describe integral roles played by the NTS, AP, and VLM in mediating cardiovascular function (Yamada et al., 2009). It seems likely that PrRP neurons in these regions may be involved. The NTS and AP receive visceral and hormonal information from peripheral cardiovascular sites (Aicher et al., 1995), so PrRP and GPR10 in these sites may be in a position to modify the ascending and descending efferent connections mediating blood pressure homeostasis (Willette et al., 1984; Aicher et al., 1995). Site specific administration of PrRP directly into the caudal VLM (where a population of PrRP neurons are localized) results in a dose-dependent increase in mean arterial blood pressure, heart rate, and renal sympathetic activity (Horiuchi et al., 2002). Interestingly however, PrRP has no effect when injected directly into the rostral VLM, AP, or the NTS. How PrRP modulates blood pressure homeostasis in an area of minimal GPR10 receptor expression such as the VLM and not in regions of high receptor expression such as the AP and NTS remains enigmatic (Chen et al., 1999; Roland et al., 1999).

Although the mechanisms underlying the pressor effects of PrRP are undefined, a recent study by Yamada et al. (2009) suggests the involvement of CRH neurons in the PVN. PrRP neurons from the VLM project to the PVN where they synapse on CRH positive cells. Central CRH has a known effect of elevating blood pressure in response to stressors (i.e., CRH stimulates sympathetic nerves via the CRH_1 receptor) (Vale et al., 1983; Spina et al., 2000). Yamada et al. (2009) show that pressor- and tachycardia-inducing doses of PrRP activate oxytocin-, vasopressin-, and CRH-producing neurons in the PVN. Furthermore, the elevation of blood pressure and heart rate elicited by PrRP administration are completely suppressed by treatment with a CRH antagonist. PrRP neurons in the VLM may, therefore, mediate CRH release to regulate the cardiovascular system via the sympathetic nervous system.

Finally, the receptor mediating PrRP pressor and tachycardia effects remains unclear. Epidemiological human studies show an association of polymorphisms in the GPR10 receptor with blood pressure, thus implying a potential role of the GPR10 receptor in blood pressure regulation (Bhattacharyya et al., 2003). Contrastingly, PrRP can still elicit effects on mean arterial blood pressure and heart rate in Otsuka Long-Evans Tokushima Fatty (OLETF) rat strain, in which the GRP10 receptor gene is naturally mutated (Ma et al., 2009). Instead, PrRP effects were blocked by administration of the NPFF-2R antagonist, RF9, suggesting that PrRP may modulate blood pressure homeostasis via the NPFF-2R (Ma et al., 2009). It will be useful to follow up these studies using other models since neither the OLETF rat (which has at least one other natural mutation, in the CCK_1 receptor gene), nor the R9 antagonist, are the best tools available. Certainly, if unwanted cardiovascular effects of PrRP are mediated solely by the NPFF-R2, there could be therapeutic potential for selective GPR10 agonists as drug targets other metabolic diseases.

EFFECTS OF PrRP AND GPR10 CIRCADIAN RHYTHMICITY AND SLEEP REGULATION

The expression of GPR10 in particular brain regions, including the preoptic area, the histaminergic ventral tuberomammillary nucleus, the noradrenergic locus ceruleus, serotonergic dorsal raphe, and suprachiasmatic nucleus suggested that PrRP-GPR10 signaling may play a part in circadian rhythmicity and/or sleep regulation (Chen et al., 1999; Roland et al., 1999). The relative importance of PrRP-GPR10 signaling in each of these specific nuclei is yet to be investigated, however, a wealth of literature exists implicating an integral role in sleep and arousal (for reviews, see Suntsova et al., 2009; Szymusiak, 2010; Brown et al., 2012; Murillo-Rodriguez et al., 2012). One region of particular interest, which has a high GPR10 receptor expression, is the Rt (Roland et al., 1999). The Rt is predominantly GABAergic and acts as a gateway for ascending inputs into the cortex that regulate the transition into sleep (Steriade, 2005; Timofeev and Chauvette, 2011). Central administration of PrRP is known to modulate sleep oscillation, and promote rapid and prolonged arousal (Zhang et al., 2000; Lin et al., 2002a). Furthermore, electrophysiological experiments on brain slices show that administration of PrRP attenuates oscillatory activity generated in the Rt, a phenomena that could underlie PrRP's modulation of circadian and sleep regulation (Lin et al., 2002a).

FUTURE PERSPECTIVES

Since the de-orphanization of GPR10, research into the physiological roles of PrRP neurotransmission has been varied and exciting. The PrRP peptide is conserved among species (fish, amphibians, birds, and mammals), pointing toward it seems both primitive and important function (Dockray, 2004; Bechtold and Luckman, 2007). Research into the physiological roles of PrRP has evolved from the initial observations as a "PrRP" (perhaps resulting in a misnomer) to a multi-functional protein integral to a number of functions. Given the current understanding of the PrRP-GPR10, it seems likely that this ancient signaling system may act in times of stress to regulate feeding behavior, induce energy expenditure and increased cardiac output, heighten arousal, and allow the systemic release of endocrine factors. It is possible that, in mammalian species, some of these functions have been modified more specifically, for example into a role in satiation and energy regulation.

To further examine the importance of PrRP-GPR10 signaling a number of outstanding questions need to be addressed.

WHAT ARE THE RELATIVE IMPORTANCE OF THE DIFFERENT POPULATIONS OF PrRP-PRODUCING CELLS IN THE BRAINSTEM, HYPOTHALAMUS, AND IN PERIPHERAL TISSUES?

This review has highlighted potential differential roles for the PrRP-expressing neuronal populations. Although currently only speculative, it seems that the VLM may play a specific role in the pressor effects of PrRP (Horiuchi et al., 2002); whereas, the NTS appears important in mediating CCK's effect on satiation (Bechtold and Luckman, 2006). Interestingly, a recent study has shown that systemic CCK acts to attenuate liver gluconeogenesis independently of insulin production (Cheung et al., 2009). Importantly, the effect requires the integration of a gut–brain–liver axis; effects that could be centrally mediated by CCK responsive PrRP neurons in the NTS.

Further speculation arises over the function of the DMN PrRP population. Takayanagi and Onaka (2010) show significant pSTAT3 co-expression following leptin administration in DMN, suggesting that DMN PrRP neurons are responsive to leptin. Although there is little doubt of the importance of leptin receptor in energy homeostasis, recent research has specifically identified leptin responsive neurons in the DMN as mediators of adaptive thermogenesis (Enriori et al., 2011; Bechtold et al., 2012). As adaptive thermogenesis and the neuronal circuitry innervating brown adipose tissue is currently topical in the domain of anti-obesity therapeutics, it is important to investigate whether the PrRP neurons play a part. Also, both PrRP and GPR10 are expressed in peripheral tissues (Roland et al., 1999). Nothing is known about the importance of peripheral PrRP-GPR10 signaling, and the exploration of these interactions could be vital to the development of viable GPR10 therapeutics.

The recent advancements in the generation of conditional transgenic mice, makes finding the answers to these questions possible. For instance the generation of mice conditionally expressing PrRP under the control of different promoters will allow the genetic dissection of specific populations.

WHAT ARE THE DOWNSTREAM AND UPSTREAM TARGETS OF PrRP – GPR10 SIGNALING?

Understanding the neurochemical make up of PrRP target neurons will help to further define and dissect out the relative importance of each neuronal population. Recent advancements in antero- and retro-grade labeling using Cre recombinase specific adenoviral vectors could advance our understanding of how specific PrRP neuronal population integrate into both the local and global neuronal circuits (Gautron et al., 2010).

There is as a potential caveat with much of the work already achieved in understanding PrRP-GPR10 signaling. As mentioned above, there is some divergence, at least in the mammalian system, between PrRP-expressing nerve fibers and the location of GPR10 receptors. Thus, an element of deliberation must be taken to understanding studies whereby PrRP is administered globally into the brain and at non-physiological doses, as this could be activating redundant receptors. Although this problem may be minimal, the use of conditional transgenic animals, conditional viral vectors, and the development of selective GPR10 agonists/antagonists will greatly enhance our understanding of this important neurotransmitter system. Although much of the ground work has been established, there is still much to learn about PrRP-GPR10 signaling and its definitive roles in the nervous system.

REFERENCES

Aicher, S. A., Kurucz, O. S., Reis, D. J., and Milner, T. A. (1995). Nucleus tractus solitarius efferent terminals synapse on neurons in the caudal ventrolateral medulla that project to the rostral ventrolateral medulla. *Brain Res.* 693, 51–63.

Bechtold, D. A., and Luckman, S. M. (2006). Prolactin-releasing peptide mediates cholecystokinin-induced satiety in mice. *Endocrinology* 147, 4723–4729.

Bechtold, D. A., and Luckman, S. M. (2007). The role of RFamide peptides in feeding. *J. Endocrinol.* 192, 3–15.

Bechtold, D. A., Sidibe, A., Saer, B. R., Li, J., Hand, L. E., Ivanova, E. A., et al. (2012). A role for the melatonin-related receptor GPR50 in leptin signaling, adaptive thermogenesis, and torpor. *Curr. Biol.* 22, 70–77.

Bhattacharyya, S., Luan, J., Challis, B., Schmitz, C., Clarkson, P., Franks, P. W., et al. (2003). Association of polymorphisms in GPR10, the gene encoding the prolactin-releasing peptide receptor with blood pressure, but not obesity, in a U.K. Caucasian population. *Diabetes* 52, 1296–1299.

Blevins, J. E., Eakin, T. J., Murphy, J. A., Schwartz, M. W., and Baskin, D. G. (2003). Oxytocin innervation of caudal brainstem nuclei activated by cholecystokinin. *Brain Res.* 993, 30–41.

Brown, R. E., Basheer, R., McKenna, J. T., Strecker, R. E., and McCarley, R. W. (2012). Control of sleep and wakefulness. *Physiol. Rev.* 92, 1087–1187.

Buck, L., and Axel, R. (1991). A novel multigene family may encode odorant receptors: a molecular basis for odor recognition. *Cell* 65, 175–187.

Chen, C., Dun, S. L., Dun, N. J., and Chang, J. K. (1999). Prolactin-releasing peptide-immunoreactivity in A1 and A2 noradrenergic neurons of the rat medulla. *Brain Res.* 822, 276–279.

Cheung, G. W., Kokorovic, A., Lam, C. K., Chari, M., and Lam, T. K. (2009). Intestinal cholecystokinin controls glucose production through a neuronal network. *Cell Metab.* 10, 99–109.

Denver, R. J., Bonett, R. M., and Boorse, G. C. (2011). Evolution of leptin structure and function. *Neuroendocrinology* 94, 21–38.

Dockray, G. J. (2004). The expanding family of -RFamide peptides and their effects on feeding behaviour. *Exp. Physiol.* 89, 229–235.

Duggan, A. W., Hope, P. J., Jarrott, B., Schaible, H. G., and Fleetwood-Walker, S. M. (1990). Release, spread and persistence of immunoreactive neurokinin A in the dorsal horn of the cat following noxious cutaneous stimulation. Studies with antibody microprobes. *Neuroscience* 35, 195–202.

Ellacott, K. L., Lawrence, C. B., Rothwell, N. J., and Luckman, S. M. (2002). PRL-releasing peptide interacts with leptin to reduce food intake and body weight. *Endocrinology* 143, 368–374.

Engstrom, M., Brandt, A., Wurster, S., Savola, J. M., and Panula, P. (2003). Prolactin releasing peptide has high affinity and efficacy at neuropeptide FF2 receptors. *J. Pharmacol. Exp. Ther.* 305, 825–832.

Enriori, P. J., Sinnayah, P., Simonds, S. E., Garcia Rudaz, C., and Cowley, M. A. (2011). Leptin action in the dorsomedial hypothalamus increases sympathetic tone to brown adipose tissue in spite of systemic leptin resistance. *J. Neurosci.* 31, 12189–12197.

Flower, D. R. (1999). Modelling G-protein-coupled receptors for drug design. *Biochim. Biophys. Acta* 1422, 207–234.

Fredriksson, R., Lagerstrom, M. C., Lundin, L. G., and Schioth, H. B. (2003). The G-protein-coupled receptors in the human genome form five main families. Phylogenetic analysis, paralogon groups, and fingerprints. *Mol. Pharmacol.* 63, 1256–1272.

Fujii, R., Fukusumi, S., Hosoya, M., Kawamata, Y., Habata, Y., Hinuma, S., et al. (1999). Tissue distribution of prolactin-releasing peptide (PrRP) and its receptor. *Regul. Pept.* 83, 1–10.

Fujiwara, K., Matsumoto, H., Yada, T., and Inoue, K. (2005). Identification of the prolactin-releasing peptide-producing cell in the rat adrenal gland. *Regul. Pept.* 126, 97–102.

Garfield, A. S., Patterson, C., Skora, S., Gribble, F. M., Reimann, F., Evans, M. L., et al. (2012). Neurochemical characterization of body weight-regulating leptin receptor neurons in the nucleus of the solitary tract. *Endocrinology* 153, 4600–4607.

Gautron, L., Lazarus, M., Scott, M. M., Saper, C. B., and Elmquist, J. K. (2010). Identifying the efferent projections of leptin-responsive neurons in the dorsomedial hypothalamus using a novel conditional tracing approach. *J. Comp. Neurol.* 518, 2090–2108.

Gouarderes, C., Puget, A., and Zajac, J. M. (2004). Detailed distribution of neuropeptide FF receptors (NPFF1 and NPFF2) in the rat, mouse, octodon, rabbit, guinea pig, and marmoset monkey brains: a comparative autoradiographic study. *Synapse* 51, 249–269.

Gu, W., Geddes, B. J., Zhang, C., Foley, K. P., and Stricker-Krongrad, A. (2004). The prolactin-releasing peptide receptor (GPR10) regulates body weight homeostasis in mice. *J. Mol. Neurosci.* 22, 93–103.

Hay-Schmidt, A., Helboe, L., and Larsen, P. J. (2001). Leptin receptor immunoreactivity is present in ascending serotonergic and catecholaminergic neurons of the rat. *Neuroendocrinology* 73, 215–226.

Hinuma, S., Habata, Y., Fujii, R., Kawamata, Y., Hosoya, M., Fukusumi, S., et al. (1998). A prolactin-releasing peptide in the brain. *Nature* 393, 272–276.

Horiuchi, J., Saigusa, T., Sugiyama, N., Kanba, S., Nishida, Y., Sato, Y., et al. (2002). Effects of prolactin-releasing peptide microinjection into the ventrolateral medulla on arterial pressure and sympathetic activity in rats. *Brain Res.* 958, 201–209.

Ibata, Y., Iijima, N., Kataoka, Y., Kakihara, K., Tanaka, M., Hosoya, M., et al. (2000). Morphological survey of prolactin-releasing peptide and its receptor with special reference to their functional roles in the brain. *Neurosci. Res.* 38, 223–230.

Iijima, N., Kataoka, Y., Kakihara, K., Bamba, H., Tamada, Y., Hayashi, S., et al. (1999). Cytochemical study of prolactin-releasing peptide (PrRP) in the rat brain. *Neuroreport* 10, 1713–1716.

Iijima, N., Matsumoto, Y., Yano, T., Tanaka, M., Yamamoto, T., Kakihara, K., et al. (2001). A novel function of prolactin-releasing peptide in the control of growth hormone via secretion of somatostatin from the hypothalamus. *Endocrinology* 142, 3239–3243.

Kalliomaki, M. L., Pertovaara, A., Brandt, A., Wei, H., Pietila, P., Kalmari, J., et al. (2004). Prolactin-releasing peptide affects pain, allodynia and autonomic reflexes through medullary mechanisms. *Neuropharmacology* 46, 412–424.

Kawakami, A., Okada, N., Rokkaku, K., Honda, K., Ishibashi, S., and Onaka, T. (2008). Leptin inhibits and ghrelin augments hypothalamic noradrenaline release after stress. *Stress* 11, 363–369.

Lawrence, C. B., Celsi, F., Brennand, J., and Luckman, S. M. (2000). Alternative role for prolactin-releasing peptide in the regulation of food intake. *Nat. Neurosci.* 3, 645–646.

Lawrence, C. B., Ellacott, K. L., and Luckman, S. M. (2002). PRL-releasing peptide reduces food intake and may mediate satiety signaling. *Endocrinology* 143, 360–367.

Lawrence, C. B., Liu, Y. L., Stock, M. J., and Luckman, S. M. (2004). Anorectic actions of prolactin-releasing peptide are mediated by corticotropin-releasing hormone receptors. *Am. J. Physiol. Regul. Integr. Comp. Physiol.* 286, R101–R107.

Lee, Y., Yang, S. P., Soares, M. J., and Voogt, J. L. (2000). Distribution of prolactin-releasing peptide mRNA in the rat brain. *Brain Res. Bull.* 51, 171–176.

Lin, S. H. (2008). Prolactin-releasing peptide. *Results Probl. Cell Differ.* 46, 57–88.

Lin, S. H., Arai, A. C., Espana, R. A., Berridge, C. W., Leslie, F. M., Huguenard, J. R., et al. (2002a). Prolactin-releasing peptide (PrRP) promotes awakening and suppresses absence seizures. *Neuroscience* 114, 229–238.

Lin, S. H., Leslie, F. M., and Civelli, O. (2002b). Neurochemical properties of the prolactin releasing peptide (PrRP) receptor expressing neurons: evidence for a role of PrRP as a regulator of stress and nociception. *Brain Res.* 952, 15–30.

Luckman, S. M. (1992). Fos-like immunoreactivity in the brainstem of the rat following peripheral administration of cholecystokinin. *J. Neuroendocrinol.* 4, 149–152.

Ma, L., MacTavish, D., Simonin, F., Bourguignon, J. J., Watanabe, T., and Jhamandas, J. H. (2009). Prolactin-releasing peptide effects in the rat brain are mediated through the Neuropeptide FF receptor. *Eur. J. Neurosci.* 30, 1585–1593.

Marchese, A., Heiber, M., Nguyen, T., Heng, H. H., Saldivia, V. R., Cheng, R., et al. (1995). Cloning and chromosomal mapping of three novel genes, GPR9, GPR10, and GPR14, encoding receptors related to interleukin 8, neuropeptide Y, and somatostatin receptors. *Genomics* 29, 335–344.

Maruyama, M., Matsumoto, H., Fujiwara, K., Kitada, C., Hinuma, S., Onda, H., et al. (1999). Immunocytochemical localization of prolactin-releasing peptide in the rat brain. *Endocrinology* 140, 2326–2333.

Maruyama, M., Matsumoto, H., Fujiwara, K., Noguchi, J., Kitada, C., Fujino, M., et al. (2001). Prolactin-releasing peptide as a novel stress mediator in the central nervous system. *Endocrinology* 142, 2032–2038.

Matsumoto, H., Maruyama, M., Noguchi, J., Horikoshi, Y., Fujiwara, K., Kitada, C., et al. (2000). Stimulation of corticotropin-releasing hormone-mediated adrenocorticotropin secretion by central administration of prolactin-releasing peptide in rats. *Neurosci. Lett.* 285, 234–238.

Matsumoto, H., Murakami, Y., Horikoshi, Y., Noguchi, J., Habata, Y., Kitada, C., et al. (1999a). Distribution and characterization of immunoreactive prolactin-releasing peptide (PrRP) in rat tissue and plasma. *Biochem. Biophys. Res. Commun.* 257, 264–268.

Matsumoto, H., Noguchi, J., Horikoshi, Y., Kawamata, Y., Kitada, C., Hinuma, S., et al. (1999b). Stimulation of prolactin release by prolactin-releasing peptide in rats. *Biochem. Biophys. Res. Commun.* 259, 321–324.

Mera, T., Fujihara, H., Kawasaki, M., Hashimoto, H., Saito, T., Shibata, M., et al. (2006). Prolactin-releasing peptide is a potent mediator of stress responses in the brain through the hypothalamic paraventricular nucleus. *Neuroscience* 141, 1069–1086.

Minami, S., Nakata, T., Tokita, R., Onodera, H., and Imaki, J. (1999). Cellular localization of prolactin-releasing peptide messenger RNA in the rat brain. *Neurosci. Lett.* 266, 73–75.

Morales, T., Hinuma, S., and Sawchenko, P. E. (2000). Prolactin-releasing peptide is expressed in afferents to the endocrine hypothalamus, but not in neurosecretory neurones. *J. Neuroendocrinol.* 12, 131–140.

Morales, T., and Sawchenko, P. E. (2003). Brainstem prolactin-releasing peptide neurons are sensitive to stress and lactation. *Neuroscience* 121, 771–778.

Moriyama, S., Ito, T., Takahashi, A., Amano, M., Sower, S. A., Hirano, T., et al. (2002). A homolog of mammalian PRL-releasing peptide (fish arginyl-phenylalanyl-amide peptide) is a major hypothalamic peptide of PRL release in teleost fish. *Endocrinology* 143, 2071–2079.

Murillo-Rodriguez, E., Arias-Carrion, O., Zavala-Garcia, A., Sarro-Ramirez, A., Huitron-Resendiz, S., and Arankowsky-Sandoval, G. (2012). Basic sleep mechanisms: an integrative review. *Cent. Nerv. Syst. Agents Med. Chem.* 12, 38–54.

Olson, B. R., Drutarosky, M. D., Stricker, E. M., and Verbalis, J. G. (1991). Brain oxytocin receptor antagonism blunts the effects of anorexigenic treatments in rats: evidence for central oxytocin inhibition of food intake. *Endocrinology* 129, 785–791.

Onaka, T. (2004). Neural pathways controlling central and peripheral oxytocin release during stress. *J. Neuroendocrinol.* 16, 308–312.

Onaka, T., Takayanagi, Y., and Leng, G. (2010). Metabolic and stress-related roles of prolactin-releasing peptide. *Trends Endocrinol. Metab.* 21, 287–293.

Osugi, T., Ukena, K., Sower, S. A., Kawauchi, H., and Tsutsui, K. (2006). Evolutionary origin and divergence of PQRFamide peptides and LPXRFamide peptides in the RFamide peptide family. Insights from novel lamprey RFamide peptides. *FEBS J.* 273, 1731–1743.

Palkovits, M., Zaborszky, L., Feminger, A., Mezey, E., Fekete, M. I., Herman, J. P., et al. (1980). Noradrenergic innervation of the rat hypothalamus:experimental biochemical and electron microscopic studies. *Brain Res.* 191, 161–171.

Paxinos, G., and Watson, C. (1998). *The Rat Brain in Stereotaxis Coordinates.* San Diego: Academic Press.

Probst, W. C., Snyder, L. A., Schuster, D. I., Brosius, J., and Sealfon, S. C. (1992). Sequence alignment of the G-protein coupled receptor superfamily. *DNA Cell Biol.* 11, 1–20.

Roland, B. L., Sutton, S. W., Wilson, S. J., Luo, L., Pyati, J., Huvar, R., et al. (1999). Anatomical distribution of prolactin-releasing peptide and its receptor suggests additional functions in the central nervous system and periphery. *Endocrinology* 140, 5736–5745.

Sakamoto, T., Oda, A., Yamamoto, K., Kaneko, M., Kikuyama, S., Nishikawa, A., et al. (2006). Molecular cloning and functional characterization of a prolactin-releasing peptide homolog from *Xenopus laevis. Peptides* 27, 3347–3351.

Samson, W. K., Resch, Z. T., and Murphy, T. C. (2000). A novel action of the newly described prolactin-releasing peptides: cardiovascular regulation. *Brain Res.* 858, 19–25.

Saper, C. (2004). "Central autonaomic system," in *The Rat Nervous System*, ed. G. Paxinos (San Diego, CA: Elsevier Academic Press), 761–794.

Seal, L. J., Small, C. J., Dhillo, W. S., Kennedy, A. R., Ghatei, M. A., and Bloom, S. R. (2002). Prolactin-releasing peptide releases corticotropin-releasing hormone and increases plasma adrenocorticotropin via the paraventricular nucleus of the hypothalamus. *Neuroendocrinology* 76, 70–78.

Seale, A. P., Itoh, T., Moriyama, S., Takahashi, A., Kawauchi, H., Sakamoto, T., et al. (2002). Isolation and characterization of a homologue of mammalian prolactin-releasing peptide from the tilapia brain and its effect on prolactin release from the tilapia pituitary. *Gen. Comp. Endocrinol.* 125, 328–339.

Spina, M. G., Basso, A. M., Zorrilla, E. P., Heyser, C. J., Rivier, J., Vale, W., et al. (2000). Behavioral effects of central administration of the novel CRF antagonist astressin in rats. *Neuropsychopharmacology* 22, 230–239.

Steriade, M. (2005). Sleep, epilepsy and thalamic reticular inhibitory neurons. *Trends Neurosci.* 28, 317–324.

Sun, B., Fujiwara, K., Adachi, S., and Inoue, K. (2005). Physiological roles of prolactin-releasing peptide. *Regul. Pept.* 126, 27–33.

Suntsova, N., Kumar, S., Guzman-Marin, R., Alam, M. N., Szymusiak, R., and McGinty, D. (2009). A role for the preoptic sleep-promoting system in absence epilepsy. *Neurobiol. Dis.* 36, 126–141.

Szymusiak, R. (2010). Hypothalamic versus neocortical control of sleep. *Curr. Opin. Pulm. Med.* 16, 530–535.

Takayanagi, Y., Matsumoto, H., Nakata, M., Mera, T., Fukusumi, S., Hinuma, S., et al. (2008). Endogenous prolactin-releasing peptide regulates food intake in rodents. *J. Clin. Invest.* 118, 4014–4024.

Takayanagi, Y., and Onaka, T. (2010). Roles of prolactin-releasing peptide and RFamide related peptides in the control of stress and food intake. *FEBS J.* 277, 4998–5005.

Timofeev, I., and Chauvette, S. (2011). Thalamocortical oscillations: local control of EEG slow waves. *Curr. Top. Med. Chem.* 11, 2457–2471.

Uchida, K., Kobayashi, D., Das, G., Onaka, T., Inoue, K., and Itoi, K. (2010). Participation of the prolactin-releasing peptide-containing neurones in caudal medulla in conveying haemorrhagic stress-induced signals to the paraventricular nucleus of the hypothalamus. *J. Neuroendocrinol.* 22, 33–42.

Vale, W., Rivier, C., Brown, M. R., Spiess, J., Koob, G., Swanson, L., et al. (1983). Chemical and biological characterization of corticotropin releasing factor. *Recent Prog. Horm. Res.* 39, 245–270.

Watanabe, T. K., Suzuki, M., Yamasaki, Y., Okuno, S., Hishigaki, H., Ono, T., et al. (2005). Mutated G-protein-coupled receptor GPR10

19

RFRP neurons are critical gatekeepers for the photoperiodic control of reproduction

Valérie Simonneaux* and Caroline Ancel

Neurobiologie des Rythmes, Institut des Neurosciences Cellulaires et Intégratives, UPR CNRS 3212, Strasbourg, France

Edited by:
Hubert Vaudry, University of Rouen, France

Reviewed by:
Lance Kriegsfeld, University of California, USA
Iain J. Clarke, Monash University, Australia

****Correspondence:***
Valérie Simonneaux, Neurobiologie des Rythmes, Institut des Neurosciences Cellulaires et Intégratives, UPR CNRS 3212, 5, rue Blaise Pascal, 67084 Strasbourg, France.
e-mail: simonneaux@inci-cnrs.unistra.fr

Seasonally breeding mammals rely on the photoperiodic signal to restrict their fertility to a certain time of the year. The photoperiodic information is translated in the brain via the pineal hormone melatonin, and it is now well-established that it is the variation in the duration of the nocturnal peak of melatonin which synchronizes reproduction with the seasons. The Syrian hamster is a long day breeder, and sexual activity is therefore promoted by exposure to a long day photoperiod and inhibited by exposure to a short day photoperiod. Interestingly, in this species electrolytic lesion of the mediobasal hypothalamus abolishes the short day-induced gonadal regression. We have shown that the expression of a recently discovered neuronal population, namely *RFamide-related peptide* (*rfrp*) neurons, present in the mediobasal hypothalamus, is strongly down-regulated by melatonin in short day conditions, but not altered by circulating levels of sex steroids. The role of *rfrp* and its product RFRP-3 in the regulation of reproductive activity has been extensively studied in mammals, and our recent findings indicate that this peptide is a potent stimulator of the reproductive axis in the Syrian hamster. It induces a marked increase in GnRH neuron activity and gonadotropin secretion, and it is able to rescue reproductive activity in short day sexually inactive hamsters. Little is known about the localization of the RFRP-3 receptor, GPR147, in the rodent brain. Accumulating evidence suggests that RFRP-3 could be acting via two intermediates, the *GnRH* neurons in the preoptic area and the *Kiss1* neurons in the arcuate nucleus, but future studies should aim at describing the localization of *Gpr147* in the Syrian hamster brain. Altogether our data indicate that the *rfrp* neuronal population within the mediobasal hypothalamus might be a serious candidate in mediating the photoperiodic effects of melatonin on the regulation of the reproductive axis.

Keywords: RFamide peptide, RFRP-3, GPR147, kisspeptin, seasonal reproduction, melatonin

MAMMALS USE THE RHYTHMIC SECRETION OF THE PINEAL HORMONE MELATONIN TO SYNCHRONIZE REPRODUCTION WITH THE SEASONS

A large number of species restrict their fertility to a particular time of the year to ensure that the birth of the offspring occurs during the most favorable season. To determine the time of the year and synchronize their reproductive activity accordingly, mammals use the highly reproducible annual variations in light duration (or photoperiod). Photoperiod is transduced by a photoneuroendocrine system composed of the retina, the suprachiasmatic nucleus (seat of the master circadian clock) and the pineal gland which releases the hormone melatonin exclusively at night, so that the duration of the secretion varies according to night length. Therefore, the photoperiodic variations in circulating levels of melatonin throughout the year provide the body with a robust and reproducible representation of the seasons (Simonneaux and Ribelayga, 2003). It has long been established that photoperiodic variations in the duration of the nocturnal peak of melatonin synchronize reproduction in seasonal species like sheep or hamsters (Hoffman and Reiter, 1965; Carter and Goldman, 1983; Pevet, 1988; Bartness et al., 1993; Malpaux et al., 2001).

Syrian hamsters are long day breeders, meaning that they are sexually active in long day (LD: 14 light/10 h dark) conditions. Upon exposure to short day (SD: 10 light/14 h dark) conditions, they undergo a dramatic inhibition of reproductive activity within 8–10 weeks manifested by a marked atrophy of the gonads and accessory organs resulting in low levels of circulating sex steroids. Surgical removal of the pineal gland before exposure to SD conditions prevents hamsters from undergoing sexual inactivation. Conversely, exogenous melatonin injections mimicking SD conditions in hamsters raised in LD conditions induce sexual inactivation. In contrast to small rodents, large mammals with a longer gestation time like sheep are SD-breeders; they are sexually active in SD conditions and become quiescent after transfer to LD conditions. Although the reproductive timing is opposite in hamsters and sheep, in both cases the circulating levels of melatonin synchronize reproduction with photoperiod. However, why the reproductive systems of LD- and SD-breeders respond in opposite ways to the same melatonin signal is not known.

MELATONIN ACTS ON THE PARS TUBERALIS TO TRANSMIT PHOTOPERIODIC INFORMATION

It is clear that melatonin does not act directly on GnRH neurons and responsiveness to GnRH does not change with photoperiod (Urbanski et al., 1991). Melatonin binding sites are found in a number of brain structures but with considerable species differences (Masson-Pevet et al., 1994). Besides, a high density of melatonin receptors has been identified in the pars tuberalis of the adenohypophysis in a large number of mammalian species (Masson-Pevet and Gauer, 1994). Notably, the pars tuberalis cells expressing melatonin receptors synthesize thyroid-stimulating hormone (TSH) in a photoperiod/melatonin-dependent manner, with a higher level of expression in LD conditions (Klosen et al., 2002; Dardente et al., 2003, 2010). TSH produced by the pars tuberalis has been recently recognized as a key messenger through which melatonin acts on the gonadotropic axis for the seasonal control of reproduction. TSH acts on a specialized glial cell type of the hypothalamic ependymal wall, the tanycytes, to induce a marked up-regulation of the thyroid hormone-activating enzyme deiodinase 2 (Dio2) which in turn increases local concentrations of the bioactive T3 thyroid hormone (Yoshimura et al., 2003; Hanon et al., 2008, 2010; Nakao et al., 2008). In quail (Yoshimura et al., 2003) and Siberian hamsters (Barrett et al., 2007) local T3 administration was reported to increase reproductive activity although through unknown mechanisms.

Altogether these observations point to the pars tuberalis as a key site for the integration of the endocrine melatoninergic message for the seasonal regulation of reproductive activity. However, the central reproductive site(s) actually controlled by the melatonin/TSH system is(are) still unknown. Various structures in the mediobasal hypothalamus have been proposed to be direct or indirect sites of action for melatonin, particularly in the sheep (Malpaux et al., 1998) and hamster (Maywood and Hastings, 1995).

RFRP-3 NEURONS LOCATED IN THE MEDIOBASAL HYPOTHALAMUS ARE STRONGLY REGULATED BY MELATONIN

In the Syrian hamster, the dorsal part of the mediobasal hypothalamus appears as a key structure for the photoperiodic regulation of reproductive activity since it contains melatonin binding sites and its ablation by electrolytic lesion prevents the inhibitory effect of melatonin on reproductive activity (Maywood et al., 1996). Recently, we reported that neurons located in this hypothalamic area express the *RFamide-related peptide* (*rfrp*) gene in a photoperiodic-dependent manner in Siberian and Syrian hamsters (Revel et al., 2008).

The *rfrp* gene was discovered in 2000 in mammals (Hinuma et al., 2000), concurrently with the discovery of its avian ortholog *gonadotropin-inhibitory hormone* (*gnih*; Tsutsui et al., 2000). The *rfrp* and *gnih* genes were found to produce new peptides of the RFamide family of peptides, which share a common C-terminal LPXRFamide (X = L or Q) motif. In the quail, GnIH was shown to act directly at the level of the pituitary to inhibit gonadotropin release (Tsutsui et al., 2000). In mammals, the *rfrp* gene is expressed in neurons located in the mediobasal hypothalamus and encodes a precursor that produces two peptides, RFRP-1 and RFRP-3 (Ukena and Tsutsui, 2001; Kriegsfeld et al., 2006; Clarke et al., 2008; Dardente et al., 2008; Revel et al., 2008; Smith et al., 2008; Rizwan et al., 2009). The demonstration that GnIH is a potent inhibitor of gonadotropin release in birds spurred great interest in the roles of RFRP-1 and particularly RFRP-3 in the regulation of endocrine functions in mammals (Bentley et al., 2010; Kriegsfeld et al., 2010; Smith and Clarke, 2010; Tsutsui et al., 2010 for reviews).

In Syrian and Siberian hamsters, we observed that the level of *rfrp* mRNA is strongly down-regulated in sexually inactive SD-adapted animals (Revel et al., 2008). This variation is solely photoperiodic as there are no daily changes in *rfrp* mRNA levels either in LD or SD conditions. In both species, the SD-induced decrease in *rfrp* gene expression is associated with a similar decrease in peptide immunoreactivity in perikarya and fibers (Revel et al., 2008; Mason et al., 2010; Ubuka et al., 2012; **Figure 1**). We have recently found a similar SD-induced inhibition of *rfrp* expression in other LD-breeders, notably the European hamster (**Figure 1**) and the jerboa (Janati et al., 2012). Strikingly, in sheep, a SD-breeder, two studies reported that hypothalamic *rfrp* mRNA levels and RFRP immunoreactivity are also reduced in SD conditions while animals are sexually active (Dardente et al., 2008; Smith et al., 2008). In contrast, in the non-photoperiodic rat *rfrp* mRNA levels are not modified by photoperiodic conditions (Revel et al., 2008).

In the Syrian hamster, we demonstrated that the SD down-regulation of *rfrp* expression is not due to the lower levels of

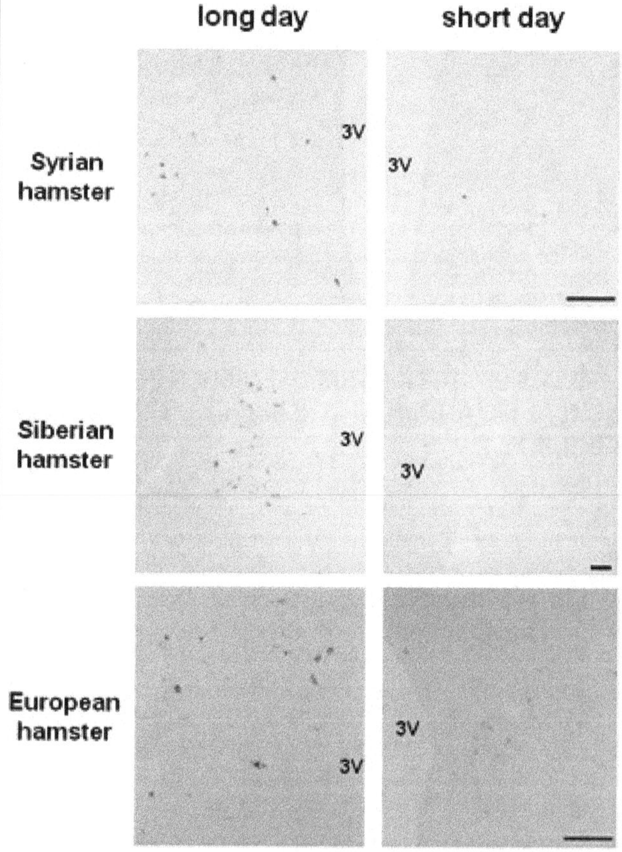

FIGURE 1 | Photoperiodic variations in RFRP immunoreactivity in the dorsomedial hypothalamus of male Syrian, Siberian, and European hamsters raised in long day or short day conditions. Scale bar = 100 μM, 3V: third ventricle. RFRP antibody was generously provided by Dr. Greg Anderson; Syrian and Siberian hamster pictures were kindly provided by Julien Bartzen and European hamster pictures by Cristina Saenz de Miera.

circulating sex steroids since neither testosterone implants in sexually inactive SD hamsters, nor testis ablation in LD-adapted hamsters altered the levels of *rfrp* mRNA. This lack of major sex steroid feedback on *rfrp* expression is in agreement with other studies conducted in rats, mice, Siberian hamsters, and sheep (Smith et al., 2008; Quennell et al., 2010; Poling et al., 2012; Ubuka et al., 2012). Of note however, studies in female Syrian hamsters reported that RFRP neurons contain Er-α and respond to estrogen administration (Kriegsfeld et al., 2006; Gibson et al., 2008) and RFRP expression in ewe is reduced during the preovulatory period (Clarke et al., 2012).

Importantly, we found that pineal gland ablation before transferring hamsters to SD conditions, a protocol which prevents the SD-induced inhibition of reproductive activity, prevented the decrease in *rfrp* mRNA levels (Revel et al., 2008). Conversely, repeated melatonin injections during the late afternoon to LD-adapted hamsters, a protocol known to inhibit reproductive activity, also induced a marked decreased in *rfrp* mRNA levels (Revel et al., 2008). In the Siberian hamster as well, the down-regulation of *rfrp* expression in SD conditions is induced by melatonin (Ubuka et al., 2012). Remarkably, in the quail, melatonin also regulates GnIH expression but in an opposite manner compared to mammals. Melatonin binds to Mel1c receptors located on GnIH neurons to increase GnIH synthesis and release, and as a consequence, expression of this inhibitory peptide is increased under SD conditions (Ubuka et al., 2005).

Altogether these observations indicate that in a number of seasonal mammalian species, *rfrp* expression is decreased in SD conditions regardless of whether the species is a LD- or a SD-breeder. Experiments with melatonin manipulation carried out in Syrian and Siberian hamsters demonstrate that *rfrp* down-regulation results from the larger production of melatonin in SD conditions. It is tempting to speculate that melatonin may act primarily on RFRP neurons in the mediobasal hypothalamus to control seasonal reproduction. Several observations, however, indicate that this central effect of melatonin is probably indirect. Melatonin binding sites are found in the area where RFRP neurons are located in the Syrian hamster, but this is not the case in the other seasonal species like the Siberian and European hamsters or the sheep. Furthermore, in the Syrian hamster, we found that at least 3 weeks of daily melatonin administration is required to induce a significant reduction in the level of *rfrp* mRNA (Revel et al., 2008) whereas the pineal hormone is much faster to control the expression of other photoperiodically regulated genes like *tsh* in the pars tuberalis or *deiodinase 2* in the tanycytes (Revel et al., 2006a; Yasuo et al., 2007; Dardente, 2012). Therefore, it appears likely that there is an intermediate between the endocrine melatoninergic message and the photoperiodic regulation of RFRP expression, and it might be interesting to investigate whether it is the melatonin-driven TSH/T3 signal.

RFRP-3 STIMULATES THE GONADOTROPIC AXIS AND RESCUES REPRODUCTIVE ACTIVITY IN PHOTO-INHIBITED HAMSTERS

An increasing number of studies now indicate that RFRP-3 is implicated in the regulation of mammalian reproductive function (Bentley et al., 2010; Tsutsui et al., 2010 for reviews). In mice RFRP-3 was found to exhibit rapid and repeatable inhibitory effects on the firing rate of a subpopulation of GnRH neurons (Ducret et al., 2009). In male rats, intracerebroventricular (icv) RFRP-3 significantly suppresses all facets of sex behavior and also significantly reduces plasma levels of luteinizing hormone (LH; Johnson et al., 2007; Pineda et al., 2010). In female rats, chronic icv infusion of RFRP-3 causes a dose-dependent inhibition of GnRH neuronal activation at the LH surge peak and also suppresses neuronal activation in the anteroventral periventricular region, which provides stimulatory input to GnRH neurons (Anderson et al., 2009). In ovariectomized mature rats, intravenous administration of RFRP-3 significantly reduces plasma LH concentrations (Murakami et al., 2008). Finally, in the ovine and bovine species, RFRP-3 administration inhibits gonadotropin release (Clarke et al., 2008; Kadokawa et al., 2009; Sari et al., 2009) although this is still controversial (Caraty et al., 2012).

Until recently, and based on the plethora of publications supporting this hypothesis, it was assumed that RFRP-3 functioned in mammals as GnIH functioned in birds and served as an inhibitory component regulating the hypothalamic–pituitary–gonadal axis. However, this statement was somehow contradictory with our observation of an increased synthesis of RFRP in LD-adapted sexually active hamsters. We have recently reported novel findings in the male Syrian hamster (Ancel et al., 2012) which have led to call this assumption into question, concurrently with another group working on the male Siberian hamster (Ubuka et al., 2012). In the male Syrian hamster, we reported that acute icv administration of RFRP-3 stimulates GnRH cell activity, gonadotropin release, and testosterone production under LD conditions (**Figure 2**; Ancel et al., 2012). In the same manner, in SD-adapted male Syrian hamsters a single central injection of RFRP-3 increases gonadotropin release [LH (ng/ml) vehicle 1.72 ± 0.31 vs. RFRP-3 4.36 ± 0.82; $n = 6$; $p < 0.05$]. Furthermore, under the same photo-inhibitory conditions, 5 weeks of continuous central administration of RFRP-3 to male Syrian hamsters produces a complete reactivation of the reproductive axis, manifested by increased testis weight and circulating levels of testosterone, similar to those observed in LD conditions (**Figure 3A**; Ancel et al., 2012). In the Siberian hamster, while administration of RFRP-3 in LD conditions inhibits gonadotropin release, the same protocol stimulates gonadotropin secretion in SD conditions (Ubuka et al., 2012). Remarkably, these findings of a stimulatory action of RFRP-3 on the male hamster reproductive axis are in sharp contrast with a previous study reporting an inhibitory effect of icv GnIH in ovariectomized female Syrian hamsters (Kriegsfeld et al., 2006). In LD conditions, reproductive activity of female rodents displays a well-described estrous cycle, characterized by varying levels of circulating gonadotropins and sex steroids. It has been hypothesized that RFRP-3 might be an inhibitory component of the negative feedback loop which regulates the estrous cycle, since RFRP cellular activity is decreased at the time of the LH surge in the Syrian hamster (Gibson et al., 2008). In this context it would be interesting to determine whether the effect of RFRP-3 on the female reproductive axis depends on the stage of the estrous cycle at which it is administered.

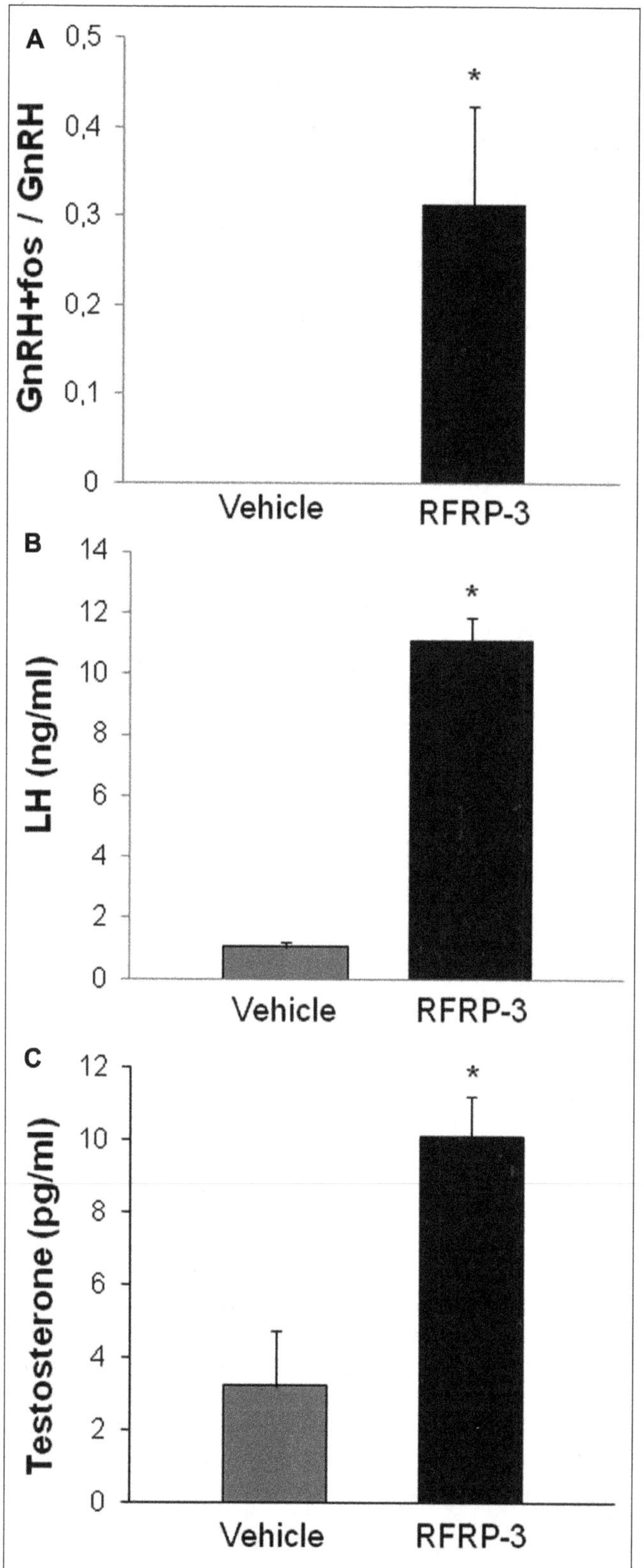

FIGURE 2 | Acute intracerebroventricular administration of RFRP-3 (1500 ng) activates c-FOS expression in GnRH neurons (A) and increases LH production (B) and circulating levels of testosterone (C) in sexually active long day-adapted male Syrian hamsters. *$p < 0.05$ when compared to vehicle-treated animals. Adapted from Ancel et al. (2012).

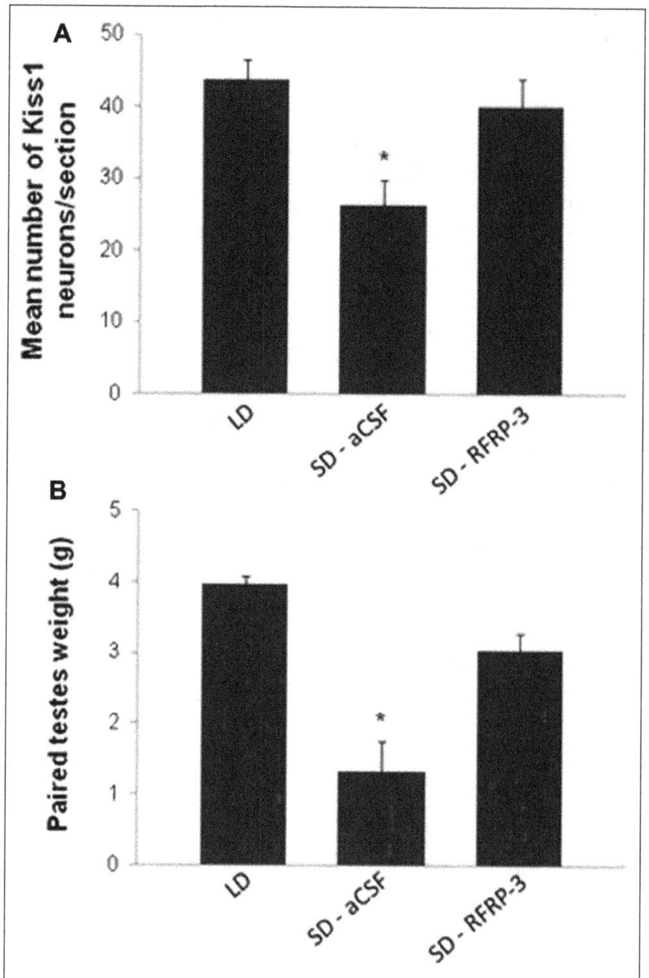

FIGURE 3 | Chronic intracerebroventricular administration of RFRP-3 [12 μg/day for 5 weeks in artificial cerebrospinal fluid (aCSF)] in sexually inactive short day (SD)-adapted male Syrian hamsters increases kisspeptin expression in the arcuate nucleus (A) and testicular weight (B) up to values comparable to animals kept in long day (LD) conditions. *$p < 0.05$ when compared to LD or RFRP-3 treated SD animals. Adapted from Ancel et al. (2012).

Taken together, these data indicate that there are certainly species- and gender-dependent differences in the involvement of RFRP-3 in the regulation of reproductive activity. As a consequence one might be cautious when calling the mammalian peptide "GnIH" based on its effect in birds, and in the light of the recent reports on work carried out in male hamsters the peptide should be termed "RFRP-3." From a seasonal point of view, when considering LD- (hamster) and SD- (sheep) breeders, it is remarkable to find that while the expression of the peptide in increased in LD conditions in both kinds of breeders, the effect of the peptide on the gonadotropic axis is opposite, as it is stimulatory in hamsters and inhibitory in sheep. This suggests a non-conserved role and/or site of action for RFRP-3 across seasonally breeding species. It is tempting to speculate that RFRP neurons may play a key role in discriminating between long and short day breeders because RFRP expression is down-regulated by a short day profile of melatonin in both kinds of seasonal breeders but the peptide appears to have an opposite effect on the reproductive axis, being stimulatory in long day and inhibitory in short day breeders. Complementary experiments will have to be carried out in other species to test this hypothesis and fully understand the role of RFRP-3 in the seasonal control of reproduction.

Interestingly, the RFRP peptides were shown to have a modulatory action on feeding behavior (Bechtold and Luckman, 2007; Johnson et al., 2007; Clarke et al., 2012) thus it might be worth investigating whether the photoperiodic variation in RFRP expression might also impact on food intake and body weight regulation in seasonal species.

RFRP-3 MODES AND SITES OF ACTION

The complex involvement of RFRP peptides in the regulation of the hypothalamic–pituitary–gonadal axis has raised a number of questions regarding the sites of action of the peptides. In various mammalian species including humans, RFRP fiber networks are found in multiple brain regions including the preoptic area, the arcuate nucleus, the lateral septum, the anterior hypothalamus, and the bed nucleus of the stria terminalis (Ukena and Tsutsui, 2001; Kriegsfeld et al., 2006; Johnson et al., 2007; Mason et al., 2010). Notably, RFRP-immunoreactive fibers make apparent contact with a subpopulation of GnRH neurons in rodents and sheep (Kriegsfeld et al., 2006; Smith et al., 2008; Poling et al., 2012; Rizwan et al., 2012; Ubuka et al., 2012) suggesting that RFRP-3 acts centrally to control the reproductive axis.

There is still uncertainty as to whether RFRP-3 also exerts a hypophysiotropic effect in mammals as reported in birds. A large body of evidence now reports the absence of fibers in the median eminence of rodents (Ukena and Tsutsui, 2001; Yano et al., 2003; Kriegsfeld et al., 2006; Rizwan et al., 2009; Smith et al., 2010; Ubuka et al., 2012). However, there are controversial data as to whether RFRP-3 acts (Kriegsfeld et al., 2006; Murakami et al., 2008; Pineda et al., 2010) or not (Anderson et al., 2009; Rizwan et al., 2009; Ubuka et al., 2012) on the rodent pituitary to regulate LH secretion. In the male hamster we reported no effect of the peptide on LH secretion when injected peripherally, nor on the basal and GnRH-stimulated production of LH from isolated pituitary glands (Ancel et al., 2012). In contrast in the sheep, RFRP fibers terminating in the median eminence have been identified and the peptide is released into the portal blood and appears to induce a marked inhibition of gonadotropin secretion (Clarke et al., 2008; Sari et al., 2009; Smith et al., 2012).

The RFRP peptides bind with high affinity to GPR147 (also known as NPFF1R) and with a lower affinity to GPR74 (also known as NPFF2R), which were first identified as neuropeptide FF receptors (Hinuma et al., 2000; Liu et al., 2001; Engstrom et al., 2003). The GPR147 receptor couples with $G\alpha_{i3}$ and $G_{\alpha s}$ proteins (Gouarderes et al., 2007) suggesting that GPR147 can have both inhibitory and stimulatory downstream effects on cellular activity. However, in CHO cells, activation of the receptor inhibits forskolin-stimulated cAMP accumulation (Mollereau et al., 2002).

NPFF receptors have been detected in rodent, lagomorph, and monkey brains suggesting that they are phylogenetically conserved (Gouarderes et al., 2004a). Importantly, however, remarkable variations in GPR147 and GPR74 receptor contents exist from one species to another and from one strain to another among the same species (Gouarderes et al., 2004a,b). Early studies describing the autoradiographic distribution of GPR147 in mice and rats indicated that the receptor was present throughout the hypothalamus (Gouarderes et al., 2002, 2004a,b). More recently, the use of *in situ* hybridization facilitated precise localization and made it possible to show that about 25% of GnRH neurons express *Gpr147*, but not *Gpr74*, in various rodent species (Poling et al., 2012; Rizwan et al., 2012; Ubuka et al., 2012). This is in agreement with the observation that RFRP-3 fibers are in contact with 20–40% of GnRH neurons (Rizwan et al., 2012; Ubuka et al., 2012). Furthermore, in mice expressing GnRH-green fluorescent protein-tagged neurons, RFRP-3 was found to exert a direct inhibitory effect on the firing rate of 41% of GnRH neurons, while 12% increased their firing rate, and the remainder were unaffected (Ducret et al., 2009). These observations support the hypothesis that RFRP-3 may exert its effects on reproduction directly via GnRH neurons. However, the peptide may also act indirectly, via upstream regulators of GnRH. This hypothesis is supported by data in rats indicating that RFRP-3 fibers are in contact with kisspeptin neurons, a subpopulation (20%) of which expresses the *Gpr147* gene (Rizwan et al., 2012).

In the Syrian hamster, RFRP-ir fibers project throughout much of the brain, including into the preoptic area and the arcuate nucleus (Kriegsfeld et al., 2006). We demonstrated that central injection of RFRP-3 to Syrian hamsters induces c-Fos expression in 30% of the GnRH neurons (**Figure 2A**) suggesting that the effects observed on the reproductive axis are mediated via these neurons (Ancel et al., 2012). Whether this effect is due to a direct action of RFRP-3 on GnRH neurons or whether it is linked to an effect on upstream regulators of the reproductive axis remains to be determined. Indeed, in the same study, although c-Fos expression was not observed in kisspeptin neurons following acute administration, the continuous central administration of RFRP-3 led to an increase in *Kiss1* expression in the arcuate nucleus together with an increase of testicular activity (**Figure 3**; Ancel et al., 2012). It is therefore possible that the RFRP-3 neuronal system regulates reproductive activity by acting at two levels of the reproductive axis: the GnRH and the kisspeptin neurons. In order to answer this question, it seems essential to carry out a detailed mapping of the *gpr147* in the Syrian hamster.

Altogether, a large amount of evidence now indicates that in various mammalian species RFRP-3 regulates reproductive activity by acting via its receptor located on GnRH neurons. This is supported by results showing that RFRP-3 fibers are in contact with a subpopulation of GnRH neurons and that *Gpr147* is expressed in GnRH neurons in rodents. However, another line of evidence points to *Kiss1* neurons as possible intermediates between RFRP peptides and the regulation of the reproductive function. Indeed, in rats RFRP-3 fibers are in contact with kisspeptin neurons which express *Gpr147* and in Syrian hamsters the reactivation of the reproductive function following continuous RFRP-3 administration goes alongside with an increase in *Kiss1* expression. Future studies using Kiss1R and GnRHR antagonists could help to understand the role of each one of these neuronal populations in mediating the effects of RFRP peptides on the reproductive axis.

RFRP-3 AND KISSPEPTIN ACT IN CONCERT TO SYNCHRONIZE RODENT REPRODUCTION WITH THE SEASONS

There is strong evidence that RFRP neurons are regulated by photoperiod/melatonin to adapt reproductive activity to the seasons. A few years ago, the same supposition was made for kisspeptin, another member of the large RFamide family of peptides. In 2003, milestone studies reported that loss-of-function mutations of the kisspeptin receptor (KiSS1R/GPR54) in humans and rodents (de Roux et al., 2003; Seminara et al., 2003) prevented pubertal development and caused infertility, leading to a large number of studies aiming at investigating the role of kisspeptins in Vertebrate reproduction (Pinilla et al., 2012 for review). The *Kiss1* gene is mainly expressed in the arcuate nucleus and the anteroventro-periventricular nucleus of the hypothalamus, and kisspeptin neurons project specifically onto the GnRH cell bodies in the preoptic area and nerve terminals in the median eminence. In all mammalian species studied to date, kisspeptin appears as a powerful stimulator of the gonadotropic axis, acting primarily on GnRH neurons.

In the male Syrian hamster, we demonstrated that kisspeptin expression in the arcuate nucleus is down-regulated by melatonin in SD conditions, despite a negative feedback effect of testosterone on these neurons (Revel et al., 2006b). In the anteroventro-periventricular nucleus, kisspeptin expression is also decrease in SD conditions, but as a result of the absence of the positive feedback of testosterone consecutive to testicular regression (Ansel et al., 2010). Importantly, we demonstrated that chronic infusion of kisspeptin in SD-adapted sexually inactive male hamsters rescues reproductive activity to levels comparable to animals kept in photo-stimulatory LD conditions (Revel et al., 2006b; Ansel et al., 2011; Simonneaux et al., 2012). In the Siberian hamster as well, kisspeptin expression displays photoperiod variations and the peptide stimulates LH release (Greives et al., 2008a,b). Interestingly in the sheep, kisspeptin expression is also regulated by photoperiod, with a higher level of expression in SD conditions when animals are sexually active, and kisspeptin infusion in LD-adapted anestrous ewes induces ovulation in a majority of treated animals (Franceschini et al., 2006; Caraty et al., 2007; Smith et al., 2007, 2009). These observations indicate that kisspeptin expression, like RFRP, is regulated by photoperiod in seasonal species but, unlike RFRP, the direction of the regulation is different according to whether animals are LD- or SD-breeders.

To make things more complicated, other parameters also influenced by seasons regulate kisspeptin expression. This is particularly true for sex steroids which inhibit kisspeptin expression in the arcuate nucleus and increase it in the anteroventro-periventricular nucleus in various species including the Syrian (Revel et al., 2006b; Ansel et al., 2010) and the Siberian (Mason et al., 2007) hamsters. Additionally, metabolic factors that are also under the influence of seasonal changes were shown to impact on kisspeptin expression (Castellano et al., 2010). Therefore, although kisspeptin has been identified as an essential component of the photoperiodic regulation of reproductive activity in seasonal breeders (Revel et al., 2007; Simonneaux et al., 2009, 2012 for reviews) recent observations indicate that kisspeptin neurons are not the primary target of melatonin action but are controlled upstream by seasonally regulated intermediates.

Our current findings in the Syrian, Siberian, and European hamsters (Revel et al., 2008; **Figure 1**), in the jerboa (Janati et al., 2012), and other reports in the sheep (Dardente et al., 2008; Smith et al., 2008) suggest that RFRP-3 expression undergoes a conserved down-regulation by the SD melatonin signal irrespective of the reproductive response to seasons. In contrast, kisspeptin expression is increased when animals become sexually active, irrespective of the photoperiod. On the other hand, kisspeptin is always stimulatory of reproductive activity whereas RFRP-3 displays species-specific effects, being stimulatory in the Syrian hamster and inhibitory in the sheep.

These observations have led us to propose a working model for the seasonal control of reproduction in rodents (**Figure 4**). We propose that in LD conditions, RFRP-3 would activate GnRH neuronal activity directly and/or indirectly via the kisspeptinergic neurons. The former pathway is supported by the report of RFRP-3 fibers apposed to subpopulations of GnRH neurons (Kriegsfeld et al., 2006) whereas the latter

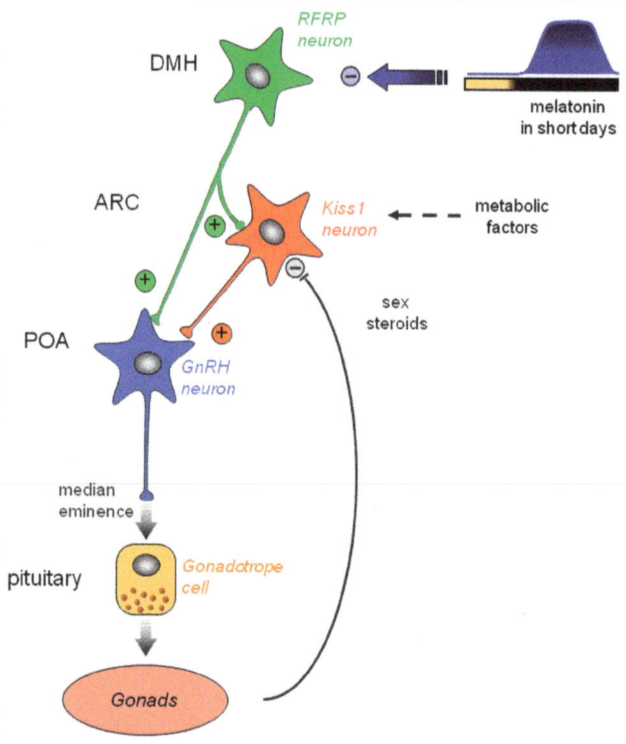

FIGURE 4 | Working model indicating how the photo-inhibitory melatonin message in short day conditions in integrated in the hypothalamus to further regulate the gonadotropic axis of the male Syrian hamster. In long day conditions, RFRP-3 activates GnRH neuron activity directly in the preoptic area (POA) and/or indirectly via the kisspeptinergic neurons in the arcuate nucleus (ARC). In short day conditions, the large production of melatonin inhibits RFRP expression in the dorsomedial hypothalamus, which in turn decreases gonadotropic activity. *Kiss1* expression in the ARC is reduced in short day conditions, but it is also inhibited by the testosterone feedback and may be regulated by metabolic factors.

is supported both by a report in rats indicating that RFRP-3 fibers are in contact with subpopulations of kisspeptin neurons (Rizwan et al., 2012) and by our observation that chronic central infusion of RFRP-3 increases arcuate *Kiss1* expression together with a reactivation of testicular function in the Syrian hamster (Ancel et al., 2012). In SD conditions, the melatoninergic signal would be primarily integrated by the hypothalamic RFRP neurons leading to a decreased expression of the peptide, but whether melatonin acts directly or not on RFRP neurons has yet to be determined. Current studies do not support a major feedback effect of sex steroids on RFRP neurons. In contrast, kisspeptinergic neurons integrate other factors related to the sexual and metabolic status of the animal in order to finely tune reproductive activity with the seasons. From studies in sheep, a SD-breeder, it appears that an increased production of RFRP-3 in LD conditions would inhibit reproductive activity by acting directly on the GnRH neurons and/or on the pituitary (Smith et al., 2008; Sari et al., 2009).

CONCLUSION

In regard to the seasonal regulation of reproductive activity, recent data have shed light on the involvement of two hypothalamic peptides of the RFamide family, RFRP-3 and kisspeptin. Clearly both peptides are regulated by the photoperiodic melatoninergic signal but may also be sensitive to other seasonally regulated factors. Our current hypothesis is that RFRP expression undergoes a conserved inhibition in short photoperiod but the peptide may be stimulatory or inhibitory according to the reproductive physiology of the species; on the other hand, kisspeptin has a conserved stimulatory action on the gonadotropic axis but its seasonal regulation shows species differences. Whether RFRP-3 and kisspeptin act on each other's expression or independently to regulate reproductive activity has yet to be clarified in different species. In the years to come, we believe that thorough comparative analyses on the effects and sites of action of both peptides between LD- and SD-breeders should help to resolve the yet unanswered question of why the same photoperiodic cue induces opposite behavioral responses.

REFERENCES

Ancel, C., Bentsen, A. H., Sebert, M. E., Tena-Sempere, M., Mikkelsen, J. D., and Simonneaux, V. (2012). Stimulatory effect of RFRP-3 on the gonadotrophic axis in the male Syrian hamster: the exception proves the rule. *Endocrinology* 153, 1352–1363.

Anderson, G. M., Relf, H. L., Rizwan, M. Z., and Evans, J. J. (2009). Central and peripheral effects of RFamide-related peptide-3 on luteinizing hormone and prolactin secretion in rats. *Endocrinology* 150, 1834–1840.

Ansel, L., Bentsen, A. H., Ancel, C., Bolborea, M., Klosen, P., Mikkelsen, J. D., et al. (2011). Peripheral kisspeptin reverses short photoperiod-induced gonadal regression in Syrian hamsters by promoting GnRH release. *Reproduction* 142, 417–425.

Ansel, L., Bolborea, M., Bentsen, A. H., Klosen, P., Mikkelsen, J. D., and Simonneaux V. (2010). Differential regulation of kiss1 expression by melatonin and gonadal hormones in male and female Syrian hamsters. *J. Biol. Rhythms* 25, 81–91.

Barrett, P., Ebling, F. J., Schuhler, S., Wilson, D., Ross, A. W., Warner, A., et al. (2007). Hypothalamic thyroid hormone catabolism acts as a gatekeeper for the seasonal control of body weight and reproduction. *Endocrinology* 148, 3608–3617.

Bartness, T. J., Powers, J. B., Hastings, M. H., Bittman, E. L., and Goldman, B. D. (1993). The timed infusion paradigm for melatonin delivery: what has it taught us about the melatonin signal, its reception, and the photoperiodic control of seasonal responses? *J. Pineal Res.* 15, 161–190.

Bechtold, D. A., and Luckman, S. M. (2007). The role of RFamide peptides in feeding. *J. Endocrinol.* 192, 3–15.

Bentley, G. E., Tsutsui, K., and Kriegsfeld, L. J. (2010). Recent studies of gonadotropin-inhibitory hormone (GnIH) in the mammalian hypothalamus, pituitary and gonads. *Brain Res.* 1364, 62–71.

Caraty, A., Blomenröhr, M., Vogel, G. M., Lomet, D., Briant, C., and Beltramo, M. (2012). RF9 powerfully stimulates gonadotrophin secretion in the ewe: evidence for a seasonal threshold of sensitivity. *J. Neuroendocrinol.* 24, 725–736.

Caraty, A., Smith, J. T., Lomet, D., Ben Said, S., Morrissey, A., Cognie, J., et al. (2007). Kisspeptin synchronizes preovulatory surges in cyclical ewes and causes ovulation in seasonally acyclic ewes. *Endocrinology* 148, 5258–5267.

Carter, D. S., and Goldman, B. D. (1983). Antigonadal effects of timed melatonin infusion in pinealectomized male Djungarian hamsters (*Phodopus sungorus sungorus*): duration is the critical parameter. *Endocrinology* 113, 1261–1267.

Castellano, J. M., Bentsen, A. H., Mikkelsen, J. D., and Tena-Sempere, M. (2010). Kisspeptins: bridging energy homeostasis and reproduction. *Brain Res.* 1364, 129–138.

Clarke, I. J., Sari, I. P., Qi, Y., Smith, J. T., Parkington, H. C., Ubuka, T., et al. (2008). Potent action of RFamide-related peptide-3 on pituitary gonadotropes indicative of a hypophysiotropic role in the negative regulation of gonadotropin secretion. *Endocrinology* 149, 5811–5821.

Clarke, I. J., Smith, J. T., Henry, B. A., Oldfield, B. J., Stefanidis, A., Millar, R. P., et al. (2012). Gonadotropin-inhibitory hormone is a hypothalamic peptide that provides a molecular switch between reproduction and feeding. *Neuroendocrinology* 95, 305–316.

Dardente, H. (2012). Melatonin-dependent timing of seasonal reproduction by the pars tuberalis: pivotal roles for long daylengths and thyroid hormones. *J. Neuroendocrinol.* 24, 249–266

Dardente, H., Birnie, M., Lincoln, G. A., and Hazlerigg, D. G. (2008). RFamide-related peptide and its cognate receptor in the sheep: cDNA cloning, mRNA distribution in the hypothalamus and the effect of photoperiod. *J. Neuroendocrinol.* 20, 1252–1259.

Dardente, H., Klosen, P., Pevet, P., and Masson-Pevet, M. (2003). MT1 melatonin receptor mRNA expressing cells in the pars tuberalis of the European hamster: effect of photoperiod. *J. Neuroendocrinol.* 15, 778–786.

Dardente, H., Wyse, C. A., Birnie, M. J., Dupre, S. M., Loudon, A. S., Lincoln, G. A., et al. (2010). A molecular switch for photoperiod responsiveness in mammals. *Curr. Biol.* 20, 2193–2198.

de Roux, N., Genin, E., Carel, J. C., Matsuda, F., Chaussain, J. L., and Milgrom, E. (2003). Hypogonadotropic hypogonadism due to loss of function of the KiSS1-derived peptide receptor GPR54. *Proc. Natl. Acad. Sci. U.S.A.* 100, 10972–10976.

Ducret, E., Anderson, G. M., and Herbison, A. E. (2009). RFamide-related peptide-3, a mammalian gonadotropin-inhibitory hormone ortholog, regulates gonadotropin-releasing hormone neuron firing in the mouse. *Endocrinology* 150, 2799–2804.

Engstrom, M., Brandt, A., Wurster, S., Savola, J. M., and Panula, P. (2003). Prolactin releasing peptide has high affinity and efficacy at neuropeptide FF2 receptors. *J. Pharmacol. Exp. Ther.* 305, 825–832.

Franceschini, I., Lomet, D., Cateau, M., Delsol, G., Tillet, Y., and Caraty, A. (2006). Kisspeptin immunoreactive cells of the ovine preoptic area and arcuate nucleus co-express estrogen receptor alpha. *Neurosci. Lett.* 401, 225–230.

Gibson, E. M., Humber, S. A., Jain, S., Williams, W. P. III, Zhao, S., Bentley, G. E., et al. (2008). Alterations in RFamide-related peptide expression are coordinated with the preovulatory luteinizing hormone surge. *Endocrinology* 149, 4958–4969.

Gouarderes, C., Mazarguil, H., Mollereau, C., Chartrel, N., Leprince, J., Vaudry, H., et al. (2007). Functional differences between NPFF1 and NPFF2 receptor coupling: high intrinsic activities of RFamide-related peptides on stimulation of [35S]GTPgammaS binding. *Neuropharmacology* 52, 376–386.

Gouarderes, C., Puget, A., and Zajac, J. M. (2004a). Detailed distribution of neuropeptide FF receptors (NPFF1 and NPFF2) in the rat, mouse, octodon, rabbit, guinea pig, and marmoset monkey brains: a comparative autoradiographic study. *Synapse* 51, 249–269.

Gouarderes, C., Faura, C. C., and Zajac, J. M. (2004b). Rodent strain differences in the NPFF1 and NPFF2 receptor distribution and density in the central nervous system. *Brain Res.* 1014, 61–70.

Gouarderes, C., Quelven, I., Mollereau, C., Mazarguil, H., Rice, S. Q., and Zajac, J. M. (2002). Quantitative autoradiographic distribution of NPFF1 neuropeptide FF receptor in the rat brain and comparison with NPFF2 receptor by using [125I]YVP and [(125I]EYF as selective radioligands. *Neuroscience* 115, 349–361.

Greives, T. J., Humber, S. A., Goldstein, A. N., Scotti, M. A., Demas, G. E., and Kriegsfeld, L. J. (2008a). Photoperiod and testosterone interact to drive seasonal changes in kisspeptin expression in Siberian hamsters (*Phodopus sungorus*). *J. Neuroendocrinol.* 20, 1339–1347.

Greives, T. J., Kriegsfeld, L. J., and Demas, G. E. (2008b). Exogenous kisspeptin does not alter photoperiod-induced gonadal regression in Siberian hamsters (*Phodopus sungorus*). *Gen. Comp. Endocrinol.* 156, 552–558.

Hanon, E. A., Lincoln, G. A., Fustin, J. M., Dardente, H., Masson-Pevet, M., Morgan, P. J., et al. (2008). Ancestral TSH mechanism signals summer in a photoperiodic mammal. *Curr. Biol.* 18, 1147–1152.

Hanon, E. A., Routledge, K., Dardente, H., Masson-Pevet, M., Morgan, P. J., and Hazlerigg, D. G. (2010). Effect of photoperiod on the thyroid-stimulating hormone neuroendocrine system in the European hamster (*Cricetus cricetus*). *J. Neuroendocrinol.* 22, 51–55.

Hinuma, S., Shintani, Y., Fukusumi, S., Iijima, N., Matsumoto, Y., Hosoya, M., et al. (2000). New neuropeptides containing carboxy-terminal RFamide and their receptor in mammals. *Nat. Cell Biol.* 2, 703–708.

Hoffman, R. A., and Reiter, R. J. (1965). Pineal gland: influence on gonads of male hamsters. *Science* 148, 1609–1611.

Janati, A., Talbi, R., Klosen, P., Mikkelsen, J., Magoul, R., Simonneaux, V., et al. (2012). Distribution and seasonal variation in hypothalamic RF-amide peptides in a semi-desert rodent, the jerboa. *J. Neuroendocrinol.* (in press).

Johnson, M. A., Tsutsui, K., and Fraley, G. S. (2007). Rat RFamide-related peptide-3 stimulates GH secretion, inhibits LH secretion, and has variable effects on sex behavior in the adult male rat. *Horm. Behav.* 51, 171–180.

Kadokawa, H., Shibata, M., Tanaka, Y., Kojima, T., Matsumoto, K., Oshima, K., et al. (2009). Bovine C-terminal octapeptide of RFamide-related peptide-3 suppresses luteinizing hormone (LH) secretion from the pituitary as well as pulsatile LH secretion in bovines. *Domest. Anim. Endocrinol.* 36, 219–224.

Klosen, P., Bienvenu, C., Demarteau, O., Dardente, H., Guerrero, H., Pevet, P., et al. (2002). The mt1 melatonin receptor and RORbeta receptor are co-localized in specific TSH-immunoreactive cells in the pars tuberalis of the rat pituitary. *J. Histochem. Cytochem.* 50, 1647–1657.

Kriegsfeld, L. J., Gibson, E. M., Williams, W. P. III, Zhao, S., Mason, A. O., Bentley, G. E., et al. (2010). The roles of RFamide-related peptide-3 in mammalian reproductive function and behaviour. *J. Neuroendocrinol.* 22, 692–700.

Kriegsfeld, L. J., Mei, D. F., Bentley, G. E., Ubuka, T., Mason, A. O., Inoue, K., et al. (2006). Identification and characterization of a gonadotropin-inhibitory system in the brains of mammals. *Proc. Natl. Acad. Sci. U.S.A.* 103, 2410–2415.

Liu, Q., Guan, X. M., Martin, W. J., McDonald, T. P., Clements, M. K., Jiang, Q., et al. (2001). Identification and characterization of novel mammalian neuropeptide FF-like peptides that attenuate morphine-induced antinociception. *J. Biol. Chem.* 276, 36961–36969.

Malpaux, B., Daveau, A., Maurice-Mandon, F., Duarte, G., and Chemineau, P. (1998). Evidence that melatonin acts in the premammillary hypothalamic area to control reproduction in the ewe: presence of binding sites and stimulation of luteinizing hormone secretion by in situ microimplant delivery. *Endocrinology* 139, 1508–1516.

Malpaux, B., Migaud, M., Tricoire, H., and Chemineau, P. (2001). Biology of mammalian photoperiodism and the critical role of the pineal gland and melatonin. *J. Biol. Rhythms* 16, 336–347.

Mason, A. O., Duffy, S., Zhao, S., Ubuka, T., Bentley, G. E., Tsutsui, K., et al. (2010). Photoperiod and reproductive condition are associated with changes in RFamide-related peptide (RFRP) expression in Syrian hamsters (*Mesocricetus auratus*). *J. Biol. Rhythms* 25, 176–185.

Mason, A. O., Greives, T. J., Scotti, M. A., Levine, J., Frommeyer, S., Ketterson, E. D., et al. (2007). Suppression of kisspeptin expression and gonadotropic axis sensitivity following exposure to inhibitory day lengths in female Siberian hamsters. *Horm. Behav.* 52, 492–498.

Masson-Pevet, M., and Gauer, F. (1994). Seasonality and melatonin receptors in the pars tuberalis in some long day breeders. *Biol. Signals* 3, 63–70.

Masson-Pevet, M., George, D., Kalsbeek, A., Saboureau, M., Lakhdar-Ghazal, N., and Pevet, P. (1994). An attempt to correlate brain areas containing melatonin-binding sites with rhythmic functions: a study in five hibernator species. *Cell Tissue Res.* 278, 97–106.

Maywood, E. S., Bittman, E. L., and Hastings, M. H. (1996). Lesions of the melatonin- and androgen-responsive tissue of the dorsomedial nucleus of the hypothalamus block the gonadal response of male Syrian hamsters to programmed infusions of melatonin. *Biol. Reprod.* 54, 470–477.

Maywood, E. S., and Hastings, M. H. (1995). Lesions of the iodomelatonin-binding sites of the mediobasal hypothalamus spare the lactotropic, but block the gonadotropic response of male Syrian hamsters to short photoperiod and to melatonin. *Endocrinology* 136, 144–153.

Mollereau, C., Mazarguil, H., Marcus, D., Quelven, I., Kotani, M., Lannoy, V., et al. (2002). Pharmacological characterization of human NPFF(1) and NPFF(2) receptors expressed in CHO cells by using NPY Y(1) receptor antagonists. *Eur. J. Pharmacol.* 451, 245–256.

Murakami, M., Matsuzaki, T., Iwasa, T., Yasui, T., Irahara, M., Osugi, T., et al. (2008). Hypophysiotropic role of RFamide-related peptide-3 in the inhibition of LH secretion in female rats. *J. Endocrinol.* 199, 105–112.

Nakao, N., Ono, H., Yamamura, T., Anraku, T., Takagi, T., Higashi, K., et al. (2008). Thyrotrophin in the pars tuberalis triggers photoperiodic response. *Nature* 452, 317–322.

Pevet, P. (1988). The role of the pineal gland in the photoperiodic control of reproduction in different hamster species. *Reprod. Nutr. Dev.* 28, 443–458.

Pineda, R., Garcia-Galiano, D., Sanchez-Garrido, M. A., Romero, M., Ruiz-Pino, F., Aguilar, E., et al. (2010). Characterization of the inhibitory roles of RFRP3, the mammalian ortholog of GnIH, in the control of gonadotropin secretion in the rat: in vivo and in vitro studies. *Am. J. Physiol. Endocrinol. Metab.* 299, E39–E46.

Pinilla, L., Aguilar, E., Dieguez, C., Millar, R. P., and Tena-Sempere, M. (2012). Kisspeptins and reproduction: physiological roles and regulatory mechanisms. *Physiol. Rev.* 92, 1235–1316.

Poling, M. C., Kim, J., Dhamija, S., and Kauffman, A. S. (2012). Development, sex steroid regulation, and phenotypic characterization of RFamide-related peptide (Rfrp) gene expression and RFamide receptors in the mouse hypothalamus. *Endocrinology* 153, 1827–1840.

Quennell, J. H., Rizwan, M. Z., Relf, H. L., and Anderson, G. M. (2010). Developmental and steroidogenic effects on the gene expression of RFamide related peptides and their receptor in the rat brain and pituitary gland. *J. Neuroendocrinol.* 22, 309–316.

Revel, F. G., Ansel, L., Klosen, P., Saboureau, M., Pevet, P., Mikkelsen, J. D., et al. (2007). Kisspeptin: a key link to seasonal breeding. *Rev. Endocr. Metab. Disord.* 8, 57–65.

Revel, F. G., Saboureau, M., Pevet, P., Mikkelsen, J. D., and Simonneaux, V. (2006a). Melatonin regulates type 2 deiodinase gene expression in the Syrian hamster. *Endocrinology* 147, 4680–4687.

Revel, F. G., Saboureau, M., Masson-Pevet, M., Pevet, P., Mikkelsen, J. D., and Simonneaux, V. (2006b). Kisspeptin mediates the photoperiodic control of reproduction in hamsters. *Curr. Biol.* 16, 1730–1735.

Revel, F. G., Saboureau, M., Pevet, P., Simonneaux, V., and Mikkelsen, J. D. (2008). RFamide-related peptide gene is a melatonin-driven photoperiodic gene. *Endocrinology* 149, 902–912.

Rizwan, M. Z., Poling, M. C., Corr, M., Cornes, P. A., Augustine, R. A., Quennell, J. H., et al. (2012). RFamide-related peptide-3 receptor gene expression in GnRH and kisspeptin neurons and GnRH-dependent mechanism of action. *Endocrinology* 153, 3770–3779.

Rizwan, M. Z., Porteous, R., Herbison, A. E., and Anderson, G. M. (2009). Cells expressing RFamide-related peptide-1/3, the mammalian gonadotropin-inhibitory hormone orthologs, are not hypophysiotropic neuroendocrine neurons in the rat. *Endocrinology* 150, 1413–1420.

Sari, I. P., Rao, A., Smith, J. T., Tilbrook, A. J., and Clarke, I. J. (2009). Effect of RF-amide-related peptide-3 on luteinizing hormone and follicle-stimulating hormone synthesis and secretion in ovine pituitary gonadotropes. *Endocrinology* 150, 5549–5556.

Seminara, S. B., Messager, S., Chatzidaki, E. E., Thresher, R. R., Acierno, J. S., Shagoury, J. K., et al. (2003). The

GPR54 gene as a regulator of puberty. *N. Engl. J. Med.* 349, 1614–1627.

Simonneaux, V., Ansel, L., Revel, F. G., Klosen, P., Pevet, P., and Mikkelsen, J. D. (2009). Kisspeptin and the seasonal control of reproduction in hamsters. *Peptides* 30, 146–153.

Simonneaux, V., Bur, I., Ancel, C., Ansel, L., and Klosen, P. (2012). A kiss for daily and seasonal reproduction. *Prog. Brain Res.* 199, 423–437.

Simonneaux, V., and Ribelayga, C. (2003). Generation of the melatonin endocrine message in mammals: a review of the complex regulation of melatonin synthesis by norepinephrine, peptides, and other pineal transmitters. *Pharmacol. Rev.* 55, 325–395.

Smith, J. T., Clay, C. M., Caraty, A., and Clarke, I. J. (2007). KiSS-1 messenger ribonucleic acid expression in the hypothalamus of the ewe is regulated by sex steroids and season. *Endocrinology* 148, 1150–1157.

Smith, J. T., Saleh, S. N., and Clarke, I. J. (2009). Seasonal and cyclical change in the luteinizing hormone response to kisspeptin in the ewe. *Neuroendocrinology* 90, 283–291.

Smith, J. T., Shahab, M., Pereira, A., Pau, K. Y., and Clarke, I. J. (2010). Hypothalamic expression of KISS1 and gonadotropin inhibitory hormone genes during the menstrual cycle of a non-human primate. *Biol. Reprod.* 83, 568–577.

Smith, J. T., Young, I. R., Veldhuis, J. D., and Clarke, I. J. (2012). Gonadotropin-inhibitory hormone (GnIH) secretion into the ovine hypophyseal portal system. *Endocrinology* 153, 3368–3375.

Smith, J. T., and Clarke, I. J. (2010). Gonadotropin inhibitory hormone function in mammals. *Trends Endocrinol. Metab.* 21, 255–260.

Smith, J. T., Coolen, L. M., Kriegsfeld, L. J., Sari, I. P., Jaafarzadehshirazi, M. R., Maltby, M., et al. (2008). Variation in kisspeptin and RFamide-related peptide (RFRP) expression and terminal connections to gonadotropin-releasing hormone neurons in the brain: a novel medium for seasonal breeding in the sheep. *Endocrinology* 149, 5770–5782.

Tsutsui, K., Bentley, G. E., Bedecarrats, G., Osugi, T., Ubuka, T., and Kriegsfeld, L. J. (2010). Gonadotropin-inhibitory hormone (GnIH) and its control of central and peripheral reproductive function. *Front. Neuroendocrinol.* 31:284–295. doi: 10.1016/j.yfrne.2010.03.001

Tsutsui, K., Saigoh, E., Ukena, K., Teranishi, H., Fujisawa, Y., Kikuchi, M., et al. (2000). A novel avian hypothalamic peptide inhibiting gonadotropin release. *Biochem. Biophys. Res. Commun.* 275, 661–667.

Ubuka, T., Bentley, G. E., Ukena, K., Wingfield, J. C., and Tsutsui, K. (2005). Melatonin induces the expression of gonadotropin-inhibitory hormone in the avian brain. *Proc. Natl. Acad. Sci. U.S.A.* 102, 3052–3057.

Ubuka, T., Inoue, K., Fukuda, Y., Mizuno, T., Ukena, K., Kriegsfeld, L. J., et al. (2012). Identification, expression, and physiological functions of Siberian hamster gonadotropin-inhibitory hormone. *Endocrinology* 153, 373–385.

Ukena, K., and Tsutsui, K. (2001). Distribution of novel RFamide-related peptide-like immunoreactivity in the mouse central nervous system. *Neurosci. Lett.* 300, 153–156.

Urbanski, H. F., Doan, A., and Pierce, M. (1991). Immunocytochemical investigation of luteinizing hormone-releasing hormone neurons in Syrian hamsters maintained under long or short days. *Biol. Reprod.* 44, 687–692.

Yano, T., Iijima, N., Kakihara, K., Hinuma, S., Tanaka, M., and Ibata, Y. (2003). Localization and neuronal response of RFamide related peptides in the rat central nervous system. *Brain Res.* 982, 156–167.

Yasuo, S., Yoshimura, T., Ebihara, S., and Korf, H. W. (2007). Temporal dynamics of type 2 deiodinase expression after melatonin injections in Syrian hamsters. *Endocrinology* 148, 4385–4392.

Yoshimura, T., Yasuo, S., Watanabe, M., Iigo, M., Yamamura, T., Hirunagi, K., et al. (2003). Light-induced hormone conversion of T4 to T3 regulates photoperiodic response of gonads in birds. *Nature* 426, 178–181.

Feeding and the rhodopsin family G-protein coupled receptors in nematodes and arthropods

João C.R. Cardoso*, Rute C. Félix, Vera G. Fonseca and Deborah M. Power

Molecular Comparative Endocrinology, Centre of Marine Sciences, Universidade do Algarve, Faro, Portugal

Edited by:
Hubert Vaudry, University of Rouen, France

Reviewed by:
Pei-San Tsai, University of Colorado, USA
Liliane Schoofs, Catholic University of Leuven, Belgium
Lindy Holden-Dye, University of Southampton, UK

****Correspondence:***
João C.R. Cardoso, Molecular Comparative Endocrinology, Centre of Marine Sciences, Universidade do Algarve, Campus de Gambelas, Faro 8005-139, Portugal.
e-mail: jccardo@ualg.pt

In vertebrates, receptors of the rhodopsin G-protein coupled superfamily (GPCRs) play an important role in the regulation of feeding and energy homeostasis and are activated by peptide hormones produced in the brain-gut axis. These peptides regulate appetite and energy expenditure by promoting or inhibiting food intake. Sequence and function homologs of human GPCRs involved in feeding exist in the nematode roundworm, *Caenorhabditis elegans* (*C. elegans*), and the arthropod fruit fly, *Drosophila melanogaster* (*D. melanogaster*), suggesting that the mechanisms that regulate food intake emerged early and have been conserved during metazoan radiation. Nematodes and arthropods are the most diverse and successful animal phyla on Earth. They can survive in a vast diversity of environments and have acquired distinct life styles and feeding strategies. The aim of the present review is to investigate if this diversity has affected the evolution of invertebrate GPCRs. Homologs of the *C. elegans* and *D. melanogaster* rhodopsin receptors were characterized in the genome of other nematodes and arthropods and receptor evolution compared. With the exception of bombesin receptors (BBR) that are absent from nematodes, a similar gene complement was found. In arthropods, rhodopsin GPCR evolution is characterized by species-specific gene duplications and deletions and in nematodes by gene expansions in species with a free-living stage and gene deletions in representatives of obligate parasitic taxa. Based upon variation in GPCR gene number and potentially divergent functions within phyla we hypothesize that life style and feeding diversity practiced by nematodes and arthropods was one factor that contributed to rhodopsin GPCR gene evolution. Understanding how the regulation of food intake has evolved in invertebrates will contribute to the development of novel drugs to control nematodes and arthropods and the pests and diseases that use them as vectors.

Keywords: rhodopsin GPCR, feeding, conservation, evolution, invertebrates

INTRODUCTION

Feeding is the process by which food is obtained to provide energy. It must satisfy growth, survival, and reproductive requirements and has driven the evolution of specialized feeding behaviors and apparatus in metazoan. Regulation of feeding is a complex mechanism, which involves a combination of physical, chemical, and nutritional factors (Neary et al., 2004; Coll et al., 2007; Woods et al., 2008). Food-taking behavior is dependent on environmental signals (odors and taste), hunger signals (metabolic signals), and also endocrine satiety signals that via the blood stream or the vagal afferent terminals act on the hypothalamus, brain stem, or afferent autonomic nerves to modulate feeding response (**Figure 1**; Konturek et al., 2004; Stanley et al., 2005; Chaudhri et al., 2006; Woods et al., 2006, 2008). In mammals, psychological factors such as mood (emotions) and food reward have also been shown to affect eating behavior (Christensen, 1993; Berridge, 1996). In vertebrates, a group of small regulatory peptides that are produced by the brain-gut axis play a major role in the endocrine regulation of feeding and control of energy homeostasis (**Figure 1**; Coll et al., 2007; Chaudhri et al., 2008). These peptide hormones are divided into two groups, those that stimulate appetite (orexigenic peptides) and induce food intake and those that cause loss of appetite (anorexigenic peptides) and reduce food consumption and increase energy expenditure (Ahima and Osei, 2001; Wilding, 2002; Suzuki et al., 2010). The action of such peptides involves the activation of specific G-protein coupled receptors (GPCRs), which undergo conformational changes and promote the activation of intracellular signaling mechanisms that ultimately lead to a cellular response (**Table 1**; Marinissen and Gutkind, 2001; Xu et al., 2004; Fredriksson and Schioth, 2005).

The involvement of GPCRs in the regulation of vertebrate feeding and appetite is well recognized (Shioda et al., 2008). Much less is known about their homologs and cognate activating peptides in non-vertebrates. However, comparative sequence approaches and functional studies suggest that the involvement of GPCRs in metazoa feeding behavior emerged early and has been maintained during the species radiation (Brody and Cravchik, 2000; Hewes and Taghert, 2001; Fredriksson and Schioth, 2005; Teng et al., 2008). GPCRs have emerged via gene or genome duplication events followed by selection of the gene duplicates. Understanding the origin of GPCRs represents a valuable tool for the characterization of basic physiological functions that have been

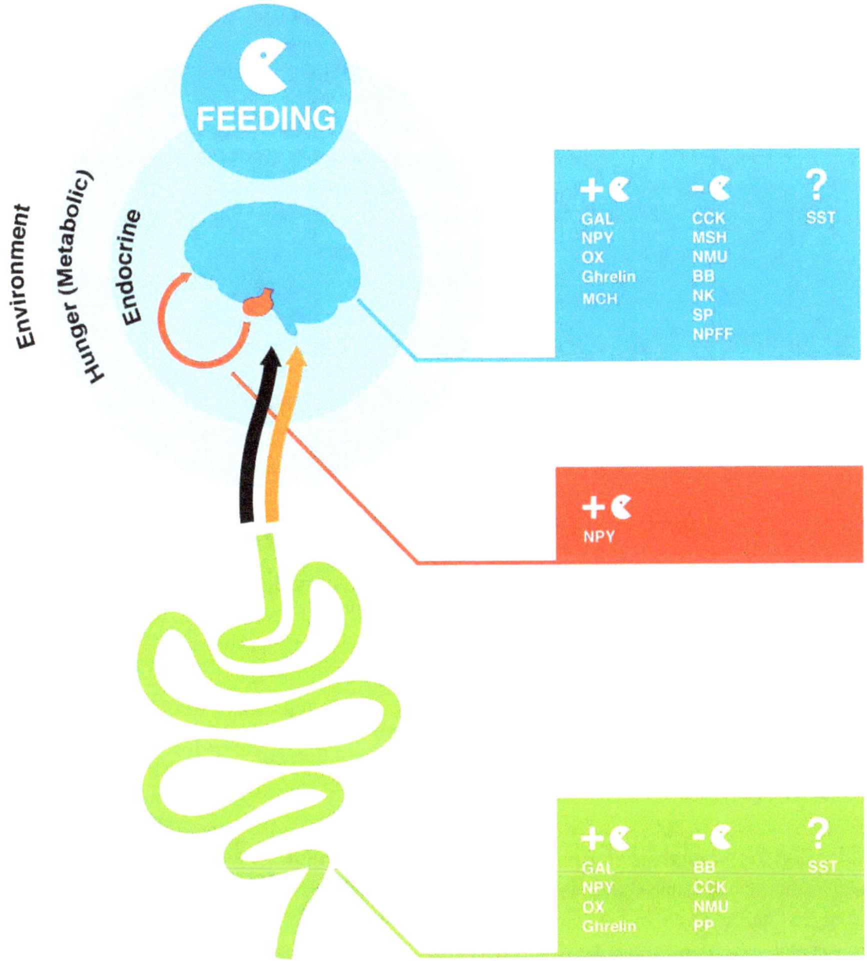

FIGURE 1 | Overview of endocrine factors that regulate feeding behavior in the human brain-gut axis. In humans and other vertebrates, feeding is regulated by signals from the environment (odor and taste), hunger (metabolic signals), and endocrine signals produced by the gut and brain. The orange arrow represents the blood connection between gut and brain and the black arrow the nervous connection via the vagal afferent terminals through which peptides produced by the gut modulate the feeding response in the brain. GAL, NPY, OX, Ghrelin, and MCH are orexigenic peptides and promote appetite and feeding. CCK, MSH, NMU, BB, NK, SP, NPFF are anorexigenic. The role of SST peptides in feeding is unclear. The full peptide names are indicated in **Table 1**.

maintained during evolution. The present review takes a comparative approach and targets rhodopsin GPCR subfamily members in the model species, *C. elegans* (a nematode) and *D. melanogaster* (a arthropod) that are sequence and function homologs of vertebrate GPCRs implicated in feeding regulation. To enrich the data and provide insight into how divergent life style and feeding strategies may have shaped receptor evolution in invertebrates the sequence of the target GPCRs were identified in other nematodes and arthropods with available genome data.

THE VERTEBRATE GPCRs SUPERFAMILY AND THEIR ROLE IN FEEDING

G-protein coupled receptors are one of the largest groups of receptors present in cells. Based upon their structure and sequence similarity five distinct superfamilies have been defined in human: glutamate (G), Rhodopsin (R), Adhesion (A), Frizzled (F), and Secretin (S) and are collectively known as GRAFS (Fredriksson and Schioth, 2005; **Figure 2**). GPCRs are characterized by a signature motif of seven conserved transmembrane spanning helix domains (TM) in vertebrates and non-vertebrates. Receptor activation is mediated by the extracellular N-terminal domain and also by TM and extracellular loops (receptor core domain) that interact with diverse types of molecules. The cellular response is provoked by the receptor C-terminal domain which activates a series of intracellular signaling cascades via the G-protein coupled pathway complex (Bockaert and Pin, 1999; Marinissen and Gutkind, 2001). Other molecular mechanisms such assembly of receptor heterodimers and allosteric receptor–receptor interactions in the cell membrane are also involved in GPCR regulation, activation and signaling (Prinster et al., 2005; Langmead and Christopoulos, 2006; Fuxe et al., 2012).

Table 1 | Rhodopsin GPCR family members and activating peptides that regulate food intake in mammals.

Receptor	Subfamily	Members	Activating peptides	Effect on feed
α-Group	Melanocortin (MCR)	MC1R to 5R	Melanocortin peptides (MSH, ACTH, LPH)	Reduce
β-Group	Gastrin-cholecystokinin (CCKR)	CCK1R, 2R	Cholecystokinin (CCK), Gastrin	Reduce
	Neurokinin (NKR)	NK1R to 3R	Substance P (SP), substance K (SK), neuromedin K (NK)	Reduce
	Neuropeptide FF (NPFFR)	NPFF1R, 2R	Neuropeptide FF (NPFF), neuropeptide AF (NPAF)	Reduce
	Orexin (OXR)	OX1R, 2R	Orexin-A and B (OXA, B)	Stimulate
	Neuropeptide Y (NPYR)	NPYRY1 to 6	Neuropeptide Y (NPY), peptide YY (PYY), pancreatic polypeptide (PP)	Stimulate/reduce
	Bombesin (BBR)	BB1R to 3R	bombesin (BB), gastrin-releasing peptide (GRP), neuromedin C and B	Reduce
	Ghrelin/obestatin (GHSR/GPR39)	GHSR, GPR39	Ghrelin (GHS), obestatin	Stimulate/reduce
	Neuromedin U (NMUR)	NMU1R, 2R	Neuromedin U (NMU) and S (NMS)	Reduce
γ-Group	Somatostatin (SSTR)	SST1R to 5R	Somatostatin (SST)	Not clear
	Galanin (GALR)	GAL1R to 3R	Galanin (GAL), galanin-like peptide (GALP)	Stimulate
	Melanin concentrating hormone (MCHR)	MCH1R, 2R	Melanin concentrating hormone (MHC)	Stimulate

Receptor subfamily members, activating peptides and their effect on feed (stimulation or reduction) are indicated. For references please consult the text.

G-protein coupled receptors are ubiquitous and involved in many different physiological functions. The glutamate receptors are involved in synaptic plasticity and participate in numerous functions in the central nervous system (CNS; Niswender and Conn, 2010). Rhodopsin receptors include receptors for hormones, neurotransmitters and photons and they are involved in taste, smell, and also regulate metabolism, reproduction, and neural function (Simoni et al., 1997; Murdoch and Finn, 2000; Gaillard et al., 2004; Waldhoer et al., 2004). Adhesion receptors participate in cell adhesion, signaling, and immune function (Bjarnadottir et al., 2007; Yona et al., 2008). Frizzled receptors are involved in the Wnt signaling pathway and in the control of cell proliferation and embryogenesis (van Amerongen and Nusse, 2009; Schulte, 2010). In contrast to other GPCRs, secretin family members are only activated by peptide hormones and they are implicated in brain-gut functions, calcium homeostasis, and in the stress response (McDermott and Kidd, 1987; Harmar, 2001; Bale and Vale, 2004; Moody et al., 2011). Due to their conserved structure and presence in many phyla, GPCRs are suggested to have a common evolutionary origin and to have arisen via gene/genome duplication early in the species radiation (Krishnan et al., 2012). With the exception of the glutamate family members, they are proposed to share a common ancestor with the cAMP receptors of primitive eukaryote species (Nordstrom et al., 2011).

In humans, more than 700 GPCR genes are predicted and a large proportion are orphans with unknown function (**Figure 2**). The rhodopsin family (a.k.a family A or class 1 GPCRs) comprise the most diverse receptor group and in humans they account for more than 80% of GPCRs and include members that are involved in regulation of feeding (Joost and Methner, 2002; Fredriksson et al., 2003). Rhodopsin family members possess a short N-terminal domain and are characterized by the presence of several conserved amino acid motifs such as N-S-x-x-N-P-x-x-Y within TM7 and the DRY (D(E)-R-Y(F)) motif between TM3 and intracellular loop (IL) 2 (Schioth and Fredriksson, 2005; Suwa et al., 2011). Based upon sequence similarity the human rhodopsin receptors are sub classified into four main groups (α, β, γ and δ; **Figure 2**; Fredriksson et al., 2003). The α-group contains clusters for the prostaglandin, amine, opsin, melatonin, melanocortin, endothelial, cannabinoid, and adenosine binding receptors. Members of the β-group include a subfamily of receptors for which known ligands are peptides such as orexin (OX), neuropeptide FF (NPFF), neurokinin (NK), gastrin-cholecystokinin (CCK), neuropeptide Y (NPY), endothelin-related (EDN), bombesin and related peptides (BB), neurotensin (NTS), ghrelin and obstatin, neuromedin (NMU), thyrotropin releasing hormone (TRH), arginine vasopressin (AVP), gonadotropin-releasing hormone (GNRH), and oxytocin (OXT). The γ group includes receptors for somatostatin (SST), opioids, galanin (GAL), melanin concentrating hormone (MCH), and chemokine peptides. The δ group contains the olfactory receptors (highly diverse > 400 members) as well as the glycoprotein, purine, and the MAS-related receptor clusters. In humans, twelve members of the rhodopsin family, which are activated by peptide hormones, play an important role in feed intake and stimulate or reduce food consumption (**Table 1**). The majority of these receptors are β group members and their role in the regulation of feed intake in mammals will now be briefly considered.

Receptors for melatonin (MT), gastrin-cholecystokinin (CCK), neurokinin (NK), neuropeptide FF (NPFF), bombesin and related peptides (BB), and neuromedin (NMU) have an inhibitory role in feed intake in vertebrates. Melanocortin receptors (MCR) are activated by melanocortin (ACTH, MSH, and lipotropin) peptides and administration of receptor agonists significantly reduces food consumption in rats (Irani and Haskell-Luevano, 2005). In addition mutant MC3R mice have increased fat mass (Coll et al., 2007) and ablation of the MC4R gene results in severe obesity (Coll et al., 2004; Millington, 2007). In rats, mutations of CCK1R are associated with obesity (Kopin et al., 1999) and peripheral administration of an NK1R antagonist leads to reduced weight gain after a high-fat diet (Karagiannides et al., 2011). Injection of NPFF provokes anorexia in mice and induces satiety (Murase et al., 1996; Bechtold and Luckman, 2006, 2007; Cline et al., 2009).

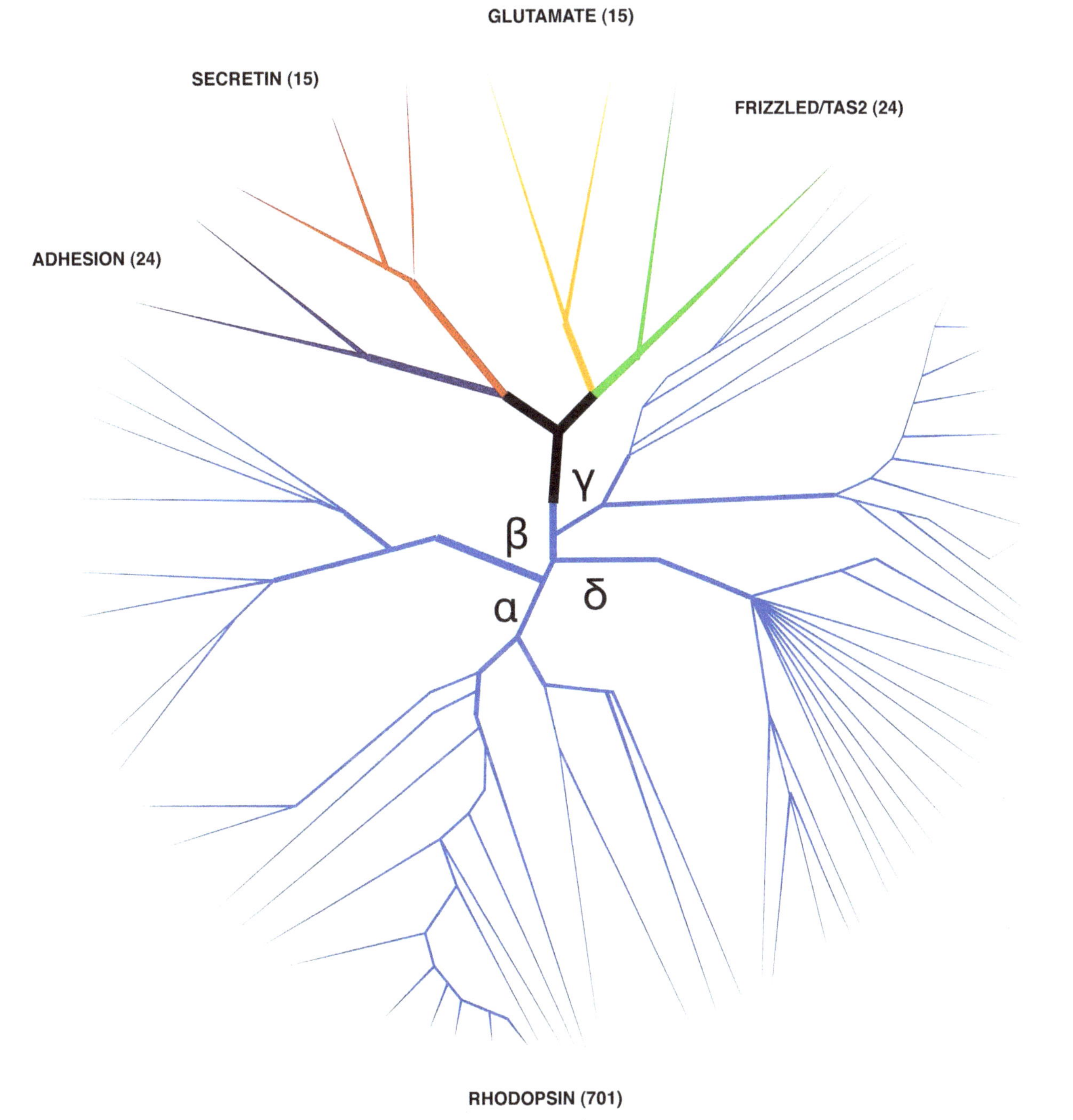

FIGURE 2 | Stylized phylogenetic tree showing the relationship between human GRAFS. The number of human representatives identified within each superfamily is indicated within brackets (Fredriksson et al., 2003). Rhodopsin family members (which are represented by the blue branch) are the most numerous and their members are classified into four main sub-branches (α, β, γ, and δ). Human receptors, which are activated by peptides and have a role in feeding regulation, are members of the rhodopsin and secretin families.

BB peptides also mediate satiety (Hampton et al., 1998; Yamada et al., 2002; Gonzalez et al., 2008) and knockout BB2R mice have increased body weight (Ladenheim et al., 2002) and BB3R-deficient mice exhibit a mild obesity phenotype and increased food intake (Ohki-Hamazaki et al., 1997). Mice lacking the NMU gene are hyperphagic and have increased adiposity and obesity and amino acid variants in NMU are associated with human obesity (Brighton et al., 2004; Hainerova et al., 2006).

In contrast, orexin (OXs), neuropeptide Y (NPYs), galanin (GAL), and melanin concentrating hormone (MCH) receptors are activated by orexigenic peptides which stimulate feeding (Sakurai, 1999; Branchek et al., 2000; Chamorro et al., 2002; Lecklin et al., 2002; Lang et al., 2007; Wong et al., 2011). Administration of orexin-A and B stimulates food consumption in a dose-dependent manner (Sakurai et al., 1998; Matteri, 2001). NPY is one of the most potent orexigenic factors and NPY-induced feeding is markedly reduced in Y1-knockout mice and NPY Y1 receptor deficient mice lack appetite (Mercer et al., 2011; Pjetri et al., 2012). GAL1R-KO mice display increased food intake and body weight gain in response to an acute 3 day high-fat challenge (Zorrilla et al., 2007). MCH is a hypothalamic appetite-stimulating peptide that is high in obese mice (Kawauchi, 2006; Coll et al., 2007) and deletions in MCH1R confer resistance to diet-induced obesity (DIO) and MCH1R antagonists are effective in reducing body weight (Chung et al., 2011).

The role of SSTR and their activating peptides in vertebrates is unclear. In rats SSTR can stimulate or inhibit appetite although peptide injections in chickens have an orexigenic effect (Tachibana et al., 2009). In addition receptors for ghrelin-obestatin have opposing effects on feeding and ghrelin is associated with hunger scores and plasma ghrelin levels increase during fasting and decrease after food intake (Rocha-Sousa et al., 2010). Treatment of rats with obestatin suppresses food intake and decreases body weight gain (Zhang et al., 2005).

Other GPCR families activated by peptide hormones may also play a role in food intake and include members of the secretin receptor family: pituitary Adenylate-Cyclase Activating Peptide/Vasoactive Intestinal Peptide (PACR/VIPR; Morley et al., 1992; Chance et al., 1995); Glucagon and related peptide (GCGR/GLPR; McMahon and Wellman, 1997, 1998; Tang-Christensen et al., 2001; Woods et al., 2006); Calcitonin (CTR; Riediger et al., 2004) and Corticotrophin Releasing Factor (CRFR) receptors (Heinrichs and Richard, 1999; Bradbury et al., 2000; Richard et al., 2002). However, the secretin receptor family will not be considered in the present review.

THE INVERTEBRATE GPCRs SUPERFAMILY

Invertebrates are one of the most diverse animal groups and they represent more than 95% of the species on Earth. Protostomia comprise the majority of the species identified and are of both ecological and economic importance as they are involved in the nutrient cycle, plant fertilization, and include agricultural pests and vectors of human disease, such as malaria and sleeping sickness. The divergence of Protostomes from Deuterostomes occurred more than 700 million years ago (MYA) and their success is associated with adaptations to a variety of ecological niches and modifications in their feeding habits that allow them to live, survive and reproduce in many different environments. Invertebrates can be herbivores (eating plant tissue, nectar, and pollen), carnivores (feeding on other invertebrates as well as larger animals), parasites (living on plant and animals), and detritus feeders (eating dead animal and plants). Surprisingly few studies exist about the regulation of feed intake in invertebrates, despite its importance for their success and this is also a neglected target for alternative control strategies. The genome of several invertebrates has been sequenced and in the metazoan Ensembl genome database (www.ensemblgenomes.org) 48 invertebrate genomes are available. Comparative molecular studies represent an invaluable mechanism to better understand invertebrate biology and to characterize endocrine factors associated with feeding.

Homologs of the vertebrate GPCR repertoire have been described in many invertebrates and representatives of the five distinct human GRAFS families are proposed to have emerged before the split of nematodes from the chordate lineage (**Table 2**; Fredriksson and Schioth, 2005). The model organisms, the nematode roundworm *C. elegans* and the fruit fly *D. melanogaster* are the most studied Prostostomes. Their genomes have been completely sequenced and are fully annotated and a vast range of functional resources exists and numerous GPCRs have been characterized (Consortium, 1998; Adams et al., 2000; Keating et al., 2003). In the roundworm, GPCRs account for approximately 5% of the genome (there are more than 1000) and the chemoreceptor genes, which are involved in chemoreception of environmental stimuli are unique in nematodes and are also the most abundant and diverse (Schioth and Fredriksson, 2005; Robertson and Thomas, 2006; Nagarathnam et al., 2012). In the fruit fly, approximately 200 GPCRs (1% of the genome) are predicted and the gustatory/taste receptors (Montell, 2009) are specific to insects although a quarter share sequence homology with vertebrate neurohormone receptors (Keating et al., 2003; Fredriksson and Schioth, 2005; Hauser et al., 2006; Nagarathnam et al., 2012). Recently GPCRs were also characterized in the genome of two Platyhelminthes, the blood fluke *Schistosoma mansoni* and the planarian *Schmidtea mediterranea* and a similar gene repertoire to vertebrates has been characterized. A platyhelminth-specific rhodopsin subfamily (PROF1) and a planarian-specific Adhesion-like family (PARF1)

Table 2 | Gene number and receptor subfamilies of the human rhodopsin GPCRs involved in feeding and the sequence homologs identified in *C. elegans* and *D. melanogaster*.

Rhodopsin	Subfamily	Human	*C. elegans*	*D. melanogaster*
α-Group	Melanocortin	5	ni	ni
β-Group	Gastrin-cholecystokinin	2	2	2
	Neurokinin	3	6	5
	Neuropeptide FF	2		
	Orexin	2		
	Neuropeptide Y	6	12	4
	Bombesin	3	ni	2
	Ghrelin/obestatin	2	6	5
	Neuromedin U	2		
γ-Group	Somatostatin	5	6	2
	Galanin	3	3	2
	Melanin concentrating hormone	2	ni	ni
Total		37	35	22

The total number of receptor genes in human, C. elegans and D. melanogaster is indicated. In C. elegans and D. melanogaster the homologs of the human Neurokinin/Neuropeptide FF/Orexin receptors and Ghrelin-Obestatin/Neuromedin U receptors were grouped due to their high sequence relatedness (Hewes and Taghert, 2001). ni, not identified.

have been identified suggesting lineage specific GPCRs evolved in invertebrates (Suwa et al., 2011; Zamanian et al., 2011).

Comparison of the neuroendocrine GPCR complement in the fruit fly and the honey bee *Apis mellifera* (*A. mellifera*) revealed that a similar gene complement is present (Hauser et al., 2006). In the malaria vector, the mosquito *Anopheles gambiae* (*A. gambiae*) genome, a total of 276 GPCRs are predicted and approximately 30 correspond to putative neuropeptide receptors (Hill et al., 2002). With the exception of *C. elegans*, very little is known about GPCRs in other nematodes despite availability of molecular data in public databases. The activating molecules for the roundworm and fruit fly GPCRs in common with other organisms are in general neurohormones (biogenic amines, protein hormones, and neuropeptides) and they play a central role in the control of behavior, reproduction, development, feeding, and many other physiological processes. This suggests that GPCR signaling has been conserved during evolution and that neuropeptide signaling plays a key role in both Proto and Deuterostomes (Grimmelikhuijzen and Hauser, 2012).

The present review provides a general overview of the evolution of the rhodopsin GPCR members that are implicated in feeding regulation. It will start by identifying and describing sequence homologs of human rhodopsin GPCRs in the model invertebrate organisms *C. elegans* and *D. melanogaster* followed by the characterization of their homologs in other nematodes and arthropods with distinctive feeding habits and life styles (**Table 4**). The *C. elegans* and *D. melanogaster* rhodopsin GPCR repertoire was obtained from published data and to enrich and confirm the dataset it was complemented with appropriate database searches using the human homologs (**Table 3**). A total of 35 rhodopsin

Table 3 | The human *C. elegans* and *D. melanogaster* rhodopsin GPCRs used for comparative sequence analysis and their accession numbers.

Human		*C. elegans*		*D. melanogaster*	
Type	**Accession number**	**Type**	**Accession number**	**Type**	**Accession number**
BB1R	AAH95542.1	*ckr-1*	T23B3.4	AICR2	CG13702
BB2R	AAA88050.1	*ckr-2*	Y39A3B.5	capaR	CG14575
BB3R	AAT79496.1	*nmur-1*	C48C5.1	CCHa1r	CG30106
CCK1R	NP_000721.1	*nmur-2*	K10B4.4	CCHa-2r	CG14593
CCK2R	NP_795344.1	*nmur-3*	F02E8.2A	CCKL-R17D3	CG32540
GALR1	NP_001471.2	*nmur-4*	C30F12.6	CCKL-R17D1	CG42301
GALR2	NP_003848.1	*npr-1*	C39E6.6	DAR-1	CG2872
GALR3	NP_003605.1	*npr-2*	T05A1.1A	DAR-2	CG10001
GHSR	AAI13548.1	*npr-3*	C10C6.2	DTKR	CG7887
GPR39	AAC26082.1	*npr-4*	C16D6.2	LKR	CG10626
MC1R	AAD41355.1	*npr-5*	Y58G8A.4	NepYr	CG5811
MC2R	NP_000520.1	*npr-6*	F41E7.3	NPFR1	CG1147
MCHR1	NP_005288.3	*npr-7*	F35G8.1	NKD	CG6515
NK1R	AAR23925.1	*npr-8*	C56G3.1B	PK-1R	CG9918
NK2R	AAH96842.1	*npr-9*	ZK455.3	PK-2-R2	CG8795
NK3R	AAR23926.1	*npr-10*	C53C7.1A	PK-2-R1	CG8784
NMUR-1	AAH51914.1	*npr-11*	C25G6.5	SNPFR	CG7395
NMUR-2	EAW61653.1	*npr-12*	T22D1.12	Star1-RA	CG7285
NPFF1R	NP_071429.1	*npr-13*	ZC412.1	CG10823	CG10823
NPFF2R	NP_004876.2	*npr-14*	W05B5.2	CG30340	CG30340
NPY1R	AAA59947.1	*npr-15*	T27D1.3	CG32547	CG32547
NPY2R	AAO92062.1	*npr-16*	F56B6.5	CG34381	CG34381
NPY4R	NP_005963.3	*npr-17*	C06G4.5		
NPY5R	NP_006165.1	*npr-18*	C43C3.2		
OX1R	AAC39601	*npr-20*	T07D4.1		
OX2R	AAC39602.1	*npr-21*	T23C6.5		
SSTR1	AAP84349.1	*npr-22*	Y59H11AL.1		
SSTR2	AAO92064.1	*npr-24*	R106.2		
SSTR3	AAP84354.1	*tkr-1*	C38C10.1		
SSTR4	AAS55648.1	*tkr-3*	AC7.1		
SSTR5	EAW85687.1	C49A9.7	C49A9.7		
		C50F7.1	C50F7.1		
		T02E9.1	T02E9.1		
		Y116A8B.5	Y116A8B.5		
		Y54E2A.1	Y54E2A.1		

Table 4 | Nematodes and arthropods used to analyze the rhodopsin GPCRs.

	Life style	Feeding type	Databases
NEMATODES			
Caenorhabditis elegans	Free-living	Bacteria	http://metazoa.ensembl.org http://www.wormbase.org
Caenorhabditis briggsae	Free-living	Bacteria	http://metazoa.ensembl.org
Caenorhabditis japonica	Free-living	Bacteria, dead eggs and adult bugs	http://metazoa.ensembl.org
Pristionchus pacificus (necromenic nematode)	Parasitic	Bacteria, fungi and other nematodes	http://metazoa.ensembl.org
Haemonchus contortus (red stomach worm)	Parasitic	Bacteria, blood and tissue	http://www.sanger.ac.uk
Brugia malayi (filariasis worm)	Parasitic	Blood and lymphatic tissue	http://blast.ncbi.nlm.nih.gov
Trichinella spiralis (pork worm)	Parasitic	Mammalian cells and blood	http://metazoa.ensembl.org
Meloidogyne incognita (root-knot plant parasite)	Parasitic	Plant tissue	http://meloidogyne.toulouse.inra.fr
ARTHROPODS			
Drosophila melanogaster (fruit fly)	Free-living	Yeast	http://metazoa.ensembl.org http://www.flybase.org
Apis mellifera (honeybee)	Free-living	Nectar and pollen	http://metazoa.ensembl.org
Bombyx mori (silkworm)	Free-living	Plant leafs	http://metazoa.ensembl.org
Aedes aegypti (yellow fever mosquito)	Parasitic	Nectar and blood	http://metazoa.ensembl.org
Anopheles gambiae (malaria mosquito)	Parasitic	Nectar and blood	http://metazoa.ensembl.org
Ixodes scapularis (blacklegged tick)	Parasitic	Blood	http://metazoa.ensembl.org

Information about life style, feeding type and the database interrogated is indicated.

GPCRs are present in *C. elegans* and 22 in *D. melanogaster* genomes (**Table 2**) and a conserved role in feeding regulation has been demonstrated.

FEEDING IN NEMATODES AND ARTHROPODS

Feeding in invertebrates in common with other animals involves a complex combination of physical, chemical, and nutritional factors (Chapman and De Boer, 1995). Taste and smell are important for feeding behavior and provide the CNS with information on quality and quantity of food and feeding behavior occurs mainly in response to both nutrient and nutritional storage status. Once feeding has been initiated and food ingested, the alimentary canal, and its associated glands triturate, lubricate, store, digest, and absorb the food material and excrete and expel unwanted remains (Audsley and Weaver, 2009).

The Nematoda is a highly diverse, complex, and specialized group of metazoans, about 30,000 species are currently known and many are renowned parasites (15%) and have specialized life cycles that depend on their host to survive and reproduce. Their success is associated with a protective, impermeable cuticle and by the diversity of the pharynx and feeding mechanisms (Coghlan, 2005). The shape and presence or absence of teeth, lancets, stylets, or other structures in the mouth reflects their distinct feeding methods. The majority of nematodes are free-living and inhabit soil and water and feed on microorganisms (bacteria, fungi, algae) and organic debris. The parasites feed on animal and plant tissues and some on vertebrate blood.

The Arthropoda represents the most diverse animal phyla and comprises over 80% of the species identified and the Insecta class is the most specious with approximately 920,000 species. Four main classes of feeding habits are recognized: plant feeders, predators (feed on aphids and mites), scavengers (feeding on dead and decaying organic matter), and parasites (of other insects and vertebrates), some of which are hematophagous. Within each of these classes, various types of feeding can be found such as biting and chewing on leaves or animal tissue and sucking from plant or animal cells or tissues. Despite this unique ability to use almost any organic substrate, most insect species restrict themselves to a particular category of food (Posnien et al., 2010) and feed primarily on a fluid diet (Prakash and Steele, 2010). The variety of feeding habits in arthropods is the result of anatomical and physiological adaptations to distinct food sources (Chapman and De Boer, 1995). The alimentary canal is composed of specialized regions that vary according to feeding habit and life stage.

The organisms selected for analysis of rhodospin GPCRs potentially involved in invertebrate feeding are members of different nematode and arthropod lineages. The specific life style and feeding habits of the invertebrates included in the analysis are indicated in **Table 4**.

HOMOLOGS OF THE VERTEBRATE RHODOPSIN FAMILY GPCRS IMPLICATED IN FEEDING AND APPETITE REGULATION IN NON-VERTEBRATES

The following section describes the evolution and function of rhodopsin family members in nematodes and arthropods. It will start with an overview of those described in *C. elegans* and *D. melanogaster* involved in or candidates for feed intake regulation (**Tables 2** and **5**). Expression data when available from wormbase and flybase is included to provide insight into receptor function. It is followed by a section in which receptor evolution in invertebrates is discussed including homologs from non-model nematode and arthropod species.

In general, no putative melatonin peptide receptors (MCR) or melanin concentrating hormone receptor (MCHR) homologs have been described or were identified in the present study in any of the selected nematodes or arthropods (**Figure 3**). In addition,

Table 5 | An overview of the amino acid sequence similarity of the main subfamilies of *C. elegans* and *D. melanogaster* rhodopsin GPCRs and their human homologs.

Rhodopsin	Subfamily	Characterized with function assigned		Novel members with an unknown role in feeding	
		C. elegans (%)	*D. melanogaster* (%)	*C. elegans* (%)	*D. melanogaster* (%)
α-Group	Gastrin-cholecystokinin	32–36	33–37		
β-Group	Neurokinin/neuropeptide FF/Orexin	38–43	27–45	30–38	27–33
	Neuropeptide Y	32–40	12–36	29–41	12–14
	Bombesin		38–40		
	Neuromedin U	35–41	29–41	30–36	21–25
γ-Group	Somatostatin		35–41	27–35	
	Galanin	36–40	37–43		

Percentage of sequence similarity was calculated in the GeneDoc program (http://www.nr.bsc.org/gfx/genedoc/). The maximum and minimum sequence similarity of receptor subgroups between invertebrate and human homologs is indicated.

in nematodes no homolog of the vertebrate and fruit fly bombesin receptors seem to exist (**Table 2**). Duplicates of the human receptor genes were identified in the genomes of nearly all target species and phylogenetic analysis suggests specific gene duplication/deletions occurred within the nematode and arthropod lineages (**Figure 3**).

THE RHODOPSIN GPCRS IN *C. ELEGANS* AND *D. MELANOGASTER* GENOMES

Characterized and functionally assigned subfamily members

Gastrin-cholecystokinin receptor subfamily. In the genomes of *C. elegans* and *D. melanogaster* two putative Gastrin-CCK-like receptor homologs of the human members have been reported (**Figure 3A**; Keating et al., 2003; Janssen et al., 2008). In *C. elegans*, *ckr-1*, and *ckr-2* have been described and functionally characterized. The *ckr-1* is expressed in the nerve ring and functional RNAi knockdown studies reveal that loss of receptor activity provokes fat accumulation (McKay et al., 2007). However, if the receptors are ablated there is no apparent effect on feeding regulation but instead embryonic lethality and reduced brood size is observed (McKay et al., 2007). The neuropeptide *nlp-12* is the ligand of nematode *ckr-2* and the peptide receptor pair shares conserved biological activity with regards to fat storage with the human homolog (Janssen et al., 2008). A cognate peptide for nematode *ckr-1* is yet to be identified.

In *D. melanogaster* the two existent CCK-like receptors were designated CCKL-R17D3 (DSKR1) and CCKL-R17D1 (Kubiak et al., 2002). They are mainly expressed in the CNS and are activated by *Drosophila* sulfakinin (DSK; Nichols et al., 1988), which is a structurally and functionally related peptide to the vertebrate CCK (Audsley and Weaver, 2009). Their role in feeding regulation has not yet been demonstrated in *Drosophila* but in other arthropods the homolog receptor stimulation by SK causes gut emptying and satiety (Nichols, 2007). Injections of SK peptides significantly reduce meal size in locusts (*Schistocerca gregaria*; Wei et al., 2000) and cockroach (*Blattella germanica*; Maestro et al., 2001), carbohydrate feeding in the blowfly (*Phormia regina*), and inhibit female horse flies from blood feeding (Downer et al., 2007).

Neurokinin/neuropeptide FF/orexin receptor subfamily. In *C. elegans* two putative neurokinin (a.k.a. tachykinins) receptors *tkr-1* and *tkr-3* have been described (Keating et al., 2003; Greenwood et al., 2005). In *D. melanogaster* three neurokinin-like receptors have been reported: the neurokinin receptor (NKD), the tachykinin receptor (DTKR; Li et al., 1991; Monnier et al., 1992; Rosay et al., 1995; Poels et al., 2009), and the leucokinin receptor (LKR; Radford et al., 2002). Phylogenetic analysis of the invertebrate receptors suggests that they arose from an ancestral Neurokinin/neuropeptide FF/orexin-like receptor gene by species-specific duplication events prior to the Proto-Deuterostome divergence (**Figure 3B**; Hewes and Taghert, 2001). Characterization of the *C. elegans tkr-1* revealed expression is restricted to the socket cells (specialized nerve-accessory cells that act as an interface between the sensillum and hypodermis) and RNAi functional screens and the Nile Red fat assay revealed that this gene affects fat metabolism and fat droplet morphology and the pattern of fat deposition (Ashrafi et al., 2003). Knock down nematodes have a substantially lower fat content suggesting that this receptor is a key lipid storage regulator. *Tkr-3* RNAi studies caused mild sluggishness and slowed locomotion in nematodes (Keating et al., 2003), which may be related to modifications in the nervous system. *Tkr-3* is also present in the intestine but no role has yet been assigned in feeding and metabolism.

The *D. melanogaster* NKD and DTK receptors are expressed in the head of both larvae and adults and are activated by *Drosophila* tachykinin (DTK1–6) peptides, which are derived from the *drosotachykinin* (*Dtk*) gene (Birse et al., 2006; Poels et al., 2007) and also by substance P which is involved in the regulation of food intake and energy homeostasis in vertebrates (Birse et al., 2006; Poels et al., 2007). Knock down of DTKR in *D. melanogaster* modulated expression in both fed and starved flies of insulin-like peptides, which play a major role in the regulation of carbohydrates and lipid metabolism (Poels et al., 2009; Birse et al., 2011).

Neuropeptide Y receptor subfamily. In *C. elegans* four putative NPY-like receptors (*npr-1, npr-2, npr-5*, and *npr-11*) that share conserved sequence with the vertebrate NPYRs have been isolated and function characterized (de Bono and Bargmann, 1998; Keating

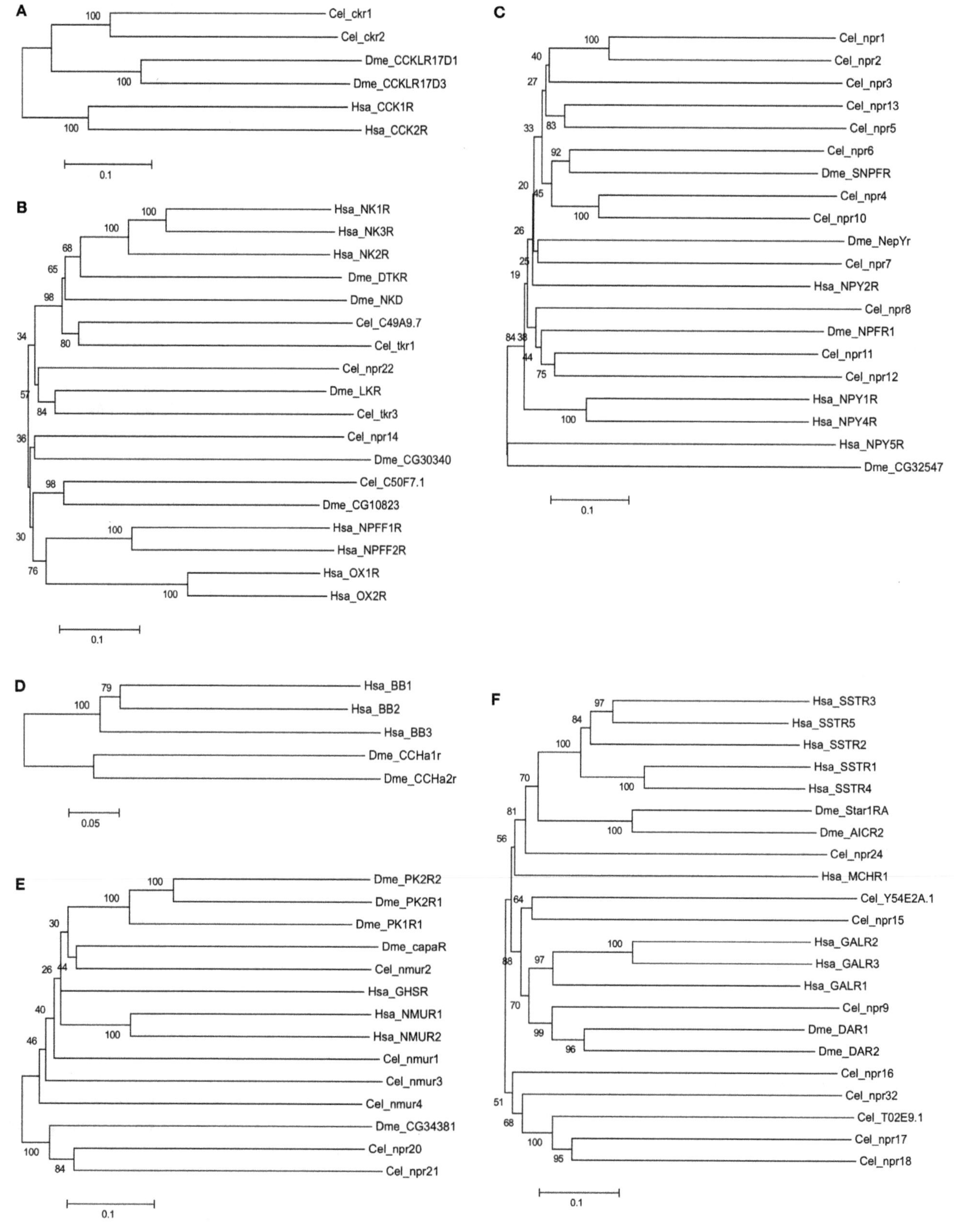

FIGURE 3 | Continued

FIGURE 3 | Phylogenetic relationship of the Human (Hsa) rhodopsin GPCRs involved in feeding with the nematode *C. elegans* (Cel) and arthropod *D. melanogaster* (Dme) sequence homologs. Trees were constructed using the neighbor joining method with 1000 bootstrap replicates (uniform rate among sites, pairwise deletion using the p-distance substitution model) built in the Mega5.1 program. Receptors were classified into six distinct subfamilies: **(A)** Gastrin-Cholecystokinin receptors; **(B)** Neurokinin/neuropeptide FF/orexin receptors, **(C)** Neuropeptide Y receptors, **(D)** Bombesin receptors, **(E)** Ghrelin/obstatin and Neuromedin U receptors, and **(F)** Somatostatin and galanin receptors. Accession numbers are described in **Table 3**.

et al., 2003; Kubiak et al., 2008; Cohen et al., 2009). Three NPY-like receptors have also been reported in *D. melanogaster*, these are the NepYr receptor and two neuropeptide F (NPF) receptors, the NPFR1 and the short NPFR (SNPFR; **Figure 3C**). The NPF peptide occurs as a long (NPF) and short (sNPF) isoform in arthropods (De Loof et al., 2001) and is the homolog of vertebrate neuropeptide Y (NPY; Li et al., 1992; de Jong-Brink et al., 2001).

In *C. elegans*, the nematode *npr-1* was the first receptor found to influence social feeding behavior and is predominantly expressed in the nervous system (de Bono and Bargmann, 1998). This receptor is activated by *flp-21* peptide (Rogers et al., 2003) and ablation of the peptide does not cause silencing of *npr-1* functions, suggesting that it can be activated by other molecules. In fact, *flp-18* peptide also activates *npr-1* and this peptide is also the ligand of *npr-5*, which is involved, in chemosensory response, foraging behavior, and fat metabolism (Rogers et al., 2003). Nematode *npr-5* is expressed in the head, neck, and body muscles and knock down and gene mutation studies revealed that in common with *npr-2* it is associated with intestinal fat storage regulation (Keating et al., 2003; Cohen et al., 2009), *dauer* formation, and other food-dependent decisions (Cohen et al., 2009). The *npr-11* has a role in reproduction and sensory dynamics of the olfactory system (Chalasani et al., 2010) but no role in feeding has yet been demonstrated (Chalasani et al., 2010).

The fruit fly NepYr and NPF receptors are expressed in the *D. melanogaster* CNS and NepYr is also present in the gut. NepYr is activated by dRYamide-1 and dRYamide-2, which has a C-terminal sequence similar to vertebrate NPY family peptides and in flies dRYamide suppresses feeding motivation (Ida et al., 2011). NPF and its receptors also modulate feeding behavior in *D. melanogaster* (Wu et al., 2003; Garczynski et al., 2005) and they promote feeding in larvae (Wu et al., 2003) and influence the effect of food deprivation in adult flies (Wu et al., 2003; Lingo et al., 2007). In other arthropods their functions have also been described and NPFR is involved in hindgut contraction in the bloodsucking bug (*Rhodnius prolixus*; Gonzalez and Orchard, 2009) and in ovarian maturation in locusts (Schoofs et al., 2001). In *D. melanogaster* sNPF is involved in the control of food intake and in the regulation of body size (Lee et al., 2004). Studies in mutant fruit flies over expressing sNPF peptide exhibit increased food intake and produce bigger and heavier flies, whereas sNPF loss-of-function mutants exhibit suppressed food intake (Lee et al., 2004). Gene expression studies with the red fire ant (*Solenopsis invicta Buren*) revealed SNPFR in brain is down-regulated during starvation (Chen and Pietrantonio, 2006) and expression of long NPF and its receptor in the malaria mosquito (*A. gambiae*) appear to be dependent on the insect nutritional status (Garczynski et al., 2005).

Bombesin receptor subfamily. Homologs of the vertebrate bombesin receptors have not been reported in nematodes and were not identified in the present study. Members of this family are only present in *D. melanogaster* and they correspond to the Allatostatin type B receptors (Stay, 2000). In *D. melanogaster*, two bombesin-like receptors have been isolated and function characterized: CCHamide-1r (CCHa1r; Johnson et al., 2003) and CCHamide-2r (CCHa-2r; Johnson et al., 2003; Hauser et al., 2008; **Figure 3D**).

In insects the function of the arthropod bombesin receptor is still poorly explored as a specific ligand has only recently been identified. CCHa-2r expression was detected in *D. melanogaster* brain and in the CNS and midgut of *B. mori* (Roller et al., 2008). Functional analysis reveals the receptors are activated by the peptides CCHamide-1 or CCHamide-2 that have been shown to suppress feeding activity in the cockroach, *Blattella germanica* (Audsley and Weaver, 2009).

Ghrelin-obestatin/neuromedin U receptor subfamily. In *C. elegans* four nmur-like receptors: *nmur-1*, *nmur-2*, *nmur-3*, and *nmur-4* have been described. In *D. melanogaster* the capaR and three pyrokinin receptors PK-1R, PK-2-R1, and PK-2-R2 are the homologs of vertebrate NMURs (Iversen et al., 2002; Park et al., 2002; **Figure 3E**). The nematode *nmur-1* is suggested to be involved in the sensory system and with processing information from specific food cues, which enables selection of different food types (Maier et al., 2010). *C. elegans nmur-2* was also shown with its ligand peptide (derived from the *nlp-44* precursor gene) to be involved in the regulation of food intake (Lindemans et al., 2009). To date no functional studies involving *nmur-3* and *nmur-4* have been reported although *nmur-4* is expressed in the pharynx and intestine suggesting it may have a role in feeding.

The *D. melanogaster* capaR is mainly expressed in the Malpighian tubules and it is involved in the increase of fluid transport and diuresis and no direct role in feeding has yet been attributed (Terhzaz et al., 2012). CapaR is activated by two neuropeptides, capa-1 and -2 that are encoded by the *capability* gene and have antidiurectic actions in insects (Pollock et al., 2004; Coast and Garside, 2005; Paluzzi et al., 2010). The *capability* gene also encodes the pyrokinin-1 (PK1) peptide that is a specific activator of PK-1R. PK-2-R1 and PK-2-R2 are activated by pyrokinin-2 (PK2) and Hug-γ that are derived from the hugin (hug) prepropeptide (Cazzamali et al., 2005).

Phylogenetic analysis of the pyrokinin receptors suggests that they share common ancestry and that PK-2-R1 and R2 are the result of a recent duplication in the fly genome. The pyrokinin peptides are involved in rhythmic motor activity in arthropods (Saideman et al., 2007) and receptors are expressed in the abdomen (carcass) and nervous tissue and involvement in modulation of feeding behavior has been suggested. Overexpression of the hugin gene was found to suppress feeding in *Drosophila*, while blockage of the synaptic activity of hugin neurons caused the opposite effect (Meng et al., 2002; Melcher and Pankratz, 2005).

Somatostatin receptor subfamily. A homolog of human SSTR in the *C. elegans* genome was predicted in the 1990's (Wilson et al., 1994). Characterization of the deduced protein revealed that the signature motif of the vertebrate SSTR was missing in TM7, suggesting that the receptor is probably activated by other ligands. Since no other homolog of vertebrate SSTR has been reported, the function of the putative SSTR-like receptors in nematodes remains to be explored. In arthropods, Allatostatin type-C receptors are the homologs of the vertebrate somastostatin receptors and in *D. melanogaster*, two receptors star1-RA and AlCR2 were described (Kreienkamp et al., 2002; Mayoral et al., 2010; **Figure 3F**).

The *D. melanogaster* star1-RA and AlCR2 receptors are detected in the CNS and they are activated by allatostatin-C peptides, which are potent modulators of hormone synthesis (Aguilar et al., 2003; Hergarden et al., 2012). These peptides inhibit or stimulate the corpora allata to synthesize juvenile hormone, which is an important regulator of development and reproduction in insects and may indirectly influence feeding behavior (Audsley and Weaver, 2009; Nassel and Winther, 2010).

Galanin receptor subfamily. In *C. elegans* and *D. melanogaster* a sequence and function homolog of vertebrate GALR has been described (**Figure 3F**). The *C. elegans* GALR-like receptor, *npr-9* in common with the vertebrate homolog may be involved in food foraging and lipid storage (Bendena et al., 2008). The *npr-9* is expressed in specific neurons around the posterior pharyngeal bulb and *C. elegans* receptor mutants are characterized by impaired food-related roaming behavior and accumulate intestinal fat as a result of fat ingestion and reduced energy expenditure (Lang et al., 2007; Bendena et al., 2008). Peptides involved in the activation of *npr-9* have not been isolated, although *nlp-5* and *nlp-6*, are candidate allatostatin-like peptides that in insects activate the GAL-like receptor (Nathoo et al., 2001).

In arthropods, the Allatostatin type-A receptors are homologs of the vertebrate GALRs (Birgul et al., 1999). Two receptors have been described in *D. melanogaster*, DAR-1 (a.k.a. AlstR) and DAR-2 (Birgul et al., 1999; Lenz et al., 2000; **Figure 3F**). AlstR is expressed in *D. melanogaster* head and CNS while DAR-2 is expressed in the gut suggesting they may have divergent functions. The receptors are activated by FGLamide neuropeptides (Pratt et al., 1991; Woodhead et al., 1994) that in arthropods inhibit food intake (Audsley and Weaver, 2009). Genetic epistasis assays in *D. melanogaster* indicate that FGLamide neuron activation inhibits or limits starvation-induced changes in feeding behavior (Hergarden et al., 2012).

Novel subfamily members with an unknown role in feeding regulation

Neurokinin/neuropeptide FF/orexin-like receptor subfamily. In *C. elegans* four additional NKRs members may exist: *npr-14*, *npr-22* and the genes C49A9.7 and C50F7.1 (Keating et al., 2003). In *D. melanogaster* the SIFamide receptor and the gene CG10823 (Hewes and Taghert, 2001) also seem to be novel receptor members (**Table 5**, **Figure 3B**). In the phylogenetic tree, the *C. elegans* gene C49A9.7 clusters with *tkr-1* suggesting they may be duplicates and the nematode *npr-14* and C50F7.1 genes group with the fruit fly CG30340 and SIFamide receptor genes suggesting that they may have emerged from the same gene prior to the nematode-arthropod divergence. Functional studies of these receptors are scarce but those that exist indicate that the *C. elegans* MVRFamide neuropeptides but not tachykinin-like peptides activate the *npr-22* receptor (Mertens et al., 2006). The function of *D. melanogaster* CG30340 gene, which is present in low abundance in the digestive and nervous system and of SIFamide receptors are unknown (Jorgensen et al., 2006).

Neuropeptide Y-like receptor subfamily. In *C. elegans* at least eight putative novel NPYR gene members are predicted: *npr-3*, *npr-4*, *npr-6*, *npr-7*, *npr-8*, *npr-10*, *npr-12*, and *npr-13* and all remain to be validated and functionally characterized (Keating et al., 2003; **Figure 3C**). The receptors share between 30–40% amino acid sequence similarity with their human counterparts (**Table 5**) and are approximately 20% identical to the *C. elegans* homologs with a characterized function. The high sequence similarity and phylogenetic relationship between *npr-5* and *npr-13* (43%), *npr-4* and *npr-10* (50%) and *npr-11* and *npr-12* (44%) suggests that they may have arisen as a result of a recent duplication event in the nematode genome. These receptors are expressed in nervous tissue and intestine and their function is incompletely described and a specific role in feeding has not been demonstrated (Keating et al., 2003; Styer et al., 2008). In the *D. melanogaster* genome a putative novel insect NPY-like gene of unknown function (CG32547) may also exist (Hewes and Taghert, 2001) and seems to be expressed in the CNS (**Figure 3C**). The CG32547 gene shares less than 14% similarity with the human NPYR members (**Table 5**) and with the other insect family members, although this is probably due to its atypical size of 1008 amino acids, which makes family annotation ambiguous.

Ghrelin-obestatin/neuromedin U receptor subfamily. Two putative additional *C. elegans* nmur-like receptor genes the *npr-20* and *npr-21* were retrieved in the present study (**Figure 3E**). They share 30–36% amino acid sequence similarity with human homologs and are probably duplicates (**Table 5**). Expression of *npr-21* in *C. elegans* occurs in nerves of the head, tail, and ventral nerve cord and also in the posterior intestine suggesting that it may have a role in brain-gut function associated with feeding regulation. Similarly in *D. melanogaster* a putative member of this family was also retrieved, the gene CG34381 (**Table 5**) and it clusters with nematode *npr-20* and *npr-21* suggesting that it may have shared common ancestry (Hewes and Taghert, 2001). Expression of the CG34381 gene occurred in the fruit fly head but so far no functional studies have been reported.

Somatostatin receptor subfamily. In the *C. elegans* genome at least eight putative SST-like receptor genes are predicted: *npr-15*, *npr-16*, *npr-17*, *npr-18*, *npr-24*, *npr-32*, and the Y54E2A.1 (Vashlishan et al., 2008) and T02E9.1 genes (Keating et al., 2003; **Figure 3F**). No additional putative SST-like receptors were identified or have been reported for *D. melanogaster*. Characterization of the nematode putative SST-like receptors revealed the *C. elegans* members share between 27–35% amino acid sequence similarity with the human SSTRs and that the *npr-24* gene is the most closely related to the insect and human homologs suggesting that they may share a common ancestry (**Table 5**). Comparisons of the putative SSTR in *C. elegans* revealed they are highly divergent suggesting that after their emergence from an ancestral gene they underwent considerable change. Nematode *npr-17* is most similar to *npr-18* and to the T02E9.1 gene with which it shares 23% sequence identity and the three receptors tend to cluster with *npr-16* and *npr-32* suggesting they emerged in the nematode lineage.

The physiological role of the nematode SST-like receptors is poorly characterized but a role in metabolism and feeding behavior is probable. RNAi knockdown studies of *npr-16*, found to be expressed in head/tail neurons and the ventral nerve cord, increased fat deposition (Ashrafi et al., 2003). Ligand binding studies revealed that the peptide *nlp-3* activates the receptor *npr-17*, which seems to be involved in food aversion and has a role in serotonergic modulation via ASH sensory neurons to modulate nematode behavior in response to an external stimuli (Harris et al., 2010). Deletion of the T02E9.1 gene resulted in an uncoordinated phenotype and nematodes moved slowly and with an increase in circular movement, although feeding was apparently unaffected (Keating et al., 2003). The function of *npr-15*, *npr-18*, *npr-24*, *npr-32*, and Y54E2A.1 remain to be explored.

EVOLUTION OF RHODOPSIN GPCR HOMOLOGS IN INVERTEBRATES

The evolution of the rhodopsin GPCRs in invertebrates was established (**Figure 4**) by identifying homologs in different nematode and arthropod lineages of the receptors present in *C. elegans* (**Figure 5** and **Table 6**) and *D. melanogaster* (**Figure 6** and **Table 7**). In general, the invertebrate GPCRs with a documented role in feeding or that are sequence homologs of mammalian seem to have evolved differently in nematodes and arthropods. A similar gene complement to that identified in *C. elegans* and *D. melanogaster* was identified in non-model nematodes and arthropods, respectively (**Figure 4**). Nematodes of the superfamily Rhabditoidea generally have more genes than other nematodes (**Table 6**). Gene duplicates in *C. elegans* and *C. brigssae* are more abundant than in arthropods (Lynch and Conery, 2000; Cutter et al., 2009) and a higher number of homologs of the human NPYRs and SSTRs occur

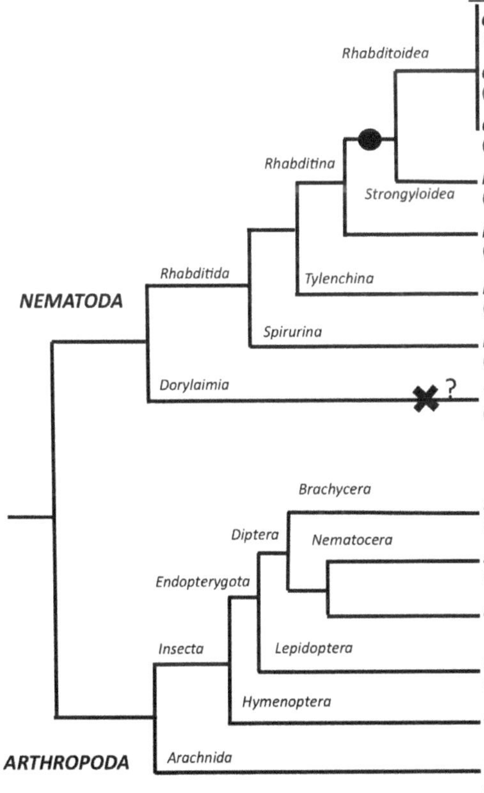

	CCKR	NKR	NPYR	BBR	NMUR	SSTR	GALR
Caenorhabditis elegans (bacteria)	2	6	12	*ni*	6	6	3
Caenorhabditis briggsae (bacteria)	2	6	11	*ni*	6	6	3
Caenorhabditis japonica (dead eggs, bugs)	1	6	12	*ni*	6	5	2 (1)
Haemonchus contortus P (bacteria, blood tissue)	2	5 (1)	6 (2)	*ni*	5	5	1
Pristionchus pacificus P (bacteria, fungi, nematodes)	1	1	6	*ni*	2 (1)	4	1
Meloidogyne incognita P (plant tissue)	(1)	1	6	*ni*	4	2 (1)	1 (1)
Brugia malayi P (blood, lymphatic tissue)	1 (1)	1	5	*ni*	*ni*	1	*ni*
Trichinella spiralis P (blood tissue, cells)	(1)	1 (1)	3	*ni*	1	1	1
Drosophila melanogaster (yeast)	2	5	4	2	5	2	2
Aedes aegypti P (sugar, mammalian blood)	2	5	6	3	4	2	2
Anopheles gambiae P (sugar, mammalian blood)	2	4	6	2	4	2	2
Bombyx mori (plant tissue)	*ni*	4	7	3	2	1	1
Apis mellifera (nectar, pollen)	1	6	3	2	5	1	1
Ixodes scapularis P (blood tissue)	3	4	5	1	1 (1)	2	3

FIGURE 4 | Distribution of rhodopsin subfamily members in nematodes and arthropods. The phylogenetic relationship of the species analyzed is represented on the right and their feeding habits are indicated. The black circle indicates a putative gene duplication event in the nematode radiation and the black cross potential gene deletion in the *T. spiralis* genome. Genes that were identified based upon sequence similarity but that were not considered for phylogenetic analysis are indicated within brackets "()"; ni- GPCR member not identified, and P represent parasitic nematode and arthropod. The evolutionary relationship within nematodes and arthropods was obtained from (Consortium, 2006; Sommer and Streit, 2011).

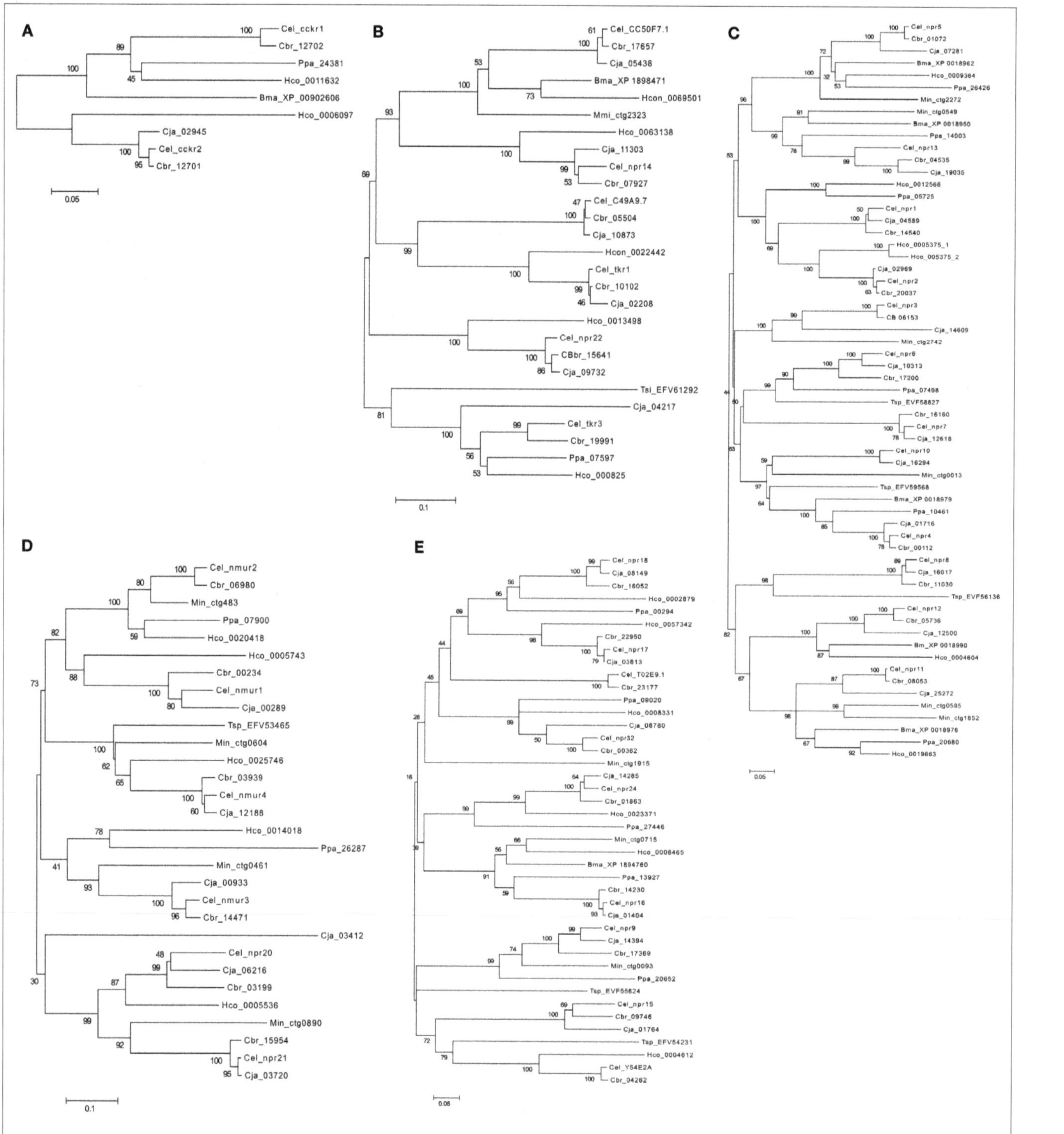

FIGURE 5 | Phylogenetic analysis of the nematode rhodopsin GPCRs. **(A)** Gastrin-cholecystokinin receptors; **(B)** Neurokinin/neuropeptide FF/orexin receptors, **(C)** Neuropeptide Y receptors, **(D)** Ghrelin-Obstatin/neuromedin U receptors, and **(E)** Somatostatin and galanin receptors. The *C.elegans* (Cel) receptors are annotated in bold. *C. briggsae* (Cbr), *C. japonica* (Cja), *P. pacificus* (Ppa) *H. contortus* (Hco) *B. malayi* (Bma), *T. spiralis* (Tsp), and *M. incognita* (Min). Accession numbers of the sequences used are indicated. Trees were constructed using the sequence alignment displayed in Figure S1 Supplementary Material using the methodology described in **Figure 3**.

in nematodes when compared to arthropods (**Figures 5C** and **6C**). In arthropods, species-specific gene duplications exist rather than a conserved gene homolog complement suggesting that, despite their common ancestry, GPCRs have had distinct evolutionary trajectories in the different lineages (**Table 7** and **Figure 6**).

Table 6 | Accession numbers of the *C. elegans* homologs in *C. briggsae, C. japonica, P. pacificus, H. contortus, B. malayi, T. spiralis*, and *M. incognita*.

Receptor subfamily	*C. elegans*	*C. briggsae*	*C. japonica*	*P. pacificus*	*H. contortus*	*B. malayi*	*T. spiralis*	*M. incognita*
Gastrin-cholecystokinin	*ckr-1*	CBG12702	CJA02945	PPA24381	Supercontig0002945	XP_001902606	EFV58901*	MiV1ctg254*
	ckr-2	CBG12701			Supercontig0006097	XP_001895620*		
Neurokinin/neuropeptide FF/orexin	*tkr-1*	CBG10102	CJA02208	PPA07597	Supercontig0022442	XP_001898471	EFV61292	MiV1ctg2323
	tkr-3	CBG19991	CJA04217		Supercontig000825		EFV59206*	
	npr-14	CBG07927	CJA11303		Supercontig0069501			
	npr-22	CBG15641	CJA09732		Supercontig0013498			
	C49A9.7	CBG05504	CJA10873		Supercontig0000067*			
	C50F7.1	CBG17657	CJA05438		Supercontig0063138			
Neuropeptide Y	*npr-1*	CBG14540	CJA04589	PPA05725	Supercontig0012566	XP_001897991	EFV58827	MiV1ctg2742
	npr-2	CBG20037	CJA02969	PPA10461	SuperContig0005375	XP_001895072	EVF56136	MiV1ctg13
	npr-3	CBG06153	CJA14609	PPA26426	Supercontig0005375	XP_001896282	EVF59568	MiV1ctg2272
	npr-4	CBG00112	CJA01716	PPA07498	Supercontig0004842*	XP_001897675		MiV1ctg595
	npr-5	CBG01072	CJA07281	PPA20680	Supercontig0009364	XP_001899021		MiV1ctg1852
	npr-6	CBG17200	CJA10313	PPA14003	Supercontig0019663			MiV1ctg549
	npr.7	CBG16160	CJA12618		Supercontig0004604			
	npr-8	CBG11030	CJA16017		Supercontig0005938*			
	npr-10	CBG08053	CJA16294					
	npr-11	CBG05736	CJA25272					
	npr-12	CBG04535	CJA12500					
	npr-13		CJA19035					
Ghrelin-obstatin/neuromedin U	*nmur-1*	GBG00234	CJA00289	PPA17766*	Supercontig0005743	ni	EFV53465	MiV1ctg483
	nmur-2	CBG06980	CJA03412	PPA07900	Supercontig0020418			MiV1ctg461
	nmur-3	CBG14471	CJA00933	PPA26287	Supercontig0014018			MiV1ctg604
	nmur-4	CBG03939	CJA12188		Supercontig0025746			MiV1ctg890
	npr-20	CBG03199	CJA06216		Supercontig0005536			
	npr-21	CBG15954	CJA03720					
Somatostatin	*npr-24*	CBG01863	CJA14285	PPA27446	Supercontig0023371	XP_001894760.1	EFV55624	MiV1ctg715
	npr-16	CBG14230	CJA01404	PPA13927	Supercontig0008465			MiV1ctg1915
	npr-17	CBG22950	CJA03613	PPA00294	Supercontig0057342			MiV1ctg1587*
	npr-18	CBG16052	CJA08149	PPA09020	Supercontig0002879			
	npr-32	CBG00362	CJA08780		Supercontig0008331			
	T02E9.1	CBG23177						
Galanin	*npr-9*	CBG17363	CJA14394	PPA20652	Supercontig0004612	ni	EFV54231	MiV1ctg93
	npr-15	CBG09746	CJA01764					MiV1ctg1567*
	Y54E2A.1	CBG04262	CJA18843*					

**Indicates sequences not used in the phylogenetic analysis due to poor sequence or non-identification of TM domains. ni, indicates gene not identified.*

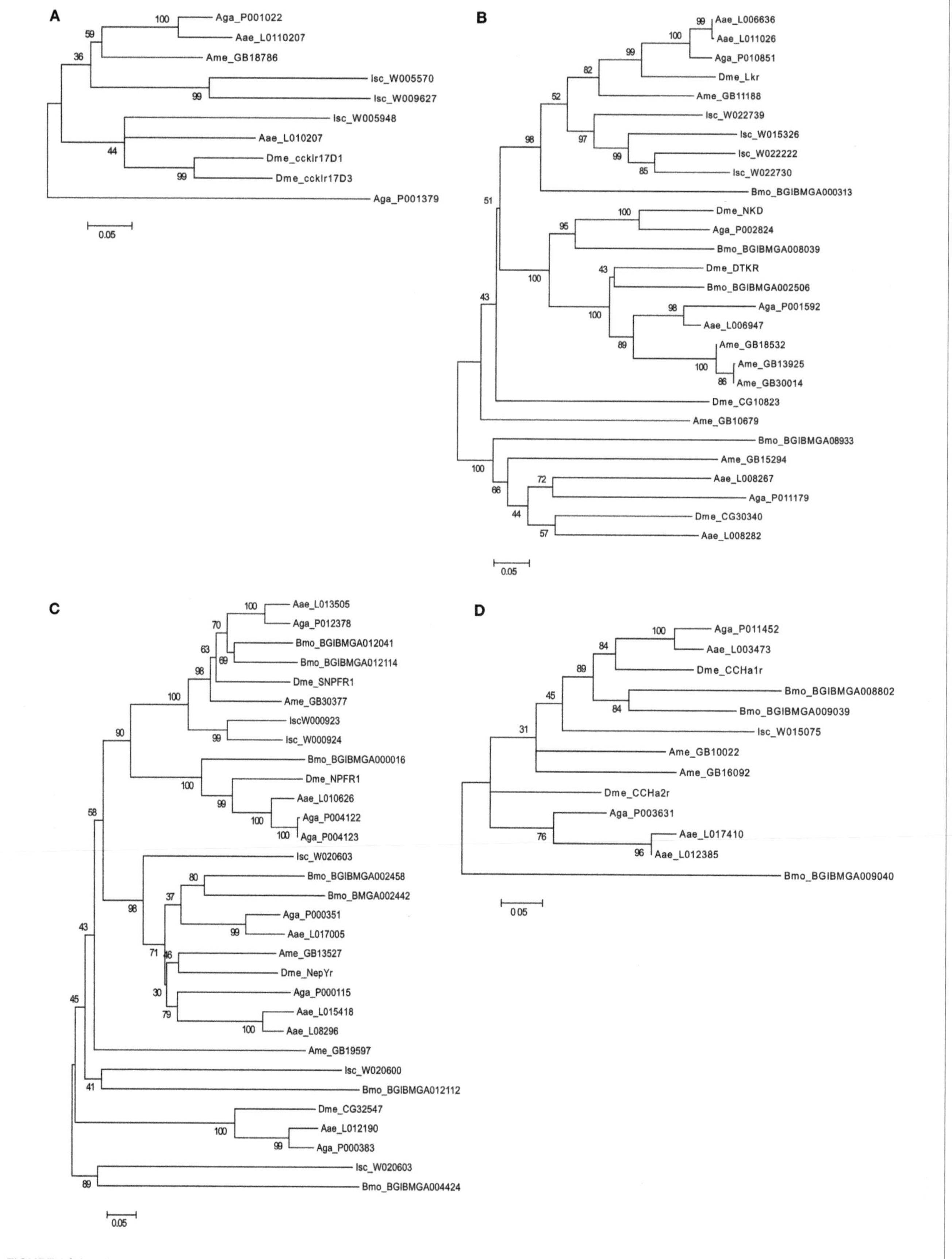

FIGURE 6 | Continued

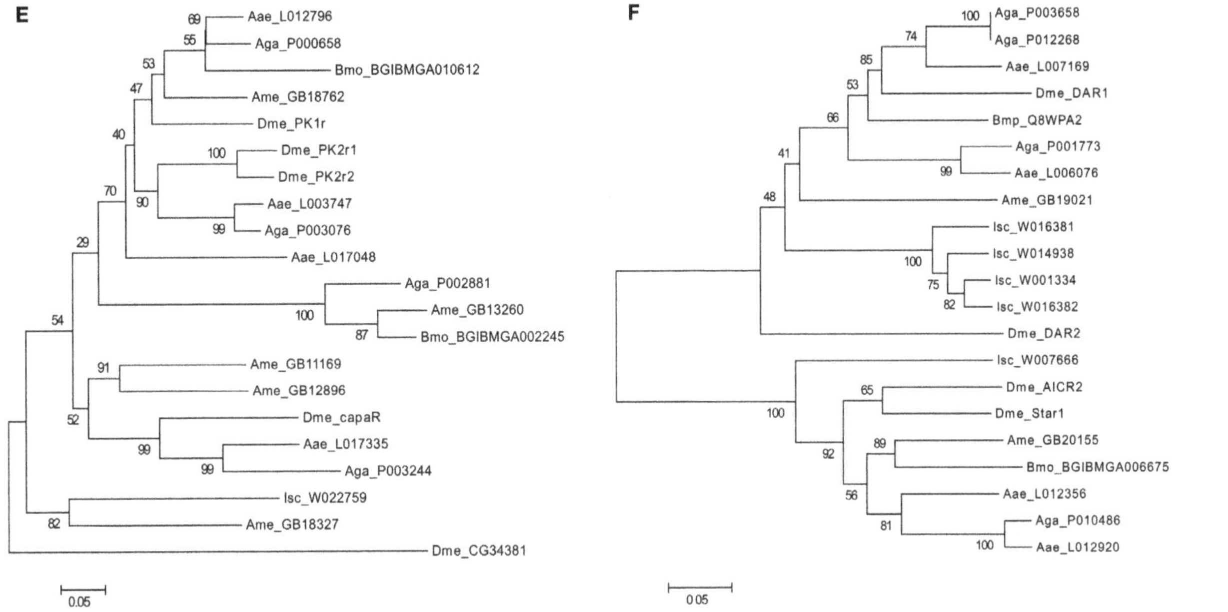

FIGURE 6 | Phylogenetic analysis of the arthropod rhodopsin GPCRs. (A) Gastrin-cholecystokinin receptors; **(B)** Neurokinin/neuropeptide FF/Orexin receptors, **(C)** Neuropeptide Y receptors, **(D)** Bombesin receptors, **(E)** Ghrelin-Obstatin/Neuromedin U receptors, and **(F)** Somatostatin and galanin receptors. The *D. melanogaster* (Dme) receptors are annotated in bold. *A. gambiae* (Aga), *A. aegypti* (Aae), *A. mellifera* (Ame), *B. mori* (Bmo), and *I. scapularis* (Isc). Accession numbers of the sequences used are indicated. Trees were constructed using the sequence alignment displayed in Figure S2 in Supplementary Material using a similar approach to that described in **Figure 3**.

A striking observation is the absence in nematodes of homologs of the arthropod bombesin receptors (BBR; **Figure 4**; **Table 5**). The reason for the loss of BBR in nematodes is unknown and their function and any link to feeding regulation remains to be established. In vertebrates, bombesin and its receptors are involved in smooth muscle contraction, exocrine, and endocrine secretion in the gut, pancreas, and pituitary and they also have a central role in food intake and energy homeostasis (Sano et al., 2004; Gonzalez et al., 2008). Three receptors have been isolated in humans and a similar number exist in arthropods and they share a common ancestry (**Figure 6D**).

A similar number of gastrin-CCK, NKR, NMUR, and GALR subfamily members were characterized in nematodes and arthropods (**Figure 4**). Two putative gastrin-CCK receptors were identified in invertebrates and in humans two gastrin-CCK receptors also exist suggesting that the evolution of the members of this family has been highly conserved. However, phylogenetic analysis suggests that the duplication, which delivered the two gene copies, was not common to all the species and occurred independently within each lineage. The two *ckr* that are present in nematodes resulted from a lineage specific duplication and homologs of the two *C. elegans* genes were identified in most nematode genomes analyzed (**Figure 5A**). In arthropods, a different situation exists and the two *D. melanogaster* genes are very similar and seem to have resulted from a species-specific duplication event (**Figure 6A**). Similarly in the blacklegged tick (*I. scapularis*) three putative gastrin-CCK receptors were also identified. In contrast, no putative homologs were identified in the plant feeding arthropod, the silkworm *B. mori*, even though they had a similar gene complement to other arthropods. It remains to be established if the absence of this receptor in *B. mori* is a consequence of its incomplete genome assembly (Xia et al., 2004) or represents an adaptation relative to feeding regulation.

Members of the NKR, NMUR, and GALR subfamilies have also evolved via lineage specific and species-specific duplication events. In nematodes, a similar number of NKR, NMUR, and GALR receptors exist in *H. contortus* and in the three representatives of the *Caernohabitis* genus analyzed (**Figures 5B,D,E**). In contrast, few genes of these families have been identified in other nematode taxa and a single NKR subfamily member was retrieved from *P. pacificus*, *M. incognita*, *B. malayi*, and *T. spiralis*. In arthropods, gene duplication of the *D. melanogaster* LKR receptor homologs was identified in the mosquito *A. aegypti* and also in *I. scapularies* in which four putative receptors exist (**Figure 6B**). In addition, in the honeybee (*A. mellifera*) three putative homologs of the fruit fly DTKR receptors were also identified. In contrast, no homologs of *D. melanogaster* NKD were detected in the honeybee and *A. aegypti* genomes. Within the NMUR family (**Figure 6E**), the *D. melanogaster* PK2Rs emerged as a consequence of a species-specific duplication event and two putative capaR were also identified in the honeybee, but only a single member was found in *I. scapulars*. In contrast, duplication of GALR occurred in the *I. scapulars* genome and four putative receptors were identified while other arthropods contained a single homolog of *D. melanogaster* DAR-1 and DAR-2 genes (**Figure 6F**).

The complete genome sequence of some of the species used in this study are not yet available, nonetheless gene representatives

Table 7 | Accession numbers of the *D. melanogaster* homologs in *A. gambiae, A. aegypti, A. mellifera, B. mori* and *I. scapularis*.

Receptor subfamily	*D. melanogaster*	*A. gambiae*	*A. aegypti*	*A. mellifera*	*B. mori*	*I. scapularis*
Gastrin-cholecystokinin	CCKLR-17D3	AGAP001022	AAEL010207	GB18786	ni	ISCW005570
	CCKLR-17D1	AGAP001379	AAEL017238			ISCW009627
						ISCW005948
Neurokinin/neuropeptide FF/orexin	NKD	AGAP002824	AAEL006947	GB13925	BGIBMGA008039	ISCW022739
	DTKR	AGAP001592	AAEL008267	GB30014	BGIBMGA002506	ISCW015326
	Lkr	AGAP011179	AAEL008282	GB18532	BGIBMGA008933	ISCW022222
	CG30340	AGAP010851	AAEL011026	GB15294	BGIBMGA000313	ISCW022730
	CG10823		AAEL006636	GB11188		
				GB10679		
Neuropeptide Y	NepYr	AGAP000351	AAEL017005	GB13527	BGIBMGA002442	ISCW020603
	NPFR1	AGAP000115	AAEL008296	GB19597	BGIBMGA002458	ISCW020600
	SNPFR1	AGAP000383	AAEL015418	GB30377	BGIBMGA000016	ISCW022779*
	CG32547	AGAP004123	AAEL012190		BGIBMGA012112	ISCW000923
		AGAP012378	AAEL010626		BGIBMGA012041	ISCW000924
		AGAP004122	AAEL007924		BGIBMGA012114	
			AAEL013505			
Bombesin	CCHa1r	AGAP003631	AAEL012385	GB10022	BGIBMGA008802	ISCW015075
	CCHa-2r	AGAP011452	AAEL017410	GB16092	BGIBMGA009039	
			AAEL003473		BGIBMGA009040	
Ghrelin-obstatin/neuromedin U	capaR	AGAP003244	AAEL017335	GB11169	BGIBMGA002245	ISCW012018*
	PK-1r	AGAP002881	AAEL012796	GB12896	BGIBMGA010612	ISCW022759
	PK2r2	AGAP000658	AAEL003747	GB18762		
	PK2r1	AGAP003076	AAEL017048	GB13260		
	CG34381			GB18327		
Somatostatin	Star1-RA	AGAP010486	AAEL012920	GB20155	BGIBMGA006675	ISCW007666
	AICR2	AGAP012268	AAEL012356			
Galanin	DAR-1	AGAP003658	AAEL007169	GB19021	Q8WPA2	ISCW001334
	DAR-2	AGAP001773	AAEL006076			ISCW014938
						ISCW016381
						ISCW016382

**Indicates sequences not used in the phylogenetic analysis due to poor sequence or non-identification of TM domains. ni: indicates gene not identified.*

identified in the selected nematodes and arthropods provides a clear idea of the GPCR evolution in invertebrates. The majority of the *C. elegans* sequence homologs were identified in the target species and an increase in gene number seems to have occurred in Rhabditoidea and Strongyloidea (Abad et al., 2008; Dieterich et al., 2008; Mitreva et al., 2011). The exception was *B. malayi* in which representatives of NMUR and GALR were not identified possibly because of its incomplete genome assembly (Ghedin et al., 2007). The absence of the majority of the *C. elegans* receptor homologs in parasitic nematode genomes and the higher number of genes present in *H. contortus* and in other representatives of the *Caernohabitis* genus is curious. A general comparison of the gene content of *T. spiralis* with *C. elegans* revealed that the parasitic nematode genome contains fewer genes (15,808 compared to 20,060 and 19,507 in *C. elegans* and *C. briggsae*, respectively) and we hypothesize that gene absence is a consequence of the selective pressures provoked by the host on which they live and depend for survival (Mitreva et al., 2011; Sommer and Streit, 2011). The genome of *P. pacificus* is predicted to contain a higher gene number than *C. elegans* and suggests that a specific GPCR gene expansion occurred in the nematode lineage after their divergence (Dieterich et al., 2008; Sommer and Streit, 2011). Comparisons between *T. spiralis* and the other blood feeding parasitic nematode *H. contortus* revealed that the latter has a higher GPCR gene number than *T. spiralis*. One explanation may be related to their life cycles and while both nematodes need blood to survive *T. spiralis* is an obligate parasite, while *H. contortus* has a non-parasitic free-living stage. Intriguingly during the parasitic stage of *H. contortus* significant changes in the active transcriptome occurs when compared to the nematode free-living stage (Hoekstra et al., 2000) and it will be of interest to establish if this affects the diversity of rhodopsin GPCRs expressed.

In arthropods, GPCR gene evolution appears species dependent and specific gene duplications and deletions have occurred despite their common ancestry. The existence of specific gene duplicates in arthropods may indicate that a divergent regulatory system evolved in different species and the origin and maintenance of duplicates in the genome remain to be explored. Gene number in the two mosquito species analyzed are very similar and may reflect their identical life styles (Klowden, 1990). In the tick, which feeds exclusively on blood, a specific expansion of NKR and GALR gene families occurred. Further studies are required to determine the significance of the specific evolution of rhodopsin family GPCRs in arthropods and to consider how life style and feeding activity may have influenced receptor evolution.

FINAL CONSIDERATIONS

In general, the physiological processes involving GPCRs are conserved and sequence and function homologs of vertebrate rhodopsin GPCRs are present in invertebrates indicating they emerged early in evolution. In Nematoda and Arthropoda the rhodopsin GPCRs have evolved differently. Gene expansion is observed in nematodes with a free-living stage and specific gene deletions seem to have affected parasitic nematode genomes. In arthropods species-specific gene duplications occurred. We hypothesize that the evolving feeding regime and life style of invertebrates was one of the pressure forcing GPCR evolution and that this may explain some of the specific gene family expansions and deletions. Comparative studies of GPCRs gained or lost in the nematodes and arthropods and their relationship to feeding regulation may provide insights into how GPCRs contributed and shaped adaptation to new ecological niche. Studies of other nematodes and arthropods coupled with experiments to assign function and potential conserved role in feeding will be needed to test this hypothesis.

ACKNOWLEDGMENTS

This study was funded by the Portuguese Science Foundation PTDC/BIA-BCM/114395/2009 and CCMAR plurianual grant. Vera G. Fonseca was supported by FCT grant SFRH/BPD/80447/2011.

SUPPLEMENTARY MATERIAL

The Supplementary Material for this article can be found online at http://www.frontiersin.org/Neuroendocrine_Science/10.3389/fendo.2012.00157/abstract

Figure S1 | Sequence of the nematodes GPCR transmembrane (TM) domains from non-model nematodes within each receptor family were extracted by sequence homology using the roundworm *C. elegans* TM regions. To facilitate visualization the TM1, 3, 5, and 7 were annotated in gray.

Figure S2 | Sequence of the Arthropod GPCR transmembrane (TM) domains used in for phylogenetic analysis. TM domains from non-model arthropods within each receptor family were extracted by sequence homology using the *D. melanogaster* TMs. To facilitate visualization the TM1, 3, 5 and 7 were annotated in gray.

REFERENCES

Abad, P., Gouzy, J., Aury, J. M., Castagnone-Sereno, P., Danchin, E. G., Deleury, E., et al. (2008). Genome sequence of the metazoan plant-parasitic nematode Meloidogyne incognita. *Nat. Biotechnol.* 26, 909–915.

Adams, M. D., Celniker, S. E., Holt, R. A., Evans, C. A., Gocayne, J. D., Amanatides, P. G., et al. (2000). The genome sequence of Drosophila melanogaster. *Science* 287, 2185–2195.

Aguilar, R., Maestro, J. L., Vilaplana, L., Pascual, N., Piulachs, M. D., and Belles, X. (2003). Allatostatin gene expression in brain and midgut, and activity of synthetic allatostatins on feeding-related processes in the cockroach Blattella germanica. *Regul. Pept.* 115, 171–177.

Ahima, R. S., and Osei, S. Y. (2001). Molecular regulation of eating behavior: new insights and prospects for therapeutic strategies. *Trends. Mol. Med.* 7, 205–213.

Ashrafi, K., Chang, F. Y., Watts, J. L., Fraser, A. G., Kamath, R. S., Ahringer, J., et al. (2003). Genome-wide RNAi analysis of Caenorhabditis elegans fat regulatory genes. *Nature* 421, 268–272.

Audsley, N., and Weaver, R. J. (2009). Neuropeptides associated with the regulation of feeding in insects. *Gen. Comp. Endocrinol.* 162, 93–104.

Bale, T. L., and Vale, W. W. (2004). CRF and CRF receptors: role in stress responsivity and other behaviors. *Annu. Rev. Pharmacol. Toxicol.* 44, 525–557.

Bechtold, D. A., and Luckman, S. M. (2006). Prolactin-releasing peptide mediates cholecystokinin-induced satiety in mice. *Endocrinology* 147, 4723–4729.

Bechtold, D. A., and Luckman, S. M. (2007). The role of RFamide peptides in feeding. *J. Endocrinol.* 192, 3–15.

Bendena, W. G., Boudreau, J. R., Papanicolaou, T., Maltby, M., Tobe, S. S., and Chin-Sang, I. D. (2008). A Caenorhabditis elegans allatostatin/galanin-like receptor NPR-9 inhibits local search behavior in response to feeding cues. *Proc. Natl. Acad. Sci. U.S.A.* 105, 1339–1342.

Berridge, K. C. (1996). Food reward: brain substrates of wanting and liking. *Neurosci. Biobehav. Rev.* 20, 1–25.

Birgul, N., Weise, C., Kreienkamp, H. J., and Richter, D. (1999). Reverse physiology in drosophila: identification of a novel allatostatin-like neuropeptide and its cognate receptor structurally related to the mammalian somatostatin/galanin/opioid receptor family. *EMBO J.* 18, 5892–5900.

Birse, R. T., Johnson, E. C., Taghert, P. H., and Nassel, D. R. (2006). Widely distributed Drosophila G-protein-coupled receptor (CG7887) is activated by endogenous tachykinin-related peptides. *J. Neurobiol.* 66, 33–46.

Birse, R. T., Soderberg, J. A., Luo, J., Winther, A. M., and Nassel, D. R. (2011). Regulation of insulin-producing cells in the adult Drosophila brain via the tachykinin peptide receptor DTKR. *J. Exp. Biol.* 214, 4201–4208.

Bjarnadottir, T. K., Fredriksson, R., and Schioth, H. B. (2007). The adhesion GPCRs: a unique family of G protein-coupled receptors with important roles in both central and peripheral tissues. *Cell. Mol. Life Sci.* 64, 2104–2119.

Bockaert, J., and Pin, J. P. (1999). Molecular tinkering of G protein-coupled receptors: an evolutionary success. *EMBO J.* 18, 1723–1729.

Bradbury, M. J., McBurnie, M. I., Denton, D. A., Lee, K. F., and Vale, W. W. (2000). Modulation of urocortin-induced hypophagia and weight loss by corticotropin-releasing factor receptor 1 deficiency in mice. *Endocrinology* 141, 2715–2724.

Branchek, T. A., Smith, K. E., Gerald, C., and Walker, M. W. (2000). Galanin receptor subtypes. *Trends Pharmacol. Sci.* 21, 109–117.

Brighton, P. J., Szekeres, P. G., and Willars, G. B. (2004). Neuromedin U and its receptors: structure, function, and physiological roles. *Pharmacol. Rev.* 56, 231–248.

Brody, T., and Cravchik, A. (2000). Drosophila melanogaster G protein-coupled receptors. *J. Cell Biol.* 150, F83–F88.

Cazzamali, G., Torp, M., Hauser, F., Williamson, M., and Grimmelikhuijzen, C. J. (2005). The Drosophila gene CG9918 codes for a pyrokinin-1 receptor. *Biochem. Biophys. Res. Commun.* 335, 14–19.

Chalasani, S. H., Kato, S., Albrecht, D. R., Nakagawa, T., Abbott, L. F., and Bargmann, C. I. (2010). Neuropeptide feedback modifies odor-evoked dynamics in Caenorhabditis elegans olfactory neurons. *Nat. Neurosci.* 13, 615–621.

Chamorro, S., Della-Zuana, O., Fauchere, J. L., Feletou, M., Galizzi, J. P., and Levens, N. (2002). Appetite suppression based on selective inhibition of NPY receptors. *Int. J. Obes. Relat. Metab. Disord.* 26, 281–298.

Chance, W. T., Thompson, H., Thomas, I., and Fischer, J. E. (1995). Anorectic and neurochemical effects of pituitary adenylate cyclase activating polypeptide in rats. *Peptides* 16, 1511–1516.

Chapman, R. F., and De Boer, G. (1995). *Regulatory Mechanisms in Insect Feeding.* New York: Chapman & Hall.

Chaudhri, O., Small, C., and Bloom, S. (2006). Gastrointestinal hormones regulating appetite. *Philos. Trans. R. Soc. Lond. B Biol. Sci.* 361, 1187–1209.

Chaudhri, O. B., Salem, V., Murphy, K. G., and Bloom, S. R. (2008). Gastrointestinal satiety signals. *Annu. Rev. Physiol.* 70, 239–255.

Chen, M. E., and Pietrantonio, P. V. (2006). The short neuropeptide F-like receptor from the red imported fire ant, Solenopsis invicta Buren (Hymenoptera: Formicidae). *Arch. Insect Biochem. Physiol.* 61, 195–208.

Christensen, L. (1993). Effects of eating behavior on mood: a review of the literature. *Int. J. Eat. Disord.* 14, 171–183.

Chung, S., Parks, G. S., Lee, C., and Civelli, O. (2011). Recent updates on the melanin-concentrating hormone (MCH) and its receptor system: lessons from MCH1R antagonists. *J. Mol. Neurosci.* 43, 115–121.

Cline, M. A., Newmyer, B. A., and Smith, M. L. (2009). The anorectic effect of neuropeptide AF is associated with satiety-related hypothalamic nuclei. *J. Neuroendocrinol.* 21, 595–601.

Coast, G. M., and Garside, C. S. (2005). Neuropeptide control of fluid balance in insects. *Ann. N. Y. Acad. Sci.* 1040, 1–8.

Coghlan, A. (2005). "Nematode genome evolution," in *WormBook*, ed. The *C. elegans* Research Community (WormBook), doi/10.1895/wormbook.1.15.1. Available at: http://www.wormbook.org

Cohen, M., Reale, V., Olofsson, B., Knights, A., Evans, P., and De Bono, M. (2009). Coordinated regulation of foraging and metabolism in C. elegans by RFamide neuropeptide signaling. *Cell Metab.* 9, 375–385.

Coll, A. P., Farooqi, I. S., Challis, B. G., Yeo, G. S., and O'Rahilly, S. (2004). Proopiomelanocortin and energy balance: insights from human and murine genetics. *J. Clin. Endocrinol. Metab.* 89, 2557–2562.

Coll, A. P., Farooqi, I. S., and O'Rahilly, S. (2007). The hormonal control of food intake. *Cell* 129, 251–262.

Consortium, T. C. E. S. (1998). Genome sequence of the nematode C. elegans: a platform for investigating biology. *Science* 282, 2012–2018.

Consortium, T. H. G. S. (2006). Insights into social insects from the genome of the honeybee Apis mellifera. *Nature* 443, 931–949.

Cutter, A. D., Dey, A., and Murray, R. L. (2009). Evolution of the Caenorhabditis elegans genome. *Mol. Biol. Evol.* 26, 1199–1234.

de Bono, M., and Bargmann, C. I. (1998). Natural variation in a neuropeptide Y receptor homolog modifies social behavior and food response in C. elegans. *Cell* 94, 679–689.

de Jong-Brink, M., Ter Maat, A., and Tensen, C. P. (2001). NPY in invertebrates: molecular answers to altered functions during evolution. *Peptides* 22, 309–315.

De Loof, A., Baggerman, G., Breuer, M., Claeys, I., Cerstiaens, A., Clynen, E., et al. (2001). Gonadotropins in insects: an overview. *Arch. Insect Biochem. Physiol.* 47, 129–138.

Dieterich, C., Clifton, S. W., Schuster, L. N., Chinwalla, A., Delehaunty, K., Dinkelacker, I., et al. (2008). The Pristionchus pacificus genome provides a unique perspective on nematode lifestyle and parasitism. *Nat. Genet.* 40, 1193–1198.

Downer, K. E., Haselton, A. T., Nachman, R. J., and Stoffolano, J. G. Jr. (2007). Insect satiety: sulfakinin localization and the effect of drosulfakinin on protein and carbohydrate ingestion in the blow fly, Phormia regina (Diptera: Calliphoridae). *J. Insect Physiol.* 53, 106–112.

Fredriksson, R., Lagerstrom, M. C., Lundin, L. G., and Schioth, H. B. (2003). The G-protein-coupled receptors in the human genome form five main families. Phylogenetic analysis, paralogon groups, and fingerprints. *Mol. Pharmacol.* 63, 1256–1272.

Fredriksson, R., and Schioth, H. B. (2005). The repertoire of G-protein-coupled receptors in fully sequenced genomes. *Mol. Pharmacol.* 67, 1414–1425.

Fuxe, K., Borroto-Escuela, D. O., Marcellino, D., Romero-Fernandez, W., Frankowska, M., Guidolin, D., et al. (2012). GPCR heteromers and their allosteric receptor-receptor interactions. *Curr. Med. Chem.* 19, 356–363.

Gaillard, I., Rouquier, S., and Giorgi, D. (2004). Olfactory receptors. *Cell. Mol. Life Sci.* 61, 456–469.

Garczynski, S. F., Crim, J. W., and Brown, M. R. (2005). Characterization of neuropeptide F and its receptor from the African malaria mosquito, Anopheles gambiae. *Peptides* 26, 99–107.

Ghedin, E., Wang, S., Spiro, D., Caler, E., Zhao, Q., Crabtree, J., et al. (2007). Draft genome of the filarial nematode parasite Brugia malayi. *Science* 317, 1756–1760.

Gonzalez, N., Moody, T. W., Igarashi, H., Ito, T., and Jensen, R. T. (2008). Bombesin-related peptides and their receptors: recent advances in their role in physiology and disease states. *Curr. Opin. Endocrinol. Diabetes Obes.* 15, 58–64.

Gonzalez, R., and Orchard, I. (2009). Physiological activity of neuropeptide f on the hindgut of the blood-feeding hemipteran, Rhodnius prolixus. *J. Insect Sci.* 9, 1–14.

Greenwood, K., Williams, T., and Geary, T. (2005). Nematode neuropeptide receptors and their development as anthelmintic screens. *Parasitology* 131(Suppl.), S169–S177.

Grimmelikhuijzen, C. J., and Hauser, F. (2012). Mini-review: the evolution of neuropeptide signaling. *Regul. Pept.* 177(Suppl.), S6–S9.

Hainerova, I., Torekov, S. S., Ek, J., Finkova, M., Borch-Johnsen, K., Jorgensen, T., et al. (2006). Association between neuromedin U gene variants and overweight and obesity. *J. Clin. Endocrinol. Metab.* 91, 5057–5063.

Hampton, L. L., Ladenheim, E. E., Akeson, M., Way, J. M., Weber, H. C., Sutliff, V. E., et al. (1998). Loss of bombesin-induced feeding suppression in gastrin-releasing peptide receptor-deficient mice. *Proc. Natl. Acad. Sci. U.S.A.* 95, 3188–3192.

Harmar, A. J. (2001). Family-B G-protein-coupled receptors. *Genome Biol.* 2, REVIEWS3013.

Harris, G., Mills, H., Wragg, R., Hapiak, V., Castelletto, M., Korchnak, A., et al. (2010). The monoaminergic modulation of sensory-mediated aversive responses in Caenorhabditis elegans requires glutamatergic/peptidergic cotransmission. *J. Neurosci.* 30, 7889–7899.

Hauser, F., Cazzamali, G., Williamson, M., Blenau, W., and Grimmelikhuijzen, C. J. (2006). A review of neurohormone GPCRs present in the fruitfly Drosophila melanogaster and the honey bee Apis mellifera. *Prog. Neurobiol.* 80, 1–19.

Hauser, F., Cazzamali, G., Williamson, M., Park, Y., Li, B., Tanaka, Y., et al. (2008). A genome-wide inventory of neurohormone GPCRs in the red flour beetle Tribolium castaneum. *Front. Neuroendocrinol.* 29, 142–165.

Heinrichs, S. C., and Richard, D. (1999). The role of corticotropin-releasing factor and urocortin in the modulation of ingestive behavior. *Neuropeptides* 33, 350–359.

Hergarden, A. C., Tayler, T. D., and Anderson, D. J. (2012). Allatostatin-A neurons inhibit feeding behavior in adult Drosophila. *Proc. Natl. Acad. Sci. U.S.A.* 109, 3967–3972.

Hewes, R. S., and Taghert, P. H. (2001). Neuropeptides and neuropeptide receptors in the Drosophila melanogaster genome. *Genome Res.* 11, 1126–1142.

Hill, C. A., Fox, A. N., Pitts, R. J., Kent, L. B., Tan, P. L., Chrystal, M. A., et al. (2002). G protein-coupled receptors in Anopheles gambiae. *Science* 298, 176–178.

Hoekstra, R., Visser, A., Otsen, M., Tibben, J., Lenstra, J. A., and Roos, M. H. (2000). EST sequencing of the parasitic nematode Haemonchus contortus suggests a shift in gene expression during transition to the parasitic stages. *Mol. Biochem. Parasitol.* 110, 53–68.

Ida, T., Takahashi, T., Tominaga, H., Sato, T., Kume, K., Ozaki, M., et al. (2011). Identification of the novel bioactive peptides dRYamide-1 and dRYamide-2, ligands for a neuropeptide Y-like receptor in Drosophila. *Biochem. Biophys. Res. Commun.* 410, 872–877.

Irani, B. G., and Haskell-Luevano, C. (2005). Feeding effects of melanocortin ligands – a historical perspective. *Peptides* 26, 1788–1799.

Iversen, A., Cazzamali, G., Williamson, M., Hauser, F., and Grimmelikhuijzen, C. J. (2002). Molecular cloning and functional expression of a Drosophila receptor for the neuropeptides capa-1 and -2. *Biochem. Biophys. Res. Commun.* 299, 628–633.

Janssen, T., Meelkop, E., Lindemans, M., Verstraelen, K., Husson, S. J., Temmerman, L., et al. (2008). Discovery of a cholecystokinin-gastrin-like signaling system in nematodes. *Endocrinology* 149, 2826–2839.

Johnson, E. C., Bohn, L. M., Barak, L. S., Birse, R. T., Nassel, D. R., Caron, M. G., et al. (2003). Identification of Drosophila neuropeptide receptors by G protein-coupled receptors-beta-arrestin2 interactions. *J. Biol. Chem.* 278, 52172–52178.

Joost, P., and Methner, A. (2002). Phylogenetic analysis of 277 human G-protein-coupled receptors as a tool for the prediction of orphan receptor ligands. *Genome Biol.* 3, RESEARCH0063.

Jorgensen, L. M., Hauser, F., Cazzamali, G., Williamson, M., and Grimmelikhuijzen, C. J. (2006). Molecular identification of the first SIFamide receptor. *Biochem. Biophys. Res. Commun.* 340, 696–701.

Karagiannides, I., Stavrakis, D., Bakirtzi, K., Kokkotou, E., Pirtskhalava, T., Nayeb-Hashemi, H., et al. (2011). Substance P (SP)-neurokinin-1 receptor (NK-1R) alters adipose tissue responses to high-fat diet and insulin action. *Endocrinology* 152, 2197–2205.

Kawauchi, H. (2006). Functions of melanin-concentrating hormone in fish. *J. Exp. Zoolog. A Comp. Exp. Biol.* 305, 751–760.

Keating, C. D., Kriek, N., Daniels, M., Ashcroft, N. R., Hopper, N. A., Siney, E. J., et al. (2003). Whole-genome analysis of 60 G protein-coupled receptors in Caenorhabditis elegans by gene knockout with RNAi. *Curr. Biol.* 13, 1715–1720.

Klowden, M. J. (1990). The endogenous regulation of mosquito reproductive behavior. *Experientia* 46, 660–670.

Konturek, S. J., Konturek, J. W., Pawlik, T., and Brzozowski, T. (2004). Brain-gut axis and its role in the control of food intake. *J. Physiol. Pharmacol.* 55, 137–154.

Kopin, A. S., Mathes, W. F., McBride, E. W., Nguyen, M., Al-Haider, W., Schmitz, F., et al. (1999). The cholecystokinin-A receptor mediates inhibition of food intake yet is not essential for the maintenance of body weight. *J. Clin. Invest.* 103, 383–391.

Kreienkamp, H. J., Larusson, H. J., Witte, I., Roeder, T., Birgul, N., Honck, H. H., et al. (2002). Functional annotation of two orphan G-protein-coupled receptors, Drostar1 and -2, from Drosophila melanogaster and their ligands by reverse pharmacology. *J. Biol. Chem.* 277, 39937–39943.

Krishnan, A., Almen, M. S., Fredriksson, R., and Schioth, H. B. (2012). The origin of GPCRs: identification of mammalian like Rhodopsin, Adhesion, Glutamate and Frizzled GPCRs in fungi. *PLoS ONE* 7:e29817. doi:10.1371/journal.pone.0029817

Kubiak, T. M., Larsen, M. J., Bowman, J. W., Geary, T. G., and Lowery, D. E. (2008). FMRFamide-like peptides encoded on the flp-18 precursor gene activate two isoforms of the orphan Caenorhabditis elegans G-protein-coupled receptor Y58G8A.4 heterologously expressed in mammalian cells. *Biopolymers* 90, 339–348.

Kubiak, T. M., Larsen, M. J., Burton, K. J., Bannow, C. A., Martin, R. A., Zantello, M. R., et al. (2002). Cloning and functional expression of the first Drosophila melanogaster sulfakinin receptor DSK-R1. *Biochem. Biophys. Res. Commun.* 291, 313–320.

Ladenheim, E. E., Hampton, L. L., Whitney, A. C., White, W. O., Battey, J. F., and Moran, T. H. (2002). Disruptions in feeding and body weight control in gastrin-releasing peptide receptor deficient mice. *J. Endocrinol.* 174, 273–281.

Lang, R., Gundlach, A. L., and Kofler, B. (2007). The galanin peptide family: receptor pharmacology, pleiotropic biological actions, and implications in health and disease. *Pharmacol. Ther.* 115, 177–207.

Langmead, C. J., and Christopoulos, A. (2006). Allosteric agonists of 7TM receptors: expanding the pharmacological toolbox. *Trends Pharmacol. Sci.* 27, 475–481.

Lecklin, A., Lundell, I., Paananen, L., Wikberg, J. E., Mannisto, P. T., and Larhammar, D. (2002). Receptor subtypes Y1 and Y5 mediate neuropeptide Y induced feeding in the guinea-pig. *Br. J. Pharmacol.* 135, 2029–2037.

Lee, K. S., You, K. H., Choo, J. K., Han, Y. M., and Yu, K. (2004). Drosophila short neuropeptide F regulates food intake and body size. *J. Biol. Chem.* 279, 50781–50789.

Lenz, C., Williamson, M., and Grimmelikhuijzen, C. J. (2000). Molecular cloning and genomic organization of a second probable allatostatin receptor from Drosophila melanogaster. *Biochem. Biophys. Res. Commun.* 273, 571–577.

Li, X., Wu, N., Ra, N., and Forte, M. (1992). Cloning, functional expression, and developmental regulation of a neuropeptide Y receptor from Drosophila melanogaster. *J. Biol. Chem.* 267, 9–12.

Li, X. J., Wolfgang, W., Wu, Y. N., North, R. A., and Forte, M. (1991). Cloning, heterologous expression and developmental regulation of a Drosophila receptor for tachykinin-like peptides. *EMBO J.* 10, 3221–3229.

Lindemans, M., Janssen, T., Husson, S. J., Meelkop, E., Temmerman, L., Clynen, E., et al. (2009). A neuromedin-pyrokinin -like neuropeptide signaling system in Caenorhabditis elegans. *Biochem. Biophys. Res. Commun.* 379, 760–764.

Lingo, P. R., Zhao, Z., and Shen, P. (2007). Co-regulation of cold-resistant food acquisition by insulin- and neuropeptide Y-like systems in Drosophila melanogaster. *Neuroscience* 148, 371–374.

Lynch, M., and Conery, J. S. (2000). The evolutionary fate and consequences of duplicate genes. *Science* 290, 1151–1155.

Maestro, J. L., Aguilar, R., Pascual, N., Valero, M. L., Piulachs, M. D., Andreu, D., et al. (2001). Screening of antifeedant activity in brain extracts led to the identification of sulfakinin as a satiety promoter in the German cockroach. Are arthropod sulfakinins homologous to vertebrate gastrins-cholecystokinins? *Eur. J. Biochem.* 268, 5824–5830.

Maier, W., Adilov, B., Regenass, M., and Alcedo, J. (2010). A neuromedin U receptor acts with the sensory system to modulate food type-dependent effects on C. elegans lifespan. *PLoS Biol.* 8:e1000376. doi:10.1371/journal.pbio.1000376

Marinissen, M. J., and Gutkind, J. S. (2001). G-protein-coupled receptors and signaling networks: emerging paradigms. *Trends Pharmacol. Sci.* 22, 368–376.

Matteri, R. (2001). Overview of central targets for appetite regulation. *J. Anim. Sci.* 79(suppl.), E148–E158.

Mayoral, J. G., Nouzova, M., Brockhoff, A., Goodwin, M., Hernandez-Martinez, S., Richter, D., et al. (2010). Allatostatin-C receptors in mosquitoes. *Peptides* 31, 442–450.

McDermott, M. T., and Kidd, G. S. (1987). The role of calcitonin in the development and treatment of osteoporosis. *Endocr. Rev.* 8, 377–390.

McKay, R. M., McKay, J. P., Suh, J. M., Avery, L., and Graff, J. M. (2007). Tripeptidyl peptidase II promotes fat formation in a conserved fashion. *EMBO Rep.* 8, 1183–1189.

McMahon, L. R., and Wellman, P. J. (1997). Decreased intake of a liquid diet in nonfood-deprived rats following intra-PVN injections of GLP-1 (7-36) amide. *Pharmacol. Biochem. Behav.* 58, 673–677.

McMahon, L. R., and Wellman, P. J. (1998). PVN infusion of GLP-1-(7-36) amide suppresses feeding but does not induce aversion or alter locomotion in rats. *Am. J. Physiol.* 274, R23–R29.

Melcher, C., and Pankratz, M. J. (2005). Candidate gustatory interneurons modulating feeding behavior in the Drosophila brain. *PLoS Biol.* 3:e305. doi:10.1371/journal.pbio.0030305

Meng, X., Wahlstrom, G., Immonen, T., Kolmer, M., Tirronen, M., Predel, R., et al. (2002). The Drosophila hugin gene codes for myostimulatory and ecdysis-modifying neuropeptides. *Mech. Dev.* 117, 5–13.

Mercer, R. E., Chee, M. J., and Colmers, W. F. (2011). The role of NPY in hypothalamic mediated food intake. *Front. Neuroendocrinol.* 32, 398–415.

Mertens, I., Clinckspoor, I., Janssen, T., Nachman, R., and Schoofs, L. (2006). FMRFamide related peptide ligands activate the Caenorhabditis elegans orphan GPCR Y59H11AL.1. *Peptides* 27, 1291–1296.

Millington, G. W. (2007). The role of proopiomelanocortin (POMC) neurones in feeding behaviour. *Nutr. Metab. (Lond.)* 4, 18.

Mitreva, M., Jasmer, D. P., Zarlenga, D. S., Wang, Z., Abubucker, S., Martin, J., et al. (2011). The draft genome of the parasitic nematode Trichinella spiralis. *Nat. Genet.* 43, 228–235.

Monnier, D., Colas, J. F., Rosay, P., Hen, R., Borrelli, E., and Maroteaux, L. (1992). NKD, a developmentally regulated tachykinin receptor in Drosophila. *J. Biol. Chem.* 267, 1298–1302.

Montell, C. (2009). A taste of the Drosophila gustatory receptors. *Curr. Opin. Neurobiol.* 19, 345–353.

Moody, T. W., Ito, T., Osefo, N., and Jensen, R. T. (2011). VIP and PACAP: recent insights into their functions/roles in physiology and disease from molecular and genetic studies. *Curr. Opin. Endocrinol. Diabetes Obes.* 18, 61–67.

Morley, J. E., Horowitz, M., Morley, P. M., and Flood, J. F. (1992). Pituitary adenylate cyclase activating polypeptide (PACAP) reduces food intake in mice. *Peptides* 13, 1133–1135.

Murase, T., Arima, H., Kondo, K., and Oiso, Y. (1996). Neuropeptide FF reduces food intake in rats. *Peptides* 17, 353–354.

Murdoch, C., and Finn, A. (2000). Chemokine receptors and their role in inflammation and infectious diseases. *Blood* 95, 3032–3043.

Nagarathnam, B., Kalaimathy, S., Balakrishnan, V., and Sowdhamini, R. (2012). Cross-Genome Clustering of Human and C. elegans G-Protein Coupled Receptors. *Evol. Bioinform. Online* 8, 229–259.

Nassel, D. R., and Winther, A. M. (2010). Drosophila neuropeptides in regulation of physiology and behavior. *Prog. Neurobiol.* 92, 42–104.

Nathoo, A. N., Moeller, R. A., Westlund, B. A., and Hart, A. C. (2001). Identification of neuropeptide-like protein gene families in Caenorhabditiselegans and other species. *Proc. Natl. Acad. Sci. U.S.A.* 98, 14000–14005.

Neary, N. M., Goldstone, A. P., and Bloom, S. R. (2004). Appetite regulation: from the gut to the hypothalamus. *Clin. Endocrinol. (Oxf.)* 60, 153–160.

Nichols, R. (2007). The first nonsulfated sulfakinin activity reported suggests nsDSK acts in gut biology. *Peptides* 28, 767–773.

Nichols, R., Schneuwly, S. A., and Dixon, J. E. (1988). Identification and characterization of a Drosophila homologue to the vertebrate neuropeptide cholecystokinin. *J. Biol. Chem.* 263, 12167–12170.

Niswender, C. M., and Conn, P. J. (2010). Metabotropic glutamate receptors: physiology, pharmacology, and disease. *Annu. Rev. Pharmacol. Toxicol.* 50, 295–322.

Nordstrom, K. J., Sallman Almen, M., Edstam, M. M., Fredriksson, R., and Schioth, H. B. (2011). Independent HHsearch, Needleman – Wunsch-based, and motif analyses reveal the overall hierarchy for most of the G protein-coupled receptor families. *Mol. Biol. Evol.* 28, 2471–2480.

Ohki-Hamazaki, H., Watase, K., Yamamoto, K., Ogura, H., Yamano, M., Yamada, K., et al. (1997). Mice lacking bombes in receptor subtype-3 develop metabolic defects and obesity. *Nature* 390, 165–169.

Paluzzi, J. P., Park, Y., Nachman, R. J., and Orchard, I. (2010). Isolation, expression analysis, and functional characterization of the first antidiuretic hormone receptor in insects. *Proc. Natl. Acad. Sci. U.S.A.* 107, 10290–10295.

Park, Y., Kim, Y. J., and Adams, M. E. (2002). Identification of G protein-coupled receptors for Drosophila PRXamide peptides, CCAP, corazonin, and AKH supports a theory of ligand-receptor coevolution. *Proc. Natl. Acad. Sci. U.S.A.* 99, 11423–11428.

Pjetri, E., Adan, R. A., Herzog, H., De Haas, R., Oppelaar, H., Spierenburg, H. A., et al. (2012). NPY receptor subtype specification for behavioral adaptive strategies during limited food access. *Genes Brain Behav.* 11, 105–112.

Poels, J., Birse, R. T., Nachman, R. J., Fichna, J., Janecka, A., Vanden Broeck, J., et al. (2009). Characterization and distribution of NKD, a receptor for Drosophila tachykinin-related peptide 6. *Peptides* 30, 545–556.

Poels, J., Verlinden, H., Fichna, J., Van Loy, T., Franssens, V., Studzian, K., et al. (2007). Functional comparison of two evolutionary conserved insect neurokinin-like receptors. *Peptides* 28, 103–108.

Pollock, V. P., McGettigan, J., Cabrero, P., Maudlin, I. M., Dow, J. A., and Davies, S. A. (2004). Conservation of capa peptide-induced nitric oxide signalling in Diptera. *J. Exp. Biol.* 207, 4135–4145.

Posnien, N., Schinko, J. B., Kittelmann, S., and Bucher, G. (2010). Genetics, development and composition of the insect head – a beetle's view. *Arthropod Struct. Dev.* 39, 399–410.

Prakash, M., and Steele, M. (2010). The hungry fly: hydrodynamics of feeding in the common house fly. *Phys. Fluids* 23, 091110–091110.

Pratt, G. E., Farnsworth, D. E., Fok, K. F., Siegel, N. R., Mccormack, A. L., Shabanowitz, J., et al. (1991). Identity of a second type of allatostatin from cockroach brains: an octadecapeptide amide with a tyrosine-rich address sequence. *Proc. Natl. Acad. Sci. U.S.A.* 88, 2412–2416.

Prinster, S. C., Hague, C., and Hall, R. A. (2005). Heterodimerization of g protein-coupled receptors: specificity and functional significance. *Pharmacol. Rev.* 57, 289–298.

Radford, J. C., Davies, S. A., and Dow, J. A. (2002). Systematic G-protein-coupled receptor analysis in Drosophila melanogaster identifies a leucokinin receptor with novel roles. *J. Biol. Chem.* 277, 38810–38817.

Richard, D., Lin, Q., and Timofeeva, E. (2002). The corticotropin-releasing factor family of peptides and CRF receptors: their roles in the regulation of energy balance. *Eur. J. Pharmacol.* 440, 189–197.

Riediger, T., Zuend, D., Becskei, C., and Lutz, T. A. (2004). The anorectic hormone amylin contributes to feeding-related changes of neuronal activity in key structures of the gut-brain axis. *Am. J. Physiol. Regul. Integr. Comp. Physiol.* 286, R114–R122.

Robertson, H. M., and Thomas, J. H. (2006). "The putative chemoreceptor families of *C. elegans*," in *WormBook*, ed. The *C. elegans* Research Community (WormBook), doi/10.1895/wormbook.1.66.1. Available at: http://www.wormbook.org

Rocha-Sousa, A., Tavares-Silva, M., Fonseca, S., Falcão, M., Falcão-Reis, F., and Leite- Moreira, A. (2010). Diabetes, ghrelin and related peptides: from pathophysiology to vasculopathy. *Open Circ. Vasc. J.* 3, 17–29.

Rogers, C., Reale, V., Kim, K., Chatwin, H., Li, C., Evans, P., et al. (2003). Inhibition of Caenorhabditis elegans social feeding by FMRFamide-related peptide activation of NPR-1. *Nat. Neurosci.* 6, 1178–1185.

Roller, L., Yamanaka, N., Watanabe, K., Daubnerova, I., Zitnan, D., Kataoka, H., et al. (2008). The unique evolution of neuropeptide genes in the silkworm Bombyx mori. *Insect Biochem. Mol. Biol.* 38, 1147–1157.

Rosay, P., Colas, J. F., and Maroteaux, L. (1995). Dual organisation of the Drosophila neuropeptide receptor NKD gene promoter. *Mech. Dev.* 51, 329–339.

Saideman, S. R., Ma, M., Kutz-Naber, K. K., Cook, A., Torfs, P., Schoofs, L., et al. (2007). Modulation of rhythmic motor activity by pyrokinin peptides. *J. Neurophysiol.* 97, 579–595.

Sakurai, T. (1999). Orexins and orexin receptors: implication in feeding behavior. *Regul. Pept.* 85, 25–30.

Sakurai, T., Amemiya, A., Ishii, M., Matsuzaki, I., Chemelli, R. M., Tanaka, H., et al. (1998). Orexins and orexin receptors: a family of hypothalamic neuropeptides and G protein-coupled receptors that regulate feeding behavior. *Cell* 92, 573–585.

Sano, H., Feighner, S. D., Hreniuk, D. L., Iwaasa, H., Sailer, A. W., Pan, J., et al. (2004). Characterization of the bombesin-like peptide receptor family in primates. *Genomics* 84, 139–146.

Schioth, H. B., and Fredriksson, R. (2005). The GRAFS classification system of G-protein coupled receptors in comparative perspective. *Gen. Comp. Endocrinol.* 142, 94–101.

Schoofs, L., Clynen, E., Cerstiaens, A., Baggerman, G., Wei, Z., Vercammen, T., et al. (2001). Newly discovered functions for some myotropic neuropeptides in locusts. *Peptides* 22, 219–227.

Schulte, G. (2010). International union of basic and clinical pharmacology. LXXX. The class frizzled receptors. *Pharmacol. Rev.* 62, 632–667.

Shioda, S., Takenoya, F., Yagi, M., Wang, L., Hori, Y., and Kageyama, H. (2008). Neural networks of several novel neuropeptides involved in feeding regulation. *Nutrition* 24, 848–853.

Simoni, M., Gromoll, J., and Nieschlag, E. (1997). The follicle-stimulating hormone receptor: biochemistry, molecular biology, physiology, and pathophysiology. *Endocr. Rev.* 18, 739–773.

Sommer, R. J., and Streit, A. (2011). Comparative genetics and genomics of nematodes: genome structure, development, and lifestyle. *Annu. Rev. Genet.* 45, 1–20.

Stanley, S., Wynne, K., McGowan, B., and Bloom, S. (2005). Hormonal regulation of food intake. *Physiol. Rev.* 85, 1131–1158.

Stay, B. (2000). A review of the role of neurosecretion in the control of juvenile hormone synthesis: a tribute to Berta Scharrer. *Insect Biochem. Mol. Biol.* 30, 653–662.

Styer, K. L., Singh, V., Macosko, E., Steele, S. E., Bargmann, C. I., and Aballay, A. (2008). Innate immunity in Caenorhabditis elegans is regulated by neurons expressing NPR-1/GPCR. *Science* 322, 460–464.

Suwa, M., Sugihara, M., and Ono, Y. (2011). Functional and structural overview of G-protein-coupled receptors comprehensively obtained from genome sequences. *Pharmaceuticals* 4, 652–664.

Suzuki, K., Simpson, K. A., Minnion, J. S., Shillito, J. C., and Bloom, S. R. (2010). The role of gut hormones and the hypothalamus in appetite regulation. *Endocr. J.* 57, 359–372.

Tachibana, T., Cline, M. A., Sugahara, K., Ueda, H., and Hiramatsu, K. (2009). Central administration of somatostatin stimulates feeding behavior in chicks. *Gen. Comp. Endocrinol.* 161, 354–359.

Tang-Christensen, M., Vrang, N., and Larsen, P. J. (2001). Glucagon-like peptide containing pathways in the regulation of feeding behaviour. *Int. J. Obes. Relat. Metab. Disord.* 25(Suppl. 5), S42–S47.

Teng, M. S., Shadbolt, P., Fraser, A. G., Jansen, G., and McCafferty, J. (2008). Control of feeding behavior in C. elegans by human G protein-coupled receptors permits screening for agonist-expressing bacteria. *Proc. Natl. Acad. Sci. U.S.A.* 105, 14826–14831.

Terhzaz, S., Cabrero, P., Robben, J. H., Radford, J. C., Hudson, B. D., Milligan, G., et al. (2012). Mechanism and function of Drosophila capa GPCR: a desiccation stress-responsive receptor with functional homology to human neuromedinU receptor. *PLoS ONE* 7:e29897. doi:10.1371/journal.pone.0029897

van Amerongen, R., and Nusse, R. (2009). Towards an integrated view of Wnt signaling in development. *Development* 136, 3205–3214.

Vashlishan, A. B., Madison, J. M., Dybbs, M., Bai, J., Sieburth, D., Ch'Ng, Q., et al. (2008). An RNAi screen identifies genes that regulate GABA synapses. *Neuron* 58, 346–361.

Waldhoer, M., Bartlett, S. E., and Whistler, J. L. (2004). Opioid receptors. *Annu. Rev. Biochem.* 73, 953–990.

Wei, Z., Baggerman, G. R. J. N., Goldsworthy, G., Verhaert, P., De

Loof, A., and Schoofs, L. (2000). Sulfakinins reduce food intake in the desert locust, Schistocerca gregaria. *J. Insect Physiol.* 46, 1259–1265.

Wilding, J. P. (2002). Neuropeptides and appetite control. *Diabet. Med.* 19, 619–627.

Wilson, R., Ainscough, R., Anderson, K., Baynes, C., Berks, M., Bonfield, J., et al. (1994). 2.2 Mb of contiguous nucleotide sequence from chromosome III of C. elegans. *Nature* 368, 32–38.

Wong, K. K., Ng, S. Y., Lee, L. T., Ng, H. K., and Chow, B. K. (2011). Orexins and their receptors from fish to mammals: a comparative approach. *Gen. Comp. Endocrinol.* 171, 124–130.

Woodhead, A. P., Khan, M. A., Stay, B., and Tobe, S. S. (1994). Two new allatostatins from the brains of Diploptera punctata. *Insect Biochem. Mol. Biol.* 24, 257–263.

Woods, S. C., Lutz, T. A., Geary, N., and Langhans, W. (2006). Pancreatic signals controlling food intake; insulin, glucagon and amylin. *Philos. Trans. R. Soc. Lond. B Biol. Sci.* 361, 1219–1235.

Woods, S. C., Seeley, R. J., and Cota, D. (2008). Regulation of food intake through hypothalamic signaling networks involving mTOR. *Annu. Rev. Nutr.* 28, 295–311.

Wu, Q., Wen, T., Lee, G., Park, J. H., Cai, H. N., and Shen, P. (2003). Developmental control of foraging and social behavior by the Drosophila neuropeptide Y-like system. *Neuron* 39, 147–161.

Xia, Q., Zhou, Z., Lu, C., Cheng, D., Dai, F., Li, B., et al. (2004). A draft sequence for the genome of the domesticated silkworm (Bombyx mori). *Science* 306, 1937–1940.

Xu, Y. L., Jackson, V. R., and Civelli, O. (2004). Orphan G protein-coupled receptors and obesity. *Eur. J. Pharmacol.* 500, 243–253.

Yamada, K., Wada, E., Santo-Yamada, Y., and Wada, K. (2002). Bombesin and its family of peptides: prospects for the treatment of obesity. *Eur. J. Pharmacol.* 440, 281–290.

Yona, S., Lin, H. H., Siu, W. O., Gordon, S., and Stacey, M. (2008). Adhesion-GPCRs: emerging roles for novel receptors. *Trends Biochem. Sci.* 33, 491–500.

Zamanian, M., Kimber, M. J., McVeigh, P., Carlson, S. A., Maule, A. G., and Day, T. A. (2011). The repertoire of G protein-coupled receptors in the human parasite Schistosoma mansoni and the model organism Schmidtea mediterranea. *BMC Genomics* 12:596. doi:10.1186/1471-2164-12-596

Zhang, J. V., Ren, P. G., Avsian-Kretchmer, O., Luo, C. W., Rauch, R., Klein, C., et al. (2005). Obestatin, a peptide encoded by the ghrelin gene, opposes ghrelin's effects on food intake. *Science* 310, 996–999.

Zorrilla, E. P., Brennan, M., Sabino, V., Lu, X., and Bartfai, T. (2007). Galanin type 1 receptor knockout mice show altered responses to high-fat diet and glucose challenge. *Physiol. Behav.* 91, 479–485.

21

Gonadotropin-releasing hormone 2 suppresses food intake in the zebrafish, *Danio rerio*

Ryo Nishiguchi[1], Morio Azuma[1], Eri Yokobori[1], Minoru Uchiyama[1] and Kouhei Matsuda[1,2]*

[1] *Laboratory of Regulatory Biology, Graduate School of Science and Engineering, University of Toyama, Toyama, Japan*
[2] *Laboratory of Regulatory Biology, Graduate School of Innovative Life Science, University of Toyama, Toyama, Japan*

Edited by:
Hubert Vaudry, University of Rouen, France

Reviewed by:
Jack Falcon, Université Pierre et Marie Curie and Centre National de la Recherche Scientifique, France
John Chang, University of Alberta, Canada

***Correspondence:**
Kouhei Matsuda, Laboratory of Regulatory Biology, Graduate School of Science and Engineering, University of Toyama, 3190 Gofuku, Toyama 930-8555, Japan.
e-mail: kmatsuda@sci.u-toyama.ac.jp

Gonadotropin-releasing hormone (GnRH) is an evolutionarily conserved neuropeptide with 10 amino acid residues, of which several structural variants exist. A molecular form known as GnRH2 ([His^5 Trp^7 Tyr^8]GnRH, also known as chicken GnRH II) is widely distributed in vertebrates except for rodents, and has recently been implicated in the regulation of feeding behavior in goldfish. However, the influence of GnRH2 on feeding behavior in other fish has not yet been studied. In the present study, therefore, we investigated the role of GnRH2 in the regulation of feeding behavior in a zebrafish model, and examined its involvement in food intake after intracerebroventricular (ICV) administration. ICV injection of GnRH2 at 0.1 and 1 pmol/g body weight (BW) induced a marked decrease of food consumption in a dose-dependent manner during 30 min after feeding. Cumulative food intake was significantly decreased by ICV injection of GnRH2 at 1 pmol/g BW during the 30-min post-treatment observation period. The anorexigenic action of GnRH2 was completely blocked by treatment with the GnRH type I receptor antagonist Antide at 25 pmol/g BW. We also examined the effect of feeding condition on the expression level of the GnRH2 transcript in the hypothalamus. Levels of GnRH2 mRNA obtained from fish that had been provided excess food for 7 days were higher than those in fish that had been fed normally. These results suggest that, in zebrafish, GnRH2 acts as an anorexigenic factor, as is the case in goldfish.

Keywords: zebrafish, GnRH2, food intake, ICV administration, Antide, anorexigenic action

INTRODUCTION

Gonadotropin-releasing hormone (GnRH) is an evolutionarily conserved decaneuropeptide that plays a crucial role in the regulation of reproduction in vertebrates (Sherwood et al., 1993; Fernald and White, 1999, Millar et al., 2004). The demonstration of GnRH structural variants in vertebrates, and even in invertebrates, has now resulted in the identification of 29 molecules (Guilgur et al., 2006; Kah et al., 2007; Roch et al., 2011). In vertebrates, these peptides are distributed in a wide range of tissues, and have diverse functions as hypophysiotropic hormones, paracrine or autocrine mediators and neuromodulators/neurotransmitters in the central and peripheral nervous systems and tissues (Gore, 2002; Millar, 2005; Kim et al., 2007; Millar et al., 2007). GnRH with substitutions at the N-terminal fifth, seventh, and eighth positions by histidine, tryptophan, and tyrosine residues, respectively, was originally purified and characterized as a second type of GnRH from chicken brain, and was named chicken GnRH II (now called GnRH2; Miyamoto et al., 1984). Subsequently, it has been found that GnRH2 is present throughout the vertebrates from cartilaginous fish to humans, but not in rodents (Conlon et al., 1993; Sherwood et al., 1993; White et al., 1998; Millar, 2003). GnRH2 has been implicated in the central regulation of reproductive behavior as well as neuroendocrine control of the gonads (Maney et al., 1997; Volkoff and Peter, 1999; Schiml and Rissman, 2000; White et al., 2002; Temple et al., 2003; Lethimonier et al., 2004; Hofmann, 2006). Recently, it has been reported that in an insectivore, the musk shrew, GnRH2 also influences feeding behavior, and that intracerebroventricular (ICV) administration of GnRH2 induces a marked decrease in food consumption, suggesting that GnRH2 controls reproduction and energy balance (Temple et al., 2003; Kauffman, 2004; Kauffman and Rissman, 2004a,b; Kauffman et al., 2005b, 2006). However, the involvement of GnRH in the regulation of feeding behavior had not been studied in other animal models.

Previous studies have indicated that ICV injection of GnRH2 also induces an anorexigenic effect in a goldfish model (Hoskins et al., 2008; Matsuda et al., 2008; Kang et al., 2011). In addition to goldfish, the zebrafish has now been widely used as an excellent animal model to investigate the effects of neuropeptides on feeding behavior (Yokobori et al., 2011, 2012; Matsuda et al., 2012). As in rodents and goldfish, it has been found that, in zebrafish, neuropeptide Y (NPY) and orexin A stimulate food intake (Yokobori et al., 2011, 2012; Matsuda et al., 2012). However, the exact role of GnRH2 is unclear, and there is no information about the effect of GnRH2 on feeding behavior in this species.

Therefore, the aim of the present study was to investigate the effect of GnRH2 on food intake in the zebrafish model, and the effect of ICV injection of Antide, a GnRH type I receptor antagonist, on the action of ICV-administered GnRH2. We also examined the effect of feeding condition on the expression level of the GnRH2 transcript in the hypothalamus.

MATERIALS AND METHODS

ANIMALS

Adult zebrafish (*Danio rerio*, 0.5–1.0 g body weight, BW) of both sexes were obtained commercially, and kept for 2 weeks under controlled light/dark conditions (12 h light/12 h dark) in a water-temperature-regulated fish tank (20–24°C) before use in experiments, since prevention of gonadal development. The fish were fed a commercially available granule diet (containing 32% protein, 4% dietary fat, 3% dietary fiber, 9% mineral, 8% water, and 44% other components; Hikari MariGold, Kyorin, Kobe, Japan) every day at noon. For 1 week before the experiments each fish was kept in a small experimental tank (24 cm in diameter) with 3.5 l of tap water. All animal experiments were conducted in accordance with the University of Toyama guidelines and the Declaration of Helsinki for the care and use of animals. Every effort was made to minimize the number of animals used and their suffering.

CHEMICALS

The zebrafish possesses two molecular forms of GnRH: GnRH2 (pGlu-His-Trp-Ser-His-Gly-Trp-Tyr-Pro-Gly-NH_2), and GnRH3 (pGlu-His-Trp-Ser-Tyr-Gly-Trp-Leu-Pro-Gly-NH_2; Powell et al., 1996; Steven et al., 2003). Therefore, in order to examine the effect of ICV injection of GnRH2 on food intake, GnRH2 was purchased from Bachem AG (Bubendorf, Switzerland) and used. Zebrafish possesses four kinds of GnRH receptors (GnRH R1–R4), GnRH R1 and R3 being of the GnRH type I receptor type whereas GnRH R2 and R4 are GnRH type III receptors (Tello et al., 2008). In the present study, we used the GnRH type I receptor antagonist, Antide (acetyl-D-Ala(2-naphthyl)-D-Phe(4-Cl)-D-Ala(3-pyridyl)-Ser-Lys(Nε-nicotinoyl)-D-Lys(Nε-nicotinoyl)-Leu-Lys(Nε-isopropyl)-Pro-D-Ala-NH_2), obtained from Sigma-Aldrich Co. (St. Louis, MO, USA). Antide was dissolved in 0.1% acetic acid and diluted with 0.6% NaCl and 0.02% Na_2CO_3 solution (saline) before use.

EFFECT OF ICV ADMINISTRATION OF GnRH2 ON FOOD INTAKE

Details of the methods used for evaluating feeding behavior in zebrafish have been reported elsewhere (Yokobori et al., 2011, 2012). Each fish was normally fed before the experiments began at noon, and placed in a wet sponge under anesthesia with MS-222 (3-aminobenzoic acid ethyl ester; Sigma-Aldrich). A small part of the parietal bone was carefully removed using a surgical blade (No. 19, Futaba, Tokyo, Japan), and then 0.5 μl/g BW of GnRH2 at doses of 0.1 and 1 pmol/g BW was injected into the third ventricle of the brain using a small Hamilton syringe. The gap in the bone was then filled with a surgical agent (Aron Alpha, Sankyo, Japan). The accuracy of the injection site was confirmed after the experiment by examining whether Evans blue dye, injected at the same time, was present in the ventricle (**Figure 1A**). Control fish in each experiment were injected with the same volume of vehicle (less than 0.01% acetic acid diluted with saline) in the same way as for the experimental group. Each fish that had received an injection was individually placed in a small experimental tank (24 cm in diameter) containing 3.5 l of tap water, and supplied with food equivalent to 3% of its BW. Food intake was measured by directly observing and recording the number of diet pellets eaten by individual fish over 15 and 30 min of commencement of feeding.

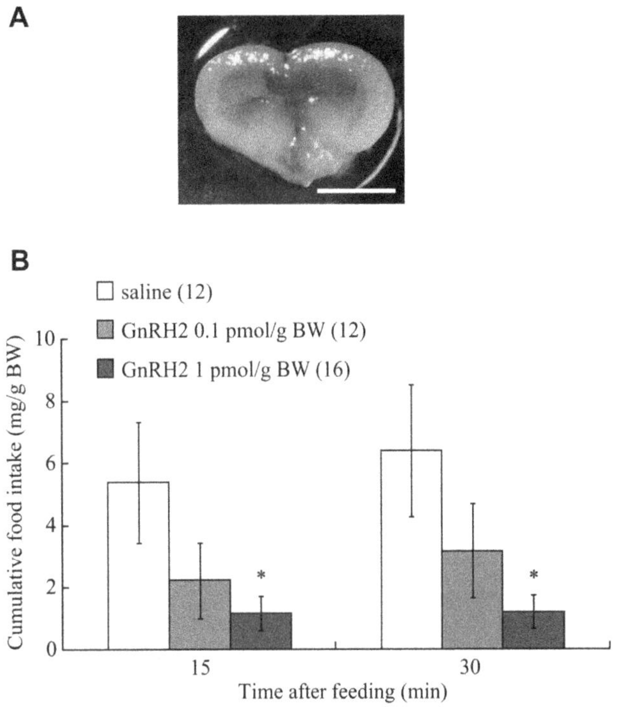

FIGURE 1 | (A) A photograph showing ICV administered-solution containing 0.05% Evans Blue into the brain. Scale bar is 1 mm. **(B)** Effect of ICV administration of GnRH2 on food intake in the zebrafish. Each column and bar represents the mean and SEM, respectively, and the numbers in parentheses in the panels indicate the number of fish in each group. Significances of differences at each time point were evaluated by one-way ANOVA with the Bonferroni's method in comparison with the vehicle-injected group (**$P < 0.01$).

EFFECT OF ICV INJECTION OF ANTIDE ON GnRH2-INDUCED ANOREXIGENIC ACTION

Because pilot experiments had shown that ICV injection of cGnRH2 at a dose of 1 pmol/g BW induced a marked decrease of food intake, Antide at 25 pmol/g BW, a dose previously determined to be sufficient to suppress the action of GnRH2 in goldfish (Matsuda et al., 2008), was delivered by ICV injection in addition to GnRH2 at 1 pmol/g BW. Control fish were injected with the same volume of vehicle (less than 0.01% acetic acid diluted with saline) in the same way as for the experimental group. Food intake was then measured over the first 15 and 30 min of commencement of feeding, as described above.

EFFECT OF FEEDING CONDITION ON GnRH2 mRNA EXPRESSION IN THE HYPOTHALAMUS

Every day for 7 days, fish were supplied an excessive amount of food corresponding to 9% of their BW. Other fish were fed an amount of food corresponding to 3% of their BW for the same period. On day 7, the fish were anesthetized with MS-222 and decapitated. Because the zebrafish brain is very small, each brain was dissected out, and the hypothalamus was collected, weighed, and immersed immediately in liquid nitrogen, before being stored at −80°C until use. Total RNA was extracted from each part of the brain with Isogen (a solution containing phenol and guanidinium isothiocyanate; Nippon Gene, Tokyo, Japan). For amplification and quantitation of the cDNA fragments encoding GnRH2 and β-actin, the one-step reverse transcription polymerase chain reaction (RT-PCR) method (SYBR Green RT-PCR Reagents Kit, Applied Biosystems, Foster City, CA, USA) was used. Reactions (including 5 μM primers, 2× SYBR Green PCR master mix, 6.25 U MultiScribe reverse transcriptase, 10 U RNase inhibitor, RNA template, and water) were set up in a 96-well reaction plate and placed in a sequence detection system for cycling (TP 800, Takara, Tokyo, Japan). Reverse transcription was carried out at 48°C for 30 min and the resulting cDNA was subsequently amplified using 40 cycles of 95°C for 15 s followed by 60°C for 60 s. The PCR products from each cycle were monitored using SYBR Green I fluorescent dye (Applied Biosystems). Gene-specific primers for amplification of the GnRH2 cDNA fragment were based on the nucleotide sequence of zebrafish GnRH2 (GenBank ID, BC162945.1, NM_181439; Ensembl ID, ENSDARG00000044754). PCR with the sense primer (5′-CAA AAT ATT AGA CTG AAG TGA TGG T-3′) and the antisense primer (5′-GGT CTA TCT CTC TCT TTC CTC CA-3′) yielded a 86-bp product encoding zebrafish GnRH2 cDNA. Zebrafish β-actin-specific primers were used as the internal control for PCR amplification (GenBank accession number, NM_181601; Ensembl ID, ENSDART00000055194). Using these primers (sense primer, 5′-GTG ATG GAC TCT GGT GAT GGT GT-3′; antisense primer, 5′-TGA AGC TGT AGC CTC TCT CGG TC-3′), a 148-bp product corresponding to a region in the central part of the β-actin cDNA sequence was obtained. The expression levels of GnRH2 mRNA were calculated quantitatively as a ratio relative to the expression of β-actin mRNA.

DATA ANALYSIS

All the results are expressed as mean ± SEM. Statistical analysis was performed by one- and two-way ANOVA with Bonferroni's method or Student's *t*-test. Statistical significance was determined at the 5% level.

RESULTS

EFFECT OF ICV ADMINISTRATION OF GnRH2 ON FOOD INTAKE

Intracerebroventricular injection of GnRH2 (at 0.1 and 1 pmol/g BW) inhibited food intake over a 30-min feeding period. A significant reduction in cumulative food consumption was observed at a dose of 1 pmol/g BW at both 15 and 30 min after commencement of feeding (**Figure 1B**). The *df*, *F*, and *P* values between treatments with saline and GnRH2 were: 2, 3.08, and 0.06 at 15 min; 2, 3.51, and 0.04 at 30 min.

EFFECT OF ICV INJECTION OF ANTIDE ON ANOREXIGENIC ACTION OF GnRH2

Intracerebroventricular administration of GnRH2 alone at 1 pmol/g BW suppressed food intake over a 30-min feeding period, and ICV-injected Antide alone at 25 pmol/g BW did not affect food intake. On the other hand, the same dose of Antide completely

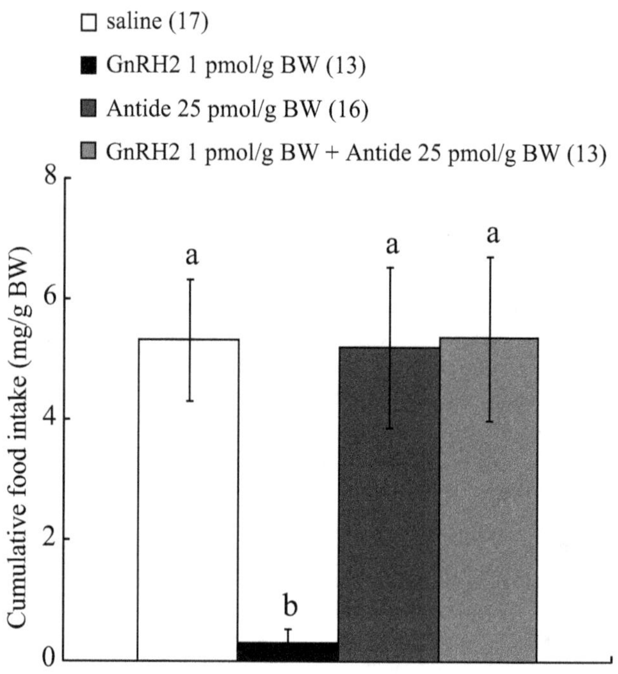

FIGURE 2 | Effect of ICV administration of Antide on the anorexigenic action of GnRH2. The results are expressed as a percentage of the control, i.e., vehicle-injected, fish. Each column and bar represents the mean and SEM, respectively, and the numbers in parentheses in the panels indicate the number of fish in each group. Significance of differences among experimental groups was evaluated by two-way ANOVA with the Bonferroni's method in comparison with the vehicle-injected group (**$P < 0.01$).

abolished the anorexigenic action of ICV-injected GnRH2 at a dose of 1 pmol/g BW, and the efficacy of the antagonist was shown to be significant by two-way ANOVA with Bonferroni's method (*df*, *F*, and *P* values, 1, 4.39, and 0.04, respectively; **Figure 2**).

EFFECT OF FEEDING CONDITION ON GnRH2 mRNA EXPRESSION IN THE HYPOTHALAMUS

Figure 3 shows the expression levels of GnRH2 mRNA in the hypothalamus of zebrafish supplied an excessive amount of food corresponding to 9% of their BW, and normal amount of food corresponding to 3% of their BW. Expression of GnRH2 mRNA was estimated quantitatively as a ratio relative to the expression of β-actin mRNA. In the hypothalamus, excessive feeding for 7 days induced a significant increase (approximately four times higher) in the level of GnRH2 mRNA compared with that in fish that had been fed normally (*t* and *P* values, 2.82 and 0.012, respectively; **Figure 3**).

DISCUSSION

We have developed methods for administering ICV test substances and for measuring food consumption in a small fish, the zebrafish, and our previous studies have demonstrated that, in this species, NPY and orexin A act as orexigenic neuropeptides (Yokobori et al., 2011, 2012). In the present study, we investigated the effect of central administration of GnRH2 on food

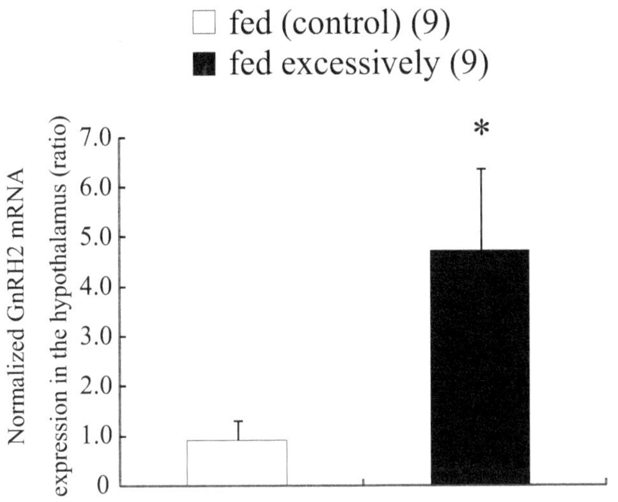

FIGURE 3 | Effect of feeding condition on the level of expression of GnRH2 mRNA in the hypothalamus. The results are expressed as the mean ± SEM, and the number of fish per group is indicated in parentheses. Statistical significance was evaluated by Student's *t*-test (**$P < 0.01$).

intake, and demonstrated for the first time that GnRH2 strongly suppresses food consumption in the zebrafish. In matured female musk shrew, an insectivore, ICV injection of GnRH2 inhibits food intake, and feeding status influences the levels of both GnRH2 mRNA expression and immunoassayable GnRH2 in the brain, which are decreased by food restriction (Kauffman and Rissman, 2004a; Kauffman et al., 2006). The present study indicates the anorexigenic action of GnRH2 in the zebrafish, as is the case in female musk shrew and goldfish (Hoskins et al., 2008; Matsuda et al., 2008; Kang et al., 2011), indicating that it may be involved generally in the regulation of feeding behavior in vertebrates. GnRH3 is widely distributed in several regions of the zebrafish brain, including the olfactory bulb, the area of the terminal nerve, and telencephalon, and GnRH3 is implicated in pituitary control (Torgersen et al., 2002; Steven et al., 2003; Palevitch et al., 2007). On the other hand, GnRH2-expressing neurons are localized mainly in the midbrain tegmentum (Palevitch et al., 2007). However, the exact role of GnRH2 in the zebrafish has been unclear. Because GnRH2 is implicated in the regulation of reproductive behavior and energy balance in the female musk shrew, sparrow, and goldfish (Maney et al., 1997; Temple et al., 2003; Kauffman, 2004; Kauffman and Rissman, 2004a; Kauffman et al., 2005a,b; Hofmann, 2006; Hoskins et al., 2008; Matsuda et al., 2008; Kang et al., 2011), it is likely that, in zebrafish, GnRH2 is involved in both feeding control and reproductive behavior. GnRH systems have been well studied in teleost fish (Lethimonier et al., 2004). The zebrafish possesses two GnRHs – GnRH2 and GnRH3 – which are encoded by two distinct genes (Steven et al., 2003), and four GnRH receptors, GnRH R1–R4 – which are members of the G protein-coupled receptor family (Tello et al., 2008). There are marked differences in structure between these two groups of GnRHRs. GnRH R1 and R3 are evolutionarily derived from the common ancestor of the GnRH type I receptor, and GnRH R2 and R4 belong to the GnRH type III receptor group (Tello et al., 2008). In the present study, ICV administration of GnRH2 at 1 pmol/g BW induced a significant decrease of food intake, and this effect was completely blocked by treatment with Antide. Antide is the GnRH type I receptor antagonist (Kauffman et al., 2005b; Matsuda et al., 2008). These results suggest that the anorexigenic action of GnRH2 is mediated by the Antide-sensitive receptor system, perhaps involving GnRH R1 and/or R3. The knowledge about the expression and the distribution of GnRH receptors in the zebrafish brain should help us to speculate on the mechanisms underlying GnRH2-induced anorexigenic effect. However, there has been no information about distribution of GnRH receptors in the hypothalamus. It is unclear which receptor type mediates the anorexigenic action of GnRH2 in zebrafish.

In mammals, several neuropeptides including CRH, galanin-like peptide, LHRH (GnRH1), kisspeptin, α-MSH, NPY, orexin, and 26RFa are implicated in the regulation of nutrition and reproduction, suggesting that feeding and reproductive functions are closely linked (Catzeflis et al., 1993; Iqubal et al., 2001; Chartrel et al., 2003; Kauffman et al., 2005a; Crown et al., 2006; Martynska et al., 2006; Navarro et al., 2006; Maeda et al., 2007). Orexin, which has crucial role in the sleep–wakefulness cycle and appetite control, affects GnRH1 release directly or via the NPY-, CRH-, and β-endorphin-signaling pathways (Li et al., 1999; Tamura et al., 1999; Irahara et al., 2001; Yang et al., 2005; Iwasa et al., 2007). In goldfish, ICV administration of orexin A suppresses spawning behavior, and ICV administration of GnRH2 reduces the level of orexin precursor mRNA in the brain (Hoskins et al., 2008). These data suggest that, in goldfish, GnRH2 and orexin have opposite roles in appetite and satiety regulation. Our previous studies have revealed that mRNA expression levels for NPY and orexin in the hypothalamus obtained from zebrafish fasted for 7 days are higher than those in zebrafish that had been fed normally, suggesting NPY and orexin in the hypothalamus act as orexigenic factors in this species. In the present study of zebrafish, we focused on the GnRH2 neuronal system, which has been implicated in the regulation of food intake in the goldfish (Matsuda et al., 2008), and demonstrated for the first time that the expression of GnRH2 mRNA in the hypothalamus is affected by feeding status. The results support the idea that GnRH2 in the hypothalamus acts as an anorexigenic neuropeptide in this species. Further investigations to clarify the regulatory mechanism of food intake by GnRH2 and other neuropeptides and factors are warranted.

In conclusion, the present study has demonstrated for the first time that ICV administration of GnRH2 suppresses food intake in the zebrafish. These results suggest that GnRH2 induces behavioral changes, and in particular acts as an anorexigenic factor in this species. The present findings also indicate that evolutionary pressure has acted to preserve the function of GnRH2 as a feeding regulator across the vertebrates.

ACKNOWLEDGMENTS

This work was supported by a Grant-in-Aid from the Japan Society for Promotion of Science (21370025 to Kouhei Matsuda), and by a research grant from the University of Toyama (to Kouhei Matsuda).

REFERENCES

Catzeflis, C., Pierroz, D. D., Rohner-Jeanrenaud, F., Rivier, J. E., Sizonenko, P. C., and Aubert, M. L. (1993). Neuropeptide Y administered chronically into the lateral ventricle profoundly inhibits both the gonadotropic and the somatotropic axis in intact adult female rats. *Endocrinology* 132, 224–234.

Chartrel, N., Dujardin, C., Anouar, Y., Leprince, J., Decker, A., Clerens, S., et al. (2003). Identification of 26RFa, a hypothalamic neuropeptide of the RFamide peptide family with orexigenic activity. *Proc. Natl. Acad. Sci. U.S.A.* 100, 15247–15252.

Conlon, J. M., Collin, F., Chiang, Y. C., Sower, S. A., and Vaudry, H. (1993). Two molecular forms of gonadotropin-releasing hormone from the brain of the frog, *Rana ridibunda*. Purification, characterization and distribution. *Endocrinology* 132, 2117–2123.

Crown, A., Clifton, D. K., and Steiner, R. A. (2006). Neuropeptide signaling in the integration of metabolism and reproduction. *Neuroendocrinology* 86, 175–182.

Fernald, R. D., and White, R. B. (1999). Gonadotropin-releasing hormone genes: phylogeny, structure, and functions. *Front. Neuroendocrinol.* 20, 224–240.

Gore, A. C. (2002). *GnRH: The Master Molecule of Reproduction.* Berlin: Springer.

Guilgur, L. G., Moncaut, N. P., Canario, A. V. M., and Somoza, G. M. (2006). Evolution of GnRH ligands and receptors in gnathostomata. *Comp. Biochem. Physiol. A Mol. Integr. Physiol.* 144, 272–283.

Hofmann, H. A. (2006). Gonadotropin-releasing hormone signaling in behavioral plasticity. *Curr. Opin. Neurobiol.* 16, 343–350.

Hoskins, L. J., Xu, M., and Volkoff, H. (2008). Interactions between gonadotropin-releasing hormone (GnRH) and orexin in the regulation of feeding and reproduction in goldfish (*Carassius auratus*). *Horm. Behav.* 54, 379–385.

Iqubal, J., Pompolo, S., Sakurai, T., and Clarke, I. J. (2001). Evidence that orexin-containing neurons provide direct input to gonadotropin-releasing hormone neurons in the ovine hypothalamus. *J. Neuroendocrinol.* 13, 1033–1041.

Irahara, M., Tamura, T., Matsuzaki, T., Saito, S., Yasui, T., Yamano, S., et al. (2001). Orexin-A suppresses the pulsatile secretion of luteinizing hormone via β-endorphin. *Biochem. Biophys. Res. Commun.* 281, 232–236.

Iwasa, T., Matsuzaki, T., Kiyokawa, M., Shimizu, F., Minakuchi, M., Kuwahara, A., et al. (2007). The type 2 corticotrophin-releasing hormone receptor mediates orexin A-induced luteinising hormone suppression in ovariectomised rats. *J. Neuroendocrinol.* 19, 732–738.

Kah, O., Lethimonier, C., Somoza, G., Guilgur, L. G., Vaillant, C., and Lareyre, J. J. (2007). GnRH and GnRH receptors in metazoa: a historical, comparative, and evolutive perspective. *Gen. Comp. Endocrinol.* 153, 346–364.

Kang, K. S., Shimizu, K., Azuma, M., Ui, Y., Nakamura, K., Uchiyama, M., et al. (2011). Gonadotropin-releasing hormone II (GnRH II) mediates the anorexigenic actions of α-melanocyte-stimulating hormone (α-MSH) and corticotropin-releasing hormone (CRH) in goldfish. *Peptides* 32, 31–35.

Kauffman, A. S. (2004). Emerging functions of gonadotropin-releasing hormone II in mammalian physiology and behaviour. *J. Neuroendocrinol.* 16, 794–806.

Kauffman, A. S., Bojkowska, K., Wills, A., and Rissman, E. F. (2006). Gonadotropin-releasing hormone-II messenger ribonucleic acid and protein content in the mammalian brain are modulated by food intake. *Endocrinology* 147, 5069–5077.

Kauffman, A. S., Buenzle, J., Fraley, G. S., and Rissman, E. F. (2005a). Effects of galanin-like peptide (GALP) on locomotion, reproduction, and body weight in female and male mice. *Horm. Behav.* 48, 141–151.

Kauffman, A. S., Wills, A., Millar, R. P., and Rissman, E. F. (2005b). Evidence that the type-2 gonadotrophin-releasing hormone (GnRH) receptor mediates the behavioural effects of GnRH-II on feeding and reproduction in musk shrews. *J. Neuroendocrinol.* 17, 489–497.

Kauffman, A. S., and Rissman, E. F. (2004a). A critical role for the evolutionarily conserved gonadotropin-releasing hormone II: mediation of energy status and female sexual behavior. *Endocrinology* 145, 3639–3646.

Kauffman, A. S., and Rissman, E. F. (2004b). The evolutionarily conserved gonadotropin-releasing hormone II modifies food intake. *Endocrinology* 145, 686–691.

Kim, H. H., Mui, K. L., Nikrodhanond, A. A., and Tamayo, N. C. R. (2007). Regulation of gonadotropin-releasing hormone in nonhypothalamic tissues. *Semin. Reprod. Med.* 25, 326–336.

Lethimonier, C., Madigou, T., Munoz-Cueto, J. A., Lareyre, J. J., and Kah, O. (2004). Evolutionary aspects of GnRH, GnRH neuronal systems and GnRH receptors in teleost fish. *Gen. Comp. Endocrinol.* 135, 1–16.

Li, C., Chen, P., and Smith, M. S. (1999). Morphological evidence for direct interaction between arcuate nucleus neuropeptide Y (NPY) neurons and gonadotropin-releasing hormone neurons and the possible involvement of NPY Y1 receptors. *Endocrinology* 140, 5382–5390.

Maeda, K., Adachi, S., Inoue, K., Ohkura, S., and Tsukamura, H. (2007). Metastin/kisspeptin and control of estrous cycle in rats. *Rev. Endocr. Metab. Disord.* 8, 21–29.

Maney, D. L., Richardson, R. D., and Wingfield, J. C. (1997). Central administration of chicken gonadotropin-releasing hormone-II enhances courtship behavior in a female sparrow. *Horm. Behav.* 32, 11–18.

Martynska, L., Polkowska, J., Wolinska-Witort, E., Chmielowska, M., Wasilewska-Dziubinska, E., Bik, W., et al. (2006). Orexin A and its role in the regulation of the hypothalamo-pituitary axes in the rat. *Reprod. Biol.* 6, 29–35.

Matsuda, K., Azuma, M., and Kang, K. S. (2012). Effects of orexin on emotional and feeding behaviors in teleost fish. *Vitam. Horm.* 89, 341–361

Matsuda, K., Nakamura, K., Shimakura, S. I., Miura, T., Kageyama, H., Uchiyama, M., et al. (2008). Inhibitory effect of chicken gonadotropin-releasing hormone II on food intake in the goldfish, *Carassius auratus.* *Horm. Behav.* 54, 83–89.

Millar, R. P. (2003). GnRH II and type II GnRH receptors. *Trends Endocrinol. Metab.* 14, 35–43.

Millar, R. P. (2005). GnRHs and GnRH receptors. *Anim. Reprod. Sci.* 88, 5–28.

Millar, R. P., Lu, Z. L., Pawson, A. J., Flanagan, C. A., Morgan, K., and Maudsley, S. R. (2004). Gonadotropin-releasing hormone receptors. *Endocr. Rev.* 25, 235–275.

Millar, R. P., Pawson, A. J., Morgan, K., Rissman, E. F., and Lu, Z. L. (2007). Diversity of actions of GnRHs mediated by ligand-induced selective signaling. *Front. Neuroendocrinol.* 29, 17–35.

Miyamoto, K., Hasegawa, Y., Nomura, M., Igarashi, M., Kangawa, K., and Matsuo, H. (1984). Identification of the second gonadotropin-releasing hormone in chicken hypothalamus: evidence that gonadotropin secretion is probably controlled by two distinct gonadotropin-releasing hormones in avian species. *Proc. Natl. Acad. Sci. U.S.A.* 81, 3874–3878.

Navarro, V. M., Fernández-Fernandez, R., Nogueiras, R., Vigo, E., Tovar, S., Chartrel, N., et al. (2006). Novel role of 26RFa, a hypothalamic RFamide orexigenic peptide, as putative regulator of the gonadotropic axis. *J. Physiol.* 573, 237–249.

Palevitch, O., Kight, K., Abraham, E., Wray, S., Zohar, Y., and Gothilf, Y. (2007). Ontogeny of the GnRH systems in zebrafish brain: in situ hybridization and promoter-reporter expression analyses in intact animals. *Cell Tissue Res.* 327, 313–322.

Powell, J. F., Krueckl, S. L., Collins, P. M., and Sherwood, N. M. (1996). Molecular forms of GnRH in three model fishes: rockfish, medaka and zebrafish. *J. Endocrinol.* 150, 17–23.

Roch, G. J., Busby, E. R., and Sherwood, N. M. (2011). Evolution of GnRH: diving deeper. *Gen. Comp. Endocrinol.* 171, 1–16.

Schiml, P. A., and Rissman, E. F. (2000). Effects of gonadotropin-releasing hormones, corticotropin-releasing hormone, and vasopressin on female sexual behavior. *Horm. Behav.* 37, 212–220.

Sherwood, N. M., Lovejoy, D. A., and Coe, I. R. (1993). Origin of mammalian gonadotropin-releasing hormones. *Endocr. Rev.* 14, 241–254.

Steven, C., Lehnen, N., Kight, K., Ijiri, S., Klenke, U., Harris, W. A., et al. (2003). Molecular characterization of the GnRH system in zebrafish (*Danio rerio*): cloning of chicken GnRH-II, adult brain expression patterns and pituitary content of salmon GnRH and chicken GnRH-II. *Gen. Comp. Endocrinol.* 133, 27–37.

Tamura, T., Irahara, M., Tezuka, M., Kiyokawa, M., and Aono, T. (1999). Orexins, orexigenic hypothalamic neuropeptides, suppress the pulsatile secretion of luteinizing hormone in ovariectomized female rats. *Bichem. Biophys. Res. Commun.* 264, 759–762.

Tello, J. A., Wu, S., Rivier, J. E., and Sherwood, N. M. (2008). Four functional GnRH receptors in zebrafish: analysis of structure, signaling, synteny and phylogeny. *Integr. Comp. Biol.* 48, 570–587.

Temple, J. L., Millar, R. P., and Rissman, E. F. (2003). An evolutionarily conserved form of gonadotropin-releasing hormone coordinates energy and reproductive behavior. *Endocrinology* 144, 13–19.

Torgersen, J., Nourizadeh-Lillabadi, R., Husebye, H., and Aleström, P. (2002). In silico and in situ characterization of the zebrafish (*Danio rerio*) gnrh3 (sGnRH) gene. *BMC Genomics* 3, 25. doi: 10.1186/1471-2164-3-25

Volkoff, H., and Peter, R. E. (1999). Actions of two forms of gonadotropin releasing hormone and a GnRH antagonist on spawning behavior of the goldfish *Carassius auratus. Gen. Comp. Endocrinol.* 116, 347–355.

White, R. B., Eisen, J. A., Kasten, T. L., and Fernald, R. D. (1998). Second gene for gonadotropin-releasing hormone in humans. *Proc. Natl. Acad. Sci. U.S.A.* 95, 305–309.

White, S. A., Nguyen, T., and Fernald, R. D. (2002). Social regulation of gonadotropin-releasing hormone. *J. Exp. Biol.* 205, 2567–2581.

Yang, Y., Zhou, L. B., Liu, S., Tang, J. F., Li, F. Y., Li, R. Y., et al. (2005). Expression of feeding-related peptide receptors mRNA in GT1-7 cell line and roles of leptin and orexins in control of GnRH secretion. *Acta Pharmacol. Sin.* 26, 976–981.

Yokobori, E., Azuma, M., Nishiguchi, R., Kang, K. S., Uchiyama, M., and Matsuda, K. (2012). Neuropeptide Y stimulates food intake in the zebrafish, *Danio rerio. J. Neuroendocrinol.* 24, 766–773.

Yokobori, E., Kojima, K., Azuma, M., Kang, K. S., Maejima, S., Uchiyama, M., et al. (2011). Stimulatory effect of intracerebroventricular administration of orexin A on food intake in the zebrafish, *Danio rerio. Peptides* 32, 1357–1362.

Permissions

All chapters in this book were first published in NGPCRSN, by Frontiers; hereby published with permission under the Creative Commons Attribution License or equivalent. Every chapter published in this book has been scrutinized by our experts. Their significance has been extensively debated. The topics covered herein carry significant findings which will fuel the growth of the discipline. They may even be implemented as practical applications or may be referred to as a beginning point for another development.

The contributors of this book come from diverse backgrounds, making this book a truly international effort. This book will bring forth new frontiers with its revolutionizing research information and detailed analysis of the nascent developments around the world.

We would like to thank all the contributing authors for lending their expertise to make the book truly unique. They have played a crucial role in the development of this book. Without their invaluable contributions this book wouldn't have been possible. They have made vital efforts to compile up to date information on the varied aspects of this subject to make this book a valuable addition to the collection of many professionals and students.

This book was conceptualized with the vision of imparting up-to-date information and advanced data in this field. To ensure the same, a matchless editorial board was set up. Every individual on the board went through rigorous rounds of assessment to prove their worth. After which they invested a large part of their time researching and compiling the most relevant data for our readers.

The editorial board has been involved in producing this book since its inception. They have spent rigorous hours researching and exploring the diverse topics which have resulted in the successful publishing of this book. They have passed on their knowledge of decades through this book. To expedite this challenging task, the publisher supported the team at every step. A small team of assistant editors was also appointed to further simplify the editing procedure and attain best results for the readers.

Apart from the editorial board, the designing team has also invested a significant amount of their time in understanding the subject and creating the most relevant covers. They scrutinized every image to scout for the most suitable representation of the subject and create an appropriate cover for the book.

The publishing team has been an ardent support to the editorial, designing and production team. Their endless efforts to recruit the best for this project, has resulted in the accomplishment of this book. They are a veteran in the field of academics and their pool of knowledge is as vast as their experience in printing. Their expertise and guidance has proved useful at every step. Their uncompromising quality standards have made this book an exceptional effort. Their encouragement from time to time has been an inspiration for everyone.

The publisher and the editorial board hope that this book will prove to be a valuable piece of knowledge for researchers, students, practitioners and scholars across the globe.

List of Contributors

Isabelle Franceschini and Elodie Desroziers
UMR8 Physiologie de la Reproduction et des Comportements, Institut National de Recherche Agronomique, Nouzilly, France
UMR7247, Centre National de la Recherche Scientifique, Nouzilly, France
Université François Rabelais de Tours, Tours, France
Institut Français du Cheval et de l' Equitation, Nouzilly, France

Pierre-Olivier Barrette and Adel Giaid Schwertani
Division of Cardiology, Department of Medicine, McGill University Health Center, Montreal, QC, Canada

SatoshiHirako, Eiji Ota, Nobuhiro Wada and SeijiShioda
Department of Anatomy, Showa University School of Medicine, Tokyo, Japan

Fumiko Takenoya
Department of Anatomy, Showa University School of Medicine, Tokyo, Japan
Department of Exercise and Sports Physiology, Hoshi University School of Pharmacy and Pharmaceutical Science, Tokyo, Japan

Haruaki Kageyama
Department of Anatomy, Showa University School of Medicine, Tokyo, Japan
Faculty of Health Care, Kiryu University, Gunma, Japan

Tomoo Ryushi
Department of Anatomy, Showa University School of Medicine, Tokyo, Japan
Department of Sports and Health Science, Daito Bunka University, Saitama, Japan

Takayoshi Ubuka, You Lee Son, Yasuko Tobari and Kazuyoshi Tsutsui
Laboratory of Integrative Brain Sciences, Department of Biology, Center for Medical Life Science, Waseda University, Tokyo, Japan

Joëlle Cohen-Tannoudji, Charlotte Avet, Ghislaine Garrel, Raymond Counis and Violaine Simon
Equipe Physiologie de l'Axe Gonadotrope, Unité de Biologie Fonctionnelle et Adaptative, CNRS-EAC4413, Sorbonne Paris Cité, Université Paris Diderot-Paris 7, Paris, France

Mathieu Méquinion and Fanny Langlet
UMR INSERM 837, Development and Plasticity of Postnatal Brain, Lille, France

Sara Zgheib and Christophe Chauveau
Pathophysiology of inflammatory of bone diseases, Université Lille Nord de France-ULCO - Lille 2, Boulogne sur Mer, France

Suzanne Dickson
Department of Physiology, Institute of Neuroscience and Physiology, The Sahlgrenska Academy, University of Gothenburg, Gothenburg, Sweden
Department of Endocrinology, Institute of Neuroscience and Physiology, The Sahlgrenska Academy, University of Gothenburg, Gothenburg, Sweden

Bénédicte Dehouck
UMR INSERM 837, Development and Plasticity of Postnatal Brain, Lille, France
Université Lille Nord de France - Université d'Artois, Liévin, France

Odile Viltart
UMR INSERM 837, Development and Plasticity of Postnatal Brain, Lille, France
Université Lille Nord de France-USTL (Lille1), Villeneuve d'Ascq, France

Rim Hassouna, Alexandra Labarthe, Philippe Zizzari, Catherine Videau Jacques Epelbaum and Virginie Tolle
UMR-S 894 INSERM, Centre de Psychiatrie et Neurosciences, Université Paris Descartes, Sorbonne Paris Cité, Paris, France

Michael Culler
IPSEN, Milford, MA, USA

Nancy Sabatier, Gareth Leng and John Menzies*
Centre for Integrative Physiology, School of Biomedical Sciences, The University of Edinburgh, Edinburgh, UK

Céline Cansell, Raphaël G.P.Deniz, Aurélie Joly-Amado
Unité de Biologie Fonctionnelle et Adaptative, CNRS-EAC 4413, Sorbonne Paris Cité, Université Paris Diderot-Paris 7, Paris, France

Julien Castel and Serge Luquet
Unité de Biologie Fonctionnelle et Adaptative, CNRS-EAC 4413, Sorbonne Paris Cité, Université Paris Diderot-Paris 7, Paris, France
Centre National de la Recherche Scientifique EAC 4413, Paris, France

Andreas Stengel
Division Psychosomatic Medicine and Psychotherapy, Department of Medicine, Obesity Center Berlin, Charité, Universitätsmedizin Berlin, Berlin, Germany

YvetteTaché
Digestive Diseases Division, CURE: Digestive Diseases Research Center, Center for Neurobiology of Stress and Women's Health, Department of Medicine, VA Greater Los Angeles Health Care System, University of California at Los Angeles, Los Angeles, CA, USA

Berengere Coupe and Sebastien G. Bouret
Neuroscience Program, The Saban Research Institute, Children's Hospital Los Angeles, University of Southern California, Los Angeles, CA, USA
U837, Neurobese Lab, INSERM, Jean-Pierre Aubert Research Center, University Lille 2, Lille, France

Yves Mear and Sylvie Thirion
CNRS, CRN2M UMR7286, Aix Marseille University, Marseille, France

Alain Enjalbert
CNRS, CRN2M UMR7286, Aix Marseille University, Marseille, France
Molecular Biology Laboratory, Conception Hospital, AP-HM, Marseille, France

Jean Mazella, Sophie Béraud-Dufour, Christelle Devader, Fabienne Massa and Thierry Coppola*
Institut de Pharmacologie Moléculaire et Cellulaire, UMR 7275, Centre National de la Recherche Scientifique, Université de Nice-Sophia Antipolis, Valbonne, France

Douglas J. MacNeil
Department of In Vitro Pharmacology, Merck Research Laboratories, Kenilworth, NJ, USA

Renjitha Gopurappilly, Satoshi Ogawa and Ishwar S. Parhar
Brain Research Institute, School of Medicine and Health Sciences, Monash University Sunway Campus, Selangor, Malaysia

Odile Della-Zuana, Viviane Levenez and Alain Ktorza
Maladies Métaboliques, Institut de Recherches SERVIER, Suresnes, France

Valérie Audinot and Jean A.Boutin
Biotechnologie, Pharmacologie Moléculaire et Cellulaire, Institut de Recherches SERVIER, Croissy-sur-Seine, France

Françoise Presse and Jean-Louis Nahon
Genomics and Evolution in Neuroendocrinology, Institut de Pharmacologie Moléculaire et Cellulaire, UMR7275, Centre National de la Recherche Scientifique, Valbonne, France
Genomics and Evolution in Neuroendocrinology, Université de Nice Sophia Antipolis, Nice, France

Peilin Chen, Daniel Lindberg and Chien Li
Department of Pharmacology, University of Virginia Health System, Charlottesville, VA, USA

Christine Van Hover
Department of Neuroscience, University of Virginia Health System, Charlottesville, VA, USA

Garron T.Dodd and Simon M. Luckman
Faculty of Life Sciences, AV Hill Building, University of Manchester, Manchester, UK

Valérie Simonneaux and Caroline Ancel
Neurobiologie des Rythmes, Institut des Neurosciences Cellulaires et Intégratives, UPR CNRS 3212, Strasbourg, France

João C.R. Cardoso, Rute C. Félix, Vera G. Fonseca and Deborah M. Power
Molecular Comparative Endocrinology, Centre of Marine Sciences, Universidade do Algarve, Faro, Portugal

Ryo Nishiguchi, Morio Azuma, Eri Yokobori and Minoru Uchiyama
Laboratory of Regulatory Biology, Graduate School of Science and Engineering, University of Toyama, Toyama, Japan

Kouhei Matsuda
Laboratory of Regulatory Biology, Graduate School of Science and Engineering, University of Toyama, Toyama, Japan
Laboratory of Regulatory Biology, Graduate School of Innovative Life Science, University of Toyama, Toyama, Japan

Index

www.ingramcontent.com/pod-product-compliance
Lightning Source LLC
LaVergne TN
LVHW081029210926
848485LV00004B/982